THERAPEUTIC EXERCISE PRESCRIPTION

THERAPEUTIC EXERCISE PRESCRIPTION

Kim Dunleavy, PT, PhD, MOMT, OCS, FNAP
Board-Certified Orthopedic Clinical Specialist
Clinical Associate Professor
Department of Physical Therapy
College of Public Health and Health Professions
University of Florida
Gainesville, Florida

Amy Kubo Slowik, PT, CSCS
Senior Physical Therapist
Rehabilitation Institute of Michigan
Detroit, Michigan
Equilibrium Studio
Bloomfield Hills, Michigan

ELSEVIER

ELSEVIER

1600 John F. Kennedy Blvd.
Ste 1600
Philadelphia, PA 19103-2899

THERAPEUTIC EXERCISE PRESCRIPTION ISBN: 978-0-323-28053-2

Notice

Library of Congress Control Number: 2018962331

Content Strategist: Lauren Willis
Content Development Manager: Laura Schmidt
Publishing Services Manager: Catherine Albright Jackson
Senior Project Manager: Doug Turner
Designer: Bridget Hoette

Printed in Canada

Last digit is the print number: 9 8 7 6 5 4 3 2 1

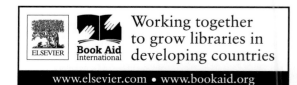

When we seek to discover the best in others, we somehow bring out the best in ourselves.

–William Arthur Ward

To all the teachers and students: Writing this textbook has been a journey for us that we could not have done alone. The process has enriched our friendship and shaped our teaching and practice. We hope that the information presented will help you on your professional journey and bring out the best in each other and the patients that we serve.

We dedicate this book to our families for their support, patience, and energy during this long and time-intensive process.

To Greg and the Dunleavy, Johnstone, and Smith families.

Kim

To Ken, Miye, and Tyler.

Amy

CONTRIBUTORS

Kim Dunleavy, PT, PhD, MOMT, OCS, FNAP
Board-Certified Orthopedic Clinical Specialist
Director of Community Engagement and Professional Education
Clinical Associate Professor
Department of Physical Therapy
College of Public Health and Health Professions
University of Florida
Gainesville, Florida

Krissa Gorman, PT, DPT*
Physical Therapist
UF Health Rehab Center at the Orthopaedic and Sports Medicine
    Institute
Gainesville, Florida

Kevin Lulofs-MacPherson, PT, DPT, FAAOMPT
Board-Certified Orthopedic Clinical Specialist
Clinical Lecturer
Department of Physical Therapy
College of Public Health and Health Professions
University of Florida
Gainesville, Florida

William F. McGehee, PT, PhD
DPT Program Director
Department of Physical Therapy
College of Public Health and Health Professions
University of Florida
Gainesville, Florida

Jason Roberts, PT, CSCS
Senior Physical Therapist
Rehabilitation Institutes of Michigan
Detroit, Michigan
Equilibrium Studio
Bloomfield Hills, Michigan

Amy Kubo Slowik, PT, CSCS
Senior Physical Therapist
Rehabilitation Institute of Michigan
Detroit, Michigan
Equilibrium Studio
Bloomfield Hills, Michigan

---

* Contributed Case Study 11.3.

As specialists in human activity and movement, one of the unique and essential roles that physical therapists have is prescribing therapeutic exercise. In the era of chronic health conditions, opioid abuse, and tightening reimbursement, it is becoming increasingly imperative to be able to select, modify, teach, and evaluate exercises chosen specifically for an individual patient in a short amount of time and with limited visits. Countless variations of exercises can be used for rehabilitation, and choosing the appropriate type and intensity of exercise to meet a patient's needs is complex. Teaching and adjusting therapeutic exercise can be surprisingly challenging, and the complexities are often difficult to navigate without application of theoretical content to practical scenarios.

This text grew out of the challenges of teaching therapeutic exercise in entry-level and continuing education settings, and its presentation developed from questions asked by students who wanted to understand the reasoning behind therapeutic prescriptions more clearly and expand their toolbox of alternative exercises and teaching tips. We watched students struggle with the paradox of viewing the task of choosing and teaching exercise as being simple but at the same time having difficulty fine-tuning their abilities to translate foundational knowledge into appropriate selections and modifications that would help their patients address impairments and regain function. *Therapeutic Exercise Prescription* addresses this issue by presenting foundational concepts in a summarized form, using examples and illustrations to apply the content to patient scenarios, and providing the reader with compare-and-contrast clinical examples, with an emphasis on safety and precautions, progression, and application of content throughout the book.

The text is divided into two parts, each organized in a different format. The first eight chapters summarize relevant foundational content and concepts, and the last three chapters act as workbooks with detailed exercise descriptions. We have tried to present the content in a succinct and useful format. We have incorporated common patient examples that use the International Classification of Functioning (ICF) model to help the reader engage in clinical reasoning by applying such concepts as precautions, SINS (severity, irritability, nature, and stage), tissue healing, biomechanics, and categories of conditions to clinical scenarios.

The concepts of tissue healing and biomechanics and the application of the ICF model are introduced in Chapters 1 through 3, followed by a summary of relevant examination and exercise parameters in Chapters 4 and 5. In Chapter 6, categories are used to contrast circumstances in which mobility either is lacking (hypomobility) or exceeds normal limits and requires additional neuromuscular support (hypermobility). Contrasting patterns of injury for repetitive strain and trauma or surgical history, also discussed in this chapter, reflects the importance of psychological factors in recovery after musculoskeletal injury. Principles of teaching or relearning movement in the presence of compensations, abnormal movement patterns, or pain are presented in Chapter 7. Chapter 8 covers methods to evaluate the outcomes of therapeutic exercise choices. The concepts in the first eight chapters are illustrated with short clinical examples, including comparisons of different diagnoses, patient characteristics, stages of recovery, progressions, and rationale for choices. The application of content is further supported with videos and illustrations.

The last three chapters, which are presented in a workbook format, deal with the lower extremity, the upper extremity, and the spine. Regional biomechanics and other important concepts are followed by presentations of exercises that are frequently used for rehabilitation purposes and are organized by mobility categories and trauma categories. Exercises are described, along with modifications, progressions, alternatives, teaching tips, and common compensations. Full case studies are presented at the end of each section in the workbooks, with explanations of choices and application of the concepts and principles as a platform to start developing and practicing these skills with patients.

We sincerely hope that the material in this book provides the reader with the opportunity to view exercise prescription from multiple perspectives, integrate clinical reasoning processes using foundational concepts, and in turn, facilitate patient outcomes.

Kim Dunleavy, PT, PhD, MOMT, OCS, FNAP
Amy Kubo Slowik, PT, CSCS

ACKNOWLEDGMENTS

This book would not have been possible without the contributions from a long list of colleagues, friends, and family who have generously provided time and expertise. We hope that we have acknowledged all these individuals who have given so freely of their time and opinions.

Thank you to the contributors to the chapters: Kevin Lulofs-MacPherson, PT, DPT, OCS, FAAOMPT; William McGee, PT, PhD; and Jason Roberts, PT, CSCS; as well as Krissa Gorman, PT, DPT, for the case study in Chapter 11. We are also indebted to the following individuals who reviewed chapters: Mark Bishop, PT, PhD, FAPTA; Alaine Blessman, PT, DPT; Brittany Britt, PT, DPT; Melissa Clarke, PT, DPT; Brooke Denninghoff, PT, DPT; Kelsey Diaz, PT, DPT; Brittany Forster, PT, DPT; Steven George, PT, PhD, FAPTA; Margaret Halsey, PT, DPT; Kelly Hardesty, PT, DPT; Jessica Herring, PT, DPT; Jaclyn Jefferson, PT, DPT; Heather Kalafarski, PT, DPT; Kristi Kirby, PT, DPT; Monica Lim, PT, DPT; Gloria Miller, PT, PhD; Jeffrey Peckins, PT, DPT; Alexandra Perry, PT, DPT; Savannah Smith, PT, DPT; Rachael Studer-Byrnes, PT, DPT, NCS; Scott Venkatamaran, PT, DPT; and especially to Dr. Derrick Sueki, PT, PhD, OCS, who provided comprehensive reviews for the foundational chapters of the book.

We would also like to thank and acknowledge the impact that our colleagues, students, and patients have had on the content and format of this book. The privilege of teaching both entry-level and post-graduate students has shaped our thoughts and guided the presentation of the concepts we have used to illustrate the reasoning processes in the book. The opportunities provided by Equilibrium Pilates Studio and Merrithew Stott Pilates provided the inspiration, structure, and format to build our repertoire while working with clients and teaching rehabilitation Pilates and Pilates certification courses. We acknowledge that the information provided in these courses shaped some of the explanations, exercise alternatives, and teaching tips in the workbook chapters. Our patients have stimulated thoughts and directions, trusted us with their goals, and supported us during this journey. We would also like to thank our mentors and instructors during post-graduate training: Dr. William Bandy, Dr. Rob Tillman, and numerous continuing education instructors.

We also appreciate the support from the departments of physical therapy at Wayne State University and University of Florida, as well as Kinetix Physical Therapy for providing space and audiovisual support for the media and photographs. This book would not have been possible without the encouragement, support, and vision of Kathy Falk, Jolyn Gower, and Christie Hart, who initiated the book proposal. Thanks to Linda Wood, who provided editorial assistance for the foundational chapters, and to Laura Schmidt, Lauren Willis, and Doug Turner from Elsevier for their help in the later stages of production.

A very special thank you to Erick Sprout, PT, DPT, at Wayne State University and Thad Boucher, PT, DPT, at the University of Florida, who were responsible for a large number of the photographs and videos.

To all the individuals who served as models or assisted with the media shoots, thank you!

- At Wayne State University: Mathew Briscoe, Susan Clayton, Shauna Cook, Ann Duff, Timothy Duff, Dale Knuth, Melissa Kutchek-Potts, Peter Lichtenberg, Selim Mahutomvic, Eric Sanders, Mathew Schwartz, Rachael Stebbins-Billingsley, and Tim Wiater.
- At the University of Florida: Lynne Arthur, Erik Black, Thad Boucher, Christopher Bruscato, Jonathan Castro, Christina Chan-Pong, Sung Cho, Robert Christy, Melissa Clarke, Ashleigh Coffman, Katie Dewar, Josh Elam, John Evanich, Kim Fasano, Abigail Garner, Ashley Gibbens, Macy Gill, Jodi Gilles, Paula Gomes, Rebecca Gordon, Mark Green, Sarah Guidry, Kelly Hardesty, Josh Hare, Jessica Herring, Jaclyn Jefferson, Karen Kilgore, Kristi Kirby, Stephen Lagor, Kevin Lulofs-MacPherson, Mark Miller, Gabriela Nunez, Jeffrey Peckins, Kamryn Pederson-Buck, Ganga Sheth, Brittny Silke, Gregory Smith, Savannah Smith, Minsuk Song, Jeremy Steiner, Alex Wietrzykowski, and Brandon Wilson.

Also thanks to Josh Cooper, Theresa Chmielewski, David Cox, Derek Drake, Cleone Dunleavy, Ian Dunleavy, Nina Dunleavy, Roxy Dunleavy, Mathew Ford, CJ Gonzalez, Anna Heinzman, Jessica MacWilkinson, Janie Ottenbreit, Arthur Smith, and Zari Whittaker, who provided media or served as the subjects for courtesy media contributions.

Kim Dunleavy, PT, PhD, MOMT, OCS, FNAP
Amy Kubo Slowik, PT, CSCS

CONTENTS

VIDEO CONTENTS

PART I

Foundations for Therapeutic Exercise Prescription

The first eight chapters of *Therapeutic Exercise Prescription* provide a summary of the foundational concepts necessary for selecting, modifying, teaching, and evaluating therapeutic exercise. The scope of the foundational chapters expands progressively by integrating and applying information introduced earlier in the book. These chapters are not intended to provide a comprehensive discussion but rather serve as summaries of available and professionally accepted practices. Readers are referred to other texts for more detailed coverage of physical examination procedures and pathology. This content is supported by brief clinical examples that illustrate concepts presented in the chapter or reinforce content from preceding chapters, along with summary boxes for easy reference. Cases illustrate reasoning processes, use of the International Classification of Functioning model, phases of recovery, and progression. The clinical examples refer to specific exercises found in the workbooks (see Chapters 9–11), where full case studies are presented at the end of each section. Videos and illustrations further demonstrate the exercises detailed throughout the text.

Chapter 1 introduces the importance of determining precautions and contraindications and assessing the severity, irritability, nature, and stage of tissue damage from patient history and subjective complaints before starting the objective examination and testing.

Chapter 2 presents the differences between tissue damage resulting from trauma versus repetitive strain, as well as phases of healing and tissue recovery for different types of tissue. The application of several concepts—stress-strain, distribution, direction and type of forces, open and closed chain movement, and balance—to limit excessive tissue load while applying optimal stimulus for regeneration is also presented.

The American Physical Therapy Association's patient management model and the International Classification of Functioning—both introduced in Chapter 3—are used as frameworks for discussing the links between impairments, activity limitations, and participation restrictions.

In Chapter 4, selected examination techniques are outlined, with discussion of implications for evaluation using tissue tension testing, static and dynamic alignment, and movement compensation analysis. Exercise testing for muscle activation, strength, power, endurance, balance, and coordination is also presented.

Chapter 5 expands on concepts introduced earlier, including exercise testing and choices regarding exercise type and parameters (i.e., position, dosage, and functional requirements).

In Chapter 6, the content is grouped into five categories to assist with the reasoning behind exercise prescription. Choices concerning mobility impairments (hypomobility versus hypermobility), related mechanism of injury (repetitive strain versus trauma/surgery), and individuals with psychological factors that affect management more than other categories are discussed.

Teaching and learning strategies and motor learning are used in Chapter 7 to emphasize the importance of developing skills to explain exercise prescription, modify movement patterns, and motivate patients.

Chapter 8 concludes the foundational section with a presentation of methods to evaluate outcomes.

1

Introduction to Therapeutic Exercise for Rehabilitation

Kim Dunleavy

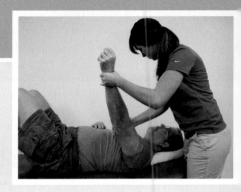

OBJECTIVES

Upon completion of this chapter, the reader will be able to:

1. Describe the role of therapeutic exercise in a patient's rehabilitation process for promoting maximal functional recovery and preventing further injury.
2. Define the components of the patient management model.
3. Describe the phases of healing.
4. Define and provide examples for the terms *precautions* and *contraindications*.
5. Define SINS (severity, irritability, nature, stage) components and explain how information from subjective complaints, patient history, and diagnoses are used to guide the choice of therapeutic exercise and modify techniques.
6. Define and explain types of exercise.

USE OF THERAPEUTIC EXERCISE FOR REHABILITATION

Therapeutic exercise is an essential component of any rehabilitation program following injury, deconditioning, or disease. This textbook will emphasize the use of therapeutic exercise for musculoskeletal conditions to promote recovery and restoration of function. Therapeutic exercise is often used in conjunction with other interventions and taught in the clinical setting. After discharge from individual management, patients may continue performing the exercises in the clinic or at home, alone, or in organized groups. While some exercises seem simple, patients often have difficulty learning how to perform them correctly. Exercising using poor form will render less than optimal results, substituting strong muscles for the targeted weak muscle and movement patterns that place continued stress on the injured area. Safe, effective therapeutic exercise requires skilled instruction and teaching strategies.

Prescribing exercise is often a complex process and requires constant monitoring and clinical reasoning. As movement specialists, therapists should select the exercises to meet each individual's needs and adjust the prescription based on their responses. Some essential aspects of therapeutic exercise prescription include (1) setting individualized goals that are repeatedly adjusted as a patient progresses, (2) selecting appropriate exercises based on foundational concepts, (3) assessing the patient's ability to perform exercise and choosing appropriate dosage, (4) teaching patients to perform the exercises safely and efficiently, and (5) monitoring and evaluating responses to exercise. The therapist also functions as a coach, encouraging patients to reach their highest potential. There are countless variations of exercises, and therapists have the unique opportunity to create exercise programs that are matched to the patient's needs rather than only using established exercise protocols. Protocols provide helpful guidelines and healing time frames, but applying the principles of safe exercise prescription will allow the therapist to prescribe tailored, inspiring exercise programs for their patients. This text is not intended to be an all-inclusive, exhaustive list of exercises and does not include rigid guidelines. Rather, the aim of the content and concepts and their application to case study examples is to provide a framework for the thought processes and decision-making required for exercise prescription, instruction, and evaluation.

PATIENT MANAGEMENT MODEL

Elements of the Patient Management Model described in the American Physical Therapy Association's *Guide to Physical Therapy Practice* will be used in this text (Table 1.1), with the major focus on the Intervention category.[1] The physical therapist will perform an **examination** including taking a history, a **review of systems,** and performing **tests and measures** to determine the extent of impairments and activity or participation limitations. Some examination techniques are covered in Chapter 4; however, because this is not the emphasis of this textbook, the reader is referred to other textbooks such as Magee's *Orthopedic Physical Assessment,*[2] Magee and Sueki's *Orthopedic Physical Assessment Atlas and Video,*[3] Reese and Bandy's *Joint Range of Motion and Muscle Length Tested,*[4] and Netter's *Orthopaedic Clinical Examination: An Evidence-Based Approach*[5] for details on specific examination techniques. The **evaluation process** involves interpreting results from the examination while considering pathology to formulate a physical therapy **diagnosis.** The medical diagnosis is often described using standardized International Classification of Disease (ICD) codes,[6] which are now used in all healthcare settings for data records.

The diagnosis helps describe patient problems and suggests a possible **prognosis** for recovery based on evidence and knowledge of a typical pathology or injury. The diagnosis also assists with identifying movements, forces, or positions that should be completely avoided (**contraindications**) or limited and monitored (**precautions**). Identifying contraindications and precautions is the key to patient safety and must occur before performing certain tests, including initial exercise testing.

This text will emphasize using knowledge of pathology-specific information related to disease, disorders, or injuries and results of tests and measures to develop therapeutic exercise interventions. During the **evaluation** process, the physical therapist identifies the relevant impairments contributing to the patient's functional deficits or disability. The text will use the International Classification of Functioning, Disability and Health (ICF) model as a framework.[7] The **impairments** (problems with body functions) that are hypothesized to have direct influence on the patient's **activity limitations** (difficulties in performing tasks) and **participation restrictions** (difficulties with activities related to life situations) affecting the patient's ability to interact socially) are then prioritized, and goals are set to direct treatment. All the evaluation findings, including the impairments, activity limitations, and participation restrictions, assist with determining a more detailed physical therapy diagnosis, a patient problem list, and patient-specific goals (Fig. 1.1 and Box 1.1). These relationships are discussed in Chapter 3.

In addition to the diagnosis, the therapist should also consider the relative severity, irritability, nature, and the stage of the condition to guide choice of **interventions** (see the section on SINS (Severity, Irritability, Nature, Stage) later in the chapter). The extent and relationship of impairments and activity limitations are considered when developing **short-term** and **long-term goals** and guide choices regarding the **type of therapeutic exercise** and **exercise parameters,** which will be discussed in Chapter 5. Finally, the patient's impairments and functional activity restrictions will help determine what type of **outcome measure** (discussed in Chapter 8) will be used to reflect improvement at specific intervals or before discharge.

Element	Process	Result
Examination	Process of collecting data from the patient using tests and measures including: • Subjective history • Systems review • Test and measures • Functional assessment	Diagnosis Precautions and contraindications are determined, along with deciding if there is a need to refer or consult with other medical providers Determining relative priorities and linkages among impairments, activity limitations, and participation restrictions (see Box 1.1 for definitions and Chapter 3 for description of components)
Evaluation	Clinical judgment and interpretation of results of tests and measures	Formulating a prognosis (potential for improvement) Developing timelines, goals, and a plan of care
Intervention	Choice, delivery, and adjustment of exercise Skilled education and coaching of patient performance	Individual exercise prescription is devised from initial evaluation results, then continuously monitored to determine if the exercises should be progressed or modified based on tolerance
Outcomes	Measurement of results including resolution of impairments and improvement in functional ability or ability to participate in society	Outcomes allow comparison to normative data and to results for patients with similar dysfunction Outcomes also assist with decisions to progress to the next phase and for reflection on the effectiveness of the intervention

TABLE 1.1   Elements of the Patient Management Model for Therapeutic Exercise Prescription[1]

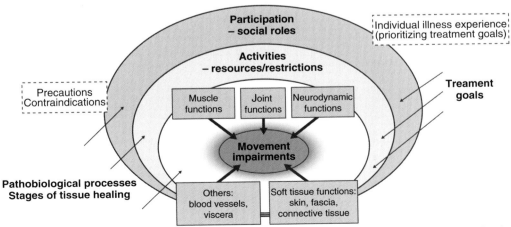

Fig. 1.1 Impairments, activity limitations, and participation restrictions. (From Hengeveld E, Banks K. *Maitland Peripheral Manipulation.* 5th ed. Edinburgh: Churchill Livingstone Elsevier; 2014)

BOX 1.1   Impairments, Activity Limitations, and Participation Restrictions[7]

Impairments: Problems with body functions (physiological) or structure (anatomical)
Activity limitations: Difficulties performing tasks
Participation restrictions: Difficulties an individual has with involvement in life situations (social interaction, work, family, or community activities)

CONTRAINDICATIONS AND PRECAUTIONS

One of the most important tasks is to identify any **contraindications** (resulting in stopping the examination and referring to other providers) or **precautions** (requirements to prevent further or new damage of tissue) (Table 1.2 and Box 1.2). Contraindications and precautions should be determined early in the evaluation process. A thorough review of symptoms and medical history should be used to rule out any serious pathology or reasons for referral to other professionals.[8] Contraindications are elements indicating that severe

---

TABLE 1.2   Examples of Precautions and Contraindications

Type of Precautions	Diagnosis	Precautions	Methods/Actions
Cardiovascular Contraindications and Precautions			
Cardiovascular contraindications	Acute angina	Do not exercise or discontinue exercise with signs of extreme fatigue, sweating, shoulder or chest pain	Do not start to exercise or discontinue; refer for medical attention
	Severe hypertension	Exercise is contraindicated if systolic blood pressure is above 200 mm Hg or below 80 mm Hg or if diastolic blood pressure is greater than 100 mm Hg[8,9]	Do not start to exercise; refer for medical attention
Cardiovascular precautions	Hypertension (150/90)	Discontinue exercise with signs of extreme fatigue, sweating, shoulder or chest pain Discontinue exercise if blood pressure increases >10 mm Hg	Monitor cardiovascular responses before, during, and after exercise
Postsurgical Precautions			
Total hip replacement precautions	Posterior total hip replacement[a]	Avoid hip flexion >90 degrees, adduction crossing midline, and internal rotation	Choose exercises that do not involve hinging at the hip past 90 degrees No gluteal or hamstring stretching past 90 degrees of hip flexion or flexion-adduction combinations Care with functional transitions (sit-to-stand, transfers to the floor) Exercise equipment settings may require adjustments (raise seat on stationary bike) See Fig. 1.2.
Weight bearing	Bi-malleolar fracture treated with internal fixation[b]	Non–weight bearing for 8 weeks, cast boot, and partial weight bearing (50%) after sufficient healing is present at 8 weeks	Use scale to ensure amount of force Use assistive device or parallel bars to reduce and distribute forces

TABLE 1.2 Examples of Precautions and Contraindications—cont'd

Type of Precautions	Diagnosis	Precautions	Methods/Actions
Fall prevention	High fall risk after bedrest	Monitor dizziness or lightheadedness during changes in position Fall prevention precautions	Monitor blood pressure pre-exercise and with transitions Monitor patient symptoms during transitions or changes in position Guarding and gait belt if any symptoms or blood pressure drops with transitions
Posttrauma Contraindications			
Screen for contraindications related to structural damage	Potential fracture after fall	Full examination to rule in or out the possibility of fracture in the presence of swelling, inability to bear weight, extreme pain, or positive screening tests Possible ligamentous laxity after whiplash Possible vertebral artery syndrome	Refer for further medical clearance Cervical ligament laxity tests (alar ligament test, upper cervical mobility tests) Vertebral artery tests
Protection of Healing Structures: Precautions			
Prevent angular forces	Knee medial collateral ligament moderate tear	Avoid valgus forces during weight-bearing exercises	Monitor for angulation (therapist) Teach patient to observe for valgus using mirror Bracing[c] Choose single-plane motion in sagittal plane to avoid localized forces to the medial structures
Avoid specific directions of force	Ankle lateral ligament moderate tear	Avoid full stretch of ligaments (plantarflexion and inversion: the direction of force causing the injury)[d] 	Ranges and movements that do not stress lateral ligaments (neutral starting position, mid-position, moving into full eversion) with exercise against elastic resistance, avoiding the full stretch of the ligament into inversion and plantarflexion—the position that resulted in the injury (see Clinical Examples 2.1 and 2.2) Use bracing or taping to assist with limiting movement in full range (see Clinical Examples 2.1 and 2.2)
Limit tensile forces	Achilles tendon partial tear	Avoid full stretch of tendon with forces exceeding tissue strength	Limit range to mid-position of the tendon length (see Clinical Example 2.3) Limit amount of force (see stress-strain curve in Chapter 2)

[a]Figure from Patton K, Thibodeau G. *The Human Body in Health and Disease*. 6th ed. St. Louis, MO: Elsevier; 2014, p 193.
[b]Figure from Rynders SD, Hart JA. *Orthopaedics for Physician Assistants*. St. Louis, MO: Elsevier Saunders; 2013, Fig 8.15.
[c]Figure from Manske RC. *Fundamental Orthopedic Management for the Physical Therapist Assistant*. 4th ed. St. Louis, MO: Mosby; 2016, Fig. 9.1.
[d]Figure from Manske RC. *Fundamental Orthopedic Management for the Physical Therapist Assistant*. 4th ed. St. Louis, MO: Mosby; 2016, Fig. 17.1.

No!	Yes

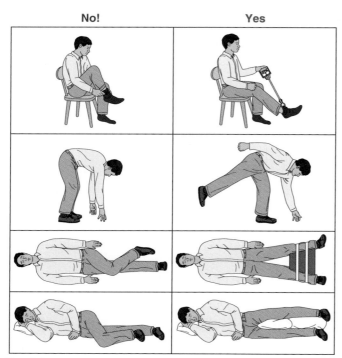

Fig. 1.2 Exercises for total hip replacement. (Cameron MH, Monroe LG. *Physical Rehabilitation Evidence-based Examination, Evaluation and Intervention.* Philadelphia: Saunders; 2007, Fig. 10.5.)

BOX 1.2   Contraindications and Precautions

Contraindication: Direction and degree of motion, extent of force, or other force-related factors that should be *completely* avoided to prevent further damage and allow structures to heal. Cardiovascular contraindications are used to prevent excessive stress on the cardiovascular system.

Precaution: Direction and degree of motion, amount of force, or other force-related factors that should be *limited* in order to allow structures to heal. Precautions can also be related to the need to rule out more serious damage or to evaluate responses to exercise. Other precautions are to *prevent* damage, injury, or adverse event, such as fall prevention.

---

consequences could result from movement or exercise. As an example, if a patient has symptoms consistent with acute angina or extremely high blood pressure, all exercise would be contraindicated and the patient would be referred for medical attention. If a patient has moderate spinal osteoporosis, spinal flexion against resistance or for long durations is contraindicated, but exercise in supported positions with low resistance may be possible.

Identifying precautions during the subjective history can result in modifying or avoiding examination procedures. An example of a precaution is limiting hip flexion to no more than 90 degrees in patients who recently had a total hip replacement with a posterior surgical approach to avoid stretching the posterior hip capsule. Therefore, the physical therapist would not attempt to measure hip flexion range of motion beyond 90 degrees during this patient's initial

---

BOX 1.3   SINS

The acronym SINS is useful for judging the intensity and difficulty of the initial exercise.

- **S** = Severity (greater severity – use more caution in the choice of exercise)
- **I** = Irritability (greater irritability – use more caution in the choice of exercise)
- **N** = Nature (observe precautions and contraindications related to diagnosis and comorbidities, elements of the pathology that influence type of forces allowed or avoided)
- **S** = Stage (phase of healing – use to determine type of exercise and focus on impairments or functional recovery)

---

evaluation. The precautions and contraindications are formulated based on subjective information reported by the patient, knowledge of pathology, and the possible identification of additional diagnoses or pathologies derived from the patient's medical and surgical histories (see Table 1.2). There are common precautions that are based on postsurgical healing requirements for incisions, while others are related to the type and extent of tissue damage. Fall and weight-bearing precautions prevent injury (see Table 1.2). Contraindications and precautions can also be related to comorbidities (other medical conditions) such as hypertension or cardiac disease.[8,9,10] While most contraindications and precautions are extremely important during the early stages of healing, precautions related to medical comorbidity are followed throughout the rehabilitation process.

SEVERITY, IRRITABILITY, NATURE, STAGE

The acronym SINS (Box 1.3) can be used to help determine the intensity and difficulty of the initial choice of exercise. In the subjective interview, the therapist collects information from the patient, including medical history, relevant medical tests, symptoms, and the relationships with movement. The therapist will use the interview findings as well as intake forms and validated tools to supplement the patient interview and determine an initial hypothesis to help plan further examination. The SINS acronym can assist with an early clinical judgment of whether the examination needs to be cautious or can be somewhat more aggressive.

Severity

Severity is usually determined by the amount of pain reported, but it can also be based on the extent of physical damage. The greater the severity of the symptoms or damage, the more cautious the initial exercise choice should be and the slower the exercise progression (Clinical Example 1.1). For example, a patient who is recovering after a fracture that required surgical fixation will be progressed cautiously, taking into account the amount of bone healing. A patient with a mild ankle sprain can be progressed faster than a patient with a moderate ankle ligament tear.

Irritability

The concept of irritability describes how easily the patient's symptoms are aggravated (Clinical Example 1.2). A patient who has easily reproducible symptoms will benefit from a conservative initial exercise plan and slow progression until his or her symptoms are not as responsive to specific movements or positions. Conversely, a patient with low irritability may be tested at a higher level of exercise or progressed more rapidly. Irritability can be defined as the degree of activity resulting in symptoms (pain, tingling, numbness, or other subjective complaints) and the length of time taken for symptoms to subside.[11] The clinical judgment of irritability also takes into account the severity

of the complaints. Questions that will help with the judgment about the degree of irritability include:

1. How easily are symptoms reproduced?

   If mild activity (specific movement, exercise, or position) results in increased symptoms, the condition can be regarded as a highly irritable. Symptoms that are only reproduced with more aggressive activity would be regarded as less irritable.

2. How long do the symptoms last?

   If the symptoms increase substantially and last for a long time after being exacerbated, the symptoms can be regarded as more irritable.

CLINICAL EXAMPLE 1.1   Severity: Degrees of Ankle Ligament Tears

Patient A

Patient A is a 26-year-old man who sustained a mild ankle sprain (Grade I; see Fig. A) while jogging. He was referred to physical therapy for progressive exercise.

Evaluation: Low Severity

The patient may be able to start weight-bearing exercises in a double-leg standing position almost immediately but should be monitored closely for swelling and pain.

Patient B

Patient B is a 30-year-old woman who sustained a complete ankle ligament tear (Grade III; see Fig. B) during an accident 3 months ago. The ligament was surgically repaired and she was non–weight bearing on crutches with the ankle immobilized in a cast for 6 weeks, followed by protection using a walking boot for 2 weeks. The patient was referred to physical therapy for progressive exercise 8 weeks after surgery and was allowed to begin partial weight-bearing exercises.

Evaluation: High Severity

The repaired ligaments should still be protected from high levels of force until there is sufficient tissue healing and muscle support. This is particularly important in the planes of movement that would increase tension on the ligaments and pull on the fracture. Initially, non–weight-bearing exercises are preferred in order to limit forces and protect the patient from poor balance responses after using crutches for 6 weeks. Equipment such as the leg press machine is used to initiate weight bearing with reduced vertical compression forces.

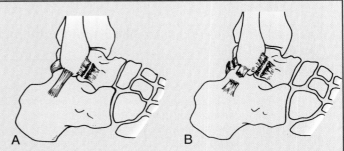

A   B

(A) Partial tear of the anterior talo-fibular ligament. A mild Grade I tear may only result in some of these fibers being disrupted. (B) Complete tear of all three ligaments of the ankle (anterior and posterior talo-fibular ligament, calcaneofibular ligament) results in complete instability. (From Manske RC. *Fundamental Orthopedic Management for the Physical Therapist Assistant*. 4th ed. St. Louis, MO: Mosby; 2016, Fig. 17.2.)

Comparison of Patients A and B

Both patients will require the same precautions to allow ligament healing (i.e., limit the length of the lateral ankle ligaments and the amount of force on the ligament; avoid full inversion and full plantarflexion). However, the severity of the damage is greater in Patient B than in Patient A, and thus the surgical repair requires strict precautions with immobilization for 2 months and slow progression once the cast is removed. Patient A will be able to start progressive movement in the sagittal plane and limited movement into eversion as soon as the effusion resolves, often within 3–5 days.

CLINICAL EXAMPLE 1.2   Irritability

Two patients, A and B, complain of neck pain and occasional referred pain and tingling into the upper extremity at their initial physical therapy appointment. They report the following symptoms on their second visit.

Patient A

Patient A reports increased neck and tingling pain down the arm that started 4 hours after the exercise session; the symptoms are still at the increased level 3 days later.

Evaluation

Patient A is exhibiting signs of high irritability and would need a more conservative approach. The patient would be asked to report any symptoms that increase after the exercise session. If any pain or other symptoms are reproduced after the session, exercise choices would be reevaluated and the type and dosage changed.

Patient B

Patient B reports slightly increased neck pain while performing the exercise in the clinic but that the pain was immediately reduced after the exercise was stopped; the patient has not returned to the clinic since.

Evaluation

Patient B is exhibiting signs of low irritability.

Comparison of Patients A and B

Patient A's symptoms can be characterized as more irritable than those of Patient B. Therefore exercise choices are more conservative, progressed more cautiously, and if symptoms are exacerbated, exercise would be adjusted promptly.

Nature

The nature of the problem is related to the medical and physical therapy diagnosis and is determined from the medical history, the type of symptoms, diagnosis, and prognosis. The information is collated from a combination of symptoms, general patterns, and specific tests. The medical and surgical history is vital when considering precautions, appropriate exercise choices, and timelines for progression. Specific modifications for postsurgical protocols are based on the physician's recommendations as well as the therapist's consideration of the extent of damage, tissue type, and comorbidities. Two categories related to the type of trauma—repetitive strain and major traumatic injury (see Chapters 2 and 6)—and two categories related to extremes of mobility (see Chapters 3 and 6) will be described later in the text.

The impact of disease will also influence the choice of exercise. For example, if a patient has rheumatoid arthritis with major joint destruction and chronic edema, lower forces and limited weight-bearing exercise is indicated (Clinical Example 1.3). The therapist will also determine impairments that influence function (discussed in Chapters 3 and 4).

Stage

Stage can refer to the phases of inflammation, tissue repair, and functional recovery or describe the progression of a disease process. Disease processes are often described in terms of stage; for example, Stage IV breast cancer is more advanced than Stage I breast cancer. The phases of tissue repair will play a significant role in guiding the exercise goals, selection, and progression. Stages often follow time guidelines, but exercise management can be initiated at any stage, and the progression

---

CLINICAL EXAMPLE 1.3   Nature of Problem: Influence of Diagnosis and Extent of Pathology on Exercise Choices

Patient A

A 60-year-old journalist with a history of chronic rheumatoid arthritis was referred for management of hand and wrist dysfunction , which lead to difficulty with dressing, bathing, writing, and grasping objects. Radiographs show joint damage resulting from synovial inflammation and loss of cartilage with joint space narrowing, subluxations, and deformities. She has had a recent exacerbation of her symptoms, and there is some redness, swelling, and heat in the hand. She is scheduled for joint replacements. The goal of physical therapy is to teach the patient active exercise, joint protection techniques, and ways to modify her activities of daily living that will limit further progression of deformity.

Precautions

The evaluation requires a conservative approach because rheumatoid arthritis, which is a systemic connective tissue disease, has a high risk of initiating inflammatory responses. In addition, the anti-inflammatory medications the patient is taking contribute to weakness of the connective tissue. Thus active movement is evaluated without any overpressure and with special consideration to the patient's tolerance level.

Minimal force is applied to the wrist joints during the examination and no hands-on techniques are used on the fingers until the heat and redness have dissipated.

Exercise Implications

Severe damage to the ligaments and joint structures restricts the amount of force and directions of force that can be used, and exercise will focus on improving functional movement using joint protection techniques. Splinting is used initially with the exercise emphasis on proximal shoulder, elbow, and wrist motion until the inflammatory processes are less active. Once the inflammatory process has decreased, exercise choices that assist movement with lower forces, such as aquatic therapy, would be useful.

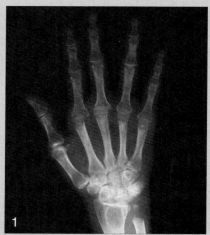

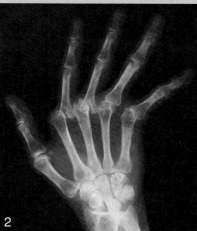

(1) Normal hand radiograph. (2) Hand radiograph for a patient with rheumatoid arthritis, similar to Patient A. Note the metacarpal phalangeal joint destruction and ulnar drift in the index through fifth fingers with extreme damage and dislocation at the second and third metacarpal phalangeal joints. The examination would need to be extremely cautious, with minimal forces on the fingers to limit further damage. (From Eisenberg R. *Comprehensive Radiographic Pathlogy.* 5th ed. St. Louis: Mosby; 2012, Fig. 4.28.)

CLINICAL EXAMPLE 1.3 Nature of Problem: Influence of Diagnosis and Extent of Pathology on Exercise Choices—cont'd

Patient B

A 53-year-old administrative assistant was referred to the clinic for management of pain in her hands. She has been diagnosed with osteoarthritis.

Precautions

Forces that increase the angulation of the index or fifth fingers would be adjusted in this patient. Excessive force is limited for the proximal and distal interphalangeal joints.

Exercise Implications

Active or passive movement may be limited by bony changes. Functional movement and exercise would need to be evaluated, keeping in mind the need to distribute forces and avoid excessive angulation.

Comparison of Patients A and B

The amount of force applied to both patients would need to be monitored, but Patient A's inflammatory disease condition requires very strict precautions and extremely limited loads. Patient B might be able to start with functional movement reeducation and with exercises at a slightly higher level than Patient A. Both patients will need to be monitored for joint effusion and exacerbation of symptoms, but the expectation for the speed of exercise progression would be higher for Patient B.

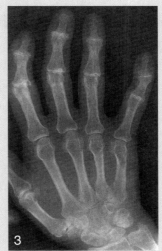

Radiograph showing osteoarthritic changes similar to Patient B. There is generalized osteopenia with joint space narrowing at the proximal and distal interphalangeal joints and osteophytic changes. While range of motion at the second and third proximal interphalangeal joints and distal fifth interphalangeal joint may be restricted, there is less need for caution here than with Patient A, and exercise would be progressed as tolerated. (From Eisenberg R. *Comprehensive Radiographic Pathlogy*. 5th ed. St. Louis: Mosby; 2012, Fig. 4.23.)

---

through stages varies. This chapter will briefly summarize each phase. Chapter 2 will cover the goals for each phase, the characteristics of various tissue types, and how these characteristics impact exercise prescription.

Phase I: Inflammation (Immediately to Approximately 10 Days)

Inflammation is the normal initial response to injury and is necessary for healing; it is typified by redness, swelling, increased warmth, and pain. Resolving the inflammation as soon as possible can help prevent the ill effects of prolonged immobility and disuse. The forces that the tissue is normally designed to withstand may need to be decreased to allow resolution of the inflammatory process. Exercises during this phase can be used to reduce inflammatory by-products while avoiding increasing the inflammatory responses. Chronic inflammation related to inflammatory arthritis, infection, or connective tissue disorders may continue for longer than 10 days, and there are occasions where aggravation of a chronic condition results in low-grade chronic inflammation for longer periods.

Phase II: Tissue Repair (10 Days to 3 Months, Variable According to Tissue Type)

Fibroblasts lay down tissue to repair the injured site and macrophages remove waste tissue. The new tissue is organized in response to stresses placed on it by a slow progression of either stress or strain (usually separately). Too much stress can reinitiate the inflammatory process and result in damage to the newly formed tissue. Exercises during this phase should address impairments.

Phase III: Functional Recovery (6 Weeks to 2 Years, Variable by Tissue Type)

Mature tissue is able to withstand the demands of functional activities. Exercises during this phase help restore the patient's functional deficits, or activity and participation limitations.

TYPES OF EXERCISE

The types of exercise are characterized by the amount of muscle activation and by the assistance provided for movement or the specificity of exercise to address impairments while providing optimal support for healing (Box 1.4).

Passive

Passive movement is performed by someone other than the patient (Video 1.1), by a mechanical device, or using gravity. Patients can also perform passive movement using another limb, without active muscle contraction of the affected area. Passive range of motion exercises are used to maintain range of motion in two instances: if a patient is unable to actively move the body part or if muscle activity at the time is likely to cause further damage.

Active-Assisted

Active-assisted exercise is conducted by the patient using some assistance from the other limb (Video 1.2), another person, mechanical devices, or gravity (Video 1.3). Active-assisted exercise may be used to help the patient achieve full range of motion when weakness or pain is limiting the range of motion or as a progression during the recovery when limited muscle force on structures is preferable.

BOX 1.4   Types of Exercise

Passive: Movement is performed by the therapist or a mechanical device or by the patient without active muscle contraction

Active: Movements are performed by the patient, with or without assistance or resistance

- **Active-assisted:** Movement is performed by the patient with assistance from therapist, mechanical devices, or the patient using another limb
- **Active:** Performed without any assistance from the therapist or mechanical devices, against gravity or external forces

- **Isometrics:** Muscle contractions performed without joint motion
- **Isotonic concentric:** Performed with joint motion with a shortening muscle contraction
- **Isotonic eccentric:** Performed with joint motion with a lengthening contraction
- **Resisted:** Movement against gravity or external resistance, such as weights

---

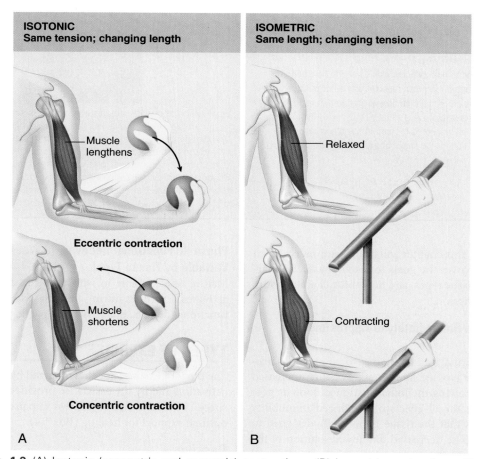

Fig. 1.3 (A) Isotonic (concentric and eccentric) contractions. (B) Isometric contractions. (From Thibodeau GA. *Structure and Function of the Body.* 14th ed. St. Louis, MO: Elsevier; 2012.)

Active

Active exercise is performed by the patient without any assistance from the therapist or mechanical devices (Videos 1.3 and 1.4).

Resisted

The patient moves limbs or the body against some form of resistance such as gravity, external forces from free weights, pulley systems (Video 1.5), mechanical equipment, or therapist-applied manual resistance. Isokinetic exercise is a type of resisted exercise using specialized equipment to maintain a constant velocity of motion while the resistance adjusts throughout the range of motion.

TYPES OF MUSCLE CONTRACTION

Isometric

Isometric contractions are performed without joint motion and the muscle length remains constant. The use of isometric contractions may be indicated when there is joint damage and joint motion is contraindicated or likely to increase pain (Video 1.6), during early strengthening when the limb is supported, or to promote circulation through alternating contractions. Isometric contractions are also required for some functional activities (Fig. 1.3).

Isotonic: Concentric

Isotonic contractions are performed with joint motion and the muscle length changes. A concentric contraction occurs with a shortening action of the muscle and results in joint motion (Video 1.7 and 1.8).

Isotonic: Eccentric

Eccentric contractions are also a form of isotonic contraction and occur when the muscle controls movement against resistance (including gravity) by lengthening or slowing the movement (Videos 1.2 and 1.5). Eccentric contractions occur during functional activities to control, counterbalance, or resist motion. The noncontractile components of the muscle (tendon, connective tissue components of muscle fibers) absorb a greater amount of the tensile forces than do concentric contractions.

SUMMARY

- Precautions and contraindications related to tissue damage and comorbidities need to be established and followed throughout the course of the evaluation and treatment.
- Elements that influence choice of exercise include severity, irritability, nature, and stage (including phase of inflammation, tissue repair, and functional recovery). This information is gathered from the subjective history and the medical background.
- Evaluation of SINS can assist with deciding on how cautious or aggressive the exercise approach will be before starting the examination.
- Type of exercise is defined based on amount of muscle activity and type of contraction.

REVIEW QUESTIONS

1. Differentiate between a precaution and contraindication and provide an example of each.
2. List and describe the four factors used to determine how cautious or aggressive the initial exercise and examination process will be.
3. Differentiate among passive, active-assisted, and active movement.
4. Explain the difference between isometric and isotonic muscle contractions.
5. Explain the difference between concentric and eccentric movement.

REFERENCES

1. American Physical Therapy Association. Guide to Physical Therapy Practice. http://guidetoptpractice.apta.org.
2. Magee DJ. *Orthopedic Physical Assessment*. 6th ed. St. Louis: Elsevier Saunders; 2014.
3. Magee DJ, Sueki D. *Orthopedic Physical Assessment Atlas and Video: Selected Special Tests and Movements*. St. Louis: Elsevier Saunders; 2011.
4. Reese NB, Bandy WD. *Joint Range of Motion and Muscle Length Testing*. 3rd ed. St. Louis: Elsevier Saunders; 2017.
5. Cleland J, Koppenhaver S, Su J. *Netter's Orthopaedic Clinical Examination: An Evidence-Based Approach*. 3rd ed. Philadelphia: Elsevier; 2016.
6. World Health Organization. *International Classification of Diseases*. http://www.who.int/classifications/icd/en/.
7. World Health Organization. *Towards a Common Language for Functioning, Disability and Health ICF*. 2002. http://www.who.int/classifications/icf/icfbeginnersguide.pdf?ua=1.
8. Boissonnault WG. *Primary Care for the Physical Therapist. Examination and Triage*. 2nd ed. St. Louis, MO: Elsevier Saunders; 2011.
9. American College of Sports Medicine. *ACSM Guidelines for Exercise Testing and Prescription*. 9th ed. Philadelphia: American College of Sports Medicine Lippincott Williams and Wilkins; 2014.
10. Smirnova I. The cardiovascular system. In: Goodman CC, Fuller KS, eds. *Pathology: Implications for the Physical Therapist*. 4th ed. St. Louis, MO: Elsevier Saunders; 2015.
11. Hengeveld E, Banks K. *Maitland's Peripheral Manipulation*. 5th ed. Edinburgh: Churchill Livingstone Elsevier; 2014.

2

Review of Foundational Concepts

Kim Dunleavy

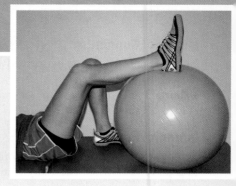

OBJECTIVES

Upon completion of this chapter, the reader will be able to:

1. Compare the causes, signs, and symptoms of traumatic versus repetitive strain injuries.
2. Describe the implications of the history of the damage on the examination and treatment using exercise.
3. List and describe the phases of tissue repair and recovery and factors for promotion of optimal recovery.
4. Describe how tissue healing concepts for bone, muscle, tendon, ligament, and cartilage influence goals for exercise therapy.
5. Describe the forces that should be limited or applied through exercise therapy to allow optimal tissue recovery.
6. Describe the biomechanical concepts that will influence functional movement and therapeutic exercise techniques during exercise therapy rehabilitation.

TISSUE DAMAGE: TRAUMATIC VERSUS REPETITIVE STRAIN INJURIES

Musculoskeletal injuries can be categorized as either **traumatic** or **repetitive strain** injuries (Box 2.1 and Table 2.1). **Traumatic injuries** occur when *major* forces are applied beyond the body part's capacity to withstand (Fig. 2.1). The individual can identify a *specific incident* when the injury occurred and often complains of immediate functional difficulty. Signs include inflammation (swelling, pain, redness) and inability to use the region. The sooner the symptoms appear, the greater the likelihood of major damage. Examples of traumatic injuries are fractures, cartilage tears, tendon ruptures, or complete muscle tears. Traumatic injuries are related to excessive load (stress), excessive tensile force (strain), or combinations of both types of forces. These injuries often occur with high-speed, uncontrolled movements, or when the individual is unable to avoid or withstand external force (Fig. 2.1A). Another possible mechanism of injury is when a patient attempts to move one body part in one direction while stabilizing another body part, such as when the foot is firmly planted and the individual attempts to turn or move the body in another direction (Fig. 2.1B).

BOX 2.1 Traumatic Versus Repetitive Strain Injury

- *Traumatic injury:* An injury resulting from a major force in a single, identifiable event.
- *Repetitive strain injury:* An injury occurring over time, from the cumulative effect of repeated minor trauma to an area.

TABLE 2.1 Traumatic Versus Repetitive Strain Injury

	Traumatic Injury (or Resultant Surgery)	Repetitive Strain Injuries
Extent of forces causing damage	Major forces (speed, torque, localized direction)	Minor forces (repeated, concentrated)
History	Sudden onset: History of an identifiable incident	Gradual onset: slow build up and multiple minor incidents, OR patient is not able to identify an incident
Signs of inflammation	Signs of inflammation (redness, heat, swelling, pain) appear *immediately* or shortly after incident, constant pain and limited function	Low-grade inflammation or no visible redness, heat, swelling; pain experienced with movement, specific positions, or after onset of movement not constant, symptoms can be due to fibrosis
Implications for evaluation	Need to identify extent of tissue damage (for possible referral) and to identify precautions and contraindications After surgical management, evaluation may need to be adjusted based on surgical technique and postoperative contraindications and precautions	Need to identify extent of damage and possible contributing factors

	Traumatic Injury (or Resultant Surgery)	Repetitive Strain Injuries
Implication for choice of exercise	Contraindications and precautions determine which exercises cannot be used during Phases I and II and would be progressed slowly throughout recovery Post injury recovery or surgical guidelines may be used	More complex choices related to initial starting point for exercise program Exercise program will need to address contributing factors Biomechanical alignment analysis and constant observation during progression is important. Functional movement reeducation will be important to prevent recurrence Assess need for external support (bracing/taping/orthotic/assistive device)

TABLE 2.1 **Traumatic Versus Repetitive Strain Injury—cont'd**

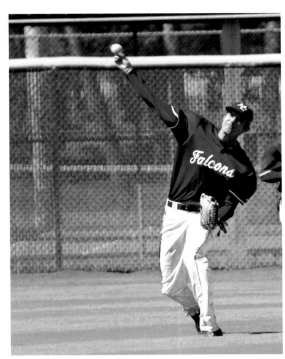

Fig. 2.2 Repetitive strain injuries. There is often no specific incident for repetitive strain injuries: patients report a slow onset over a period of time or after an intense period of activity. There are also contributing impairments that contribute to microfailure. Throwing injuries, such as shoulder impingement, labral tears, and anterior laxity of the shoulder, are examples of repetitive strain injuries. (Courtesy of Derek Drake and David Cox.)

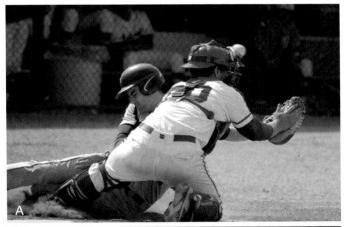

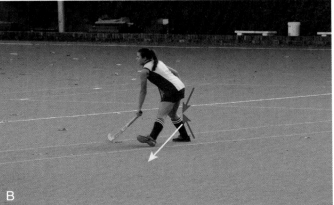

Fig. 2.1 Traumatic injury involves either (A) impact or (B) rapid movement away from a stabilized body segment (*yellow arrow*) with localized stress such as angulation (*red arrows*). ([A] Courtesy of Derek Drake and David Cox.)

Repetitive strain injuries occur *over time* when *minor* forces are applied to an area of the body and the structures are unable to an area of the body and the structures are unable to withstand the *repeated* forces. Repetitive injuries result from an accumulation of forces due to overuse, insufficient time to replenish tissue strength, or the concentration of force on one area of a joint, region, or tissue. One or more factors, such as lack of joint range of motion or flexibility, insufficient muscle strength or endurance, coordination inefficiencies, or structural malalignments, can contribute to excessive force concentration (Fig. 2.2). Forces contributing to repetitive strain injuries include (1) compressive forces, (2) angulation, (3) rotation, (4) tensile strain, or combinations of force directions. Examples of repetitive strain injuries are stress fractures, cartilage degeneration in osteoarthritis, or tendinopathy (Videos 2.1 and 2.2).

ABILITY TO WITHSTAND FORCES (STRESS-STRAIN RELATIONSHIPS)

Each tissue has the capacity to withstand **load** (amount of external force or forces applied to the tissue). The larger the cross-sectional area, the greater the area available to distribute force and the more force the tissue can withstand. **Stress** is defined as the amount of force per cross-sectional area, while **strain** describes the tensile forces resulting in change in length (Fig. 2.3 and Box 2.2). The direction of the load can be described as a **compressive** (causing tissue to condense) or **tensile** (causing tissue to lengthen or expand) force.

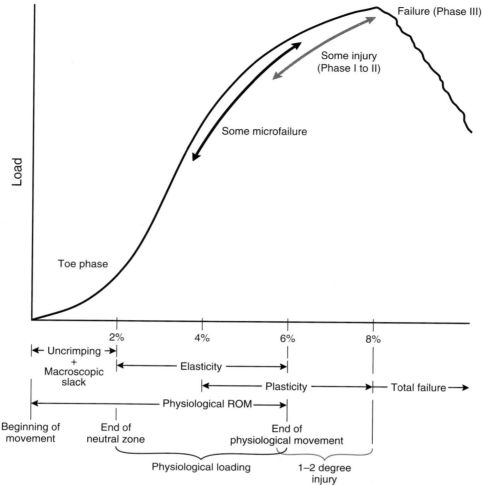

Fig. 2.3 Stress-strain curve showing microfailure and macrofailure. (Fig. 1.1 from Magee DJ, Zachazewski J, Quillen S. *Scientific Foundations and Principles of Practice in Musculoskeletal Rehabilitation*. St. Louis, MO: Saunders Elsevier; 2007.)

BOX 2.2 Stress-Strain Definitions

- *Load*: The amount of external stress applied to tissue
- *Stress*: The ability to withstand a given amount of force per cross-sectional area
- *Strain*: The ability to resist lengthening.
- *Elasticity*: The ability to return to original length after application of force
- *Plasticity*: Ability to deform with permanent changes (sometimes often desired for improvements in mobility)
- *Failure*: Tissue damage
  - *Microfailure* of small amounts of tissue occurs after the yield point in the plastic range
  - *Macrofailure* of entire tissue complex occurs after the failure point with rupture

---

Each tissue has a different stress-strain relationship depending on the material properties of the tissue. Tissue also has some ability to deform and return to its initial position (**elasticity**), ability to deform over time and retain the new position (**plasticity**), or slowly return to its initial position (**viscoelasticity**) (see Fig. 2.3). All of these properties are determined by (1) the alignment of the collagen fibers, (2) the percentage of elastin versus collagen fibers, (3) the amount of ground substance, and (4) the strength of cross-links. Each tissue differs in the extent to which it can deform and return to its normal length.[1–3] Collagen can return to normal after reaching of 2–3% of initial length, while increases of 4–6% result in *microfailure*, and 6–10% is likely to result in *macrofailure* (see Fig. 2.3).[1,3]

The stress-strain curve varies slightly for different tissues but essentially consists of the same components: a *toe phase* where the connective tissue slack is taken up, followed by a linear relationship between the amount of stress and the strain until the maximum elasticity (**yield point**) is reached. Up to this point, if the stress is removed, the tissue will return to its previous length without any permanent changes. If the stress is increased past this point, plastic or permanent changes will occur. In some instances, tissue plasticity is desirable, such as with stretching or joint mobilization. The threshold or **failure point** may be reached with lower stress or strain in healing tissue or after immobilization (see Fig. 2.3).[1,2] The stress and strain concepts are important considerations for establishing precautions to effectively limit further damage and when adjusting exercises to provide sufficient forces for promoting optimal regeneration.

If the tissue reaches the endpoint of the ability to withstand the forces, **failure** will occur. Partial damage of tissue results in **microfailure**, while **macrofailure** is a complete tissue tear. Microfailure can occur after the yield point when the loads reach the plastic region of the stress-strain curve and tissue is unable to return to the initial length after the force is removed. Application of repeated forces without sufficient time for the tissue to recover and mild damage after a traumatic incident can both result in failure of some fibers and are both described as microfailure. Macrofailure occurs when the failure point is reached and permanent rupture of collagen occurs.[1,2]

Ligament, tendon, and muscle tears are often classified according to the extent of damage, such as Grade I (mild), Grade II (moderate), and Grade III (complete disruption) (Box 2.3).[4,5] Grade I damage is the result of microfailure. More fibers reach the failure point in Grade II. In Grade III, complete macrofailure and disruption occurs.[4] The greater the tissue damage, the greater the inflammatory response and the risk of further structural damage to the affected or nearby tissues.

After diagnosis of the location and degree of damage, appropriate medical or surgical management should follow.

Precautions or contraindications are determined based on the extent of damage and the need to protect healing structures. The process of orthopedic physical therapy examination and diagnosis is described extensively in other texts.[4–6] The extent of the damage is considered when determining the severity of the injury (Clinical Example 2.1; see Chapter 1), which guides the aggressiveness of the exercise choices and progression. If tissue is partially torn, the amount of stress or strain that will result in further damage is less than for intact tissue. The anatomical plane and tissue type are used to establish precautions related to which directions of movement and forces are safe and promote optimal healing (see Box 2.1 and Clinical Example 2.1; Videos 2.3 and 2.4).

BOX 2.3 **Classifications of Tissue Damage**

- *Grade I:* Mild tear (microfailure)
- *Grade II:* Moderate tear
- *Grade III:* Complete disruption (macrofailure)

CLINICAL EXAMPLE 2.1 **Precautions During Healing After Grades I–III Ankle Sprain**

The types of precautions will depend on the structure and function of the damaged tissue. The degree and length of time required for precautions increase based on the extent of tissue damage (see the following figures).

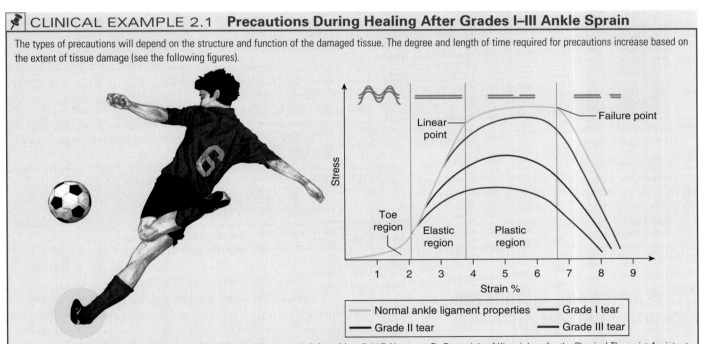

Stress and strain need to be limited more for Grade III tears. (Image on left from Mansfield P, Neumann D. *Essentials of Kinesiology for the Physical Therapist Assistant.* 2nd ed. St. Louis, MO: Mosby; 2014.)

Grade I Ankle Sprain:
- Brace or taping is used to limit inversion for 6 weeks for walking, up to 3 months or longer for running and sports.
- Avoid placing the anterolateral ligaments in the fully stretched position (full combined plantarflexion and inversion). Midrange plantarflexion and dorsiflexion or isometrics are used to assist with resolution of the inflammatory by-products.

- While the ligament heals, full stretch of the ligaments in plantarflexion and inversion and outer range of the peronei is avoided, especially with high forces in weight-bearing positions. Often the position and direction of force of the injury is the same as the directions that need to be avoided.

Continued

CLINICAL EXAMPLE 2.1   Precautions During Healing After Grades I–III Ankle Sprain—cont'd

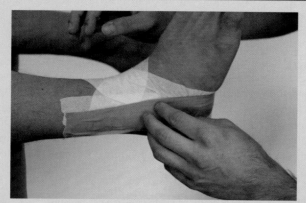

Ankle taping to limit inversion.

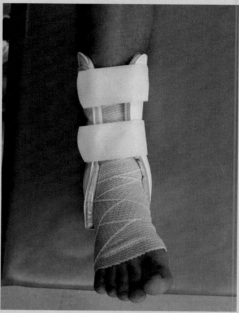

An Aircast brace is used to limit frontal plane motion while still allowing sagittal plane movement. The compressive bandage is used to assist resolving edema.

- Take care with excessive stress or strain for additional 6–8 weeks Exercise is introduced and progressed in the sagittal plane first before the frontal plane.

Grade III Ankle Ligament Tear:

- No stress on the ligament until sufficient healing. Treatment is either full immobilization or surgical management. Weight-bearing precautions: Non–weight-bearing for 6–8 weeks with cast boot; partial weight-bearing with cast boot for additional 6 weeks.
- Continued movement limitation precautions similar to Grade II after allowed to bear weight at 3 months.
- Care with excessive stress or strain for additional 6–8 weeks dependent on muscle activation and function recovery.

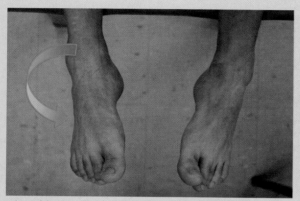

Direction of force to be avoided the most is the combination of plantarflexion and inversion for an anteriorlateral ligament sprain.

Grade II Ankle Ligament Tear:

- Avoid any stress on the ligament; the ankle is maintained in neutral position using a cast boot until sufficient healing (approximately 6–8 weeks), followed by air cast or ankle brace (consistently for additional 6 weeks, longer for running and sports). Isometric contractions are indicated to assist with resolution of inflammatory by-products.

TISSUE REPAIR AND FACTORS FOR PROMOTING OPTIMAL RECOVERY

The degree of healing and repair are important considerations when selecting exercises and setting appropriate parameters. The phases of tissue repair will direct the goals, type, intensity, and progression of exercises. General guidelines for exercise selection, progression, and goals are presented here; however, personal factors (age, genetics, comorbidities) will influence both the initial starting point and the rate of progression through exercise programs.

Phases of Tissue Repair and Recovery

Therapeutic exercises can enhance tissue repair and recovery. Understanding the events, time frames, and objectives of each phase will guide exercise selection and progression. It is the therapist's responsibility to prescribe exercises during the appropriate time frame that will promote resolution of inflammatory by-products, provide sufficient forces to stimulate healing, and provide activities to challenge neuromuscular recovery while respecting the limits of each tissue.

Phase I: Inflammation (Immediately to 3–10 Days)

The inflammatory process is the body's response to damage, infection, or abnormal cellular mechanisms, and is a necessary process for healing and repair (Box 2.4). Inflammation is the first response to tissue damage and is responsible for removing damaged tissue and initiating cellular mechanisms to promote repair and avoid further damage (Box 2.5).[1] The early process of tissue damage includes bleeding and fluid release into joint (**effusion**) and extracellular spaces (**edema**) (Fig. 2.4), which also results in redness and heat in the inflamed area (Fig. 2.5).

BOX 2.4 Symptoms of Inflammation

- *Edema*: An accumulation of excessive extracellular tissue fluid outside a joint
- *Effusion*: Increased intraarticular fluid in a synovial joint
- *Heat and redness*: Increased local vasodilation in region
- *Pain*: From damage to tissue, inflammatory mediators, hypoxia, pressure from edema and effusion

BOX 2.5 Phase I Goals

- Limit inflammation and protect the injured tissue
- Assist with removal of by-products of inflammation (edema, effusion, metabolites), increase circulation to the area, and decrease pain related to hypoxia, muscle spasm, and vasoactive mediators
- Exercise can minimize the effects of immobility or deconditioning without placing excessive stress on injured structures.

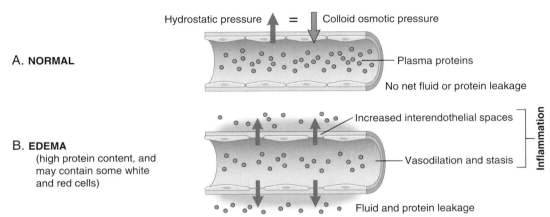

Fig. 2.4 Edema resulting from increased blood flow to damaged tissue. (A) Under normal circumstances, capillaries contain blood plasma and cells with a continuous exchange of fluid and nutrients based on the osmotic and hydrostatic pressure balance within the vessel and the extracellular space. (B) After trauma there is a rapid increase in blood flow, and the inflammatory responses extend the vasodilation and stress on the endothelium due to the increase in hydrostatic pressure. Water escapes into the surrounding extracellular space, resulting in effusion. If there is more severe trauma plasma proteins leak into the extracellular space, and, finally, blood cells leak into the surrounding tissue. The resulting increase in colloid osmotic pressure further increases fluid motion. The external pressure on the blood vessels also causes pain. (From Kumar et al., *Robbins and Cotran Pathologic Basis of Disease*. 8th ed. Philadelphia, PA: Saunders Elsevier, 2010.)

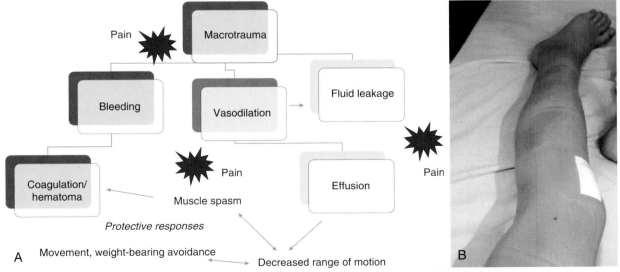

Fig. 2.5 (A) Immediate and secondary responses to traumatic injury. (B) Bruising, edema, and effusion after an anterior cruciate ligament (ACL) reconstruction.

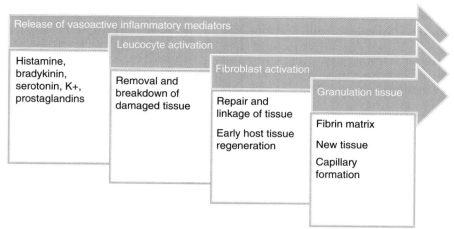

Fig. 2.6 Secondary responses to traumatic injury.[1]

TABLE 2.2	Goals of Exercise During Phase I (Acute Inflammation)	
Goals	**Exercise Choices**	**Elements to Consider**
Protect injured structures	Avoid placing excessive load (stress or strain) on injured tissue where microfailure or macrofailure is likely to occur (see stress-strain curve) Additional protection may be provided by use of assistive devices, bracing, or taping	Motion without strain may be possible in planes other than the plane controlled by the injured tissue
Increase circulation to region Assist with removal of edema and effusion Maintain muscle activation without excessive stress on injured structures	Active low-intensity exercise of other joints around the injured region Alternating active muscle contraction within available range (low intensity)	Muscle activity will assist with venous return, particularly if the limb is elevated Only used if likelihood of bleeding is small
	Isometric muscle contraction for short durations followed by relaxation	Active contractions are likely to provide mechanical "pumping" actions for circulation as well as promote movement of extracellular edema or intraarticular effusion
	Generalized movement of the affected limb or trunk as well as localized muscle contractions listed above will help with motion of edema and effusion	Motion of proximal or distal joint or other areas of the body can increase overall circulatory flow and challenge
	Small-range active movement without stress on injured structures to maintain range or assist with removal of effusion. Decreasing effusion helps restore range if caused by increased intraarticular volume or pain at the end of range	Motion may increase immediately if effusion is the cause of limited range
Minimize effects of lack of activity or immobilization	Minimizing muscle atrophy and cardiovascular effects of immobility for the uninvolved regions and general body systems; may need to be adapted to follow precautions and allow adequate healing of the affected structure	Allow movement in other regions and joints, include equipment and unloaded exercise such as bike, aquatic therapy, upper body ergometer, upper body and trunk exercise, or resistance exercise with uninvolved body regions

Stimulation of nociceptive pathways occurs with the tissue damage and continues with the release of inflammatory mediators such as histamine and bradykinin (Fig. 2.6). Inflammatory responses also include a secondary vasoconstriction to reduce bleeding and muscle spasm to avoid further motion and damage. The inflammatory cycle is intended to restrict further damage and is completed by the removal of the damaged cellular debris and stimulation of fibroblastic activity. Scar tissue is formed to repair the structures.

During Phase I, the primary rehabilitation goals are to limit excessive forces to protect the damaged area and assist with resolution of inflammatory by-products (Table 2.2). Exercises can target the injured area or uninvolved areas and can assist with promoting circulation to the area, limiting pain, and assisting with resolution of edema.

Phase I exercises directed toward the injured joint should avoid excessive loads (stress) or stretching (strain), or the inflammatory phase can reinitiated. Movement in directions that do not place stress on the injured tissue is used to assist with removal of edema and effusion. The patient can exercise uninvolved areas to help deter the effects of disuse or inactivity, or, if the therapist has identified compensations or other areas of dysfunction likely to impact recovery, these impairments can also be addressed during Phase I.

If excessive load or tension is placed on tissue during Phase I, bleeding may continue and edema and effusion may increase, resulting in excessive hematoma formation. Extensive bleeding results in a greater likelihood of excessive fibrotic tissue and pressure on surrounding tissue, further increasing pain responses. The therapist should monitor the patient's injured region for signs of inflammation: increased redness, pain, heat, swelling, or bruising. These signs indicate the need for caution and further evaluation. If present, the precautions should be strictly enforced, and load or tension on the area during exercises and activities of daily living reassessed and modified accordingly.

While the damaged tissue must be protected following acute inflammation, chronic inflammation related to repetitive strain injury calls for identifying and training to correct faulty biomechanics and compensations. If excessive forces on the joint are not resolved or other factors limit resolution of inflammation, chronic inflammation can result. Chronic inflammation due to excessive forces can lead to edema, effusion, and prolonged proliferation of fibroblasts, causing thickened connective tissue and mobility limitations (Fig. 2.7 and Box 2.6).[2] Pain, deconditioning, and compensations can also further complicate and contribute to excess stress and decreased ability to withstand strain.

Not all patients will enter the rehabilitation process while in Phase I of healing. During the initial evaluation, the physical therapist should determine where the patient's injury falls

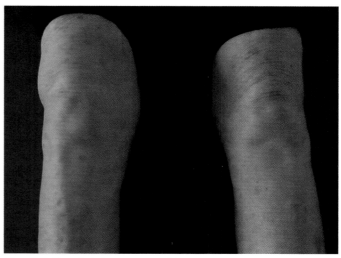

Fig. 2.7 Chronic inflammation, effusion, and thickening in a patient with knee osteoarthritis.

BOX 2.6 Differences Between Acute and Chronic Inflammation

- Acute inflammation occurs with immediate trauma.
- Chronic inflammation can be a result of accumulation of forces, repeated microtrauma, or inadequate resolution of acute inflammation.

---

in the tissue healing process, before prescribing the appropriate type and intensity of exercise based on the state of the injured tissue. Each tissue has unique healing time frames, and these time frames can be influenced by other factors such as age, genetics, nutrition, medication, and comorbidities[1-3] (Clinical Example 2.2).

CLINICAL EXAMPLE 2.2 Phase II and Phase III Exercise for an Ankle Ligament Injury

Precautions

As the patient progresses to Phase II, the injured tissue is still protected in the plane of the ligament. Stress is increased slowly in shortened positions without placing strain on the ligament, and impairments such as diminished neuromuscular activation and endurance are addressed.

Phase II exercises are the same for all grades of injury; however, contraindications for stress and strain are in place for 6–8 weeks for Grade II injuries and 8–12 weeks for Grade III ligament tears. Phase II rehabilitation is only started once sufficient healing has taken place to lift complete contraindications for motion in the frontal plane or in the line of the ligament. Precautions are still required until further healing has taken place.

Exercise Choice

Exercise choices are related to the need to protect the ligament from excess strain and to progressive return to function.

A patient with a Grade I ankle sprain is progressed relatively rapidly while a patient with a Grade II or III injury is progressed slowly once there is adequate

healing. Exercises address impairments (limited mobility from the effusion, decreased muscle activation) and are designed to help protect the ligament using proprioceptive training and neuromuscular coordination.

Exercises are progressed from non–weight-bearing (Video 2.3) to weight-bearing (Video 2.4) in Phase II to promote frontal plane stability and balance reactions (Video 2.5), with additional proprioceptive input or support from taping or bracing if needed.

In Phase III, activities are progressed to meet goals to return to the individual's pre-injury function. Exercises are chosen to address activity limitations and impairments taking into account personal factors (athletic hobbies) and environmental needs (uneven surfaces). Running in place (Video 2.6) forward and backward is introduced before sideways (Video 2.7) or cutting. Changing directions rapidly and running on uneven surfaces is added last in the progression. The timelines to progress to Phase II are slower for more severe ligament damage in Grades II and III damage. The relative speed of exercise progression is also slower with Grades II and III injuries as the threshold for damage has decreased due to the injury and the immobilization/lack of normal activity.

Continued

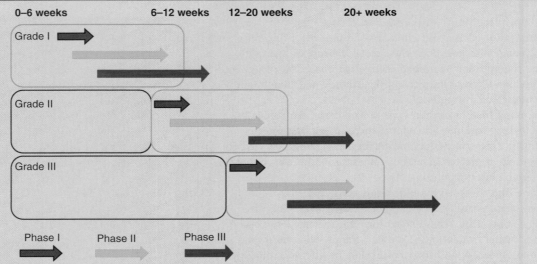

Phases of rehabilitation for Grades I–III ankle ligament injury. Precautions for a Grade II or III tear are in place during early stages (*red box*). Rehabilitation (*yellow box*) may be started in Phase I or II, depending on the extent of inflammation.

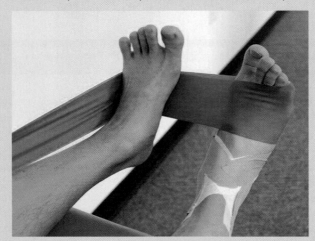

Isometric eversion activation, endurance, and strengthening using elastic resistance (Phase I and II).

Eversion muscle activation in supine against elastic resistance through isometrics or small-range to neutral exercise is used in Phase I to promote muscle activation. The peronei are often stretched and may be painful in the early phases after an inversion injury; therefore, muscle activation is used to improve circulation, remove inflammatory by-products, and decrease pain.

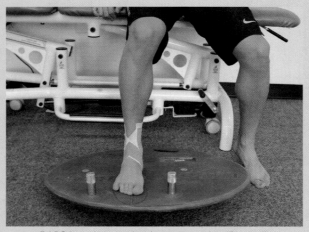

BAPS board strengthening progression (Phase II)

In Phase II, the resistance may be increased, and isotonic control is promoted using a balance board with a weight.

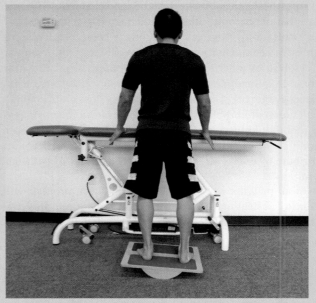

Double-leg balance activities on a balance board (Phase II).

Double-leg balance activities are started with some hand support. The balance board can be placed to allow plantar and dorsiflexion range first, followed by controlled weight shift from side to side to activate the lateral muscles.

Weight transference from foot to foot is started in the sagittal plane or without movement in space by running on the spot (Video 2.6). Movement is progressed as the patient tolerates the activity, with slower progression for lateral movements and changes of direction (Video 2.7; see Fig. 3.6B). Transitional movements, such as cutting and changing direction to train the neuromuscular responses for weight acceptance and change of directions at high speeds, are included in late Phase III.

Phase II: Tissue Repair and Early Tissue Regeneration (5–10 Days to 3 Months, Depending on Tissue Type)

The primary mechanism for tissue repair occurs through fibrous tissue bridging the gap in damaged tissue. The amount of fibrous tissue is proportional to the amount of damage and the length of time that fibroblasts remain active. Phase II normally begins around 5–10 days after injury and can last through 3 months, depending on the tissue type (Box 2.7 and Table 2.3). The rate of production of new collagen fibers is greatest between 7 and 14 days post injury.[1] The repair phase will overlap with the removal of inflammatory products.

The ability to monitor and evaluate a patient's tolerance to load is an essential skill for therapists. Therapists should verify that there is adequate distribution of forces, graded load, and activity, and monitor responses to exercise (delayed-onset pain, edema, effusion, or other abnormal symptoms). Adverse responses warrant constant reevaluation and reduction of exercise load. If excessive load or tension is placed on tissue during Phase II, damage to the immature collagen or regenerated tissue results in inflammation and increased fibrosis. The subsequent edema and pain can also result in the patient avoiding use of the region and compensating with other movement strategies. This can cause muscle atrophy, weaker connective tissue, and, ironically, further stresses on the damaged region. If additional stress occurs and damage of the immature collagen or the injured tissue ensues, the inflammatory cycle is reinitiated (see Phase I, Fig. 2.8).

The organization and strength of fibrous tissue is remodeled in response to stress applied to the structures during Phases II and III.[1-3] Phase II exercises should promote tissue repair with targeted, smaller loads specific to the tissue type and function without reaching the ultimate failure point of the tissue. In addition, impairments such as muscle atrophy, joint restrictions, muscle tightness, pain, and compensatory mechanisms should be addressed during this phase (see Fig. 2.8 and Clinical Example 2.2). Exercises may target the impairments that are in the primary, injured area or in secondary regions that are contributing to biomechanical accumulation of forces.

Phase III: Tissue Maturation and Remodeling (6 Weeks to 2 Years, Depending on Tissue Type)

Phase III involves maturation and remodeling of the involved tissue as well as removal of excessive fibrotic tissue (Table 2.4 and Box 2.8). Tissue is remodeled by organizing the direction of collagen fibers to promote tissue capable of withstanding the forces needed for function. This process occurs in response to the appropriate type and direction of force for a particular tissue (see the section "Factors Influencing Healing: Tissue Characteristics"). The entire process may take up to 2 years, depending on the type of tissue.[1-3] If necessary, Phase III treatment should

---

BOX 2.7 Phase II Goals

- Address impairments
- Provide optimal stimulus for tissue regeneration
- Minimize the effects of inactivity or immobilization
- Protect injured structures
- Improve muscle function without placing undue stress on injured tissues

---

TABLE 2.3 Goals for Healing in Phase II

Goals	Exercise Choices	Elements to Consider
Protect injured structures	Avoid placing excessive load on injured tissue or stretching to lengths where microfailure or macrofailure is likely to occur (see stress-strain curve). Load (stress) is increased slowly in planes of movement of the injured structures, and range is limited to avoid maximum tension (strain).	Load can be increased using isometric contractions or contractions in the inner or mid-range of injured structures to avoid extreme strain. Midrange is determined by available range and not necessarily by normative values. Other diagnoses, comorbidities, and higher severity or irritability are indications for stricter monitoring and extending periods of contraindications and precautions.
Improve muscle function without excessive stress on injured structures Minimize effects of inactivity or immobilization	Target other joints around the injured region with active, moderate-intensity exercise to assist with overall aerobic conditioning, improving muscle function and distributing forces.	Positioning and choice of exercise can be adjusted to avoid excessive stress on injured structure with slow reapplication of stress. Allow and progress movement in other regions and joints.
Address specific impairments Provide optimal stimulus for regeneration	Mobility, strength, specific muscular endurance, aerobic conditioning, coordination, or balance exercise	Tissue will regenerate in response to appropriate loads and strains placed on the structure. Initial loads should be light and directed in a way that places little stress on the healing tissue. Monitor for adverse responses (delayed-onset muscle soreness, pain, effusion, or regression of improvements).

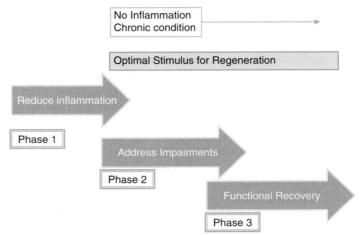

FIG. 2.8 Overlapping phases of tissue recovery.

TABLE 2.4 **Goals for Tissue Recovery in Phase III**		
Goals	**Exercise Choices**	**Elements to Consider**
Address remaining impairments required for function	Continue to progress mobility, strength, specific muscular endurance, aerobic conditioning, coordination, or balance exercise.	Load (stress or strain) is increased related to functional requirements (see Chapter 3). Specific emphasis on strength, power, coordination, speed with increased complexity and multi-planar movement.
Progress forces for optimal stimulus for regeneration and tissue remodeling and restore the ability to withstand forces	Progressive exercise to promote injured tissue regeneration and remodeling Exercise addressing causative factors	
Return to function	Functional training	

continue to address any remaining impairments influencing the specific functional requirements of the individual. Exercises are progressed to address causative factors, with the major focus on functional exercise. This phase should include progressions from uni- to multi-planar movements that match the complexity and speed of the functional activities that the patient wants to address. Monitoring the patient's tolerance and performance of exercises is important during all phases of tissue repair, including Phase III. If the patient requires higher level functional preparation, Phase III can be extended into advanced activities to return to sport or work requirements (see Clinical Example 2.2). Some postsurgical protocols will list these stages as Phase IV or V. Postsurgical or recovery protocols may divide phases based on specific tissue recovery time frames and can include targets for progression from one phase to the next.

BOX 2.8 **Phase III Goals**
• Restore functional movement.
• Restore the ability to withstand forces required for function.
• As specific impairments are resolved, exercises are progressed to meet functional strength, power, coordination, and speed.
• Activities need to be progressed to multi-planar movement with appropriate complexity and intensity to achieve the patient's goals.

FACTORS INFLUENCING HEALING: FORCE CONSIDERATIONS FOR TISSUE CHARACTERISTICS

All types of tissue contribute to the complexities of normal movement and each tissue has unique characteristics that assist with the specialized function of the tissue (Box 2.9). These characteristics influence the precautions, choice of exercise type, and parameters for therapeutic exercise. The provision of **optimal stimulus for regeneration** refers to adjusting the stress and strain to match the target tissue's function, alignment, and physiological characteristics to stimulate tissue repair or regeneration and avoid forces that reinitiate an inflammatory responses or cause further damage. Connective tissue adapts to imposed demands with tissue remodeling in response to the direction, type, and level of forces applied to it. These force characteristics are therefore important to consider when choosing exercises to promote tissue stimulus for healing and for functional demands.

While the patient may report pain as a protective mechanism, it is the therapist's responsibility to prescribe exercises that promote resolution of by-products of inflammation, stimulate healing, and promote neuromuscular recovery while still respecting the limits of each tissue. In Phase I, the forces that the tissue is normally designed to withstand may need to be limited to allow adequate fibrosis formation to bridge the gap in the damaged tissue. During Phase II, the damaged tissue should be stimulated by slow progression of either stress or strain (usually separately). Motions in other planes or types of motion that do not stress the tissue may be progressed more rapidly. During Phase III, the damaged tissue is further challenged to promote optimal adaptations and alignment.

Immobilization or bed rest causes rapid deterioration of connective tissue, muscle atrophy, and neuromuscular adaptations.[1-3] Tissue changes are characterized by a lower volume of ground substance in connective tissue along with increased concentration of collagen fibers and weaker cross-links. The resulting tissue may be less mobile and vulnerable to further injury. Sufficient gliding and extensibility of the scar tissue is essential to allow adequate motion while still withstanding external forces (Video 2.8). The challenge is to provide enough motion and force to promote fiber organization in a similar manner to the original tissue, but without allowing too much force or motion beyond the tissue's capability.[1-3]

If insufficient forces are placed on the tissue, the tissue is susceptible to further injury. However, too much stress (or strain) will result in reinitiation of the inflammatory cycle and can result in further damage or excessive fibrosis (Box 2.10).[1,2] Adjusting forces to match the individual's tissue status is therefore a key consideration. The ability of tissue to resist the forces required for normal function is influenced by individual patient factors such as age, nutritional status, overall activity level, pregnancy, and genetic characteristics.[1,2] Comorbidities and disease processes influence metabolic rate and connective tissue composition, as do some medications used to treat the health conditions. The factors listed in Table 2.5 are obtained from the patient's demographics and medical history, and they impact the overall healing potential and therefore result in more cautious exercise selection and progression (Box 2.11).

Each tissue has approximate time frames for resolution of inflammatory responses and partial and full healing. While no time frame is exact, postsurgical and trauma protocols provide approximate time frames for healing of the injured structures, surgical incisions, and any surgical support systems, but timelines may need to be adjusted based on individual characteristics.[7] Physical therapists will use this information during an initial evaluation to estimate exercise intensity for initial testing, expectations for prognosis, and anticipation of exercise responses. Exercise selection, dosage, progression, and type of outcome measures are also influenced by the status of the tissue, and the therapist must respect the healing time frames and precautions at all times.

Skin, fascia, and other connective tissue provide linkages and respond to forces in multiple directions. Tendons and ligaments have specialized connective tissue function and will be discussed in more detail. Cartilage and intervertebral discs provide additional linkage for some joints, are designed to absorb shock, and have additional force considerations. Each tissue has unique a biochemistry, functions, and approximate healing time frames, but, as mentioned previously, these are influenced by a patient's individual characteristics and medical comorbidities.

BOX 2.9 Optimal Stimulus for Regeneration

- *Optimal stimulus for regeneration*: Specific application of stress and strain to match the target tissue's function, alignment, and physiological characteristics to stimulate tissue repair or regeneration and to avoid forces that result in excessive inflammatory responses or further damage.
- *Davis's law*: Soft tissue adapts to imposed demands.
- *Wolff's law*: Bone adapts to imposed demands.

BOX 2.10 Consequences of Inadequate or Excessive Load During Exercise Progression

- Inadequate load (stress or strain):
  - Weak connective tissue with potential for further damage
  - Disorganized or excessive scar tissue that limits motion
- Excessive load (stress or strain):
  - Further damage
  - Excessive fibrosis

Connective Tissue

Connective tissue (Box 2.12) structures function to enclose organs and tissues, support joints, and attach muscle to bone. Skin is a type of connective tissue with specific characteristics. A comparison of types of connective tissue and the forces that each is designed to withstand is presented in Table 2.6. Connective tissue consists of elastin and collagen fibers suspended within a matrix of fluid, salts, and glycosaminoglycans (protein-sugar molecules) (Fig. 2.9A). The consistency of the matrix varies with type of tissue and functions

TABLE 2.5   Factors Influencing Healing and Ability to Reverse Changes [1–3]

Factor	Type of Change	Reversible?
Immobilization	Decreased ground substance	Yes; depends on length of immobilization for time of return of glycosaminoglycan concentration and ground substance, movement, and functional requirements of tissue
	Scar tissue/fibrosis	Depends on extent of scar tissue and organization
	Increased cross-bridges decrease extensibility	Needs motion between layers of tissue, and tissue must
	Disorganization decreases ability to resist strain or stress	adapt to required length for function
	Replacement of elastin fibers with collagen decreases stress capability	
Increased biomechanical stresses on specific areas due to alignment	Increased strength and density of collagen fibers in certain areas, less in others	Yes; rate depends on application of force suitable for tissue type and amount/direction of forces without damage that initiates inflammatory cycle
	Adaptation to specific length of tissue	
Preexisting fitness level and exposure to forces	Increased collagen strength and ability to resist stress or strain related to patterns of loads	Yes; whether tissue is able to return to pre-injury status depends on the extent of tissue damage
Hormonal influence (e.g., pregnancy)	Relaxin decreases cross-linkage capability	Yes; depends on absence of relaxin or resolution of other hormonal imbalances
Medications (corticosteroids/nonsteroidal anti-inflammatory drugs)	Decreased ability to resist force (stress) and poor healing response when damage occurs	Local steroids: Occasional Systemic steroids: Long term
Nutrition (including specific deficits; vitamin deficiencies, vitamins K, B, C)	Strength of collagen diminished and slow regeneration	With adequate nutrition, restoration of tissue properties might be possible
Genetic predisposition	Increased collagen formation or cross-linkages (keloid formation)	Poor response to strain
	Decreased elastin percentage	
	Decreased collagen formation	Poor response to stress
	Autoimmune diseases; chronic inflammation that is easily triggered increases fibrosis (scleroderma, lupus erythematosus)	Low threshold to stress and strain
Age	Pediatrics; relatively greater percentage of elastin versus collagen	Lower threshold for load stress, relative higher threshold for tensile stress related to increased elasticity
	Geriatrics; decreased elastin, decreased cross-links, decreased ground substance collagen	Lower threshold for load stress, lower threshold for tensile stress, decreased elastic responses
	Decreased muscle fiber cross-sectional diameter, increased relative percentage of fat and collagen within muscle	Lower ability to produce force, lower muscle flexibility

BOX 2.11   Personal Factors and Health Conditions Affecting Tissue Strength

- Immobilization
- Age
- Nutritional status
- Genetics
- Comorbidities
- Medications
- Pregnancy or hormonal imbalances
- Alignment
- Overall activity and fitness levels

BOX 2.12   Connective Tissue Healing: Force Considerations

- To heal, damaged connective tissue requires protection or limitation of forces in the plane of the injured structure for varying time frames.
- The amount of stress or strain tolerated is based on extent of injury and connective tissue structure.
- Stress-strain forces need to be maintained within the toe or elastic regions during the early phase of healing (precaution).
- Stress-strain forces may be progressed past the yield point into the plastic range if improvements in tissue mobility are needed during recovery.
- Stress-strain past the failure point is avoided (contraindication).

TABLE 2.6 Connective Tissue Function Forces to be Considered for Precautions and Optimal Stimulus[1-3]

Tissue	Function	Forces That Tissue Is Able to Withstand	Forces to be Limited During Healing
Skin	Barrier to infection Superficial tissue that protects and encloses other tissues Encloses sensory receptors (touch, pain, pressure) Controls release of body heat	Generalized planar motion in multiple directions Minimal strength	Direct sustained pressure
Generalized connective tissue: fascia	Contains organs Provides division and orientation of muscle structures Distributes forces Muscle origins and attachments	Direction specific	Excessive tension Directions with less collagen fiber alignment
Ligament	Limits joint range of motion in specific directions Connects bone to bone	Resists excessive strain in one or more joint plane/direction of motion Threshold for stress varies based on particular ligament and individual characteristics	Excessive strain in plane of ligament at full length OR with additional directions (angulation and rotation)
Tendon	Attaches muscle to bone Provides elastic responses for muscle control Contains stretch receptors	Ability to lengthen or resist tensile forces from muscle contractions or stretch of the muscle tendon complex	Excessive strain at full tendon length If both ends of tendon are stretched or if muscle contraction occurs with the opposite end stabilized (often multi-joint muscles) maximal strain is placed on tendon
Cartilage	Hyaline cartilage protects bone surfaces from friction Conforms joint surfaces to allow joint motion Fibrous cartilage changes articular surface alignment (meniscus) or links bones in syndesmotic joints	The superficial layer provides a barrier that requires translatory gliding for collagen fiber alignment Vertical compression and decompression is needed for fluid replenishment	Compression, rotation, and translation combination Sustained high loads in weight-bearing positions
Intervertebral disc	Links spinal segments Annulus contains nucleus and resists rotation Nucleus pulposus absorbs shock and compression	Compression and decompression promotes fluid transfer Annular fibers limit rotation	Extreme flexion and rotation with compression of disc

to withstand deformation and support the collagen fibers.[1,2] The ratios of collagen and elastin vary, based on tissue type. A higher percentage of elastin fibers results in a more elastic tissue with the ability to return to its initial length after being stretched. Typically, tendons have greater elastic properties than ligaments, and therefore the length change is likely to be greater for tendons than for ligaments given the same amount of stress (Fig. 2.9B).[2,3]

If force is applied to connective tissue, the toe region of the stress-strain curve (Fig. 2.10A) represents the "uncrimping" of the wave format of the collagen fibers as fibrils are able to slide past each other to produce some increase in length. Minimal levels of force can result in changes in length. In the next phase of the stress-strain curve, the linear region, collagen fibers are able to resist additional force, and the tissue is still able to return to the original length once the load is removed (see Fig. 2.10A). Following injury, the tissue is unable to withstand the same amount of stress and percentage of strain as before the injury.[1-3,8]

While recovering from injury, the goal is for exercises to limit applied forces that the healing tissue can withstand without reaching the plastic range where permanent changes in tissue length can negatively impact function. This usually occurs within the toe phase in Phase I and the elastic range during Phases I and II without reaching the new lower linear endpoint (see Fig. 2.10A). If immobilization or range of motion limitations were used to protect healing structures, the new fibrous tissue, as well as the surrounding tissue, may have adapted to a shortened length with disorganized collagen fibers (Video 2.8). Excessive cross-links between the fibers further decrease the overall mobility of the tissue. In this case, applying forces approaching the plastic range may be necessary in some directions to remodel the fibrous scar tissue and allow functional tissue mobility. This is usually only needed toward the end of Phase II or in Phase III, but stress-strain is progressed cautiously and slowly, and the amount of stress/strain is adjusted based on the extent of injury and comorbidities, age, and length of

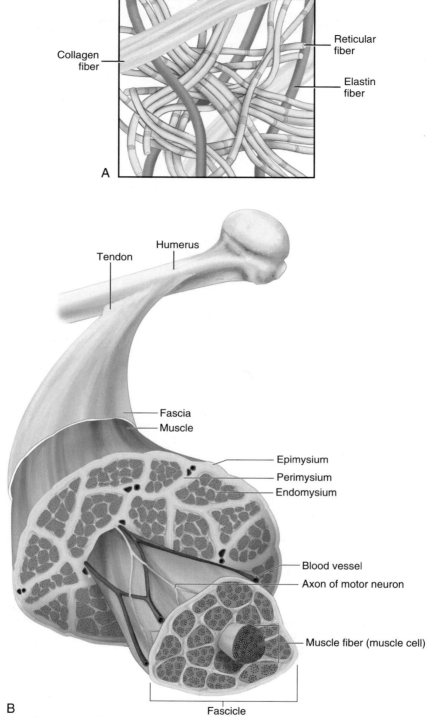

Fig. 2.9 Connective tissue structures. (A) Connective tissue consisting of collagen, elastin, and reticular fibrils and proteoglycan molecules suspended in ground substance (fluid, fibroblasts, and minerals). (From Muscolino JE. *Kinesiology: The Skeletal System and Muscle Function.* 3rd ed. Elsevier Mosby, 2017; Fig. 4.3). (B) Connective tissue organization surrounding muscle fibers and tendon attachments. (From Patton K, Thibodeau G, Douglas M. *Essentials of Anatomy and Physiology.* Mosby, 2012; Fig. 10.1.)

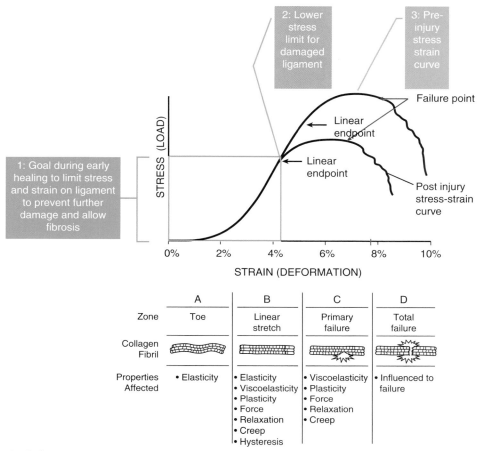

Fig. 2.10 Stress-strain curve considerations for phases of rehabilitation. *Top:* (*1*) The goal during early rehabilitation after tissue injury is to limit the stress and strain and allow fibrosis in the toe and linear stretch zones without exceeding the linear endpoint. (*2*) Note the adjusted stress (load) limits and strain (elongation) point prior to the linear endpoint where tissue changes will occur (primary failure). Bracing, taping, and limiting exercise ranges will attempt to limit both the load and the elongation. (*3*) Pre-injury stress-strain capabilities before macro (total) failure. After injury, the tissue is unable to withstand the same load (stress), particularly at extreme length (strain), and the potential for further damage is higher. Precautions and contraindications are needed to avoid reaching the failure point. The degree of protection depends on the amount of tissue damage; for example, a Grade II ligament tear will need to be protected to a greater degree than a Grade I tear. *Bottom: (A)* The goal for Phase I is to only apply stress or strain within the toe phase (the crimping of the connective tissue allows up to 2% increase in length) or into the linear range (4–6% increase in length) with loads below the new lower linear yield point. The tissue length is kept in a shortened position and low stress is applied to the tissue until inflammation and edema have resolved. (*B*) Goals for stress and strain to increase range of motion and provide load for optimal stimulus for regeneration. In Phase II, the amount of stress and strain is increased slowly, but the tissue is still protected from stress or strain that may result in further damage. Ideally, either stress or strain is progressed independently. In Phase II and III, exercise and interventions with the goal to increase range of motion will start to move toward the plastic region (*C*, primary failure) by elongating the tissue with lower load. To promote specific tissue adaptation, the amount of stress can be increased without elongation of the tissue to avoid further damage (*D*, total failure). The application of force is designed to gradually recover those properties that allow one to resist functional load and length requirements. (Modified from Magee DJ, Zachazewski JE, Quillen WS. *Scientific Foundations and Principles of Practice in Musculoskeletal Rehabilitation.* St. Louis, MO: Saunders Elsevier; 2007; Fig. 25.11.)

immobilization. The damaged tissue should not reach failure point at any point during recovery, and, in some cases, the plastic range is also contraindicated if there is major damage (see Fig. 2.10B).

Tendons

Tendons attach muscles to bone and have greater elastic properties than ligaments (Box 2.13). If the muscle-tendon complex is lengthened, both the muscle and tendon connective tissue are exposed to the tensile forces. Eccentric contractions or slow, controlled motion distribute greater forces to the tendons. Because eccentric loading is a requirement for many functional tasks, it is important to slowly introduce eccentric activities during Phases II and III, but caution should be exercised if using eccentric exercises during Phase I.[2]

Muscle tendon complexes that cross two joints (the hamstrings, for example) are important for complex functional movements such as running. In this case, both ends of the muscle are moving in opposite directions, increasing the overall tissue strain while simultaneously contracting during the late swing phase of running. Traumatic damage of a tendon is often due to uncontrolled motion at one joint when the opposite end of the muscle-tendon complex is still contracted. The combination of high external stress while the complex is at the maximum strain point leads to failure, often at the weakest point in the complex at the muscle-tendon junction (Fig. 2.11).

Another anatomical consideration is the angulation and location of the tendon with respect to bone or connective tissue pulleys that change the direction or localize forces. Excessive angulation can result in concentrated forces and localized tension on a specific area of the tendon (Fig. 2.12 and 2.13).[2] Dynamic valgus angle in a patient with patellofemoral dysfunction is an example of increased angulation with increased localization of forces (Video 2.2). A rotator cuff tendon moving over the greater tuberosity is an example of a tendon snapping over a bony prominence. This will create friction, and damage to the tendon can ensue. If the concentration of forces continues after microfailure, the repetitive loading on the remaining fibers further increases the force per unit area (stress), even with lower loads. The consistent application of force eventually results in degeneration

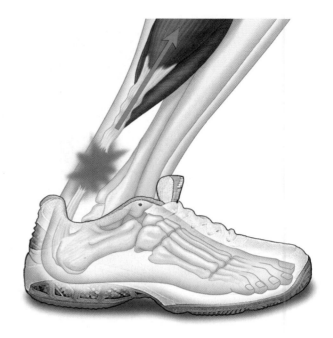

Fig. 2.11 Mechanisms of tendon damage. Achilles tendon rupture often occurs when the foot is planted firmly on the ground and the body moves away without allowing the heel to rise. The full elongation of the tendon as a result of the gastrocnemius/soleus muscle contraction (*arrow*) and the forces from the body weight moving away from the foot exceeds the stress-strain failure point, with an immediate audible sound. This is an example of macrotrauma. Arrow denotes the direction of the muscle contraction.

of the tendon.[2] *Tendonitis* is used to describe active inflammation of the tendon, while *tendinopathy* describes chronic degeneration.[2] If repeated movement patterns are contributing to the localized stress, it is important to adjust these patterns, decreasing angulation or redistributing the concentrated forces during recovery. Forces (particularly with eccentric contractions) are slowly reintroduced with the tendon aligned in the anatomical plane of the tissue.[2] Progression from isometric to isotonic exercise and concentric to eccentric exercise is used to provide optimal stimulus for recovery (Clinical Example 2.3).

Ligaments

Ligaments can withstand higher stress thresholds, but have lower percentage strain limits than tendons (Box 2.14).[3] This has implications for the amount of load (stress) and motion (strain) permitted throughout healing (see Fig. 2.10). Ligament macrofailure typically occurs at around 6–8% of starting length,[3] while tendon failure occurs slightly later at 8–10% of starting length.[2] The amount of load that the ligament can withstand is dependent on the thickness of the ligament. Normally, the position and plane of a ligament determines whether the ligament functions as a primary or secondary restraint to excess joint mobility in specific directions. If there is damage to a primary

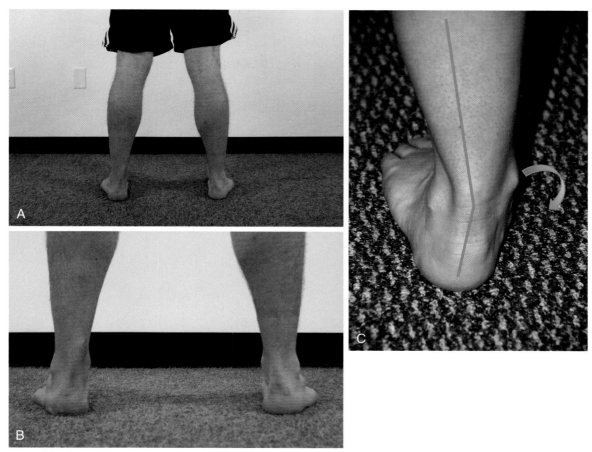

Fig. 2.12 Mechanisms of tendon microtrauma (Achilles tendinopathy). Microtrauma results from repeated application of force toward the plastic range of the stress-strain curve. Angulation of the Achilles tendon can increase elongation of the tendon through early, prolonged, or excessive pronation. This patient's genu valgus (A) with compensatory rearfoot valgus (B and C, *blue lines*), resulting in pronation (C, *blue arrow*) are contributing factors for chronic tendinopathy. He is a marathon runner, and the repeated microtrauma without time to allow healing also contributed to a prolonged history of tendon problems. He is 3 months post surgical debridement on the left side.

restraint, the secondary restraint has some ability to resist forces but is usually able to withstand less overall stress. Damage to ligaments will therefore necessitate protection from excess forces. Precautions will need to include limited stress and strain in the plane and direction that the ligament normally restrains and also in directions where the ligament normally supplements restraint provided by other structures.[3,4]

Forces causing ligament damage are often due to external forces directed toward an extremity but may be related to the excessive internal stabilization needs of one part of the lever, such as pivoting on a planted foot (see Fig. 2.1B). Combinations of forces (angulation, shear forces, and rotation) produce maximum tension of the collagen fibers of the ligament, with a higher risk of failure. Ligaments are damaged by high-velocity or high-impact injuries. During early healing, forces should be limited to one plane as much as possible, and there

may be specific ranges of joint motion that are contraindicated at least until early healing has taken place (Clinical Example 2.4).[2]

While neuromuscular coordination can assist with overall stability, loss of ligamentous support leaves a joint without the passive restraint system necessary for high-level functional activity. During progression of exercise, the healing ligament needs to be protected from excessive forces until there is sufficient stability and neuromuscular coordination. External support from braces and assistive devices can decrease overall forces placed on the healing ligament until sufficient fibrosis has linked the damaged tissue (see Clinical Example 2.4). However, immobilization weakens connective tissue,[3] and it can take up to 12 months to recover the initial properties, so movement is recommended in planes that do not cause excessive tension of the ligament. Surgery is indicated after complete Grade III injuries and, in some cases, for Grade II tears.[9]

CLINICAL EXAMPLE 2.3   **Force Considerations After Achilles Tendon Repair**

A 45-year-old runner who has chronic Achilles tendinopathy ruptures his left Achilles tendon. The progression through phases of rehabilitation is determined by the precautions and forces that should be limited to allow healing and tissue regeneration.

Achilles tendon rupture and surgical repair	Time period	Forces allowed	Precautions (forces to be limited)
Phase I: Acute inflammation	5–10 days	External compression around ankle Movement of other joints around the area to increase blood flow, remove exudate, minimize effects of immobilization	Tensile forces (dorsiflexion combined with knee extension) Tensile with angulation (inversion/eversion) Tensile forces with concentric contractions of the gastrocnemius/soleus complex Weight-bearing contraindicated No load in stretched position (protected in midrange of muscle-tendon complex: cast boot in slight plantarflexion, progressing to neutral for functional position) 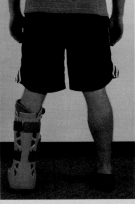 Cast boot used to protect the tendon in midrange and limit loads.
Phase II: Partial healing	6–8 weeks post op	Motion in one plane Motion in midrange Lower loads Lower velocity Protected weight-bearing (partial weight-bearing in rocker boot with heel lift) Distribute forces to proximal joints	Avoid extreme strain (use midrange or limit full loaded dorsiflexion with stretch) Protect amount of load Avoid high velocities Avoid combined planes of motion or concentrated loads (see image below on *right*) 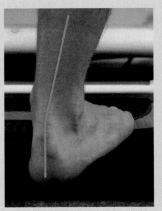 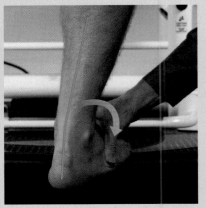

As the patient progresses, healing precautions are lifted and loads are introduced slowly. Double-leg plantarflexion from the floor is started with support. At 3 months, plantarflexion exercises with slow eccentric lowering (bilateral) from a platform are introduced. The exercise is demonstrated on his non-surgical side. Note the angulation of the Achilles tendon increases as the heel is lowered below the level of the platform and the foot pronates.

The patient is taught how to actively correct his foot position using using tactile cues to maintain supination and limit the degree of eccentric lowering below the platform.

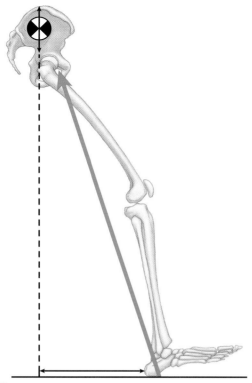

Fig. 2.13 Biomechanical movement pattern contributions to microtrauma (running injuries). If the foot is placed in front of the body during heel-strike, the distance from the line of gravity through the center of mass (*dotted line*) to the weight acceptance leg (*black arrow*) is larger than if the body moves in space and the foot is placed under the body on impact. The vertical ground reaction forces and rotational loads are greater with a larger stride and asynchronous timing of the body motion in space in the landing phase.

Cartilage and Intervertebral Discs

Cartilage and intervertebral discs (Box 2.15) are designed to promote shock absorption and provide spacing. There are two types of cartilage: hyaline articular cartilage and fibrous cartilage. **Hyaline cartilage** covers and protects synovial joint surfaces and provides smooth surfaces to decrease friction during joint motion (Fig. 2.14). The mechanical properties include the ability to withstand compression, high elasticity, and self-lubrication.[10] **Fibrous cartilage** links bones and, in certain areas, can assist with improving congruency or extending joint surfaces, such as in the knee, hip, or shoulder (Fig. 2.15). Fibrocartilage also acts as a shock absorber and transmits loads.[10] Patients with cartilage injuries are often seen in rehabilitation settings for damage to the articular surfaces (hyaline cartilage) due to macrotrauma or microtrauma resulting in osteoarthritis (Fig. 2.16) or damage

---

BOX 2.14 Ligament Healing: Force Considerations

- Ligaments are designed to withstand force from specific directions.
- Protection of the ligament in early healing phases can consist of avoiding multi-planar movements, limiting specific ranges of motion, using braces, or providing weight-bearing limitations.
- Movements can be introduced in a single plane of motion (those planes that the injured ligament does not control) and can progress to movements in the previously protected planes of motion and to multi-planar movements.
- Neuromuscular training can assist with muscular support around the joint.

CLINICAL EXAMPLE 2.4   Force Considerations After Anterior Cruciate Ligament (ACL) Grade II Tear

A 32-year-old nurse is assisting a patient who slips. While protecting the patient, the nurse sustains a Grade II ACL tear. The precautions and force considerations through the phases of rehabilitation are shown in the following table.

ACL Grade II tear	Time period	Forces/movement desired	Precautions (forces to be limited)
Phase I: Acute inflammation	5–10 days	External compression Movement of other joints around the area to increase blood flow, remove exudate, minimize effects of immobilization Flexion and extension within available range	Shear and rotary forces avoided (varus, valgus, anterior translation of tibia on femur) Immobilizer brace, non–weight-bearing on crutches to limit forces on area
Partial healing	Up to 6 months	Loads that do not stress ACL (start with frontal plane, then progress to sagittal plane movements) Strength and coordination exercises in closed chain positions to minimize shear forces Promote neuromuscular coordination to prevent excessive angulation or rotation with anterior shear during weight transfer, landing, and direction changes	Limit the amount of load, velocity Brace to limit rotary or angular motion Avoid hyperextension with load Avoid combined rotation, angulation (no pivoting)
Full healing	1–2 years	Progressive movement complexity and loading to develop muscle strength, power, motor control, coordination, and endurance to minimize and distribute passive forces on the ligament Progressive movements in all directions, loads, and velocities needed for functional requirements Activities based on neuromuscular ability to control position and produce motion	Based on functional ability

to the fibrous cartilage (knee meniscus) or labrum (hip and shoulder) (Fig. 2.17). Articular cartilage has limited potential for regeneration, but structural shape can be salvaged with surgical techniques, and there are promising advances in stem cell and tissue scaffolding.[10,11] Fibrous cartilage has very limited potential for healing, partly due to a poor blood supply (Fig. 2.18) and is often trimmed or sutured with the hope of retaining most of the joint surface.[11]

The collagen in the superficial layer of articular cartilage is aligned parallel to the joint surface to provide a barrier between the hyaline cartilage and the synovial fluid (see Fig. 2.14) and responds to gliding or translational forces. Disruption of the superficial zone leads to leakage of water and glycosaminoglycan complexes into the articular space. Uneven

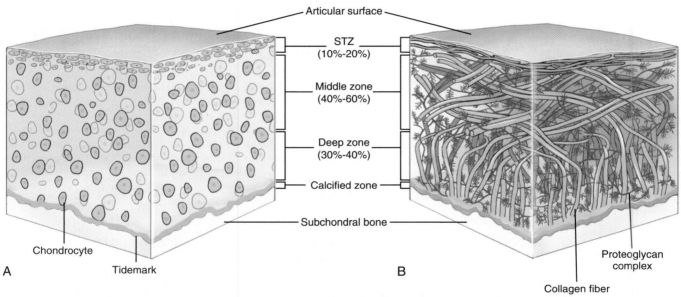

Fig. 2.14 Hyaline cartilage structure zones. (A) The distribution of chondrocytes embedded in the matrix of fluid and minerals transitions to the subchondral bone. (B) The alignment of the collagen fibers transitions from more vertical to horizontal alignment, which creates the structural integrity of the cartilage. The articular surface consists of more densely packed chondrocytes and collagen aligned to provide a barrier to retain fluid in the cartilage. (From Neumann DA. *Kinesiology of the Musculoskeletal System: Foundations for Rehabilitation*. 3rd ed. St. Louis, MO: Mosby Elsevier; 2017; Fig. 2.16.)

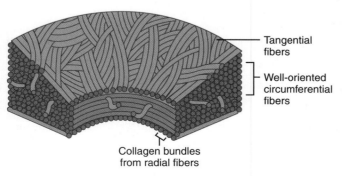

Fig. 2.15 Fibrous cartilage (meniscus) collagen arrangement. Diagrammatic representation of the distribution of collagen fibers in the meniscus of a knee. Collagen is oriented throughout the connective tissues in such a way as to maximally resist the forces placed on these tissues. The majority of the fibers in the meniscus are circumferentially arranged, with a few fibers on or near the tibial surface placed in a radial pattern. This structural arrangement enables the meniscus to resist the lateral spread that occurs during high loads generated during weight-bearing. Longitudinally arranged collagen fibers facilitate shock absorption and sustain the tension generated between the anterior and posterior attachments. (From Bullough PG. *Bullough and Vigorita's Orthopaedic Pathology*. 3rd ed. St. Louis, MO: Mosby, 1997.)

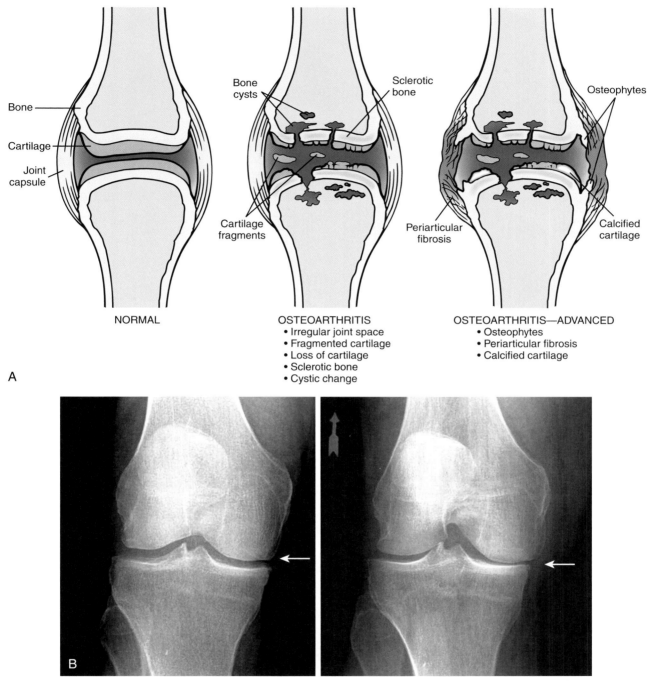

Fig. 2.16 (A) Normal knee joint space. (From Damjanov I. *Pathology for the Health-Related Professions*, 4th ed. Philadelphia, PA: WB Saunders, 2012; Fig. 19.15.) (B) Osteoarthritis. The medial compartment shows joint space narrowing with sclerotic changes on the tibial plateau. (From Harris ED. *Kelley's Textbook of Rheumatology*. 7th ed. Philadelphia: WB Saunders, 2005; Fig. 27.6.)

surfaces on the superficial surface also result in abrasion and further wearing down of both joint surfaces (see Fig. 2.16).[10] Weight-bearing compresses the articular cartilage and also moves fluid out of the cartilage into the joint space. Once weight-bearing forces are removed, the cartilage osmotic potential promotes return of water into the cartilage. Under

normal circumstances, intermittent compression and decompression facilitates exchange of nutrients and fluid. If the articular structure is damaged, the barrier is disrupted and excess fluid leaks into the articular space with limited return, resulting in effusion. Exercise considerations should include reducing weight-bearing forces while promoting joint

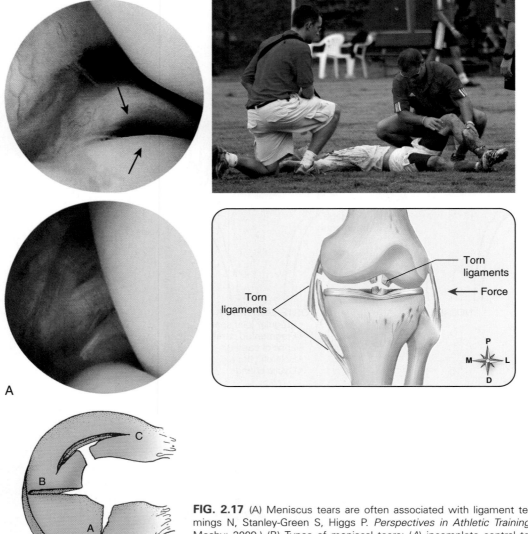

FIG. 2.17 (A) Meniscus tears are often associated with ligament tears. (From Cummings N, Stanley-Green S, Higgs P. *Perspectives in Athletic Training.* St Louis, MO: Mosby; 2009.) (B) Types of meniscal tears: (*A*) incomplete central tear, (*B*) complete tangential tear, (*C*) incomplete radial tear. (From Rothrock JC, Alexander S. *Alexander's Surgical Procedures.* Mosby: St. Louis, MO; 2012, Fig. 11.89.)

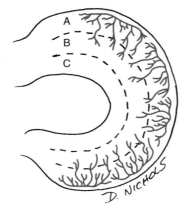

A: Red-on-red zone
B: Red-on-white zone
C: White-on-white zone

FIG. 2.18 Vascular supply in the knee meniscus. The vascular supply to the meniscus is limited to the outer circumferences, limiting the potential for healing and regeneration. (Modified from Shankman G: *Fundamental Orthopedic Management for the Physical Therapist Assistant*, 3rd ed. St Louis, MO: Mosby, 2011; Fig. 18-20A.)

CLINICAL EXAMPLE 2.5 Force Considerations After Osteochondral Defect and Repair

A patient with a history of a high-impact lacrosse injury was diagnosed with an osteochondral defect on the femoral articular surface. He was treated surgically with an arthroscopic debridement to remove loose bodies and micro-fractures to stimulate bleeding and cartilage cell production.[a,b]

Osteochondral defect	Time period	Forces/movement desired	Precautions (forces to be limited)
Phase I: Acute inflammation	0–6 weeks	External compression Movement of other joints around the area to increase blood flow, remove exudate, minimize effects of immobilization Flexion and extension within available range up to 120 degrees (continuous passive motion), active-assisted pain-free range	Immobilizer brace locked at 0 degrees and strict non–weight-bearing on crutches to limit forces on area
Partial healing	6–12 weeks	Promote neuromuscular coordination to prevent excessive vertical forces, particularly control of vertical movement, landing, and direction changes	Protect amount of vertical compression; slow progression of stairs, squats Progressive loading from supported without gravity to upright with support, followed by progression from double- to single-leg activities Care with weight-shifting in any direction in weight-bearing
Full healing	12–18 weeks	Progressive movement complexity and loading to assist with developing adequate muscle strength, power, motor control, coordination, and endurance to minimize and distribute passive forces Progressive movements in all directions, loads, velocities as needed for functional requirements	Based on functional ability and impairment status

[a]Mayman DJ, Gill TJ. Injuries to the meniscus and articular cartilage. In: Magee DJ, Zachazewski JE, Quillen WS. *Pathology and Intervention in Musculoskeletal Rehabilitation.* St. Louis, MO: Elsevier Saunders; 2009: 579–600.
[b]Cavanaugh JT, Williams HA. Microfracture procedure of the knee. In: Cioppa-Mosca J, Cahill JB, Tucker CY (eds). *Handbook of Postsurgical Rehabilitation Guidelines for the Orthopaedic Clinician.* St. Louis, MO: Elsevier Saunders; 2008: 294–302.

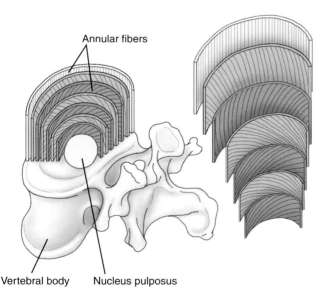

Fig. 2.19 Intervertebral disc structure. Note the outer annular fiber arrangement with diagonals in both directions to limit rotation. The inner nucleus pulposus consists of a gel-like colloid which deforms and absorbs compression with vertical loading and during flexion. (From Muscuolino JE. *Kinesiology of the Skeletal System and Muscle Function,* 2nd ed. St. Louis, MO: Elsevier Mosby, 2011; Fig. 8.12.)

Annular fibers

Vertebral body   Nucleus pulposus

movement that will facilitate fluid movement and gliding (Clinical Example 2.5). However, if there are long-standing and severe changes in the joint surface or cartilage structure, there is limited potential for recovery of the smooth surface and shock absorption properties.[12] Under these circumstances compressive forces will need to be reduced and the importance of distribution of forces through muscle support and alignment becomes a major component of symptom management.[10]

The structure of intervertebral discs is similar to fibrous cartilage, with the exception of having a central nucleus pulposus that is mostly gel-like and provides shock absorption for weight-bearing forces through the spinal column. The surrounding annular fibers contain the gel, which maintains the integrity of the disc. The fibers are aligned at 45-degree angles to resist rotational forces (Fig. 2.19). Maximal stress on the annular fibers occurs with multi-planar movements combining flexion with rotation. After an acute disc injury, combined flexion and rotation should be avoided.

The vertebral bodies are separated by the discs, and, with advancing age, the disc space narrows. Once the disc height decreases, the relative tension of the spinal ligaments becomes slack and the passive restraint system is less efficient, placing

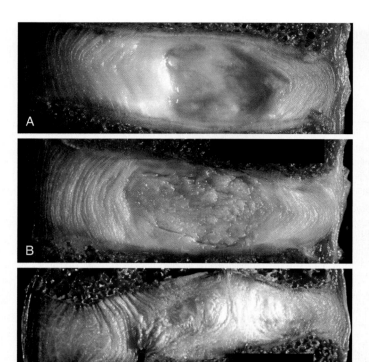

Fig. 2.20 Comparison of normal intervertebral disc, aging changes, and disc disruption. Note the changes in lumbar intervertebral disc structure related to aging and with disc pathology (mid-sagittal section; anterior on the left). (A) Young disc in a 35-year-old man. (B) Mature disc in a 47-year-old man. (C) Disrupted disc in a 31-year-old man. Note the endplate and inward collapse of the inner annulus. (From Adams MA. *The Biomechanics of Back Pain*. Edinburgh: Churchill Livingstone, 2002.)

> ### BOX 2.16   Bone Healing: Force Considerations
>
> - Healing times differ for cortical and cancellous bone.
> - Cortical bone may take up to 48 weeks for full healing.
> - Fracture healing depends on adequate callus formation to link the fracture segments.
> - Initially limit vertical weight-bearing loads until the segments are linked (union). This is followed by progressive weight-bearing to stimulate new bone growth and remodeling.
> - Equal weight-bearing promotes formation of trabeculae in areas and directions needed.
> - Muscle stimulus on the periosteum helps with new bone growth.
> - Angular, shear, or rotational forces may be contraindicated or protected during healing.
> - Bone healing takes precedence over other tissue impairments.

additional stresses on the joints and soft tissues in the area. The decreased fluid content in the disc also impacts the ability of the disc to absorb shock, thus transmitting forces to joint structures. Disc degeneration is a normal aging process, and it is not possible to restore tissue qualities from younger years (Fig. 2.20). However, the exercise prescription can promote neuromuscular adaptations for loss of stability and shock absorption (see the section "Form Closure Versus Force Closure") and limit excessive shear and rotational and compressive forces.[9,10]

Bone

Bones consist of connective tissue embedded with calcium and mineral deposits (Box 2.16). There are two major types of bone: cortical (Fig. 2.21A) and cancellous (Fig. 2.21B). In long bones, the outer cortical bone provides longitudinal and vertical support for lever systems, while the inner medullary region is responsible for producing red blood cells. Cortical bone is densely organized along lines of force in circumferential layers (Haversian systems) (Fig. 2.22).[13] Haversian systems are organized along lines of forces to withstand higher weight-bearing forces, with some additional areas of density where muscle attachments concentrate forces (Fig. 2.22C). Spongy, cancellous bone is not as resilient to larger forces and is the primary component of flat bones such as the pelvis, sternum, vertebral structures, and calcaneus. Flat bones function to protect organs, provide muscular attachments, or absorb shock (Fig. 2.21B).

During fracture healing, the hematoma (Fig. 2.23A) is replaced with granulation tissue (Fig. 2.23B), supported by early cartilaginous callus formation bridging the fracture segments. This is later replaced by bony callus (Fig. 2.23C), and the remodeling phase concludes with osteoclastic activity absorbing the callus and replacing new Haversian systems that bridge the fracture site (Fig. 2.23D).[14,15] Healing times for cortical and cancellous bone differ, with cortical bone taking longer to reform the supportive Haversian systems and restore the structural support and strong lever systems. For new systems to align, vertical weight-bearing forces promote development of the Haversian canals. If weight-bearing is unequal, the trabeculae formation leaves areas of vulnerability for functional force requirements.[13–15]

Once the callus formation is solid enough to prevent the fracture segments from displacing, slow progressive weight-bearing forces will promote bone growth and remodeling in the required directions. Although vertical compressive forces are indicated at this point, until the callus and new bone is well-developed, angular, shear, or rotational forces are contraindicated. Muscle contraction will stimulate periosteal bone growth, promoting Haversian systems that are designed to withstand the direction of the pull on the bony attachments (Clinical Example 2.6). Bone healing takes precedence over other tissue impairments until solid healing has occurred (Video 2.9). The extended healing times for fractures (Table 2.7) do result in deconditioning and connective tissue adaptations from lack of weight-bearing, immobilization, and limited use of the area.[14,15]

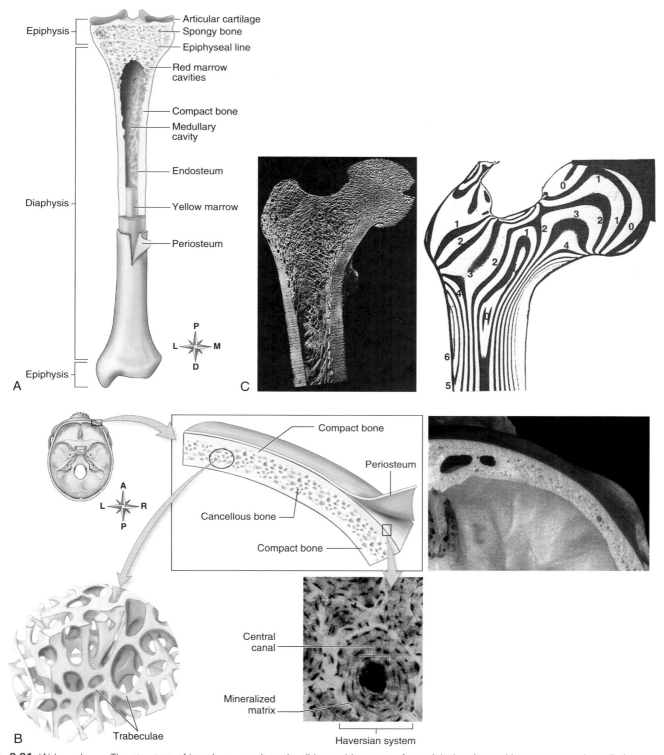

Fig. 2.21 (A) Long bone. The structure of long bones such as the tibia provide support for weight-bearing and lever systems through the compact cortical bone. Muscle attachments also require dense bone as a base for transmission of muscle forces to produce movement. The central medullary canal and cancellous (spongy) bone in the epiphysis also assist with shock absorption and production of red blood cells. (From Patton K, Thibodeau G, Douglas M. *Essentials of Anatomy and Physiology*. St. Louis, MO: Mosby, 2012; Fig. 8.2.) (B) Flat bone. Flat bones such as the skull, sternum, and pelvis provide protection for internal organs and have less compact bone and a greater percentage of cancellous bone. This figure also shows the organization of the spongy cancellous bone with a looser arrangement of trabeculae, while the cortical bone arrangement consists of circular organization of Haversian systems with dense mineralization around a central canal to resist forces. (From Moses K, Nava P, Banks J, Petersen D: *Moses Atlas of Clinical Gross Anatomy*. Philadelphia: Mosby: 2005.) (C) Cortical bone structure: femur. In the cross-section of the femur on the *left*, the dense compact cortical bone is visible on the medial and lateral aspects of the shaft, providing strong support for the limb and transmission of the vertical weight-bearing forces. In the diagram on the *right*, the areas of force concentration are illustrated. The alignment of the Haversian canals in response to the predominant vertical weight-bearing distribution (*4, 5, 6*), muscle forces from the hip abductors on the greater trochanter (*1, 2*), transmission of forces through the neck of the femur (*1, 2, 3, 4*), and related compression on the head of femur (*0*) are illustrated in the diagram. (From Patton K, Thibodeau G, Douglas M. *Essentials of Anatomy and Physiology*. St. Louis, MO: Mosby, 2012; Fig. 8.2.)

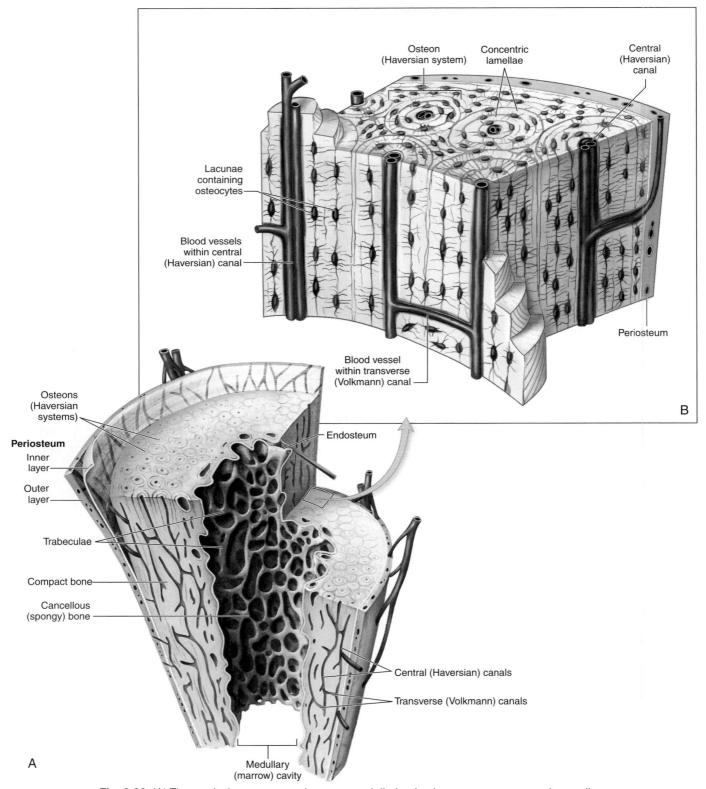

Fig. 2.22 (A) The vertical structure, periosteum, and distinction between compact and cancellous bone. (B) The central vasculature and the organization of the Haversian systems in concentric lamellae. (From Patton K, Thibodeau G, Douglas M. *Essentials of Anatomy and Physiology.* St. Louis, MO: Mosby, 2012; Fig. 8.4.)

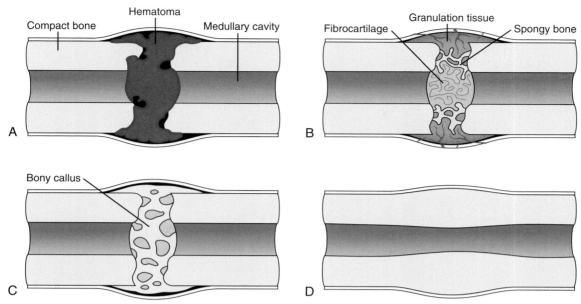

Fig. 2.23 Fracture healing. Overlapping stages of bone healing. (A) Immediate bleeding and hematoma formation. (B) Formation of granulation tissue, fibrocartilage develops in between the fracture fragments, and early spongy bone is laid down to provide a soft union. In this phase, periosteal bone formation provides an external callus that helps link the bone fragments. (C) The soft callus is replaced with harder bone deposition. (D) Remodeling occurs with resorption of some of the callus, reshaping of the medullary canal, and deposition of bone along lines of stress. (From Damjanov I. *Pathology for the Health-Related Professions*, 4th ed. Philadelphia, PA: WB Saunders, 2012; Fig. 19.10.)

TABLE 2.7	**Cortical and Cancellous Bone Healing Phases**[13,14]		
	Inflammatory Phase	**Reparative Phase**	**Remodeling Phase**
Findings	Inflammation hematoma and early granulation Osteoclastic activity to remove remnants and hematoma Blood vessels start to grow into area	Union Soft callus is produced by fibroblasts; periosteal bone growth to provide bridging callus Early woven bone is laid down between fragments	Consolidation and remodeling once mechanically stable Lamellar bone formation and alignment Resorption of extra callus Osteoblastic and osteoclastic activity Medullary canal is reshaped
Approximate percentage of entire cycle	10%	20–40%	50–70%
Timelines	Days	Weeks to months	Years
Example timelines: Cortical Cancellous	0–14 days 0–7 days	10 days–24 weeks 5 days–8 weeks	12–48 weeks 6–12 weeks

Note these are approximate timelines. The healing time is dependent on the size of the bone and requirements for function; weight-bearing bones require greater strength than non–weight-bearing bones. The type of fracture and surgical fixation also influence time frames. Additional personal characteristics such as age, weight, and nutritional status, along with comorbidities, all influence the actual time for healing.
Data from Loitz-Ramage BJ, Zernicke R. Bone biology and mechanics. In: Magee DJ, Zachazewski JE, Quillen WS. *Scientific Foundations and Principles of Practice in Musculoskeletal Rehabilitation*. St. Louis, MO: Saunders Elsevier; 2007:122–143; and Hoppenfeld S, Murthy VL. *Treatment and Rehabilitation of Fractures*. Philadelphia, PA: Lippincott Williams & Wilkins; 2000.

CLINICAL EXAMPLE 2.6   **Force Considerations After Fracture**

A 20-year-old man was hit by a car while trying to change a flat tire on the freeway and sustained an open distal tibia and fibular fracture. The fracture was reduced surgically with open reduction and internal fixation.

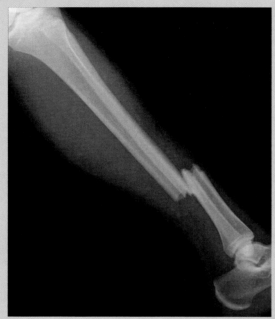

Lateral view of distal tibia/fibular fracture. The fracture of the distal one-third of the tibia and fibula is transverse with anterior displacement of the proximal fragments. The fracture is highly unstable in the anterior posterior direction.

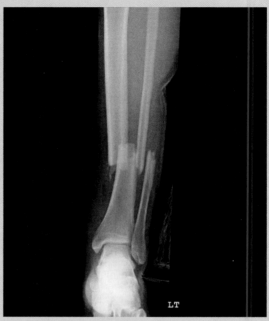

Anteroposterior view of tibia and fibular fracture showing overlap. The bleeding and muscle damage from the trauma and the position of the fragments will need to be addressed during the recovery.

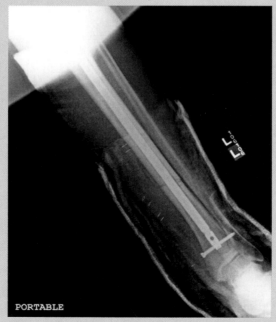

Postoperative anteroposterior view of intramedullary rod placement in tibia for fixation of distal tibia/fibular fracture (distal view including ankle). Anteroposterior view of the rod and the distal fixation screw immediately postop. The ankle is stabilized in a cast. The fracture has been reduced and is stabilized by the intramedullary rod, while the distal screw prevents the rod sliding into the ankle joint and limits rotation. Until full fracture healing is present, rotation and angulation forces will need to be limited. The angle of the fracture also indicates the need to be cautious with anteroposterior forces, although the internal fixation is extremely stable.

CLINICAL EXAMPLE 2.6 Force Considerations After Fracture—cont'd

After surgery, the contraindications and precautions override impairments and functional deficits until sufficient healing is evident. As the patient progresses, precautions are lifted and weight-bearing forces are allowed without angulation or rotation to stimulate new bone formation. Slow progression of vertical or compressive loading helps stimulate new cortical bone formation, while muscle contraction stimulates periosteal bone formation.

Tibial fracture	Time period	Forces/movement desired	Precautions (forces to be limited)
Phase I: Acute inflammation	8 weeks	Active hip and knee range of motion Isometric contractions in cast (ankle and toe muscles)	Hard cast and non–weight-bearing on crutches to limit forces on area (particularly rotation as the hardware was not limiting rotation within the intramedullary canal)
Partial healing	9–12 weeks	Partial weight-bearing Light resistance for ankle movement in midrange with remainder of leg supported Hip strengthening with application of force above knee	Full weight-bearing Rotation or angulation with weight-bearing
	12–24 weeks	Weight-bearing as tolerated; progressive load and training for weight shifting Progressive-resistance knee and ankle exercise	Care with functional activities with weight-bearing and angulation or rotation
Full healing	24–48 weeks	Progressive movement complexity and loading to assist with developing adequate muscle strength, power, motor control, coordination, and endurance to minimize and distribute passive forces Progressive movements in all directions, loads, velocities as needed for functional requirements Capabilities depend on neuromuscular ability to control position and produce motion	Based on functional ability

BOX 2.17 Specific Adaptations to Imposed Demand (SAID Principle)

- Muscle adapts to imposed demand by:
  - Alterations in connective tissue alignment
  - Improved neuromuscular activation and sequencing
  - Muscle hypertrophy
  - Increased vascularity and mitochondrial adaptations.
- Imposed demand specificity includes type of movement, required forces, aerobic demands, repetition, type of contraction (concentric/eccentric), muscle length, and direction.
  - Overload principle: Hypertrophy results from loads beyond the normal demands.
  - Delayed-onset muscle soreness (DOMS) after starting new exercise can start 8–12 hours later, peaks at 24–48 hours, and usually dissipates after 72 hours.
  - Appropriate dosage and slow progression is important to limit DOMS.

BOX 2.18 Stabilizer and Mover Function

- *Local stabilizer*: Small muscles located close to the joints that provide local positional control of joints, often for postural control against gravity or to support joints for stability in multiple directions (*stability*).
- *Global stabilizer*: Large muscles are recruited to stabilize joints or regions when greater force requirements are present and control movement toward the end of range. Global stabilizer use may be required for stability against external forces for balance (*stability in response to higher external loads*).
- *Global mover*: Large muscles often crossing more than one joint; required for rapid, phasic motion and power or precise movement (*mobility*).

Muscle

Muscle strength (Boxes 2.17–2.19) is dependent on the frequency and timing of motor unit activation as well as the amount of muscle tissue (cross-sectional diameter). **Strength** is defined as the ability to lift weight. Muscle atrophy (decreased cross-sectional diameter) results from disuse or immobilization. The loss of muscle protein and changes in connective tissue result in decreased ability to resist forces. There are also changes in neuromuscular activation and physiological changes that result in decreased endurance or ability to contract repeatedly with decreased use.[16] Exercise can be used to restore muscle strength and integrity after atrophy or to minimize atrophy during periods of immobilization.

The concept of **specific adaptations to imposed demands (SAID)** is vital for all exercise therapy.[17] Muscle responds by structural and physiological changes unique to the type of movement, amount of force, aerobic demands, and other variables such as concentric versus eccentric control, the muscle length, and direction of force. Muscle tissue adapts to imposed demand by (1) alterations in connective tissue alignment/ability to resist force, (2) improved neuromuscular activation and sequencing, (3) muscle hypertrophy (increased cross-sectional diameter), and (4) increased vascularity and mitochondrial adaptations.[17] The neurological system adapts within the first few weeks of initiating or increasing activity by increasing the efficiency of coordination and sequencing of motor unit firing. Therefore, the therapist could anticipate quick progression in ability to resist forces as a result of the neuromuscular responses.

On the other hand, muscle hypertrophy or increased cross-sectional diameter can take longer to develop (up to 6 weeks) and requires reaching **overload** (load beyond normal demands).[18] Tissue healing restrictions during rehabilitation often prohibit prescribing loads heavy enough to be considered overload, so patients will often have to continue to advance their strengthening exercises after completing therapy. Therapists will need to educate patients how to safely yet sufficiently continue to progress their load even after they have completed their rehabilitation program. Muscle strength is dependent on both neuromuscular activation and the ability to produce force related to muscle cross-sectional diameter and is defined as the ability to lift weight. The amount of weight that an individual is able to lift just once is defined as a *one-repetition maximum* (1RM), while the amount possible for 10 repetitions is a *10-repetition maximum* (10RM). Using the overload principle, weight involving 1 to 10 repetitions before fatigue is an approximate guideline for strengthening exercise.[19] However, in older or deconditioned individuals, the load that can be lifted up to 15 times is sometimes regarded as an appropriate strengthening exercise.[18] Muscle **endurance** changes occur with improvements in vascular supply and with mitochondrial adaptations and more efficient use of oxidative processes; these require higher repetitions (>15 repetitions) that are only possible with lower loads.[18]

While exercise is a key element for muscle recovery after injury or deconditioning, exercise can induce **delayed-onset muscle soreness** (DOMS) when new exercise is introduced. Typically, delayed-onset soreness starts anywhere from 8 to 12 hours after exercise, peaks between 24 and 48 hours, and usually dissipates within 72 hours. However, if severe soreness occurs, the pain may last 5 to 7 days (Clinical Example 2.7).[19-20] All forms of exercise can induce pain if the dosage exceeds the muscle's ability to withstand the forces applied to the tissue, although eccentric exercise has the potential to cause earlier onset and more intense DOMS than concentric exercise.[19,20] The resultant pain often influences adherence to exercise programs and can hinder rehabilitation progress. Therefore, DOMS should be avoided as much as possible. The appropriate exercise dosage is key to avoiding any DOMS, with slow progression of strengthening exercise.

BOX 2.19 Muscle Adaptation and Recovery: Force Considerations

- Muscle strength depends on the frequency and timing of motor unit activation, as well cross-sectional size.
- Specificity of muscle activation is important for strength gains.
- Overload principle: Hypertrophy results from loads beyond the normal demands.
- Delayed-onset muscle soreness (DOMS) after starting new exercise can start 8–12 hours later, peaks at 24–48 hours, and usually dissipates after 72 hours.
- Appropriate dosage and slow progression is important to limit DOMS.
- Muscle function depends on how much load is applied to the area and how long the muscle needs to maintain the area against the load.
- Local and global stabilizer function is related to stability or control of a joint position, with local stabilizers controlling smaller joint motion and ranges than global stabilizers.
- Global movers are responsible for producing larger forces for movement and power.
- The order of muscle recruitment is based on requirements to withstand load, with local stabilizer muscles activating at low thresholds, followed by global stabilizers at higher thresholds, and global movers at the highest threshold.
- Function is also related to physiological energy requirements, with stabilizers using aerobic metabolic pathways and movers using primarily anaerobic pathways.

CLINICAL EXAMPLE 2.7 Muscle Stimulus and Delayed-Onset Muscle Soreness

A 55-year-old executive presents with a rotator cuff tear after lifting a heavy suitcase into an overhead compartment while traveling.

Evaluation

From the subjective evaluation the therapist determines the following:

Severity: Mild (3/10 intermittent pain, pain only with higher-range shoulder flexion, lifting objects, or sustained positions)

Irritability: Mild (pain is constant, pain increases to 4/10 with overhead movement but decreases to baseline immediately afterward)

Nature: Grade I supraspinatus tear

Stage: Phase II (injury was 2 weeks ago, pain is now intermittent, impairment focus)

As part of the treatment plan, the therapist determines that there is a need to improve the rotator cuff muscle function for the patient to maintain the glenohumeral approximation while holding the arm at 70 degrees of flexion for at least 2 minutes for dressing. The patient is unable to hold the arm in this position for more than 15 seconds against gravity without any weight.

Exercise Choice

The overall exercise progression focuses on the rotator cuff (**local stabilizers**). As anti-gravity exercise is difficult, a supportive position is chosen that allows **isometric stabilization** without pain and is held to fatigue of the rotator cuff. Isometric contraction against elastic resistance is chosen as the first exercise to limit strain on the rotator cuff while providing some stimulus for muscle adaptation to stress. The patient was able to hold the position for 30 seconds for both internal and external rotation and is able to repeat the exercise twice.

The patient reports that there was no increase in pain during the exercise, but there was some mild constant muscle soreness in the rotator cuff area a day later. The pain decreased by 48 hours.

Evaluation

This pattern fits with **delayed-onset muscle soreness**. However, the soreness was mild. There are multiple options to adjust the exercise but, in this case, the patient was asked to decrease the intensity of the contraction and use less elastic resistance although the position is still held for as long as possible. After the adjustment, there was no pain the following day.

TABLE 2.8   Muscle Function, Characteristics, and Examples[21]

	Function	Characteristics	Examples	Responses to Pain or Inflammation
Local stabilizers	Provide local positional control of joints, often for postural control against gravity or to support joints for stability in multiple directions (*stability*)	Small muscles, close to joints Recruited at low thresholds of force requirements Early or anticipatory function to provide stable proximal segments Maintain position through tonic muscle activity (isometric or small midrange activity) or alternating control of muscle around the joint Endurance capabilities Primarily slow oxidative muscle fiber activation (see Fig. 2.22)	Spinal stabilizer muscles: multifidi, rotators, intertransversarii Transversus abdominis Rotator cuff muscles Cervical deep flexors Hip external rotators	Initial spasm, inactivity, and atrophy with prolonged pain Late activation, insufficient control, or poor endurance
Global stabilizers	Recruited to stabilize joints or regions when greater force requirements are present May be required for stability against gravity for balance (*stability in response to higher external loads*)	Larger intermediate layer muscles, cross multiple joints Recruited at higher thresholds than local stabilizers May be recruited throughout the range, including end range of motion (concentric or eccentric control) to protect joints or for shock absorption Used to withstand higher loads than local stabilizers Primarily fast oxidative glycolytic muscle fiber activation (see Fig. 2.22)	Erector spinae Obliques Deltoid Scalenes Gluteus medius	Initially hyperactive, later inactivity, late activation, or insufficient force generation
Global movers	Produce motion (*mobility*)	Larger or two-joint muscles Activated at highest threshold Speed, precision, or power Requires rapid phasic contractions and high-power production from primarily fast-twitch, fatigable muscle fibers (see Fig. 2.22)	Rectus abdominis Biceps Sternocleidomastoid Hamstrings	Hyperactivity, insufficient strength, power, precision, or speed

Data from Magee DJ, Zachazewski JE. Principles of stabilization training. In: Magee DJ, Zachazewski JE, Quillen WS. *Scientific Foundations and Principles of Practice in Musculoskeletal Rehabilitation.* St. Louis, MO: Saunders Elsevier; 2007:388–413.

Muscle Function

Muscles can also be described in terms of their functions as *local stabilizers, global stabilizers,* or *global movers.*[21] The degree of force required during a functional movement or exercise may result in selective recruitment of different muscles. (See Table 2.8 for function, characteristics, and examples for each category.) The physiological characteristics of the majority of the muscle fiber types for each muscle group differ based on their function: stabilizers have a higher percentage of slow oxidative fibers (local stabilizers) or fast oxidative glycolytic fibers (global stabilizers), while global movers have mostly fast fatigable properties (Fig. 2.24; see Box 2.18).[21] The threshold of force requirements is lower for the local stabilizers that also need to be able to maintain postural positions for longer periods. Global stabilizers respond to higher force requirements, including the need to maintain or control motion toward the end of range, where length-tension relationships decrease muscle efficiency. Global movers are recruited if there is a need for high force production, fast speeds, or power production. Global movers use anaerobic metabolic pathways because the requirements are phasic to produce high force or more precise movement in short time frames. The type of muscle recruited may be altered in response to injury or avoidance patterns. Altered in response to injury and avoidance patterns (see Table 2.8 and Box 2.19).[21] If the smaller, stabilizing muscles are inactive (a common response to pain, swelling, and edema), preferential use of the larger global movers can result in stresses being absorbed by the joint structures. If motor patterns are repeated, the global movers shorten with limited opposition or proximal spinal support. These postural patterns or imbalances are potential causes of localized breakdown or overuse syndromes.[21] Exercise programs can be tailored to restore the optimum use of specific muscle for function by thoughtful choice of exercise parameters and skillful instruction in motor learning concepts.

BIOMECHANICAL CONCEPTS TO APPLY, DISTRIBUTE, OR MINIMIZE FORCES TO REGIONS OR SPECIFIC TISSUES

Force and Torque

The human body is designed to be able to withstand external loads (push or pull) produced by gravity or outside objects, as

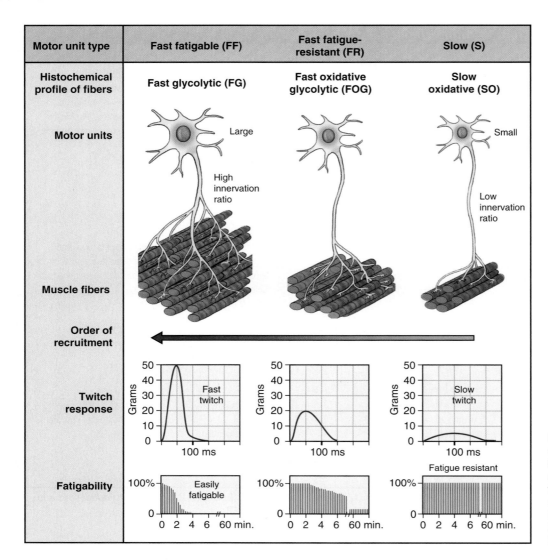

Motor unit type	Fast fatigable (FF)	Fast fatigue-resistant (FR)	Slow (S)
Histochemical profile of fibers	Fast glycolytic (FG)	Fast oxidative glycolytic (FOG)	Slow oxidative (SO)
Motor units	Large / High innervation ratio		Small / Low innervation ratio
Muscle fibers			
Order of recruitment			
Twitch response	Fast twitch		Slow twitch
Fatigability	Easily fatigable		Fatigue resistant

FIG. 2.24 Classification of motor unit types from muscle fibers based on histochemical profile, size, and contractile characteristics. (From Neumann DA. *Kinesiology of the Musculoskeletal System: Foundations for Rehabilitation*. 2nd ed. St. Louis, MO: Mosby Elsevier; 2010; Fig. 3.19.)

well as internal forces created by muscle (Box 2.20 and Fig. 2.25). The ability to counteract forces allows individuals to maintain an upright posture, avoid falling in response to gravity, and perform functional activities. The point of application of the force on the body, distance from the point of application to the axis of the motion, and the relevant muscles that oppose the resistance are important considerations when analyzing functional movements or exercise technique. Exercise dosage can be adjusted by changing the distance of applied resistance to muscle attachments or joints to make an exercise easier or more challenging. The angle of the muscle attachment to the lever arm and insertion sites will also influence the relative efficiency of the muscle to produce or counteract movement (Fig. 2.26; Video 2.10).[22]

Axis of Motion

The **axis of motion** is the point around which motion of a segment occurs. The axis of motion is important when considering

> ### BOX 2.20   Force Characteristics to Consider During Exercise Prescription
>
> - Magnitude of force (weight or load)
> - Point of application of force to the body
> - Distance of the application of force to the axis of motion
> - Goal to create movement or maintain stability by counteracting internal or external forces
> - Axis of motion and if the area is designed or intended to be the axis of movement during functional motion

the distance of the resistance from the axis (which influences the type of lever system and biomechanical advantage due to the relative moment arms) (Fig. 2.27; Video 2.11). *Torque* is the rotational magnitude of the force (force multiplied by the distance from the axis). The overall torque being applied to structures can

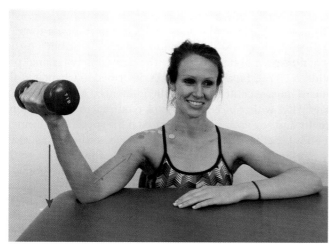

Fig. 2.25 Internal forces created by muscle opposing external forces from gravity acting on the forearm. Internal forces created by the elbow flexors (*blue arrow*) are opposing the external force from the weight of the arm and the free weight (*red arrow*). If the arm is moving toward the body, the flexors are contracting concentrically. If the arm is lowered slowly toward the table, the elbow flexors lengthen and the contraction is still opposing the gravitational pull from the weight and the forearm. The lengthening contraction is an eccentric contraction and some of the force is absorbed by the muscle connective tissue.

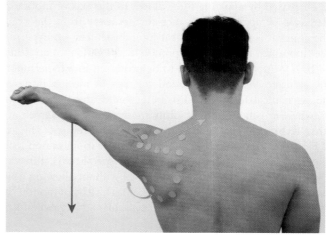

Fig. 2.26 Angular insertion of shoulder abductors at 120 degrees. The resistance from the arm weight (*red arrow*) is counterbalanced by the contraction of the deltoid, supraspinatus, and other shoulder flexors/abductors (*blue arrows*), and the position of the shoulder is reliant on the scapula support provided by the upward rotation force couple from the serratus anterior and trapezius muscles (*green arrows*). The angle of the supraspinatus muscle is oriented based on the position of the scapula relative to the humerus. The alignment of the muscle is also influenced by the glenohumeral joint rotation. If the arm is internally rotated, the tendon is at an angle relative to the scapula. The scapula upward rotation is a result of the trapezius action on the spine of the scapula and serratus anterior providing an upward and forward motion supporting the upper limb motion in higher ranges of shoulder flexion and abduction.

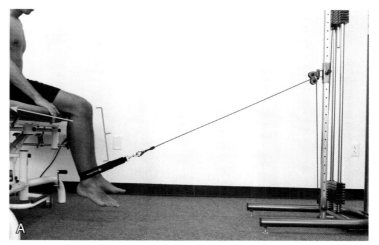

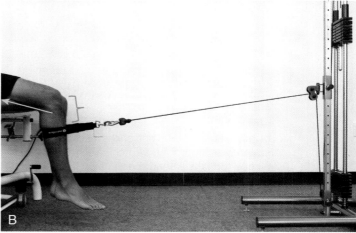

FIG. 2.27 (A) Application of force further from the axis compared with (B). The moment arm from the axis of the joint to point of the application of the force is larger than in B, thus requiring greater overall torque from the hamstrings to flex the knee against the pulley weight. (B) The moment arm from the axis of the joint to point of the application of the force is smaller than in A and decreases the overall torque required from the hamstrings to flex the knee against the pulley weight.

be decreased by applying force closer to the axis of motion or increased by applying resistance further away from the axis.[22] The concept is also important if joint structures are hypermobile (too much motion) or hypomobile (too little motion; Video 2.12). If joint structures need to be protected in a hypermobile area, muscle contraction around the axis of motion improves the mechanical advantage, distributes forces, and allows motion elsewhere during healing. If joints are hypomobile, exercise and other techniques can be used to promote movement. The axis of motion is considered during stretching or mobilization techniques to apply appropriate force to the specific structure that is shortened and needs to be addressed without allowing other more mobile regions to move (Fig. 2.28). The axis of motion can also be changed by adjusting neuromuscular strategies and timing (Video 2.13).

Direction of Force, Gravity Assistance, Elimination, and Resistance

The influence of gravity on the human body and body segments is a vital consideration for all exercises and functional movements (Box 2.21 and Fig. 2.29). External moments (the distance from the axis to the torque created by body weight) will depend on where the line of gravity falls relative to the joint axis (Fig. 2.29).[22] It is also important to consider body alignment to promote anti-gravity muscle activation or to use balance to promote or resist gravity. If the body is in a balanced static posture, the line of gravity through the center of mass projects inside the base of support. If the line of gravity falls outside the base, the body will move in response to gravity (Fig. 2.30) unless the individual alters his or her posture by activating muscles to oppose the natural gravitational pull (Videos 2.11, 2.14, and 2.15).[22] As described in Chapter 1, the type of muscle contraction will be influenced by the direction of gravity, with *concentric control* required to move against gravity and *eccentric control* required if the speed of movement or body weight is being controlled when lowering against gravity (see Fig. 2.25 and Videos 1.3 and 1.5). The muscles on the opposite side of the limb are used to counteract the weight of the limb against gravitational forces (Videos 2.10 and 2.16). Gravitational forces acting on body segments should also be considered before positioning the patient for an exercise. This is the case when gravity will be the primary force acting on the

---

BOX 2.21   Direction of Force: Gravitational Forces and Pulleys

- Direction of gravitational force on the body as well as external resistance should be considered when selecting exercise position and resistance.
- Pulley systems can be used to change direction of forces to optimize resistance for specific muscle length-tension relationships.
- Muscle length-tension is optimal in midrange; at completely contracted length, force is only generated through active mechanisms and limited once filaments overlap. At completely stretched position, passive mechanisms provide most of the force.

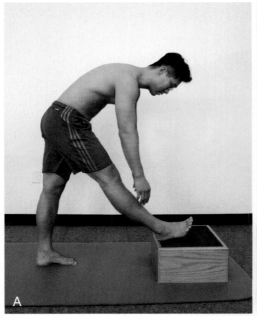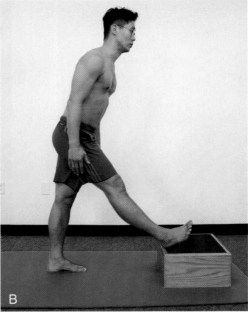

Fig. 2.28 Hip flexion (hinging) in standing. (A) If the patient flexes forward at the hips but also allows the spine to flex, motion occurs in multiple areas. If he allows the spine to move as a result of reaching the endpoint of the hamstring flexibility, additional stress is absorbed by the spinal structures rather than stretching the hamstrings. (B) If the patient keeps his spine straight and hinges forward around the hip axis, the length of the hamstrings is stretched to the maximum. Note that the amount of overall forward flexion is less than in A. If the patient has limited flexibility of the hamstrings, this option would not only be preferred to maximize the stretch, but also to limit the amount of stress on the lumbar spine.

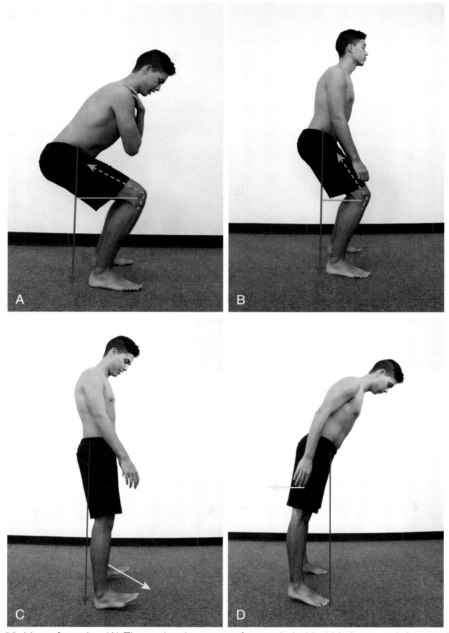

Fig. 2.29 Line of gravity. (A) The patient's center of mass is behind his base and the quadriceps muscles are controlling his knee flexion eccentrically on the lowering action and are also preventing him from falling backward. If his weight was further forward over his base, the forces would be distributed between the knee and the hip muscles, and the external moment arm for the knee joint would be smaller. (B) The distance from his center of mass to the knee (external moment arm) is smaller with less knee and hip flexion. There is less overall muscle action required to prevent him falling backward, and the center of mass is also closer to his base of support on the patellofemoral joint in this position than in B. (C) If the patient leans backward so that his center of mass is behind the base of his feet, the anterior ankle muscles are activated to bring his body back into a position of equilibrium or static balance. (D) If the patient leans forward so that his center of mass is in front of the base of his feet, the posterior leg or trunk muscles are activated to bring his body back into a position of equilibrium or static balance. The position of the body needs to be considered when targeting muscles for muscle function improvements or for safety. *Blue arrow*, quadriceps eccentric contraction to control knee position; *orange line*, external moment arm; *red arrow*, line of gravity; *yellow arrow*, muscle activity required to return body to a balanced position over the base of support.

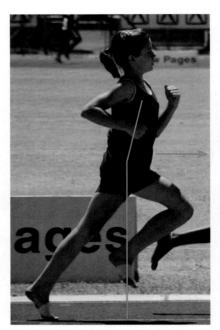

Fig. 2.30 Gravitational force implications for movement. During dynamic motion, the body is propelled through space, assisted by the center of mass placement in front of the base of support to help with forward momentum (*blue arrow*). Note that the runner has a forward trunk inclination (*top blue line*) along with a split between her push-off leg and the leading swing leg. The trunk rotation assists with dynamic counterbalance to help with the forward momentum. *Blue line* indicates line of gravity from center of mass. (Photograph courtesy of Ian Dunleavy.)

body part, but also when other forms of external forces, such as free weights (Video 2.17; see Fig. 2.25), elastic resistance (Video 2.18), pulleys (Videos 1.5 and 2.19; see Fig. 2.27A, B), or therapist-delivered resistance (Video 2.20) provide the load.

Gravity-assisted exercise uses gravitational force to promote movement with little or no muscle contraction. This form of exercise is useful to increase or maintain range of motion. **Gravity-eliminated** exercise minimizes the effect of gravity by supporting the limb to minimize the effect of gravity. Gravity-eliminated exercise may be useful when muscle strength is inadequate to exercise against gravity or to allow movement without pain. Systems that support body weight can also be used to decrease the effect of gravity in upright positions or during walking on a treadmill. Aquatic therapy is another means of decreasing the effect of gravity because the buoyancy of the water supports the limb, and additional assistance can be provided by using flotation devices.

Gravity resistance occurs when the limb or body is moving against gravity. The amount of load is influenced by the mass of the limb or trunk and the angle relative to gravitational pull (see Figs. 2.25 and 2.26; Videos 2.10 and 2.16). External resistance may be applied during exercise by use of the patient's body or limb weight, elastic resistance (Videos 2.18 and 2.21), free weights (e.g., dumbbells or weighted balls; Video 2.11), pulley resistance (Videos 1.5 and 2.19), or exercise equipment.

External pulleys provide options for directing the angle and controlling the amount of force through a suitable range of motion for muscular tension. Pulleys can be used to alter the direction and resultant torque to match the desired range of muscle length.

The mid or resting length of a muscle provides the **optimal length-tension relationship** to resist loads (Fig. 2.31).[23] A shortened length results in muscle filament overlap and limited ability to develop force through contraction. If the muscle length increases past the resting or mid-position, passive connective tissue tension increases, contributing to the ability to resist force (Fig. 2.31).[23] At this point, active force is the lowest. There is more likelihood of damage to the passive connective tissue at the extreme lengths. Resistance exercise and passive stretching toward the end of muscle length can result in muscle soreness and damage if the forces exceed the muscle complex's ability to withstand tension. Therapists can apply their knowledge of optimal muscle length and length-tension relationships to challenge or reduce the difficulty of an exercise or task.

Distribution of Force

Form Closure Versus Force Closure

Joints have varying degrees of stability provided by the anatomical structure of the bone, capsule, and ligaments or nonmuscular

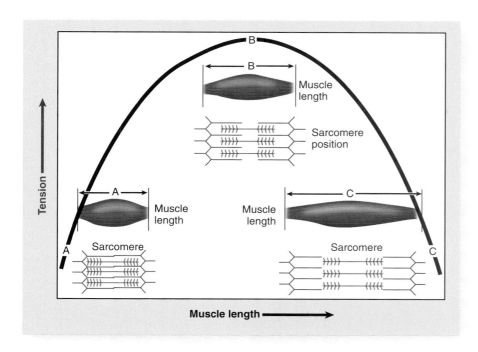

FIG. 2.31 Length-tension relationships for muscle contraction. The mid position of any muscle length is the most efficient position for length-tension relationships. The completely shortened position results in overlap of sarcomeres, decreasing the potential for development of tension, while the lengthened position creates tension on the connective tissue, also decreasing potential for contraction force. (From Patton K, Thibodeau G, Douglas M. *Essentials of Anatomy and Physiology*. St. Louis, MO: Mosby, 2012.)

BOX 2.22 Distribution of Force: Form Closure and Force Closure

- *Form closure*: Stability provided by the shape, structure, or form of a joint (noncontractile)
- *Force closure*: Stability from neuromuscular contributions (contractile) to maintaining joint relationships
- If form closure is influenced by injury, degenerative changes, or congenital structural abnormalities, there is a greater reliance on force closure

---

structures (**form closure**) and muscular activity (**force closure**) (Box 2.22).[24] The joint stability depends on form and force closure, as well as on neuromuscular control. Under optimal conditions and with normal structural alignment, the hip joint has greater form closure than the shoulder, which has less bone enclosure for the ball and socket joint (Fig. 2.32). With joint damage, congenital structural alignment, or connective tissue laxity, less joint stability is present. The use of neuromuscular control (force closure) becomes a major focus of the rehabilitation program to compensate for the loss of structural stability or to distribute forces to other areas (Fig. 2.33 and Clinical Example 2.8).

Bony Alignment

Bony alignment (Box 2.23) influences overall support for balance and movement. The ability to maintain alignment while moving, or *dynamic alignment*, is a function of bony alignment and muscular control. The more extreme the bony angulation, rotation, curvature, or limb length discrepancies are, the more difficult it becomes to support the limb or body against gravity.

Promoting neuromuscular force closure and force distribution becomes that much more important for individuals with bony malalignments. The use of positions that require less opposition against gravity (Videos 2.22 and 2.23) may therefore be preferred for initial strengthening and endurance exercise until the individual is able to improve neuromuscular recruitment patterns, endurance, and strength.

Internal forces on anatomical structures are also influenced by the angles and directions of muscles, tendons, and forces on joint structures. Overall, increased angulation of structures requires additional muscle control and strength due to the increased moment arms. The angulation and rotational forces also place excessive stress on specific areas of tendon, joints, and muscle and can contribute to repetitive strain injuries. Unfortunately, excessive angulation (varus or valgus; Fig. 2.34), extreme rotation (femoral or tibial torsion), and leg length discrepancies cannot be reversed after adolescence. As muscle attachments are established and fixed, the natural bony alignment should therefore be maintained and *not* corrected during exercise. The extent of bony alignment abnormalities will influence the prognosis for full recovery after repetitive strain injury or the potential for future problems. The natural bony alignment should not be confused with dynamic alignment abnormalities related to inadequate neuromuscular control or coordination.

Open Versus Closed Chain Motion

Open chain movement occurs when the end of a limb is free to move, and individual joint control can be produced without

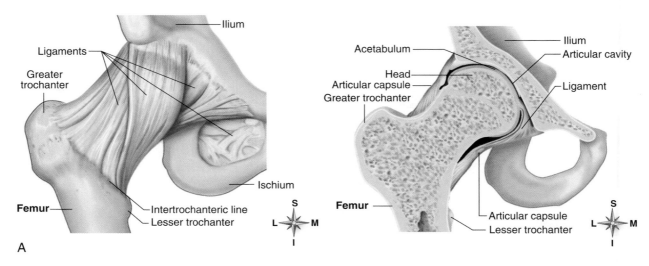

A

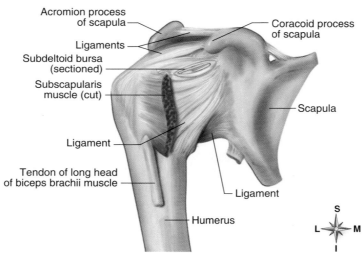

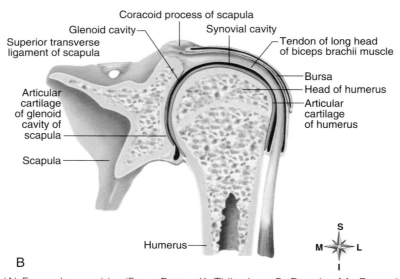

B

FIG. 2.32 (A) Form closure, hip. (From Patton K, Thibodeau G, Douglas M. *Essentials of Anatomy and Physiology*. St. Louis, MO: Mosby, 2012; Fig. 9.28B.). (B) Form closure, shoulder. Both the hip and shoulder joints have similar structural arrangements. The form closure of the hip is greater as a result of the deeper hip acetabulum and labrum enclosing the femoral head and strong capsular support, while in the shoulder the glenoid is relatively shallow and the humeral head is larger than the articular surface. (From Patton K, Thibodeau G, Douglas M. *Essentials of Anatomy and Physiology*. St. Louis, MO: Mosby, 2012; Fig. 9.26.)

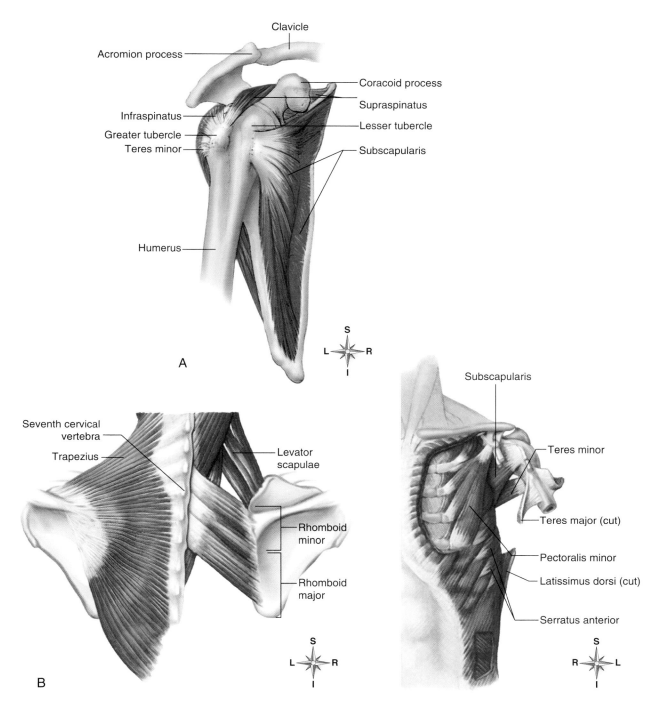

Fig. 2.33 Force closure shoulder. The shoulder complex relies on force closure for stability from the (A) shoulder local stabilizing muscles (rotator cuff), (B) posterior global stabilizing muscles (rhomboids, lattisimus dorsi, posterior deltoid, trapezius), and (C) anterior global stabilizing muscles (pectoralis minor, pectoralis major, deltoid, serratus anterior). (From Patton K, Thibodeau G, Douglas M. *Essentials of Anatomy and Physiology*. St. Louis, MO: Mosby, 2012.)

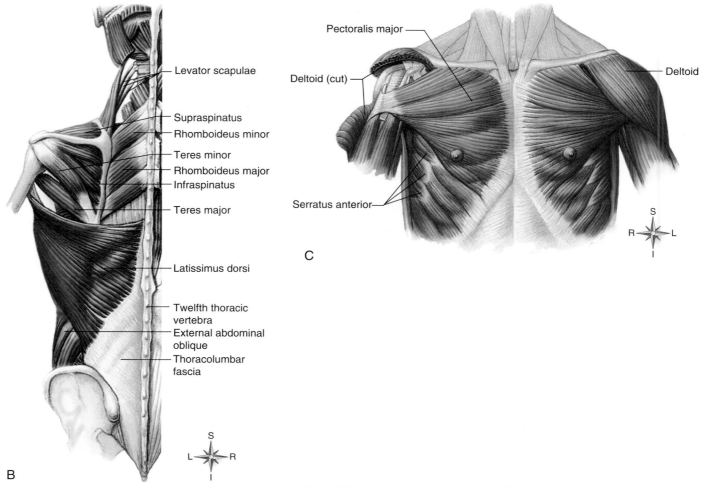

B

C

- Levator scapulae
- Supraspinatus
- Rhomboideus minor
- Teres minor
- Rhomboideus major
- Infraspinatus
- Teres major
- Latissimus dorsi
- Twelfth thoracic vertebra
- External abdominal oblique
- Thoracolumbar fascia

Pectoralis major

Deltoid (cut)

Deltoid

Serratus anterior

Fig. 2.33, cont'd

⚑ CLINICAL EXAMPLE 2.8   **Need for Additional Force Closure With Hip Dysplasia**

A 26-year-old female student and ballet teacher (former professional dancer) presents with a history of hip pain and clicking. She is now complaining of increased hip discomfort in the anterior thigh, pinching in the groin, and pain over the greater trochanter. She has had intermittent episodes of giving way. Radiographs showed (*A*) shallow acetabular angle, (*B*) coxa valga, and (*C*) sclerosis of the superior acetabulum. Trabeculae changes show weight-bearing through the medial aspect of the femur and (*D*) decreased bone density around the greater trochanter, also indicating decreased muscle pull on the greater trochanter. She is diagnosed with hip dysplasia and early arthritic changes due to the lack of form closure. The limited form closure from the congenital bony alignment requires greater muscle support from all hip muscles for stability in weight-bearing positions in comparison to other individuals with full acetabular coverage.

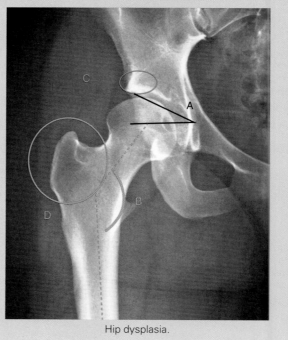

Hip dysplasia.

motion elsewhere in the chain (Box 2.24). There are minimal joint compression forces, and individual coordination of motion is possible (Fig. 2.35A).[25] **Closed chain** movement is performed when the end of the chain is in contact with a surface and weight-bearing compression forces are placed on the joints (Fig. 2.35B). Motion at one joint requires motion at all others within the chain. Closed chain movement produces greater sensory stimuli through capsular and ligamentous receptors when intraarticular pressure increases and muscular support of the local stabilizers is enhanced to help stabilize the joints in the midrange. Open chain exercise can be used to challenge individual joint coordination or when closed chain exercise is contraindicated due to precautions for cartilage or bone damage (Clinical Example 2.9). Closed chain exercise is indicated when joint stability is desired to promote muscle contraction around a joint, for functional training, or when open chain exercise is contraindicated during early healing of ligaments and excessive shear stress needs to be limited (see Clinical Example 2.9). As most functional activity requires closed chain movement in the lower extremity, closed chain exercise is often preferred for functional training in Phases II or III.

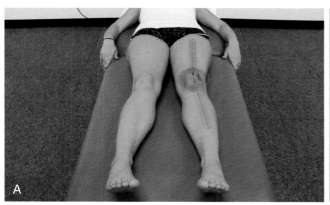

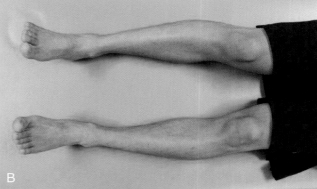

Fig. 2.34 (A) Genu valgum. (B) Genu varum.

BOX 2.23 Distribution of Force: Bony Alignment

- Extreme structural alignment increases the neuromuscular control requirements for static and dynamic balance and movement.
- Structural alignment cannot be reversed, and alignment during exercise is based on the natural bony alignment.
- Exercise positions are chosen to minimize gravitational balance requirements in Phases I and II.
- Exercise goals are to promote neuromuscular control and muscle strengthening without excessive angulation or rotation.

BOX 2.24 Distribution of Force: Open Versus Closed Chain

- Open chain movement occurs when a limb segment is free to move at one end of the lever. Individual joint motion does not automatically result in motion elsewhere.
- Closed chain movement occurs when the end of the lever chain is fixed or in contact with a surface. Motion at one joint can result in movement in other segments of the chain, and compressive forces occur to a greater or lesser extent through the joints. Closed chain movement results in greater proprioceptive input.

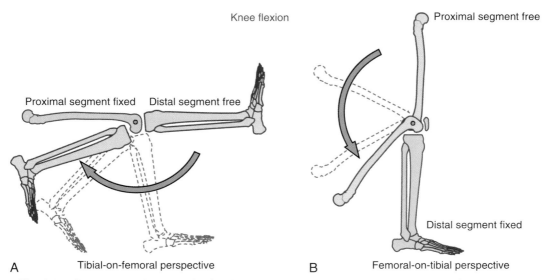

Fig. 2.35 Open versus closed chain. See Box 2.24. (From Neumann DA. *Kinesiology of the Musculoskeletal System: Foundations for Rehabilitation.* 3rd ed. St. Louis, MO: Mosby Elsevier; 2017; Fig. 1.6.)

CLINICAL EXAMPLE 2.9   Open or Closed Chain Exercise Choices: Implications for Precautions

Open chain allowed, closed chain contraindicated for intraarticular fractures: Patients with intraarticular fractures will need to avoid-weight bearing and closed chain exercises in the early phases of healing to prevent compression of the joint surface, which could result in healing with irregularities of the joint surface. However, motion of the joint *without* compressive loading promotes gliding and shaping of the new callus formation and may be allowed if it is unlikely to disrupt the fracture.

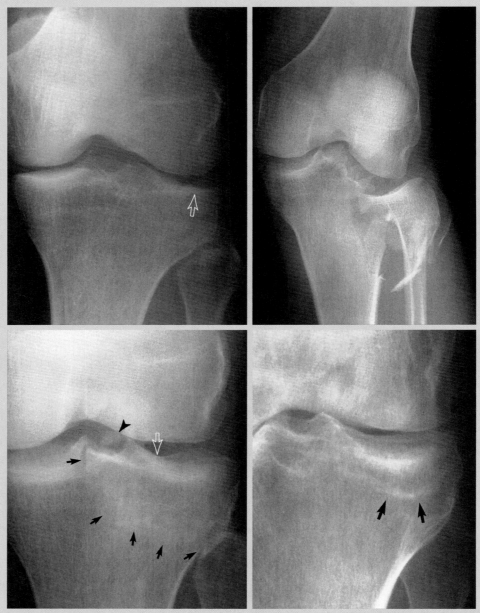

Intraarticular fracture. Fracture severity varies from minor compression (*white arrow, top left*) to complete displacement of joint congruity (top right and bottom left). In the bottom left radiograph, the black arrows show fracture lines extending into the joint, with fragments visible in the joint and depression of the tibial plateau (*white arrows*). Compression fractures below the tibial plateau (*black arrows*, bottom right) increase the risk of abnormal congruity if there is excessive load during healing. All intraarticular fractures will have weight-bearing precautions, but the extent of the fracture will change initial surgical or conservative management and timelines.

CLINICAL EXAMPLE 2.9   Open or Closed Chain Exercise Choices: Implications for Precautions—cont'd

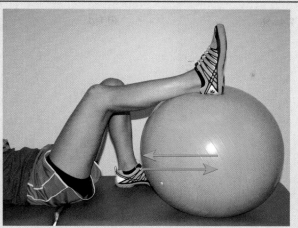

Open chain knee flexion; extension (*blue arrows*) using gym ball can be used once sufficient healing has taken place after surgical fixation of a tibial plateau fracture.

Open chain against resistance contraindicated, closed chain allowed: After ligament injury, specific shear forces may be increased with open chain exercise. For the first 6–8 weeks after anterior cruciate ligament (ACL) repair, open chain resistive extension exercise against high loads is contraindicated from 0 to 40 degrees due to the anterior shear forces on the ligament. Closed chain exercise is allowed and promotes muscle co-contraction, a centralized axis of motion, and less force on the ligament during this period (Video 2.24). Closed chain exercise can be performed using equipment allowing support of body weight and progressed to squats and isometric holds in flexion below 45 degrees (Video 2.24).

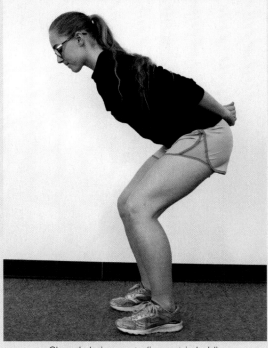

Closed chain squats (isometric hold).

Patients with patellofemoral syndrome need to stabilize the hip joint in the transverse (A) and frontal (B) planes to limit the undesirable angulation and rotational forces at the knee (Video 2.2). Hip stabilization exercises are an integral part of management for these patients (Video 2.26).

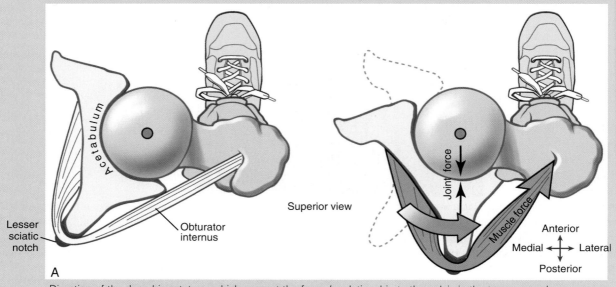

Direction of the deep hip rotators, which support the femur's relationship to the pelvis in the transverse plane.

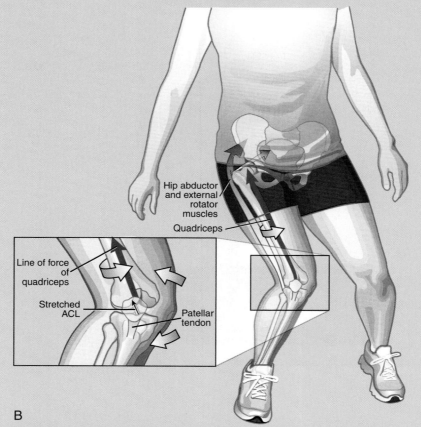

The hip external rotator and abductors need to be active to prevent dynamic valgus angulation and additional force on the patellofemoral complex.

Note that the patient's body weight is lateral to the knee and foot, the pelvis is dropped on the left, and there is relative pelvic rotation to the right. The patient is "hanging" on the lateral structures of the hip, and there is increased load on the lower extremity joints due to lack of active muscular force distribution.

Images from Neumann DA. *Kinesiology of the Musculoskeletal System: Foundations for Rehabilitation*. 3rd ed. St. Louis, MO: Mosby Elsevier; 2017, Figs. 12.44 and 13.21.

BALANCE CONCEPTS: STATIC AND DYNAMIC BALANCE

Static balance is the ability to maintain equilibrium using muscle activity to provide equal forces to oppose gravity (Box 2.25). Positions are more or less stable based on the area of the base of support and the position of the center of gravity within the perimeters of the base of support. The starting position can make an exercise more or less difficult. Neuromuscular responses and balance reactions allow individuals to maintain upright posture against gravity (see Fig. 2.29C and D). The sensory information from the vestibular system, eyes, and peripheral receptors in the skin, ligaments, joint capsule, and tendons is processed rapidly in the cerebellum to produce muscular activity for postural support and to maintain equilibrium. Visual targets can be used to promote static or dynamic balance, or balance responses can be challenged by removing one of the incoming sensory sensations. For example, closing the eyes or blindfolding the patient will remove visual input.

Dynamic balance is the ability to create motion in a controlled manner without excessive motion outside the base of support or the ability to control the speed of motion when the line of gravity is outside the base (e.g., while running). The ability to change direction, stop suddenly, and regain a balanced upright position requires complex and rapid adjustments.

Both forms of balance are important for functional activities, and balance reactions can be used to initiate muscle activation or train neuromuscular response time (Videos 2.5 and 2.15).[26] The base of support can provide an inherently more or less stable starting position to activate muscles opposing gravity for improving postural muscle support or endurance or to improve balance reactions (Video 2.25).

Perturbations or oscillations are methods used to promote muscular initiation by challenging the patient to maintain the limb or body in one place.[26] Equipment with a smaller base or moving platforms can also be used to promote balance responses.

DIRECTIONS AND PLANES OF MOVEMENT

The direction of the motion and plane of movement (Box 2.26 and Fig. 2.36) influence the muscle force requirements for stability or mobility. One of the most important foundations of movement analysis is knowledge of the muscle origins and insertions. Knowing the location of the muscles allows the therapist to determine which muscles are responsible for the direction of motion and the function of the muscle (see Clinical Example 2.10). In simple one-plane movements, the motion should not drift into multiple

---

BOX 2.25 Balance Concepts

- Exercises can be designed to improve static or dynamic balance OR balance responses can be used to promote neuromuscular initiation.
- Starting position for exercise will provide a more or less stable condition. Positions can be adjusted to promote anti-gravity muscle activity for static postural reactions.
- Perturbations or oscillations promote use of balance reactions. Balance exercise can use visual targets, unstable surfaces, equipment (balance boards, foam rollers, exercise balls).
- Removal of sensory input will challenge balance reactions and can be used to progress balance activities.

BOX 2.26 Directions and Planes of Movement

- Limiting movement to specific planes of movement will influence the direction of muscle pull to help protect injured ligaments, tendons, and muscle.
- Movements should be observed from more than one direction. This will help the therapist ensure that movement occurs in the desired plane.
- Stability can be provided by muscles in planes other than the primary movement.

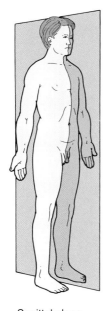   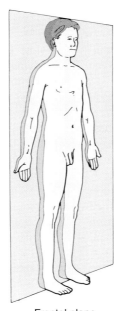   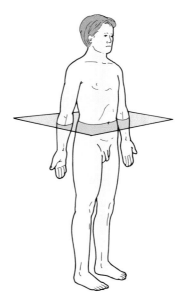

Sagittal plane   Frontal plane   Transverse plane

FIG. 2.36 Planes of movement. (From Cameron MH, Monroe LC. Physical *Rehabilitation: Evidence-Based Examination, Evaluation, and Intervention.* St. Louis, MO: Saunders Elsevier; 2007.)

directions (Videos 2.1, 2.2, and 2.26). Muscles in other planes may act to control or direct the movement or support joint areas so that efficient movement can occur. The ability to stabilize joints in one plane while producing movement in another is required for many functional tasks. Muscular support at one joint can also influence the direction of forces and, therefore, stress at another.

The planes of movement are also important when considering which forces need to be limited to protect ligaments, tendons, and muscles during healing (Videos 2.3–2.6). Precautions and contraindications may be required in one or more planes during Phases I and II. In simple, one-plane motion, the muscle activation is relatively easy to control, but functional movements often require multi-planar, multi-joint motion and also more adjustments by the therapist. Therefore, the therapist may need to educate the patient about the distinction among exercises to address strength or muscle endurance deficits versus functional movements. Some movements will be discouraged until sufficient healing has taken place and the patient has demonstrated appropriate control in less-complicated movements. In early phases of healing, muscle activation using one plane of motion is preparatory for exercise progression in a later stage, including multi-planar, functional movements.

SUMMARY

- Musculoskeletal injuries can be categorized as traumatic or repetitive strain injuries.
- The ability to withstand stress and strain is important for precautions and is used to inform the choice of range of motion and amount of resistance during healing.
- The phases of tissue repair will direct the goals, type, intensity, and progression of exercises.
- Phase I goals involve assisting with resolving inflammation, protecting the area, and minimizing deconditioning.
- Phase II goals involve resolving impairments, providing optimal stimulus for regeneration, and progressing toward functional goals.
- Phase III goals are to restore functional movement and the ability to withstand forces required for function.
- Optimal stimulus for regeneration is specific to tissue type and informs the type of exercise, direction of force, and specific exercise parameters.
- All tissues are designed to withstand specific forces and are more vulnerable to other directions of force.

- Specific adaptations to imposed demand concepts include consideration of type of movement, required forces, aerobic demands, overload, and specificity principles.
- Stabilizer and mover functions can be used to help in understanding the requirements for stability and mobility and targeting specific muscle function.
- Force considerations to consider during exercise include magnitude, point of application, distance of application from the axis, and goal of the activity of stability or mobility.
- Therapists apply their knowledge of anatomy and biomechanical concepts to prescribe safe, effective exercise programs.
- Stability can be provided by form closure or force closure, and in the presence of injury further contributions from force closure may be needed.
- Structural alignment influences the forces on specific tissues.
- Distribution of force, including open and closed chain motion, directions, and planes of motion, is important to allow healing of injured tissue.
- Balance concepts are important for choice of exercise as well as for integration into functional exercise.

REVIEW QUESTIONS

1. Differentiate between traumatic and repetitive strain injuries and use the stress-strain curve to distinguish between the forces that are likely to result in each category.
2. List the three phases of tissue healing, the time frames of each, and the primary goal to attain while in each phase.
3. List five factors that can impact tissue strength. Are these changes reversible? If so, how?
4. Describe how the concept of optimal stimulus for regeneration may influence exercise selection and progression.
5. Discuss the type of forces that connective tissue (tendon and ligament), muscle, bone, and cartilage are designed to withstand for function and how this information influences the progression of exercise in Phases II and III.
6. Discuss how injury to a specific tissue may influence the amount of load a tissue can withstand during healing. Provide examples for two types of tissue.

7. List four ways that muscle tissue responds to imposed demand.
8. Define the terms *overload*, *specificity*, and *specific adaptations to imposed demands*.
9. Describe and provide an example of a local stabilizer, global stabilizer, and a global mover muscle.
10. List the biomechanical force components that need to be considered when analyzing an exercise or selecting appropriate levels of resistance.
11. Describe how forces will impact the goal of stability or mobility.
12. Compare the structural components of a joint where stability is inherently dependent on form closure to an example of a joint where stability is more dependent on force closure.
13. Discuss when force closure is a major focus of exercise prescription.

14. Describe how the presence of a bony malalignment will influence exercise position and instructions.
15. Explain how force distribution is used to assist patients in recovering from repetitive strain injuries.
16. Provide an example of an open kinetic chain exercise and a closed kinetic chain exercise. Provide an example of a situation when each type of exercise is preferred or is not indicated.
17. Describe the difference between static and dynamic balance

REFERENCES

1. Lee AC, Quillen WS, Magee DJ, Zachazewski JE. Injury, inflammation, and repair: tissue mechanics, the healing process, and their impact on the musculoskeletal system. In: Magee DJ, Zachazewski JE, Quillen WS, eds. *Scientific Foundations and Principles of Practice in Musculoskeletal Rehabilitation.* St. Louis, MO: Saunders Elsevier; 2007:1–23.
2. Curwin SL. Tendon pathology and injuries: pathophysiology, healing and treatment considerations. In: Magee DJ, Zachazewski JE, Quillen WS, eds. *Scientific Foundations and Principles of Practice in Musculoskeletal Rehabilitation.* St. Louis, MO: Saunders Elsevier; 2007:47–78.
3. Hildebrand KA, Hart DA, Rattner JB, Marchuk LL, Frank CB. Ligament injuries: pathophysiology, healing and treatment considerations. In: Magee DJ, Zachazewski JE, Quillen WS, eds. *Scientific Foundations and Principles of Practice in Musculoskeletal Rehabilitation.* St. Louis, MO: Saunders Elsevier; 2007:23–47.
4. Magee DJ. *Orthopedic Physical Assessment.* 6th ed. St. Louis, MO: Elsevier Saunders; 2014.
5. Magee DJ, Sueki D. *Orthopedic Physical Assessment Atlas and Video: Selected Special Tests and Movements.* St. Louis, MO: Elsevier Saunders; 2011.
6. Cleland JA, Koppenhaver S. *Netter's Orthopaedic Clinical Examination: An Evidence-Based Approach.* 2nd ed. St. Louis, MO: Elsevier Saunders; 2011.
7. Cioppa-Mosca J, Cahill JB, Tucker CY, eds. *Handbook of Postsurgical Rehabilitation Guidelines for the Orthopaedic Clinician.* St. Louis, MO: Elsevier Saunders; 2008.
8. Levanjie PK, Norkin CC. *Joint Structure and Function. A Comprehensive Analysis.* 5th ed. Philadelphia, PA: FA Davis; 2011.
9. Magee DJ, Zachazewski JE, Quillen WS. *Pathology and Intervention in Musculoskeletal Rehabilitation.* St. Louis, MO: Elsevier Saunders; 2009.
10. Lundon K, Walker JM. Cartilage of human joints and related structures. In: Magee DJ, Zachazewski JE, Quillen WS, eds. *Scientific Foundations and Principles of Practice in Musculoskeletal Rehabilitation.* St. Louis, MO: Saunders Elsevier; 2007:144–174.
11. Mayman DJ, Gill TJ. Injuries to the meniscus and articular cartilage. In: Magee DJ, Zachazewski JE, Quillen WS, eds. *Pathology and Intervention in Musculoskeletal Rehabilitation.* St. Louis, MO: Elsevier Saunders; 2009:579–600.
12. Cavanaugh JT, Williams HA. Microfracture procedure of the knee. In: Cioppa-Mosca J, Cahill JB, Tucker CY, eds. *Handbook of Postsurgical Rehabilitation Guidelines for the Orthopaedic Clinician.* St. Louis, MO: Elsevier Saunders; 2008:294–302.
13. Loitz-Ramage BJ, Zernicke R. Bone biology and mechanics. In: Magee DJ, Zachazewski JE, Quillen WS, eds. *Scientific Foundations and Principles of Practice in Musculoskeletal Rehabilitation.* St. Louis, MO: Saunders Elsevier; 2007:122–143.

14. Hoppenfeld S, Murthy VL. *Treatment and Rehabilitation of Fractures.* Philadelphia, PA: Lippincott Williams & Wilkins; 2000.
15. Greenspan A. *Orthopaedic Imaging – A Practical Approach.* 5th ed. Philadelphia, PA: Lippincott Williams & Wilkins; 2011.
16. Bandy WD, Dunleavy K. Adaptability of skeletal muscle: response to increased and decreased use. In: Zachazewski JE, Magee DJ, Quillen WS, eds. *Athletic Injuries and Rehabilitation.* Philadelphia, PA: WB Saunders; 1996:55–91.
17. Matzkin E, Zachazewski JE, Garrett WE, Malone TR. Skeletal muscle: deformation, injury, repair and treatment considerations. In: Magee DJ, Zachazewski JE, Quillen WS, eds. *Scientific Foundations and Principles of Practice in Musculoskeletal Rehabilitation.* St. Louis, MO: Saunders Elsevier; 2007:97–121.
18. American College of Sports Medicine. In: Pescatello LS, ed. *ACSM's Guidelines for Exercise Testing and Prescription.* 9th ed. Baltimore, MD: Wolters Kluwer Lippincott Williams & Wilkins; 2014.
19. Tufano JJ, et al. Effect of aerobic recovery intensity on delayed-onset muscle soreness and strength. *J Strength Cond Res.* 2012;26(10):2777–2782.
20. Vila-Cha C, et al. Eccentric exercise and delayed onset muscle soreness of the quadriceps induce adjustments in agonist-antagonist activity, which are dependent on the motor task. *Exp Brain Res.* 2012;216(3):385–395.
21. Magee DJ, Zachazewski JE. Principles of stabilization training. In: Magee DJ, Zachazewski JE, Quillen WS, eds. *Scientific Foundations and Principles of Practice in Musculoskeletal Rehabilitation.* St. Louis, MO: Saunders Elsevier; 2007:388–413.
22. Blanpied PR, Nawoczenski DA. Biomechanical principles. In: Neumann DA, ed. *Kinesiology of the Musculoskeletal System: Foundations for Rehabilitation.* 2nd ed. St. Louis, MO: Mosby Elsevier; 2010.
23. Hunter SK, Brown DA. Muscle: the primary stabilizer and mover of the skeletal system. In: Neumann DA, ed. *Kinesiology of the Musculoskeletal System: Foundations for Rehabilitation.* 2nd ed. St. Louis, MO: Mosby Elsevier; 2010:47–76.
24. Lee LJ, Lee D. Integrated, multimodal approach to the thoracic spine and ribs. In: Magee DJ, Zachazewski JE, Quillen WS, eds. *Pathology and Intervention in Musculoskeletal Rehabilitation.* St. Louis, MO: Elsevier Saunders; 2009:206–337.
25. Neumann DA. Knee. In: Neumann DA, ed. *Kinesiology of the Musculoskeletal System: Foundations for Rehabilitation.* 2nd ed. St. Louis, MO: Mosby Elsevier; 2010:520–571.
26. Chmielewski TL, Hewett TE, Hurd WJ, Snyder-Mackler L. Principles of neuromuscular control for injury prevention and rehabilitation. In: Magee DJ, Zachazewski JE, Quillen WS, eds. *Scientific Foundations and Principles of Practice in Musculoskeletal Rehabilitation.* St. Louis: MO Saunders Elsevier; 2007: 375–387.

3

Relationship Between Impairments and Function

Kim Dunleavy, Kevin Lulofs-MacPherson, and Amy Kubo Slowik

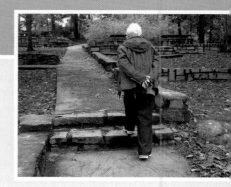

OBJECTIVE

Upon completion of this chapter, the reader will be able to:

1. Develop a clinical reasoning framework using the International Classification of Functioning (ICF) Model.
2. Define and provide examples of impairments, activity limitations, and participation restrictions.
3. List and explain common impairments and describe how impairments lead to activity and participation restrictions.
4. Define and describe mobility (hypomobility and hypermobility), muscle function (activation, muscle endurance, strength, power), aerobic endurance, balance, task-specific coordination and response efficiency, and psychological impairments.
5. Discuss the relationships among impairments, activity limitations, and participation restrictions and how these might influence exercise prescription.

FUNCTION: THE KEY FOR ESTABLISHING GOALS DURING PATIENT MANAGEMENT

In order to meet a patient's goals, the therapist needs to identify the factors contributing to the patient's problems. In 2001, the World Health Organization developed the International Classification of Functioning (ICF) model, which is a patient-centered system that considers biological, psychological, and social factors.[1,2] The ICF model can be used to help link and prioritize a patient's problems and goals as well as understand the full context influencing the patient's rehabilitation. The American Physical Therapy Association (APTA) has integrated the ICF definitions, coding categories, and theoretical constructs into the *Guide to Physical Therapy Practice* to assist practitioners with clinical reasoning and decision-making.[3] The APTA Clinical Practice Guidelines also follow the ICF model (see References). This chapter will describe the application of the ICF model and clinical reasoning strategies when choosing exercises for patients.

International Classification of Functioning Model: Overview of Impairments, Activity Limitation, and Participation Restrictions

The ICF model (Box 3.1)[2] provides a framework for describing the interrelationships among the complex factors that influence function (Fig. 3.1) or disability (Fig. 3.2) within the context of **environmental** and **personal** factors. The model links **body structures and function** to the normal **activities** and tasks that individuals need to be able to perform in order to **participate** in their communities, home, and work settings (Fig. 3.1). The model also provides standardized labels for health conditions (diagnoses) to allow comparison of clinical treatment and outcomes. The terms **impairments,**

activity limitations, and **participation restrictions** are used to refer to difficulties with any of the intertwining elements. **Impairments** are described as problems with body functions and can be related to any of the body systems, including mental, sensory (including pain), speech, cardiovascular, pulmonary, skin, musculoskeletal, and neuromuscular. Examples of impairments and the related body structure or function are provided in Table 3.1. Some of the common impairments addressed with therapeutic exercise include decreased range of motion, strength, coordination, and endurance. Impairments and medical conditions can lead to activity limitations and participation restrictions. **Activity limitations** are difficulties in performing tasks, varying from basic activities of

> ### BOX 3.1 International Classification of Functioning Concepts
>
> - The International Classification of Functioning is a model used to assist with connecting diagnosis, prognosis, patient problems, and goals.
> - The relationship between impairments and functional activity/participation limitations will influence exercise selection.
> - Goals should address activity and participation restrictions.
> - Exercises can address impairments, but the impairments should be directly linked to activity limitations and participation restrictions.
> - Personal and environmental factors also influence goals and treatment choices.

Data from Sykes C, Snyman S. International Classification of Functioning, Disability and Health (ICF) framework to facilitate interprofessional education and collaborative practice. World Health Organization. www.who.int/hrh/news/2014/hrh_icf_framwork/en/. Accessed March 21, 2016; World Health Organization. How to use the ICF. A practical manual for using the International Classification of Functioning, Disability and Health (ICF). 2013. www.who.int/classifications/drafticfpracticalmanual2.pdf. Accessed March 21, 2016.

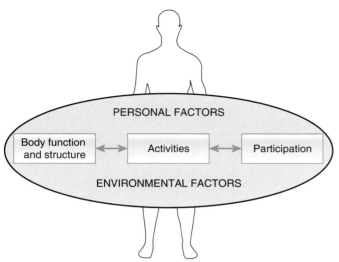

Fig. 3.1 International Classification of Functioning Model.[2]

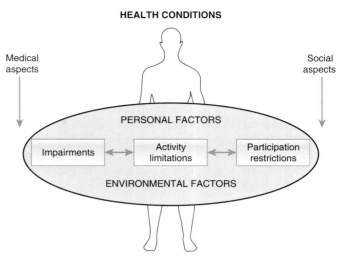

Fig. 3.2 International Classification of Functioning Model[2]: Impairments, Activity Limitations, Participation Restrictions.

TABLE 3.1 Impairments, Body Structures or Functions, and Examples		
Impairments	**Body Structures or Functions**	**Examples**
Loss of mobility (hypomobility)	Musculoskeletal Neuromuscular	Decreased joint range of motion Decreased connective tissue extensibility Decreased muscle flexibility Increased muscle tone/spasm
Excessive mobility or loss of stability (hypermobility)	Musculoskeletal Neuromuscular	Decreased joint stability (ligamentous laxity) Decreased active support due to impaired muscle function (strength, power, endurance, inefficient neuromuscular activation and coordination) Decreased neuromuscular reaction time for postural stability Inability to regain static postural balance after movement (impaired reaction time, muscle support, neuromuscular coordination)
Pain	Musculoskeletal Neurological Sensory	Early pain receptor activation or sensitization to mechanical stimuli Perception of pain in the absence of mechanical or chemical stimuli Reproduction of protective pain responses with mechanical or chemical stimuli
Muscle function (activation, muscular endurance, strength, power)	Musculoskeletal Neuromuscular Cardiovascular Respiratory Metabolic	Inability to initiate or maintain muscle contraction or movement for time required for task Inability to repeat muscle contractions or movement Difficulty producing sufficient force for functional tasks
Aerobic endurance	Musculoskeletal Neuromuscular Cardiovascular Respiratory Metabolic	Inability to repeat movement due to cardiovascular or respiratory system fatigue Inability to repeat movement or functional activities due to inefficient removal of waste products
Sensory	Integumentary Musculoskeletal Neuromuscular Vision, hearing	Lack of or altered light touch, deep pressure or joint position (proprioceptive) awareness Increased sensory information (paresthesia) Visual deficits Hearing deficits
Coordination	Neuromuscular	Slow reaction times due to muscular weakness or impaired neuromuscular activation Impaired proprioception or sensory input resulting in slow, uncoordinated motion Slow or inaccurate specificity of motor tasks due to impaired neurological integration of sensory and motor pathways Impaired integration of neuromuscular activity for functional mobility and stability tasks

daily living such as dressing, bathing, and eating to more complex activities required for work or sports. Activity limitations can be a result of physical, psychological, or social factors. The most common activity limitations that can be addressed with therapeutic exercise are listed in Table 3.2. **Participation restrictions** refer to difficulties participating in life situations including family, work, or social settings (Video 3.1). Activity limitations and participation restrictions are usually the primary reasons patients seek rehabilitation care, and these can be grouped together when setting goals or prescribing exercise. The interrelationships among health conditions, impairments, activity limitations, and participation restrictions are illustrated in Clinical Example 3.1.

TABLE 3.2 Primary Activity Limitations Applicable to Physical Therapy Practice

Mobility: Walking and moving around
Changing and maintaining body position
Carrying, moving, and handling objects
Self-care
Other primary functional limitations
Other secondary or subsequent functional limitations

Data from http://www.ptnow.org/FunctionalLimitationReporting/ScoringHelp.

🔬 CLINICAL EXAMPLE 3.1 Application of the ICF Model for a Patient With Knee Osteoarthritis

A 76-year-old woman has knee osteoarthritis with pain, range of motion, strength, and neuromuscular coordination impairments limiting her ability to participate in social activities. The ICF model can be used for clinical reasoning processes to link health conditions, impairments, activity limitations, and participation restrictions. Using this clinical reasoning model provides an opportunity to select appropriate treatment interventions that address the patient's major priorities.

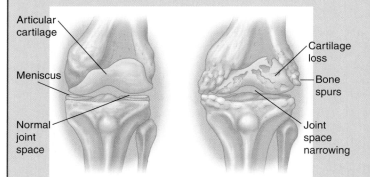

Knee osteoarthritis (health condition) is the result of cumulative stress and degeneration of the articular cartilage. As the cartilage wears down, there is a loss of joint space with increased shear forces and stress on the capsule. The synovial membrane becomes irritated and inflamed, with thickening and knee effusion resulting in a swollen and painful joint. The knee structure is altered, impacting the knee's contributions for tasks such as walking, transfers, and climbing stairs.

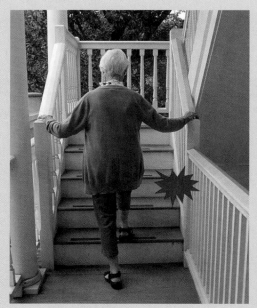

Impairments (swelling, limited knee extension, muscle inhibition, and pain) result in difficulty climbing stairs (activity limitation; Video 3.2).

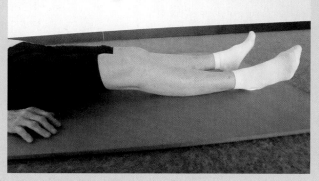

Swelling and capsular thickening result in knee extension limitations (impairment).

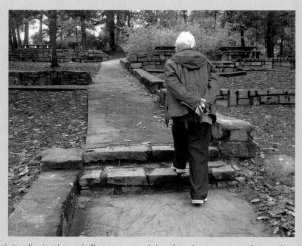

Activity limitations influence participation in events where there is a need to climb stairs, thus decreasing interaction with family and friends and resulting in isolation.

While there is often a link between impairments and activity and participation limitations, there is not always a cause-and-effect relationship. It is the therapist's responsibility to determine the relative impact of each deficit to formulate short- and long-term goals that in turn direct exercise choices. Impairments contributing toward the functional deficits are usually listed as short-term goals while functional activity and participation problems are typically listed as long-term goals. The extent of impairments and activity/participation restrictions is used to establish the initial degree of difficulty for the exercise and for developing an appropriate progression for return to activities of daily living. Planning to address activity and participation limitations should be a joint effort between the therapist and patient; addressing impairments alone does not automatically resolve activity limitations or participation restrictions.

The therapist will determine a prognosis based on results from the evaluation, knowledge of the patient's health condition and comorbidities (using available evidence), and the patient's personal and environmental factors. The prognosis will influence the expectations and goals. The more closely aligned the exercise choices are with the patient's activity and participation goals, the higher the motivation and likelihood of successful rehabilitation. Personal factors include characteristics such as age, economic status, social support, literacy, education, hobbies, and occupation—all of which are vital to consider when creating an exercise prescription. Environmental factors also influence the type of exercise choices and goals. A patient who lives in a rural area may need to be able to walk over rough terrain, whereas a patient who lives in an urban area is more likely to need to be able to cross a busy road (Video 3.1) or negotiate a subway system.

IMPAIRMENTS

Typical impairments for individuals receiving physical therapy treatment include hypomobility (loss of mobility), hypermobility (excessive mobility or loss of stabilizing restraint systems), pain, diminished muscular or aerobic endurance, diminished strength and diminished power, sensory deficits (tactile sensation, proprioception, vision, hearing), and impaired neuromuscular coordination and balance. (See Table 3.1 for impairments related to body structure and function and examples.) Trauma, repetitive strain, disease, and/or psychosocial dysfunction result in impairments of the physiological mechanisms required to produce the complex movements necessary

Mobility

Mobility is the range of motion available from articular joints, muscles, and other structures such as fascia and nerves. Therapists compare joint range of motion and muscle flexibility test results to normative values and the range of motion required for specific movements and activities to judge whether additional mobility is needed. Reese and Bandy's[4] text on joint range of motion and muscle length testing provides a very comprehensive resource for the tests and normative values. There are variations in the normative values for range of motion and flexibility across age ranges, genders, and body types. The required range of motion for different functional activities is also variable.[5] For

example, some sports-related movements require extreme ranges of motion compared to activities of daily living. For rehabilitation purposes, the ranges of motion necessary for a given functional task are often more relevant than goals to meet the normative values. Clinical Example 3.2 illustrates the typical hip range of motion requirements for lower extremity functional activities and the implications for goal setting. The typical biomechanical response to limited motion or discomfort is to compensate in other areas as soon as full tension of the restricted structures is reached or if there is pain (Videos 3.3–3.5). Therefore, movement analysis observational skills are essential for detecting and correcting compensatory strategies during the evaluation and throughout the course of treatment. The relationship between ankle range of motion impairments and the biomechanics of standing up from a chair is illustrated in Clinical Example 3.3. The Reese and Bandy text[4] also provides details of approximate ranges of motion required for a wider variety of functional tasks.

Hypomobility

If there is insufficient mobility for function, the goal of exercises is to increase the available active joint and muscle flexibility simultaneously (Box 3.2). Mobility techniques aim to reach the elastic or plastic regions of the stress-strain curve to improve available range (see Chapter 2). When mobility is the major impairment contributing to activity limitations, mobility may need to improve prior to practicing more complex functional tasks. Once range has improved, encouraging the patient to

---

🔖 CLINICAL EXAMPLE 3.3   Influence of Ankle Mobility Limitations on Sit-to-Stand Transfers

A 30-year-old man has a history of an ankle fracture with surgical fixation (12 years ago) resulting in ankle dorsiflexion range of motion limitations (0 degrees dorsiflexion) since the injury. While he does not have ankle pain, he has intermittent knee pain aggravated by steps (Video 3.6), squats (Video 3.7), and sit-to-stand (Video 3.8). During functional evaluation, the ankle range of motion limitations influence sit-to-stand mechanics.

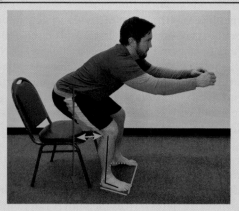

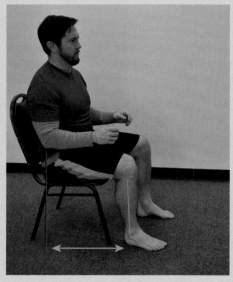

The line of gravity running through the center of mass of the trunk is posterior to the anticipated new base for standing—the double support from the feet. The ankle is in approximately 5–10 degrees of plantarflexion in the starting position.

The patient's body weight and center of mass (*red line*) are still posterior to the new base of support (*blue outline* around the foot width and length) in response to not being able to achieve more than 0 degrees of dorsiflexion. The distance from the center of mass to the base of support requires recruitment of the anterior leg muscles to prevent falling backward and to move the body forward over the feet. These movement strategies are normal during sit-to-stand, and the patient has moved his trunk and arm weight forward over his base to assist with counterbalance and anterior motion. However, the patellofemoral compression forces are increased by the moment arm due to the distance of the center of mass (*green arrow*) from the knee joint.[1] His ankle range of motion limitations (0 degrees of dorsiflexion) can therefore contribute to patellofemoral joint symptoms. He may also compensate for the lack of closed chain ankle dorsiflexion by using other joints to accomplish the task or by using a completely different strategy, such as moving toward the opposite side (see the section on altered movement strategies in this chapter).

Reference

1. Neumann DA. *Kinesiology of the Musculoskeletal System. Foundations for Rehabilitation.* 2nd ed. St. Louis, MO: Mosby Elsevier; 2010:537–558.

BOX 3.2   Hypomobility

- Hypomobility can be due to limited joint range of motion or muscle flexibility.
- Joint range of motion and muscle flexibility test results are compared to age-related normative values; requirements for functional tasks and patient-specific goals are used to determine mobility needs.
- Movement observation is important during testing and exercise to avoid compensations.
- Functional activity using the improvements is necessary for long-term changes.
- Principles of elasticity and plasticity can be used to increase tissue length, but the therapist should exercise care to avoid causing an inflammatory response.

BOX 3.3   Hypermobility

- Addressing hypermobility impairments requires use of force closure with refined muscle activation, neuromuscular coordination, and dynamic stabilization.
- Training is usually conducted within the midrange (or does not reach or exceed end range).
- Specificity principles are important for functional preparation (specific adaptations to imposed demands [SAID]).
- Overload principles are used in Phases II and III in midrange, with progression of load without increasing strain placed on tissue.

utilize the full range of motion (without excessive compensations) during functional activities is appropriate. The reinforcement and integration into functional movements is of utmost importance in retaining mobility.

Hypermobility

Supporting the body in upright positions requires resisting gravity and connecting bony lever systems to protect the body against outside forces. The complex coordination of posture and movement requires underlying passive support from ligamentous and joint structure (form closure) and active dynamic support from neuromuscular activity (force closure) (see Chapter 2). Damage or dysfunction to the passive, active, or neurological systems can all result in hypermobility (Box 3.3 and Fig. 3.3). Excessive mobility can be due to poor structural support from congenital conditions (see Clinical Example 2.8); damage to inert structures, such as previous ligament disruption, connective tissue disorders (e.g., Ehlers-Danlos syndrome), or problems with neuromuscular control. With excessive mobility, the restraints needed to protect structures against external forces are inadequate or absent, and the constant motion beyond the normal ranges results in damage to joints and soft tissues. The management of hypermobility focuses on **training the neuromuscular system** to provide control and feedback in a connected and integrated movement system (**force closure;** Video 3.9). Some individuals who have lost support from the inert stabilizing structures, such as after a complete ligament rupture, are able to control movement through highly trained neuromuscular coordination and do not present with activity or participation limitations. Skaters, dancers, and gymnasts often present with hypermobile joints, but these highly trained athletes are able to support joint structures with finely tuned neural coordination and muscular strength.

Regardless of the cause of hypermobility, excessive mobility can be managed with refined muscle activation, strength, and neuromuscular control. Exercises should focus on maintaining the body segments or trunk within a midrange of the structures without exceeding the range where inert structures would normally limit motion (Video 3.9). If the individual needs to resist higher forces, the exercise goals will include improving the ability to withstand outside forces in a timely manner using appropriate neuromuscular responses (Clinical Example 3.4).

The neuromuscular responses to stabilize body segments are complex, and the therapeutic exercise program should follow the specific adaptations to imposed demands (SAID) principles of specificity (Chapter 2). Exercises need to be specific to the desired range of motion, type of muscle contraction, speed, and functional context. While isolated muscle activation is useful during early rehabilitation (Phase I; Video 3.10 and 3.11), exercises during Phases II and III should include activities that mimic the functional requirements (Videos 3.12 and 3.13). Phase III also includes complex, multidirectional movements (Videos 3.14 and 3.15; see Clinical Example 3.4).

Typically, the muscles that are closer to a joint control the joint axis of motion, and the local postural muscles control joint position. In addition to monitoring and controlling position, the local postural muscles assist with postural endurance. The timing of the local stabilizer muscle activity is important. When the local stabilizer muscles are not firing efficiently, the larger, global stabilizer muscles often compensate by firing early or excessively. The global stabilizers are designed to resist higher torques, and the global movers are intended to produce movement. Dysfunction of any muscle group influences function. Assessment of muscle function; observation of neuromuscular coordination and sequencing; and tests and measures of muscle strength, endurance, and power are correlated to provide guidance for exercise choices.

Utilizing exercise to address excessive mobility should include progressive exercises that assist with control of *midrange* motion for resisting loads and maintaining positions for longer periods. The awareness of position (proprioception) and ability to return to a midrange is important for individuals with hypermobility as the incoming sensory information from stretch receptors is often only triggered in the extreme ranges. The SAID concepts (see Chapter 2) and **motor control principles** (Chapter 7) are important considerations when addressing muscle function deficits involving hypermobility. Exercise suggestions and progression to address primary hypermobility are presented in Chapter 6.

Muscle Function

Muscle function is a combination of the physiological ability to produce contractions and force and the neurological control of those coordinated contractions. Muscle function involves varying degrees of activation, strength, power, and endurance components (Table 3.3), and an analysis of activity and functional requirements is important for establishing goals.

Muscle activation and endurance exercises are often prescribed before strengthening exercises. Both muscle activation and endurance exercises require lower external loads and therefore place less stress on tissues than the loads needed for strengthening through muscle hypertrophy. Both types of exercise (muscle activation and endurance) are therefore appropriate in the presence of active inflammation or weak connective tissue where loads need to be slowly increased to allow tissue to accommodate and change. Typically, Phases I and II start with muscle activation and endurance exercises, and strength and power exercises are added in late Phase II and in Phase III. Impairment deficits identified during the initial evaluation are addressed in a progressive manner with the intention of providing the functional building blocks necessary to meet the patient's activity and participation needs.

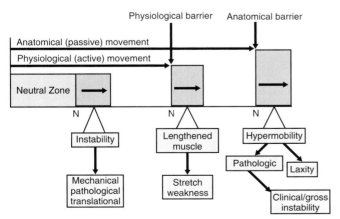

Fig. 3.3 Hypermobility and instability. *N,* Normal position. (From Magee DJ, Zacheweski JE. Principles of stabilization training. In: Magee DJ, Zacheweski JE, Quillen WS, eds. *Scientific Foundations and Principles of Practice in Musculoskeletal Rehabilitation.* St. Louis: Saunders Elsevier; 2007. Fig. 19.2.)

TABLE 3.3	Muscle Function Term Definitions[6,7]
Muscle activation	Appropriate initiation of muscle contraction
Muscle endurance	Ability of muscle to contract repeatedly with proper form until fatigue or compensations occur
Muscle strength	Ability to generate force at a specific speed of contraction; depends on the length-tension relationship
Muscle power	Force produced by muscle contraction per unit of time
Neuromuscular coordination	Timing, degree, and relative use of muscle contraction appropriate for the task

A 30-year-old woman with a generalized connective tissue disorder and shoulder hypermobility is referred for treatment. She wants to be able to lift and play with her children.

Body Structure: Impairment Related to Inability to Stabilize and Support the Glenohumeral Joint

There is increased range prior to the ligamentous "stop point" resulting in increased reliance on muscle control (force closure). In particular, the rotator cuff (local stabilizers) needs to be trained to maintain the humeral head position relative to the glenoid, and the deltoid, pectoralis major and minor, and teres major (global stabilizers) must be trained to support the glenohumeral joint throughout the range but particularly for higher loads or extreme positions (see Fig. 3.4).

Body Structure and Health Condition: Implications of Hypermobility

Precautions for Shoulder Hypermobility

Full stretch in the outer range of the shoulder in any direction is avoided, and exercises are chosen to place the glenohumeral and scapulohumeral connective tissue and muscles in mid-position. Isometric activation, endurance, and strengthening exercises are used to promote force closure.

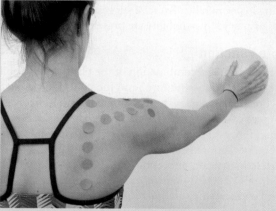

Exercises are chosen to address impairments using force closure in Phase II (scapulothoracic and glenohumeral stabilization in midrange).

Isometric scapula protraction and upward rotation along with small-range circumduction are used in a closed chain mid-position. The position takes into account precautions, as the glenohumeral joint is in the mid-position in all planes, and the scapulohumeral muscles are also in midrange in the scaption plane and mid-elevation.

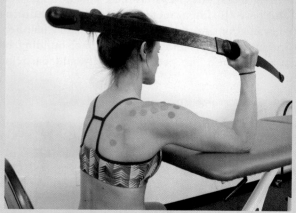

Exercises are chosen to address impairments linked to activity limitations using exercise to promote neuromuscular activation and coordination in Phase II (responses to perturbations).

Exercise is performed in mid-position with the arm positioned on a plinth, the body blade is moved through a small range of internal and external rotation. As the blade increases speed, the patient needs to activate all the local stabilizers to prevent the arm moving with the blade. The repeated activation to withstand the perturbations trains the neuromuscular system to respond to outside forces. This exercise simulates responding to unexpected movements when holding her children (linking the impairment with the activity limitation). The arm is supported with feedback from the table, and precautions are adhered to as the glenohumeral joint is in the mid-position in all planes (pink dots show the superior aspect of the humerus). The scapulohumeral and upper body muscles are reactive, and her postural alignment allows the shoulder position to be in the optimum biomechanical alignment. Note that the scapula is in a slight upward rotation and protraction (orange dots).

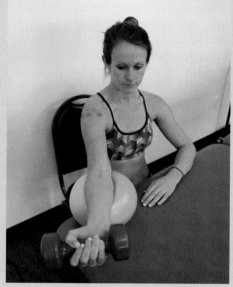

Shoulder stabilization with distal challenge.

Biceps curls are used to challenge maintaining her shoulder in mid-position, again with some arm support. The unstable surface provided by the ball requires concentration and shoulder muscle activation to prevent motion, thus facilitating isometric contractions.

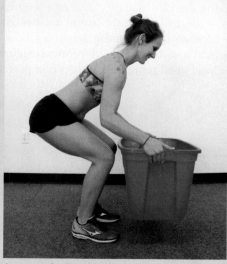

Exercises chosen to facilitate full activity and participation (Phase III).

During Phase III, functional activities are practiced with feedback to address biomechanical principles. Lifting activities are introduced with light weights to train concepts of planning to lift weight closer to the center of mass, using the lower extremities for vertical power, and establishing a solid core and scapulohumeral connection prior to lifting her child. Loads are increased to meet the goal of being able to lift her 2-year-old child who weighs 25 lbs to allow her to fully participate in her role as a mother.

Muscle Activation

The timing of muscle activation (initiation of contraction) is coordinated by the nervous system (Box 3.4). The type of muscle (local stabilizers, global stabilizers, or global movers) can be distinguished by the muscle fiber type and other morphological characteristics such as the size, location relative to joint structures, and muscle shape. These characteristics allow the muscle to support specific structures for tasks, such as postural support, or to produce movement. Efficient movement involves integrated muscle support using the *appropriate* level of muscle activation for the task. Muscle activation patterns can be altered due to pain inhibition, overuse, fatigue, or altered neurological function. During early rehabilitation, correcting neuromuscular activation may be the first priority before focusing on strength and endurance (Videos 3.9–3.11 and 3.16–3.18). If the exercise targets strengthening or endurance without appropriate activation of the specific muscles, other muscles are activated to perform the movement, and compensatory patterns develop.[6] Sometimes the reduction of effusion, pain, and inflammatory by-products will address any muscle inhibition in Phase I. Methods of promoting muscle activation include isolated exercises in supported positions (Videos 3.10 and 3.16) to limit compensations, targeted and specific instructions or cueing, simultaneous electrical stimulation (Video 3.11), and methods of providing tactile or visual feedback (such as biofeedback) (Clinical Example 3.5).

BOX 3.4 Muscle Function: Activation[1]

- Muscle activation may be the first goal prior to focusing on strength and endurance.
- Pain and edema resolution may address muscle activation in Phase I.
- Mechanisms to promote muscle activation include isolated exercises in supported positions, targeted and specific instructions, simultaneous electrical stimulation, or biofeedback.
- Long-standing muscle imbalances require use of sensory stimuli and motor learning principles to reeducate muscle timing and movement patterns.

CLINICAL EXAMPLE 3.5 Muscle Activation

A female patient is seen after an anterior cruciate ligament (ACL) reconstruction. She is still having difficulty with activating her quadriceps muscle and has a slight quadriceps lag of 10 degrees (she is only able to extend her knee to 10 degrees of flexion; her passive knee hyperextension is 5 degrees). Although she has been instructed on how to perform isometric exercises of the quadriceps, short-arc quadriceps exercises, and straight leg raises in all directions, she is still having difficulty with the terminal range.

Exercise Choices

Exercises are chosen to assist with quadriceps activation. The therapist chooses to use electrical stimulation to reeducate the neuromuscular activation and sequencing while performing static isometric quadriceps contractions (see quad sets, Exercise 9.39), short arc quads (see Exercise 9.43) with passive assistance to achieve full extension, followed by isometric or eccentric control and self-assisted terminal extension using a belt (see Exercise 9.4A) as a home program. The patient is instructed to contract the muscles actively at the same time as the electrical stimulation bursts. The timing for verbal cueing of the quadriceps muscle activation *and* the electrical stimulation is sequenced prior to lifting the lower leg for the short arc quads or the straight leg raise.

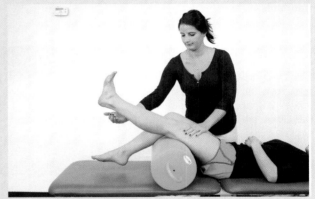

Passive assistance through terminal extension followed by isometrics and eccentric control.

The therapist assists the patient through full extension, asking the patient to perform a static isometric contraction and to hold the position. After the therapist removes support, the patient will either be able to maintain the isometric contraction or need to contract the quadriceps eccentrically to control the leg descent.

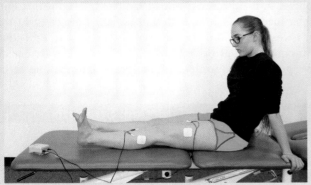

Quadriceps activation with electrical stimulation.

Electrical stimulation can be used to enhance muscle activation, train neuromuscular sequencing, or supplement activation of motor units. The patient is asked to contract actively at the same time as the electrical impulse. The patient is watching her muscle contraction and ability to lift the heel off the table to provide targets and incentives for neuromuscular reeducation.

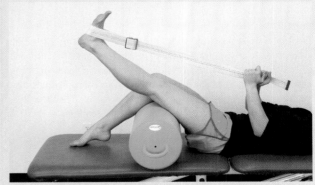

Self-assisted knee extension using a strap.

The patient assists the terminal extension using her hands but is encouraged to perform as much of the extension as possible actively. The strap allows her to perform the exercise as a home program and to practice the movement repeatedly while providing the specificity of the neuromuscular training in the terminal range.

Long-standing muscle imbalances will require neuromuscular reeducation to change established dysfunctional patterns and teach the patient how to activate muscles in a timely manner. A variety of sensory stimuli including tactile cues, visual feedback (Video 3.12), auditory explanations, and proprioceptive input (Videos 3.13, 3.18 and 3.19) can help the patient learn how to initiate and engage inhibited muscles or learn new patterns. Changing neuromuscular coordination patterns involves learning what the desired pattern is and how to sequence the movement using motor learning concepts[6] (see Chapter 7).

Muscle Endurance

Muscle endurance (Box 3.5) is the ability to contract a muscle repeatedly or for a long period and with a set amount of load before fatigue or compensations occur.[7,8] Muscle endurance is required for joint support and alignment in various postures, such as control of the hip and pelvis position when standing for long periods. Repetitive movement also requires muscle endurance. Personal factors such as posture, activities of daily living, and work requirements will also influence the need for muscular endurance (Clinical Example 3.6).

BOX 3.5   Muscle Function: Endurance[6,7]

- Muscle endurance is required to maintain postural positions for prolonged periods or to contract repeatedly prior to fatigue.
- Low-intensity muscle activity is required for muscle endurance.
- Rest periods are important to allow recovery and replenish the oxygen supplies.
- Repetitions, time held in a specific position, or number of sets are progressed prior to increasing load.

CLINICAL EXAMPLE 3.6   Functional Endurance

Functional activities that require muscle activity to support an area for longer periods will require muscle endurance. Work or hobby requirements (personal factors), as well as the muscle function for a task, will need to be considered for goals related to muscle endurance.

Patient A

Patient A is 15-year-old high school student who has chronic neck pain. His neck pain is worse after working on the computer for more than an hour and at the end of the school day. His typical seated posture is slouched, and he is unable to maintain an upright spinal posture for more than 5 minutes. He has recently gone through a major growth spurt. His ability to sit in actively supported position would require increasing his spinal muscle endurance.

Patient B

Patient B is a 45-year-old electrician who is recovering from a mild rotator cuff tear and decreased endurance of the right rotator cuff. Although he no longer has pain, he is unable to hold his arm in higher ranges of flexion or abduction above 90 degrees for more than 2 minutes. His job requires working with both arms, often in these ranges. In order to reverse the effects of specific deconditioning, endurance of the rotator cuff and scapulothoracic muscles must be improved. A goal to hold the arm in positions and ranges required for his work activities for at least 10–15 minutes might be included in the treatment plan.

Deconditioning occurs when normal activity is limited by bed rest, injury, or pain. The changes in muscle physiology as a result of lower functional demands (whether in specific areas or generalized inactivity) occur very quickly. At the capillary level, deconditioning results in reduced numbers of capillaries per cross-sectional area of the muscle. This, in turn, lowers the oxygen levels supplied to those muscle cells located furthest from the blood vessels. Oxidative enzyme levels in the muscle are also affected by lack of stimulus and are less than ideal for processing the end products of glycolysis and enhancing fatty acid use for oxidative respiration. In addition to changes in the ability to produce energy and vascularization, deconditioning also results in weaker connective tissue with more disorganization of collagen structure and a loss of overall ground substance. The connective tissue is therefore at risk for injury with lower amounts of stress or strain. Most patients will present with specific or generalized deconditioning to some extent, but reversing the effects of inactivity is especially important for those patients who need to sustain positions for extended periods or if repeated functional activities are necessary.

Endurance exercises are performed with lower resistance to allow for longer periods of muscle activity and repeated contractions that stimulate the oxidative pathways. Rest periods between contractions are important to allow adequate recovery for replenishing the oxygen supplies. Progressing muscle endurance involves increasing the repetitions, the time for sustaining a specific position, or the number of sets prior to increasing load (Video 3.20).

Muscle Strength

Strength (Box 3.6) is the ability of a muscle to exert a force against resistance that varies with the specific speed of contraction.[7,8] The amount of strength needed depends on the patient's daily activities and personal characteristics. The distance that the body segments need to be moved and the relative biomechanical advantage of the agonist muscles are all biomechanical factors that influence the relative muscle strength required for function. Therapeutic strength training is intended to restore muscle function after immobilization, deconditioning, or damage. In these cases, overload can be achieved with a much lighter load and is relative to status at the time of evaluation, not necessarily to the previous physical condition. Individuals with comorbidities or conditions such as cardiovascular disease, pulmonary disorders, or cancer, or those taking certain

---

BOX 3.6   Muscle Function: Strength[6,7]

- Therapeutic strength training restores the muscle function after immobilization, deconditioning, or damage.
- Overload can be achieved with lighter loads for therapeutic exercise.
- Medical history, including comorbidities, may suggest the need for a conservative starting point.
- Progressive resistance exercise includes slow, progressive increase in load.
- Loads include body weight resistance.
- Strengthening exercises progress from specific movements to functional movements designed by considering the patient's individual characteristics, environment, and goals.
- Specificity is key to strength training.

medications that influence muscle function (such as prednisone) should start with a more conservative load. The amount of resistance is slowly and progressively increased to match the recovery status (**progressive resistance exercise [PRE]**). While early exercise may be performed in supported positions using isolated motion, weight-bearing closed-kinetic chain exercises are more closely aligned with the loads and challenges required for functional activities. However, the therapist should be mindful that when transitioning from gravity-eliminated (Video 3.10) to closed-kinetic chain exercises, weight-bearing positions significantly increase the strength requirements to oppose body weight (Video 3.12). Exercise programs should progress from specific strengthening exercise to target weaker muscles while limiting compensations to closed-kinetic chain exercises that mimic the patient's functional requirements.

Therapeutic exercise programs should reflect the patient's personal and environmental factors along with his or her activity and functional requirements. The amount of muscle strength required for function depends on personal characteristics—age, body weight, anthropometric characteristics, and functional requirements. A patient who weighs 300 pounds will need greater knee extensor muscle strength to get out of a chair than another patient weighing 150 pounds. Exercise requirements will be different for an individual living in the city who relies on a subway system for transportation compared to an individual who works for a moving company (Clinical Example 3.7) or who wants to return to weight lifting (Video 3.21).

Strength training challenges the muscle through overload and specificity principles. The type of muscle contraction (isometric or isotonic) and the range where the muscle is loaded will determine how the connective tissue and muscle fiber adapts. The type of contraction and range required for return to function should therefore be a consideration when choosing exercises and parameters.

Muscle Power

Muscle power (Box 3.7) is the ability to produce speed or large forces in a specified amount of time—a vital component of functional performance.[8] Examples of functional activities requiring greater muscle power are jumping, snatch lifting, and sprinting. Exercises that address muscle power are performed at greater speed and can involve both initiating and stopping the movement (Clinical Example 3.8). Typically, the larger global movers, which have a higher percentage of glycolytic fibers, are capable of generating greater forces and anaerobic energy production involved in quick movements. When making adjustments in an exercise or functional activity, there is an inverse relationship between speed and resistance. Power exercise, such as plyometrics or snatch lifting, is usually included in therapeutic exercise only after other impairments have been addressed and when adequate functional strength and mobility are available with slower movement. If muscle power deficits are contributing to diminished functional performance, training speed can be increased or the resistance decreased to target physiological changes in glycolytic fibers without placing excessive stress on the connective tissue or muscle.

⚡ CLINICAL EXAMPLE 3.7 Muscle Function: Specificity of Strength Training

The specificity of exercise is influenced by both personal and environmental factors.

Patient A
Patient A lives in an urban environment and needs to be able to climb three flights of stairs to access the subway system.

Patient B
Patient B is a moving company employee who needs to be able to carry heavy furniture, sometimes up or down a flight of stairs. Both patients are recovering from knee surgery and are progressing into Phase III. Both patients have successfully progressed from equipment-based strengthening using a leg press machine to squats against body weight (see Exercise 9.30).

Comparison of Patients A and B
In Phase III, Patient A may benefit from step-ups onto a platform without weight and a goal to reach the number of repetitions consistent with the number of steps in the local subway (see Exercise 9.31), while Patient B may benefit more from squats with progressive resistance holding heavy loads (see Exercises 11.43 and 11.44) and a goal to reach the loads expected to return to work.

BOX 3.7 Muscle Function: Power[7]

- Power exercise is performed at high speed or with high load in a short period of time.
- Exercises addressing muscle power can involve initiating or stopping movement rapidly.
- Power exercise requires use of the global mover muscles and anaerobic or glycolytic energy production.
- Power exercise is usually only included in therapeutic exercise after other impairments have been addressed, with adequate functional strength and mobility for slower movement.

Aerobic Endurance

Aerobic endurance (Box 3.8) is used to describe time-based exercise with a general cardiovascular focus that enhances aerobic cellular respiration and usually includes general systemic responses in the cardiac, respiratory, and peripheral circulatory systems. All of the aspects of oxygen delivery, enzyme function, and by-product removal are interrelated and influence the ability to perform exercise for longer periods. A brief list of physiologic functions influencing aerobic conditioning includes respiratory gas exchange, cardiac pump function, and oxygen

---

CLINICAL EXAMPLE 3.8 Muscle Power

Muscle power is often associated with sports requirements, with higher speed and forces required. Different sports will require sports-specific movements and training.

Patient A

Patient A is a basketball player is recovering after a patella fracture and needs to be able to jump vertically with explosive power and safely control the return (see Exercise 9.51). A vertical jump program progresses in the following order: (1) supported jumps on equipment, (2) rapid squats with a weighted ball (Video 3.22), (3) double- or single-leg vertical jumps on a trampoline or land (Video 3.23), (4) hop jumps onto a box and drop jumps off a box, and (5) tuck jumps in Phase III. Single-leg hop for distance is also included in late stage progressions (Video 3.24).

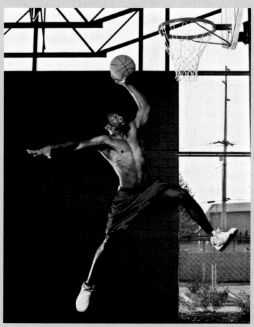

Basketball player in a vertical jump. (From Myers TW. *Anatomy Trains*. 3rd ed. Oxford, UK: Churchill Livingston, 2014, Fig. 10.14.)

Patient B

Patient B is an ice hockey player who requires power using the hip abductors and adductors for the sideways skating motion (A), to be able to resist outside forces (B), or prevent falling (C). Lateral motion against elastic resistance (Exercise 9.28) is included in Phase II, and goals are set to improve push-off speed in positions required for skating. The patient is further challenged using a sliding board for a lateral skating motion (Exercise 9.52) when he is relatively pain-free in standing and with sideways resistance.

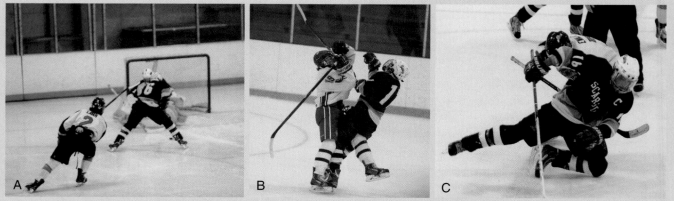

Ice hockey player using skating motion. (From Provencher M, Reider B, Davies G. *Orthopaedic Rehabilitation of the Athlete*. Philadelphia: Elsevier Saunders; 2015, Fig. 24.24.)

diffusion across capillary and cellular membranes. Aerobic endurance exercise is particularly important when there are systemic changes related to comorbidities or deconditioning. Basic concepts will be addressed in this section, but the reader is directed to Frownfelter's text[9] for a review of metabolic systems with a focus on oxidative respiration and applications for clinical practice.

The three main metabolic systems used for energy production are the phosphocreatine system, the glycolytic system, and the oxidative system. At any given time, and to varying degrees, all three of these systems are active. At rest, the predominant metabolic system is the oxidative system, which requires a significant period of time to increase energy production. With increased activity, muscles begin to rely heavily the phosphocreatine system to produce energy. After approximately 30 seconds of exercise, the glycolytic system is activated, precipitated by three events: (1) a decrease in available cellular phosphocreatine, (2) increases in transfer of blood glucose into the muscle cells, and (3) an increase in substrate concentrations required for the glycolytic process. Glycolysis remains the primary source of energy production until the oxidative system adjusts to a new, steady-state activity level, at around 1–4 minutes[9] (Table 3.4). If increased effort is required beyond steady-state level, the phosphocreatine and glycolytic systems will predominate until either a steady-state is met or the patient has reached the limit of his or her aerobic capacity. Understanding the metabolic systems allows the therapist to prescribe appropriate exercise duration and intensity dosages.

Decreased aerobic endurance due to deconditioning is common and is impacted by multiple physiological systems. Impairments in the cardiovascular system reduce the delivery of oxygenated blood to the exercising muscles, causing fatigue and decreased ability to perform prolonged or repetitive movements. Deconditioning also decreases the efficiency of the autonomic system's ability to control rate, extensibility, and contractility of the cardiac muscle. Altered autonomic system function also impacts vascular system function, decreasing the transportation of oxygen to muscles. In addition, the respiratory muscles become less efficient and there is an increased energy cost just to move oxygen into and carbon dioxide out of the lungs (Fig. 3.4 and Table 3.5).

BOX 3.8   Aerobic Endurance[7,8]

- Training for muscular endurance requires activating the glycolytic systems to provide a boost of energy production over a steady metabolic state.
- Training for aerobic function involves stimulating the oxidative system to improve the ability to take in and utilize oxygen to maintain longer term, steady-state activity levels.
- General aerobic exercise is appropriate to limit deconditioning or improve overall cardiovascular and respiratory capacity.

TABLE 3.4   Functional Tasks, Metabolic System Focus, and Exercise Duration[8]

Functional Task	Metabolic System Focus	Exercise Duration
Lifting a box and carrying it 50 m once per hour	Phosphocreatine Glycolytic	<1 minute
Climbing 5 flights of stairs once per hour (takes 3–5 minutes)	Glycolytic	>30 seconds, <4 minutes
Walking 1 hour 3 times per day	Oxidative	>4 minutes

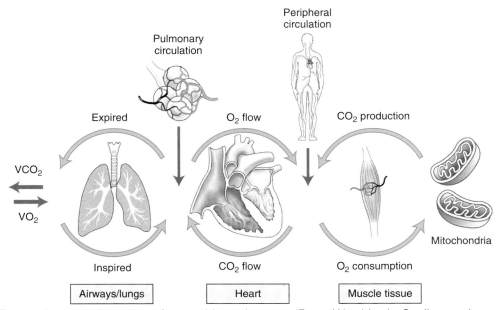

Fig. 3.4 Integrated systems for aerobic endurance. (From Watchie J. *Cardiovascular and Pulmonary Physical Therapy a Clinical Manual.* 2nd ed. St. Louis: Saunders Elsevier; 2010. Fig 1.1.)

Aerobic endurance deficits can be described as a local impairment or a systemic impairment. Local impairments involve the transportation of oxygen to muscle fibers related to changes in capillary density and decreased efficiency of oxygen transfer from the blood to the cells. The use of oxygen within the target muscle is also influenced by muscle physiology changes such as alterations in the enzyme systems and mitochondria. Systemic impairments include alterations in cardiopulmonary and circulatory mechanisms for transportation of oxygen and substrates required for energy metabolism.[9] An exercise prescription for a patient with an acute injury may include precautions limiting the amount of load that can be applied to the injured tissues, but aerobic exercise without excessive stress on the tissue is beneficial in preparing the patient for future stages of rehabilitation when the precautions are lifted. Generalized aerobic exercise is therefore useful for limiting deconditioning or improving overall cardiovascular or respiratory capacity (Clinical Example 3.9).

Balance

Balance impairments (Box 3.9) can present in all patient populations and have a major impact on activity and participation. Poor balance is a potential cause for serious injuries, and therefore preventing falls is always a fundamental physical therapy goal. Balance is also critical for athletes after injury and for injury prevention. The ability to sit upright, stand, and maintain upright postures influences all functional activities except sleeping. Balance impairments can result from disruption of the incoming sensory information (tactile, proprioceptive, vestibular or visual), balance reaction processing and coordination deficits, or from loss of motor output capability. Each of these interrelated systems will play a role in effective and timely balance responses (Fig. 3.5). If there are impairments related to one system, other sensory, motor, or coordination systems may need to be emphasized or used to enhance appropriate responses. An exercise program focusing on balance rather than

TABLE 3.5 Cardiac Function, Output, and Effect of Deconditioning

Cardiac Function	Effect on Cardiac Output	Effect of Deconditioning
Autonomic control of heart rate	Adjusts rates of contraction	Slower, less precise response of heart rate to challenge
Extensibility of cardiac muscle	Allows for precise pre-contraction filling of heart chambers	Decreased filling of chambers prior to ejection, higher heart rate needed to circulate blood
Contractility of cardiac muscle	Adjusts force of muscle contraction and velocity of blood flow with each heart beat	Decreased force of contraction, higher heart rate required to move blood flow

BOX 3.9 Balance

- Balance impairments can result from sensory, central processing, or motor output dysfunction.
- Static balance involves the ability to maintain a stable position, while dynamic balance is the ability to move from one position to another or return to a stable position after the center of gravity is perturbed.
- Balance activities may need to be adapted, and patients will need to be taught to compensate for permanent loss of sensory, motor, or coordination function.
- Personal and environmental considerations will influence the type of functional balance activities used in Phases II or III.

CLINICAL EXAMPLE 3.9 Aerobic Endurance Training

Endurance training can be used to maintain cardiac and pulmonary function during recovery after a musculoskeletal injury, for patients who are deconditioned, or for individuals with cardiopulmonary health conditions.

Patient A

Patient A is a competitive marathon runner with an Achilles tendon tear. The upper body ergometer (UBE) can be used to maintain conditioning while the patient is recovering (see Exercise 10.1).

Patient B

Patient B is a 65-year-old man who was recently hospitalized for gastrointestinal problems and is having difficulty with general endurance and difficulty walking. The UBE is used in this case to address the primary impairment of decreased aerobic endurance.

Patient C

Patient C is being seen for thoracic and neck pain but has a history of open heart surgery for cardiac bypass 3 years ago. In this case, the UBE can be used to increase thoracic rotation but also provide stimulus for improving aerobic endurance with appropriate monitoring of cardiac responses.

Comparison of Patients A, B, and C

All three patients are able to use the UBE for endurance related to cardiopulmonary function goals. Patient A is likely to use higher dosage parameters to maintain general fitness while he adheres to precautions for healing for his lower limb injury compared to both Patients B and C. Patient B may benefit from use of the UBE compared to other types of equipment if he has decreased ability to stand for longer periods, and the UBE allows him to rest if he is fatigued. Patients B and C will need close monitoring to avoid excessive cardiopulmonary stress, with Patient C adhering to strict precautions related to increasing blood pressure or pulse rate within appropriate limits. Goals for Patient C also include slow increases in the amount of thoracic rotation.

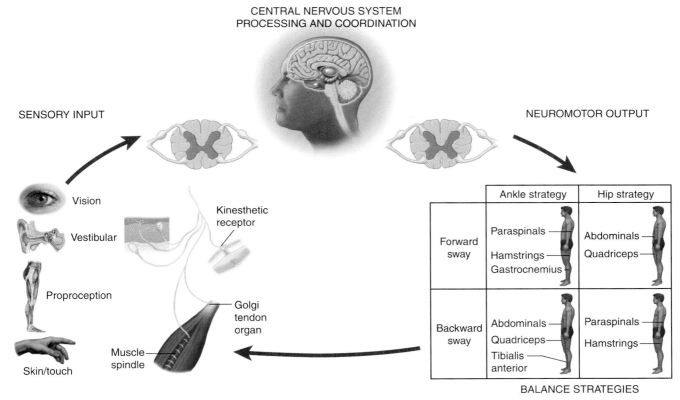

Fig. 3.5 Interactions among sensory input, balance processing, and motor output.

a straightforward prescription for mobility or stability impairment is somewhat more complex, and the prognosis may be limited in the presence of permanent neurological damage.

The causes of balance impairments will influence exercise instruction and prescription. If there is a good prognosis for full recovery after an injury, the exercises should progressively challenge balance and coordination with the expectation of a full recovery. On the other hand, if there are impairments that are likely to be permanent or progressive, the exercises will need to include mechanisms for adapting to the loss of the specific physiological mechanism, structure, or function. Training balance responses is a priority when there are afferent (incoming sensory) deficits (tactile, proprioceptive, or visual) or when the motor responses are impaired. The patient's personal and environmental factors will also influence the type of balance required for daily activities (see Clinical Examples 3.1 and 3.10). Good static *and* dynamic balance responses are required for return to full activity and participation.

Static balance is the ability to maintain an upright trunk position against gravitational forces or outside perturbations. The ability to support the body in a state of equilibrium requires both form closure from joint and ligamentous support and postural muscle activity to support the trunk or limbs. If static balance against gravity is impaired, the therapist should assess and address the patient's core or trunk stability as a fundamental building block for improving balance.

Assuming that the patient has adequate static balance in more supported positions, exercises should progressively challenge the neuromuscular system in less supported

positions (Clinical Example 3.10). The base of support and position of the center of gravity relative to the base of support become important considerations when selecting or progressing exercises to appropriately challenge balance deficits and activities (Fig. 3.6). In order to maintain balance, the patient must be able to maintain the center of gravity within the base of support (Video 3.25). If a patient is leaning forward, the muscles on the posterior aspect of the body will oppose gravitational forces and return to the most stable position using either the hip or ankle muscles (ankle and hip strategies). The opposite direction involves the anterior muscles bringing the body back to the most stable position (Fig. 3.7). In addition to responses to gravity, challenges for static and dynamic balance are increased when sensory input is removed. For example, limited visual input will make a static task more difficult. If there are permanent impairments, as in patients with low vision, other systems will need to be targeted to provide additional sensory input.

Dynamic balance refers to the ability to move from position to position without falling. The ability to return to a more stable position, change direction, stop, or continue to move in a coordinated and smooth manner relies on complex neuromuscular control using multiple motor, sensory, and coordination systems. The importance of dynamic balance increases in Phases II and III to prepare for transitional movements and appropriate functional activities. Rapid and accurate dynamic balance reactions are particularly important for older adults who are at higher risk for falls as well as for individuals wanting to return to higher level sporting and recreational activities. The patient's

Balance impairments involve both static and dynamic balance and may be addressed in patients of all ages.

Patient A

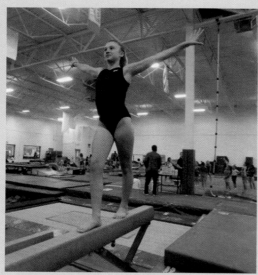

Phase II static balance training on the beam.

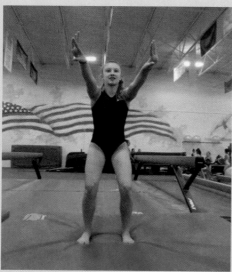

Phase III dynamic balance training during landing dismount practice.

Patient B

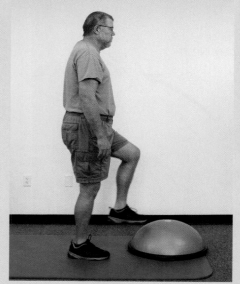

Phase II static balance training (single-leg stance) for fall prevention.

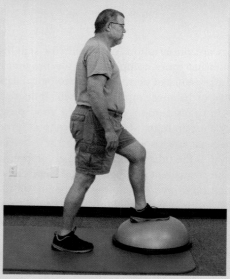

Phase III training dynamic balance training (step reactions to prepare for walking in crowds).

Comparison of Patients A and B

Both patients will need to progress from static to dynamic balance exercises. However, Patient A will start with more aggressive positions requiring a small base of support and progress to high-impact landing activities. Patient B is likely to progress slowly to dynamic balance and will be challenged to the point where the therapist is confident that the patient can recover safely. The therapist will need to be careful with choice of position and degree of instability while staying close to the patient at all times if there is any chance of falling or if the patient is unable to respond quickly using stepping reactions.

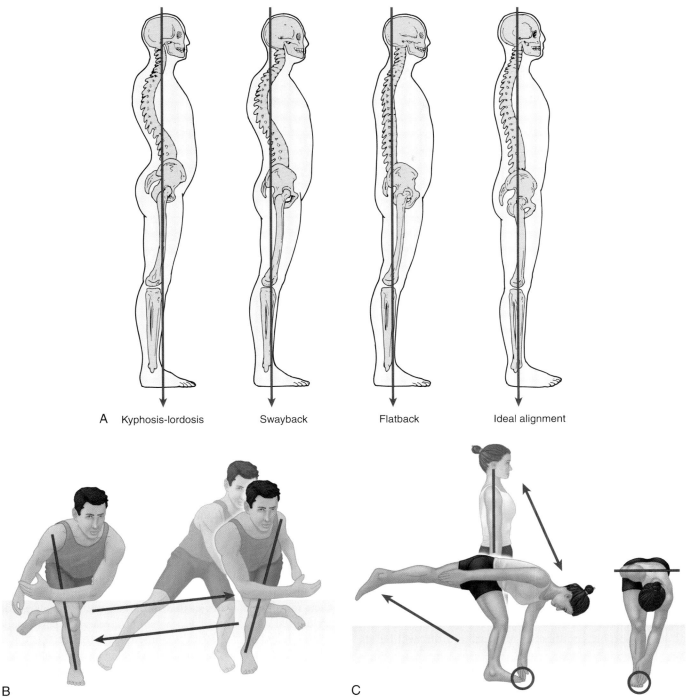

| A | Kyphosis-lordosis | Swayback | Flatback | Ideal alignment |

B

C

Fig. 3.6 Balance impairments (challenging ability to maintain the center of gravity within the base of support). (A) In a stable position, the line of gravity falls within the base; in double-leg standing within the area between the feet, slightly in front of the ankle joint. Any perturbation requires additional muscle activity to return the body segments to a state of equilibrium. (B) During movement, the body segments are moved from one foot to another, requiring muscle activity to stop the movement in the plane of the movement. In a side-stepping action, the hip abductors and adductors and ankle invertors and evertors have to be activated rapidly to limit motion of the body past the foot. The base is smaller in the frontal plane, and the width of the hip and the trunk exceeds the base at all times, increasing the challenge for frontal plane neuromuscular activation. (C) In a hip hingeing exercise, the motion occurs in the sagittal plane. The base is larger in the sagittal plane than in the frontal plane, but the mass of the trunk falls in front of the base and the leg mass falls behind the base. The patient will need to use muscle activity on the posterior aspect of the leg to oppose gravity, as well the posterior trunk muscles. As the body hinges forward and the leg is lifted, the supporting leg muscles will need to counteract and respond to maintain the center of mass over the foot. ([A] From Cameron MH, Monroe LG. *Physical Rehabilitation Evidence-Based Examination, Evaluation, and Intervention*, 1st ed. St. Louis: Saunders Elsevier; 2007. Fig. 4.19.)

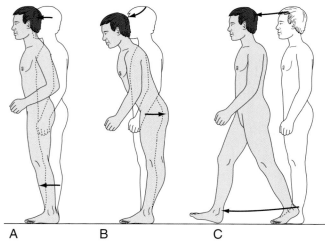

Fig. 3.7 Strategies to regain postural equilibrium when balance is disturbed. Ankle (A), hip (B), or step (C) strategies can be used to maintain equilibrium if the line of gravity falls outside the base. Ankle strategies (A) result in distal to proximal muscle recruitment, with muscles on the opposite side of the line of gravity activating to bring the body back toward the midline. Muscle recruitment for hip strategies (B) are proximal to distal, and the trunk and head move in opposite directions to the lower extremity relative to the line of gravity. Step strategies (C) are used in response to large or quick forces, with the foot placed in under the body to regain balance. One foot is placed in under the body as the trunk moves forward (or backward) to regain balance. Each of these strategies is necessary for balance reactions but can also be used to promote muscle activation as balance is a priority for function. (From Cameron MH, Monroe LG. *Physical Rehabilitation: Evidenced Based Examination, Evaluation, and Intervention*, 1st ed. St. Louis: Saunders Elsevier; 2007. Fig. 13.8.)

personal characteristics and environmental considerations are important to determine the type of transitions to be used during functional training. Transferring weight from foot to foot during running or changing directions or landing from a jump would be appropriate for an athlete. Tasks such as responding to uneven surfaces or outside stimuli may be more appropriate for an older adult (see Clinical Example 3.10). Dynamic balance responses are also influenced by movement compensations and other task-specific coordination deficits, and this will be discussed in the next section.

Task-Specific Neuromuscular Coordination and Response Efficiency

All movements and activities involve a complex sequence of events and multiple systems. The coordination of the movement needs to be appropriate for the task requirements, and individuals need to react fast enough to respond to outside challenges (Box 3.10). The fine-tuning of tasks also requires the ability to monitor, adjust, and change the degree, direction, and extent of the movement. Neuromuscular coordination includes timing of movement, sequencing, and selective activation of different muscle groups. The adjustment of movement and appropriate response efficiency is also influenced by incoming information including vision, tactile, and proprioceptive input.[10] Movement patterns and strategies vary considerably across individuals and tasks. Ideally, movement strategies for functional activities should require the least amount of energy possible. The primary

CLINICAL EXAMPLE 3.11 **Movement Compensations**

A 70-year-old patient recently had a total knee replacement and is allowed to bear weight fully on the affected limb. He has a history of knee osteoarthritis that has become progressively more painful over the past 3 years. He has sufficient range of motion and muscle strength on the affected side to ambulate, but, despite encouragement, he continues to use a walker and places 75% of his weight on his unaffected leg. One of the goals for the patient is to obtain equal weight-bearing during standing and full weight acceptance during the stance phase of gait. While the exercise plan will also address other impairments, the focus on bilateral weight-bearing activities with feedback from the therapist to help him recognize when he is drifting away from the affected leg is used to address the movement compensations. Exercises that encourage weight transference and gait training activities will be initiated in the parallel bars using a mirror to provide feedback and allow the patient to self-monitor the patterns.

requirements for human movement are to be able to maintain a balanced position against gravity (static or dynamic) and to be able to move from one position to another. Ensuring efficiency and distribution of forces is particularly important following repetitive stress injuries. If forces are not distributed throughout the kinetic chain, accumulation of forces contributes to microtrauma, and repeated stress does not allow the tissue to recover (see Chapter 6).

Response efficiency is equally important for all patient populations. Patients compensate for impairments by avoiding weight-bearing or motion of the affected area or by modifying their movement strategies and minimizing stresses placed on an injured area. Altered movement strategies are particularly common and immediate in response to pain (or anticipation of pain). While pain is a normal protective mechanism when used to avoid further injury or damage, learned pain behavior is maladaptive if reinforced and practiced after the initial tissue damage has been resolved. If pain responses are activated, muscle guarding or avoidance of positions often results in movement compensations. Similar patterns occur if there is insufficient muscle strength or endurance. Over time, maladaptive compensatory patterns become habit, and altered movement patterns become the new "normal" without the patient being aware of the changes (Clinical Example 3.11). Unfortunately if the movement patterns are not rectified, alterations in biomechanics and stress can result in secondary impairments. This cycle of adjustments can result in chronic problems despite successful treatment of local impairments. Altered patterns can also contribute to the accumulation of force in remote regions of the body and other repetitive strain injuries at a later stage. Under these circumstances, the patient will need to relearn normal movement patterns to avoid persistent pain and recurrent complaints. The motor learning concepts included in Chapter 7 are important for addressing movement compensations and should be incorporated into Phases I and II.

Psychological Contributions to Impairments

Psychological contributions (Box 3.11) are important factors to consider during exercise prescription because they can influence activity and participation both positively and negatively. Negative psychological aspects of the pain and injury experience (depression, fear, avoidance, hypervigilance, catastrophizing, and general negative affect) result in poor outcomes[11,12] (Fig. 3.8). In contrast, positive affect, an expectation of a successful outcome, and a positive therapeutic alliance with the therapist has been shown to have a positive impact on outcomes.[11,13–15] Pain normally functions as an alarm for either current injury or the risk of further injury. The process has traditionally been portrayed as an insult to bodily tissue that stimulates nociceptors and therefore the perception of pain. These nociceptors relay their signal to the brain, and the brain perceives pain. This simplistic and linear view of the pain

experience is no longer considered as the only or primary mechanism, particularly with chronic pain. The brain interprets the quality and intensity of the incoming sensory information in the context of previous memories and the perceived threat of the situation. Therefore, the intensity of the pain experience is often driven by not only nociceptors, but also by somatosensory, visual, auditory, and other reminders of the threat of further injury.[16] Fear of pain is the anticipation that pain will worsen with movement, positions, or activities and also results in exaggerated pain reports. **Catastrophizing** is a belief that the worst possible outcome is likely and that pain cannot be controlled.[17] **Kinesophobia** is defined as the avoidance of movements or positions that are perceived to cause pain regardless of whether or not the movement will actually result in the perception of pain.[18] The presence of heightened levels of negative beliefs will result in activity avoidance and decreased participation but should not be automatically interpreted as malingering behavior. **Malingering** is used to describe the behavior of an individual who is fabricating or exaggerating impairments or activity limitations for secondary gain, often financial. Most patients with elevated fear may display exaggerated responses to many types of stimuli. This is often considered as a plea for help rather than an attempt to misrepresent his or her condition. In addition to anticipating pain, a fall, or other negative consequences may cause avoidance behavior such as not wanting to perform specific movements or exercises. Addressing avoidance patterns will contribute to the long-term success of the rehabilitation outcome and help prevent further injury. If psychological contributions are identified, exercise management should be adjusted to encourage the patient to increase activity and participation levels, building on and celebrating improvements without focusing on the sensation of pain. There are also methods of

---

BOX 3.11 Fear of Pain[10–17]

- Anticipation of pain, exaggeration of pain intensity, or avoidance of any activities perceived to increase pain can greatly impact outcomes
- Identifying psychological contributions to patient problems is important as it may impact the treatment approach
- *Catastrophizing*: Belief that the worst outcome is likely and pain cannot be addressed
- *Kinesiophobia*: Avoidance of movements or positions that are perceived to cause pain
- *Malingering*: Fabrication or exaggeration of impairments for secondary gain

---

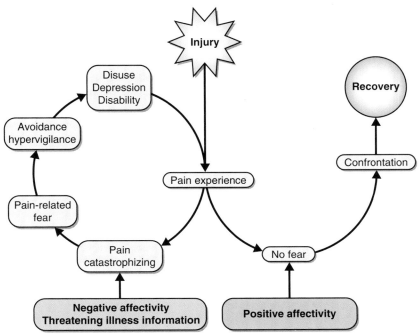

Fig. 3.8 Psychological impact on recovery from injury. (From Griensven HV, Strong J, Unruh A. *Pain: A Textbook for Health Professionals*, 2nd ed. St. Louis: Elsevier Health Sciences; 2014.)

behavior management and motivation that may be used during exercise or functional activity education. The pain experience is multifactorial and complex, and ideal treatment takes into account psychological factors during assessment, patient education, exercise selection, goals, and motivation. The integration of psychologically informed practice is discussed in Chapter 6.

RELATIONSHIP BETWEEN IMPAIRMENTS AND FUNCTION

The primary goal of therapeutic exercise is to restore, improve, or maintain functional movement required for activity and participation. The ICF model can be used to assist the clinical reasoning process and link the health condition, relevant body function and structure, impairments, activity limitations, and participation restrictions for all systems (Box 3.12 and Table 3.6). This section discusses impairments including mobility, muscle function, aerobic endurance, balance, neuromuscular coordination, and psychological impairments. Each patient is likely to have combinations of one or more of these impairments, and therefore prioritizing the impairments is essential. For example, patients with hypomobility may also present with psychological impairments. Patients with hypermobility may present with neuromuscular coordination and muscle endurance deficits. At times the exercise plan will address all impairments, but there are occasions when impairments are managed sequentially rather than concurrently. The prioritization of impairments will be important throughout recovery while considering the patient's goals and individual characteristics.

Some impairments may not be as relevant across all phases of rehabilitation, and, as one impairment is resolved, others may need to be addressed (Clinical Example 3.12). Some isolated impairments may not result in major functional loss, but the repeated redistribution of effort contributes to tissue breakdown and can lead to subsequent impairments (Table 3.7). In time, these compensations result in limited functional ability and/or pain. Addressing impairments that are directly related to the primary activity limitations and participation restrictions will assist with choosing interventions that are most likely to meet the patient's needs. The linkage also provides a framework to build relevant goals. The physical therapist should therefore determine which impairments are contributing most to a patient's functional problems and design the exercise program to address the primary problems at the different points across the phases of rehabilitation. The priorities and primary problems are likely to change as the patient progresses through rehabilitation.

The health condition allows comparison of outcomes using available literature. The International Classification of Diagnoses (ICD) codes[2] provide standardized definitions for health conditions. The therapist will need to use background knowledge of physiology, anatomy, and pathology when considering the implications of diagnoses during evaluation and treatment. The health condition (diagnosis) also informs the determination of prognosis and precautions, thereby influencing goals and exercise choices.

The surrounding context of the personal characteristics and environmental considerations also influences all aspects of exercise prescription. The patient's age, gender, family history, comorbidities, and genetics influence collagen structure and

---

BOX 3.12 Relationship Between Impairments and Function

- The ICF model can be used to assist the clinical reasoning process and link the health condition, relevant body function and structure, impairments, activity limitations, and participation restrictions for all systems.
- At times the exercise plan addresses all impairments, but there are occasions when one impairment is more important than another, or management is sequential rather than concurrent.
- Addressing impairments that are directly related to the primary activity limitations and participation restrictions will assist with choosing interventions that are most likely to meet the patient's needs.
- Using the ICF model allows the therapist to work toward functional goals while addressing precautions and preventing further injury.
- The health condition (diagnosis) also allows a comparison of outcomes to available literature and is considered when determining the prognosis and precautions.
- The surrounding context of the personal characteristics and environmental considerations also influence all aspects of exercise prescription.
- Ultimately, the ICF system provides a framework for clinical reasoning to meet the patient's unique set of needs.

TABLE 3.6 Linkage Between Health Condition, Body Structure, Impairment, Activity Restriction, and Participation Limitation

Health Condition	Body Structure	Impairment	Activity Limitation	Participation Restriction
Nerve entrapment	Peripheral nerve	Limited dynamic nerve mobility; pain and mobility limitation	Difficulty reaching forward	Unable to drive vehicle for work
Chronic obstructive airway disease	Pulmonary	Impaired pulmonary gas exchange; decreased cardiovascular endurance	Difficulty walking prolonged distances	Difficulty delivering mail as postal worker
Coronary artery disease	Cardiovascular	Impaired cardiac muscle oxygenation; decreased cardiovascular endurance	Chest pain with activity	Unable to walk family dogs
Peripheral vascular disease	Vascular	Impaired oxygen delivery; decreased muscular endurance	Fatigue with upper extremity activity	Difficulty self-propelling wheelchair in the community for social interaction
Degenerative joint disease	Articular	Joint mobility	Bending knee	Unable to climb step ladder to paint houses

CLINICAL EXAMPLE 3.12 **Evaluation of Linkage Between Impairments and Activity Limitations: Sit-to-Stand Balance Deficits**

The patient is 35-year-old engineer who sits for most of the day. He is observed having difficulty with balance when moving from sitting to standing and is consistently keeping his center of gravity behind the base of support (see Clinical Example 3.3). He is complaining of anterior knee pain after sitting for long periods and difficulty standing from the chair.

Influence of Personal and Environmental Factors

The patient's age allows the therapist to prioritize possible mobility impairments higher than other potential causes of poor balance. The expected range of motion is based on comparisons to the maximum values collected for young healthy adults.[1]

Initial examination	Interpretation
Hip flexion 120 degrees	Sufficient for sit-to-stand in healthy young adults[1,2]
Knee flexion 105 degrees	Sufficient for sit-to-stand transfer in healthy young adults[3,4]
Ankle dorsiflexion 0 degrees	Insufficient for sit-to-stand transfer (normal healthy adults 27–29 degrees)[2]

The major problem with potential to influence sit-to-stand transfer is hypothesized as insufficient dorsiflexion.

Treatment

Initial Goal

The patient will demonstrate improvements in bilateral ankle dorsiflexion to 28 degrees in order to allow sit-to-stand transfer without loss of balance within 4 weeks.[2]

Initial Plan of Care

- Stretching gastrocnemius complex in standing, joint mobilization of the ankle and foot
- Functional range of motion in supported positions holding onto table, small squats focusing on maintaining new range

Re-evaluation (4 weeks)

- Ankle dorsiflexion 25 degrees in prone
- Ankle dorsiflexion 25 degrees in standing, weight-bearing lunge holding onto table 25 degrees
- Ankle dorsiflexion during sit-to-stand transfer (using video analysis) 5 degrees

Additional Tests

- Evaluate number of sit-to-stand repetitions in 30 seconds and record the successful number of repetitions achieved with body weight over base of support. Use video analysis to determine the time taken to transfer into standing. Utilize this information to update goals. Therapist would also record quality of movement, the use of available range, and the patient's ability to safely and quickly transition the body over the base.
- Evaluate fear of movement (fear avoidance; activities, balance, confidence [ABC] questionnaires).

Assessment

The patient is not using the full, available range. There is minimal influence of fear of movement or falling.

Adjusted Plan

- Improve neuromuscular coordination using available range during functional movements (Phase III).
- Functional stretching will be continued as a home program.
- Squats will be continued with focus on maintaining body over the base, decreasing upper body support, and increasing range.
- Progress to sit-to-stand transfers through range with body weight fully over the base of support, increase repetitions and speed, improve coordination to access available range during functional movement.

Goal for Phase III

The patient will demonstrate the ability to transfer from sit-to-stand using available ankle range of motion for 80% of the repetitions during a 30-second sit-to-stand task without any fear of movement.

References

1. Reese NB, Bandy WD. *Joint Range of Motion and Muscle Length Testing.* 2nd ed. St. Louis, MO: Saunders Elsevier; 2010.
2. Ikeda ER, Schenkman ML, O Riley P, et al. Influence of age on dynamics of rising from a chair. *Phys Ther.* 1991;71:473–481.
3. Jevsevar DS, Riley PO, Hodge WA, et al. Knee kinematics and kinetics during locomotor activities of daily living in subjects with knee arthroplasty and in healthy control subjects. *Phys Ther.* 1993;73:229–276.
4. Rowe PJ, Myles CM, Walker C, et al. Knee joint kinematics in gait and other functional activities measured using flexible electrogoniometry: how much knee motion is sufficient for normal daily life. *Gait Posture.* 2000;12:143–155.

TABLE 3.7 Possible Results of Long-Term Compensations for Impairments

Health Condition	Impairment	Activity Limitation	Compensatory Strategy	Possible Sequelae
Nerve entrapment	Limited dynamic nerve mobility	Difficulty lifting objects	Lumbar extension or asymmetry to avoid neural tension	Low back pain
Chronic obstructive pulmonary disease	Impaired pulmonary gas exchange	Walking prolonged distances	Scalene contractions for respiration	Neck pain
Coronary arterial disease	Impaired cardiac muscle oxygenation	Chest pain with activity	Assistive device dependence	Deconditioning
Peripheral vascular disease	Impaired movement of metabolic materials in/out of vessels	Walking due to ischemic pain	Assistive device dependence	Deconditioning
Degenerative joint disease	Joint mobility	Bending knee	Contralateral step-to gait pattern	Contralateral knee pain

potential for healing. Height, weight, and anthropometric characteristics will impact all biomechanical factors such as leverage, body weight resistance, and balance. Muscle strength, power, and endurance, as well as aerobic endurance, are influenced by advancing age, and although all patients have the potential for improvement, the extent and rate of progression will need to be adjusted for older adults. General health habits such as smoking, drug and alcohol use, diet, activity levels, and stress all influence healing potential. Other personal characteristics that directly influence functional exercise include work and hobby requirements. Home programs and patient goals will also need to be adjusted based on the environment, type of equipment available, and potential for return to full function in the patient's social and family settings. Ultimately, the ICF system provides a framework for clinical reasoning to meet the patient's unique set of needs.

SUMMARY

- The ICF model can be used to provide a clinical reasoning framework to select appropriate impairments that are linked to difficulties with activity and participation
- Limitations in mobility (hypomobility) are addressed if the available range of motion does not allow the relevant functional activity without compensations. Hypomobility requires interventions designed to increase tissue length and elasticity.
- Hypermobility can be related to lack of structural restraints from trauma or congenital abnormalities, limited neuromuscular control, or connective tissue laxity. Interventions include improvements in muscle function and neuromuscular coordination.
- Muscle function impairments include difficulty with activation and limitations in muscle strength, power, and endurance. Each element requires different loads to target the appropriate muscle responses. Activation and endurance require low loads; muscle strength and power require higher loads to improve function. Muscle endurance requires high repetitions or longer bouts of time to challenge appropriately.
- Aerobic endurance refers to exercise that challenges aerobic oxidative metabolism including cardiovascular and respiratory components. After deconditioning, aerobic function is often diminished, and systemic exercise is beneficial to return to any activity with prolonged activity requirements.
- Static balance refers to the ability to maintain the trunk in equilibrium in gravity-resisted positions. Dynamic balance is the ability to move from one position to another and return to a stable state.
- Task-specific coordination is the ability to perform specific movements in a smooth manner to achieve the task required in a timely manner.
- Compensatory movement is likely to continue with activities in the presence of impairments and pain. Maladaptive patterns need to be addressed for full functional return and prevention of further injury.
- Psychological contributions can impact recovery negatively or positively.
- Impairments should be prioritized in order to address the most relevant impairments directly related to activity limitations and to meet the patient's needs.
- Personal and environmental considerations also impact all elements of exercise prescription including prognosis, goal-setting, and progression of exercise.

REVIEW QUESTIONS

1. Describe the relationships among impairments, activity limitations, and participation restrictions.
2. Differentiate between hypomobility and hypermobility impairments and how each type of impairment influences exercise choices.
3. Define and describe the different types of impairments affecting muscle function, and include appropriate exercise choices.
4. Differentiate between the focus of exercise for muscle activation, strength, power, and endurance.
5. Distinguish between muscle endurance and general aerobic endurance.
6. Differentiate between static and dynamic balance.
7. Describe how compensatory movement can result in long-term negative outcomes.
8. Discuss how psychological impairments impact recovery.
9. Prioritize impairments that relate to a patient's activity limitation for noncomplex case scenarios.
10. Discuss how personal and environmental considerations influence goals for treatment and exercise prescription.

REFERENCES

1. Sykes C, Snyman S. International Classification of Functioning, Disability and Health (ICF) Framework to Facilitate Interprofessional Education and Collaborative Practice. World Health Organization. www.who.int/hrh/news/2014/hrh_icf_framwork/en/.
2. World Health Organization. How to use the ICF. A practical manual for using the International Classification of Functioning Disability and Health (ICF). 2013. www.who.int/classifications/drafticfpracticalmanual2.pdf.
3. *Guide to Physical Therapist Practice 3.0*. Alexandria, VA: American Physical Therapy Association; 2014. http://guidetoptpractice.apta.org/.
4. Reese NB, Bandy WD. *Joint Range of Motion and Muscle Length Testing*. 2nd ed. St. Louis, MO: Saunders Elsevier; 2010.
5. Magee DJ. *Orthopaedic Physical Assessment*. 6th ed. St. Louis, MO: Elsevier Saunders; 2014.
6. Magee DJ, Zacheweski JE. Principles of stabilization training. In: Magee DJ, Zacheweski JE, Quillen WS, eds. *Scientific Foundations and Principles of Practice in Musculoskeletal Rehabilitation*. St. Louis, MO: Saunders Elsevier; 2007:388–413.

7. Cipriani DJ, Falkel JE. Physiological principles of resistance training and functional integration for the injured and disabled. In: Magee DJ, Zacheweski JE, Quillen WS, eds. *Scientific Foundations and Principles of Practice in Musculoskeletal Rehabilitation.* St. Louis, MO: Saunders Elsevier; 2007:432–457.

8. American College of Sports Medicine. In: Pescatello LS, ed. *ACSM's Guidelines for Exercise Testing and Prescription.* 9th ed. Baltimore, MD: Wolters Kluwer Lippincott Williams & Wilkins; 2014.

9. Frownfelter D, Dean E. *Cardiovascular and Pulmonary Physical Therapy: Evidence to Practice.* 5th ed. St. Louis, MO: Mosby; 2013.

10. Chmielewski TL, Hewett TE, Hurd WJ, Snyder-Mackler L. Principles of neuromuscular control for injury prevention and rehabilitation. In: Magee DJ, Zacheweski JE, Quillen WS, eds. *Scientific Foundations and Principles of Practice in Musculoskeletal Rehabilitation.* St. Louis, MO: Saunders Elsevier; 2007:375–387.

11. Lentz TA, et al. Development of a yellow flag assessment tool for orthopaedic physical therapists: results from the Optimal Screening for Prediction of Referral and Outcome (OSPRO) cohort. *J Orthop Sports Phys Ther.* 2016;46(5):327–343.

12. Griensven HV, Strong J, Unruh A. *Pain: A Textbook for Health Professionals.* 2nd ed. St. Louis, MO: Elsevier Health Sciences; 2014.

13. Bishop MD, et al. Patient expectations of benefit from interventions for neck pain and resulting influence on outcomes. *J Orthop Sports Phys Ther.* 2013;43(7):457–465.

14. Bishop MD, Bialosky JE, Cleland JA. Patient expectations of benefit from common interventions for low back pain and effects on outcome: secondary analysis of a clinical trial of manual therapy interventions. *J Man Manip Ther.* 2011;19(1):20–25.

15. Bialosky JE, Bishop MD, Cleland JA. Individual expectation: an overlooked, but pertinent, factor in the treatment of individuals experiencing musculoskeletal pain. *Phys Ther.* 2010;90(9): 1345–1355.

16. Sueki DG, Dunleavy K, Puentedura EJ, Spielholz NI, Cheng MS. The role of associative learning and fear in the development of chronic pain: a comparison of chronic pain and post-traumatic stress disorder. *Phys Ther Rev.* 2014;19(5):266–352.

17. Frey Law LA, George SZ. Individual differences and pain variability. In: Sluka K, ed. *Mechanisms and Management of Pain for the Physical Therapist.* 2nd ed. Philadelphia: WoltersKluwer Health IASP; 2016:83–99.

18. Vincent HK, Seay AN, Montero C, Conrad BP, Hurley RW, Vincent KR. Kinesiophobia and fear-avoidance beliefs in overweight older adults with chronic low-back pain: relationship to walking endurance: part II. *Am J Phys Med Rehab/Assoc Acad Phys.* 2013;92(5):439–445.

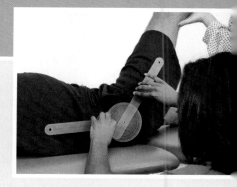

4

Examination Techniques and Evaluation

Kim Dunleavy, Kevin Lulofs-MacPherson, and Amy Kubo Slowik

OBJECTIVES

Upon completion of this chapter, the reader will be able to:

1. Describe how the subjective history and assessment of severity, irritability, nature, and stage (SINS) are used to guide the selection of examination and exercise techniques, positioning, intensity, and parameters.
2. Summarize the use of selective tissue tension principles to assist with selecting exercises.
3. Apply biomechanical principles introduced in Chapter 2 to postural alignment, movement observation, and analysis during exercise testing.

4. Identify common bony and postural malalignments and describe how static and dynamic postures influence exercise selection, positioning, and instructions.
5. Identify common movement compensations.
6. Differentiate among exercise testing for muscle activation, strength, power, endurance, balance, and coordination.
7. Describe how functional movement assessment contributes to the evaluation, choice of interventions, and goal-setting.

The specific examination techniques used to provide baseline subjective and objective information will not be covered in detail in this text. This chapter will introduce how the assessment of examination results for impairment and functional testing is used to guide exercise selection during initial exercise prescription.

SUBJECTIVE HISTORY AND EXAMINATION: INFLUENCE ON OBJECTIVE EXAMINATION TECHNIQUE SELECTION

The information a therapist gathers from the initial interview with the patient will help guide the examination techniques that will follow (Box 4.1). The therapist should ask about past and present medical history, mechanism of the injury, patient goals, and personal and social demographics to set the stage for the subjective interview.[1] The information gained about severity, irritability, nature, and stage (SINS; Chapter 1) along with special questions to determine specific diagnoses help to plan the examination. If the patient has comorbid diagnoses, additional information about these conditions will be needed to determined if there are related precautions and/or contraindications.

The subjective information, along with the objective findings during the evaluation[1-4] will be combined to help the therapist determine the treatment plan, including the type of exercise, a starting point for exercise intensity, and position. The exercise dosage will be tested and the plan adjusted accordingly (see Chapter 5). Psychological screening tools can be used during the initial evaluation and followed with more specific tools, if needed. If the patient's symptoms are more severe or highly irritable and the physical therapist has identified a number of potential

precautions or contraindications, this may be indicative of a more serious pathology or the presence of acute inflammation. This calls for a more comprehensive and careful examination if serious pathology is suspected or less intense examination procedures in the presence of acute inflammation. A chronic condition or a less severe injury with less irritability involves fewer precautions

- High severity
- High irritability
- Contraindications/precautions (nature)
- Acute

- Low severity
- Low irritability
- Limited precautions
- Chronic

Examination starting point	
Cautious examination • Start in supportive positions	More intense examination possible • Less supportive positions
Examination with least force	Examination may include stress testing, maximal range, or combined movements
Exercise testing is set for higher repetitions, lower force, tissue stress, smaller ranges of motion	Exercise testing may include repetitions to fatigue, more exercises, or larger ranges of motion
Use subjective information before, during, and after objective tests	Monitor main symptoms but may aim to reproduce main symptoms of concern
Avoid increasing symptoms • Anticipate and set stop points for testing	May aim to reproduce symptoms, accept minor increase in symptoms, or perform maximal testing

Fig. 4.1 Choice of examination techniques related to SINS categories.

CLINICAL EXAMPLE 4.1 Use of SINS for Decisions Related to Examination and Exercise Testing

Patient A

Patient A sustained multiple avulsion fractures (calcaneus and talus), 3 months ago after falling off a curb. Specifically there were avulsions of the extensor digitorum brevis and bifurcate ligament attachments from the calcaneus and the talonavicular capsule attachment from the talar neck. She is a very active 50-year-old university professor. She wants to return to working out at home on her Pilates reformer and to be able to attend Tai Chi classes.

The fracture was treated conservatively with non–weight-bearing status for 6 weeks and partial weight-bearing in a walking boot for 2 weeks. At 12 weeks, the patient is referred to physical therapy for progressive weight-bearing, ankle range of motion, and strengthening. She has low levels of pain with standing and walking for more than 30 minutes, but the pain decreases as soon as she sits down. There is no longer any effusion.

Evaluation

The multiple fractures indicate major force during the trauma: the nature of the problem requires consideration of healing status for precautions. The immobilization and weight-bearing restrictions are likely to have resulted in mobility and compensatory patterns. The examination should therefore be cautious. Edema and effusion will need to be monitored after examination and exercise techniques. Limited stress should be placed on the injured ligaments and healing fracture sites, particularly with full strain, until there is sufficient tissue healing and muscle support. Examination should be started in non–weight-bearing and progressed to weight-bearing positions if the patient can tolerate the loads. Initially supine, sitting, or supported positions are preferred for exercise to limit forces and potentially poor balance responses.

Patient B

Patient B sustained a mild ankle sprain 2 days previously; he has low levels of pain but is limping. He is able to accept weight fully on the left side during stance although he reports using crutches to be able to get to classes.

Evaluation

There is a need to establish the extent of tissue damage and if precautions are needed. However, the patient is reporting mild pain and he is able to weight-bear on the leg, indicating a lower likelihood of severe injury. The judgment of the severity and nature is delayed until after full objective testing. The patient is in Phase I.

Comparison of Patient A and Patient B

The nature of the problem for both patients is similar but the extent of damage was much more extensive for Patient A. The examination techniques chosen for both patients are the same, but the time frame for bone healing for Patient A's injury requires more caution with use of force. Precautions for Patient A during initial examination will consist of monitoring responses to force and limiting the time or degree of load at extremes of range in all directions. The amount of force used in the initial examination for Patient B can be slightly more aggressive but only after the possibility of more severe injury has been ruled out. The phase of rehabilitation for Patient A (Phase II) suggests that there is the possibility of more established connective tissue and neuromuscular adaptations related to the immobilization and limited weight-bearing, while for Patient B (Phase I), the effusion and inflammatory exudate is likely to impact mobility.

SINS, Severity, irritability, nature, and stage.

---

and allows a more vigorous and intense examination (Fig. 4.1 and Clinical Example 4.1). In addition to the history and SINS data, a review of symptoms helps screen for serious or undiagnosed medical pathology (red flags) that, if present, require referral for further medical examination.[1] Symptoms consistent with psychological impairments are also collected (yellow flags).[1]

SELECTIVE TISSUE TENSION EVALUATION

The relationship between available active, passive, and resisted range of motion is used to indicate sources of impairments

and is described as **selective tissue tension testing** (Box 4.2) Selective tissue tension testing is used to assess the integrity of each of the component tissues of a specific joint and help determine whether contractile or noncontractile structures are the most likely source of dysfunction. The range, end feel, and pain symptoms during the movement are evaluated (Table 4.1). During the examination, the patient is asked to move through range actively and the therapist conducts passive range of motion. Differences between active movement and passive range can indicate if muscle contraction or spasm is influencing movement or if range of motion limitations are more likely to be due to noncontractile structures. The use of resistive testing also provides information related to neuromuscular status. Selective tissue tension results are used in conjunction with subjective symptoms and a number of other specialized tests to guide the choice of type of exercise and parameters (Clinical Example 4.2).

Active range of motion (AROM) involves asking the patient to move actively through available motions. The amount of range is influenced by restraints of the articular structures, including capsule and intraarticular relationships as well as extraarticular limitations (muscle and connective tissue restrictions; Videos 4.1 and 4.2). Active range of motion is also influenced by neuromuscular function and strength, pain responses, and/or psychological fear reactions.

Passive range of motion (PROM) is tested by the therapist moving the limb to the endpoint without the patient performing the movement. PROM reflects the amount of motion possible without active neuromuscular control or influence (Videos 4.3 and 4.4) but can still be limited by protective pain response or psychological fear reactions. Passive motion assessment should also include the joint end feel. The quality of the end feel will suggest what type of tissue is limiting passive motion. If end feel is **firm**, limitations are more likely to be related to capsular or connective tissue limitations. If the end feel is **elastic**, limits may be more likely to be from reaching full muscle length, whereas

an **empty end feel** may be due to muscle guarding caused by pain or spasm. A **soft end feel** is normal in the presence of soft tissue interposition, while a **hard end feel** detected short of the normal joint range of motion is caused by abnormal bony alignment, abnormal bone formation, or intraarticular limitations such as meniscal or loose body impingement. Specific joint play tests compare the available end feel to the typical end feel from normal anatomical structures. Although end feel testing is not very reliable across testers, the information can provide additional information about the relative restraints to movement, particularly in relation to normative values for specific joint range of motion (Table 4.2). The relationship between active and passive range of motion, end feel, and range of motion values helps determine if there are primary mobility impairments related to hypomobility or hypermobility.

Muscle flexibility is usually tested using passive range of motion. The therapist places the muscle in the fully lengthened position with consideration of the anatomical direction of the muscle fibers (Video 4.5). If the muscle crosses more than one joint, both ends of the muscle need to be at the maximal stretch. Some muscle flexibility tests, such as the Thomas test (hip flexors; Video 4.6) or Ely's test (rectus femoris), are also listed as special tests. For a full description of muscle length testing see Reese and Bandy[4] and Magee and Sueki.[2]

Neural tension involves testing the mobility of the peripheral nervous system and is usually tested with multijoint positioning to place the specific neural complex at the maximum stretch. Joints are moved sequentially through maximal range and symptoms monitored.[2,3] Both muscle flexibility tests and neural tension test positions can be used to improve mobility. For more detail on evaluation of mobility and consideration of the structures contributing to mobility deficits see Zachazewski[5] and Magee.[1]

Resistive or **resisted range of motion** (RROM) provide information about the neuromuscular capacity and can be compared to the uninvolved limb or expected force production capabilities of individuals within similar age groups and demographics. Resisted testing can be conducted using isotonic motion through full or selected ranges of motion or isometric contractions (no motion of the joint). Usually, for selective tissue tension purposes, a neutral joint position is used for testing to avoid tension on ligaments or capsule. If pain is reproduced

---

BOX 4.2   Selective Tissue Tension and End Feel

- These tests assist with determining if contractile or noncontractile structures are contributing to impairments.
- They also help determine if there is hypomobility or hypermobility.
- AROM and PROM are used for mobility testing and muscle function (activation).
- AROM and RROM functional movement testing is used for coordination.
  - AROM and PROM painful, RROM pain-free: noncontractile
  - AROM < PROM, RROM weak: contractile
  - PROM pain-free, AROM, RROM painful: contractile
- End feel assists with determining source of mobility impairment (firm, capsule, connective tissue; hard, bone; elastic, muscle; empty, fear, severe pathology, hypermobility)

AROM, Active range of motion; *PROM*, passive range of motion; *RROM*, resisted range of motion.

TABLE 4.1   Selective Tissue Tension: Relationship of AROM, PROM, and RROM to Indicate Possible Source of Impairments

AROM	PROM	RROM	Possible Source of Impairment
Decreased, painful	Full	Normal strength + reproduced pain *OR* decreased strength	Pain from muscle or other structures
Decreased		Decreased strength + effort	Fear-related psychological responses resulting in voluntary limitation of active and resisted motion
Decreased, pain at end range	Decreased (PROM = AROM), pain or discomfort when end feel reached. Decreased when full muscle length is reached (one or more joints)	Normal strength in the midranges	Decreased extensibility of joint capsule, soft tissue, other connective tissue. Decreased muscle flexibility
Decreased, pain-free	Full	Weak, pain-free	Muscle strength limitations due to lack of activation, decreased muscle capability, or neuromotor conduction impairments

AROM, Active range of motion; *PROM*, passive range of motion; *RROM*, resisted range of motion.

🔨 CLINICAL EXAMPLE 4.2 Use of Selective Tension Testing

The therapist continues with the assessment of the patients in Clinical Example 4.1.

Patient A

The initial examination for Patient A is cautious, and range of motion is tested in supine prior to any standing tests. No overpressure is used for any of the active or passive range of motion examinations, and gentle isometric resistance is used for selective tissue tension testing. The therapist's hand position is modified to avoid direct pressure over the healing avulsion fractures. Gastrocnemius length is tested in sitting rather than in a weight-bearing standing lunge test. Joint mobility testing is cautious and discontinued if there is any pain.

Evaluation

Despite the possibility of high severity due to the avulsion fractures and the high force causing the damage, the severity and irritability of the pain symptoms in Patient A are low. The primary impairments are decreased dorsiflexion, decreased isometric strength of all of the ankle muscles, weight-bearing asymmetry, difficulty with single-leg balance, gait deviations, and pain during ambulation. The dorsiflexion mobility limitation is not severe but, along with antalgia and established movement patterns, is contributing to gait deficits and asymmetry. Although the initial examination was cautious, the patient is in Phase II and the primary focus will be on restoration of symmetry and muscle function, as well as on ankle dorsiflexion mobility.

Patient B

The therapist must determine the extent of tissue damage for Patient B. The location of the pain on the lateral aspect of the ankle and the history of rolling over on the ankle indicates a high probability of lateral ligament damage. Ankle range of motion is tested actively first with the addition of overpressure for plantarflexion, dorsiflexion, and eversion after determining that these motions result in minimal discomfort. There was pain early in the inversion range, and no overpressure is added to inversion to avoid tension or stress on the lateral ligaments. The talar tilt test[1] is performed with the hands close to the ankle joint with a shorter lever arm, and the motion is performed slowly and carefully. The range and pain help determine the grade of lateral ligament injury (Grade I). The patient was able to complete the standing lunge test, but active and passive dorsiflexion range was limited by effusion, and therefore the evaluation of gastrocnemius length is deferred to a later time. Palpation and other special tests are also performed (anterior drawer).[1]

Evaluation

Patient B's diagnosis of a Grade I calcaneofibular ligament sprain is confirmed. Impairments include decreased mobility of the ankle due to effusion (plantarflexion and dorsiflexion) and pain (plantarflexion and inversion). The mild Grade I sprain indicates the need to protect the ligament from excessive forces while assisting with resolution of effusion and promotion of muscle activation. However, progression is likely to be rapid once the effusion is resolved. Further evaluation of balance responses and proprioception is indicated as soon as the effusion resolves. Weight-bearing distribution, gait, and functional difficulty are influenced by pain and limited mobility due to edema and effusion.

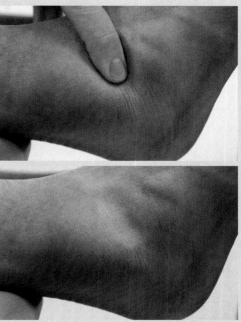

Effusion after a Grade I calcaneofibular ligament ankle sprain.

Comparison of Examination Techniques and Implications for Exercise for Patients A and B

The examination techniques chosen for both patients are similar; however, the time frame for bone healing and the severity of Patient A's injury requires more caution with use of force. The acute stage for Patient B also required evaluation of the extent of damage. Range of motion and movement patterns are more established for Patient A after her extended immobilization. Patient B has range of motion limitations due to effusion and pain. Exercise parameters will differ, and the expected time frames for improvements will be longer for Patient A.

Reference

1. Magee DJ, Sueki D. *Orthopedic Physical Assessment Atlas and Video: Selected Special Tests*. St. Louis, MO: Elsevier Saunders; 2011.

TABLE 4.2 Passive Range of Motion and End Feel

End Feel	Cause	Possible Explanations for Abnormal End Feel
Firm	Capsule Connective tissue	Full length of connective tissue: needs to be assessed relative to other limb, compared to average population and average range for specific joint.
Hard	Bone	Normal for some joints at end range of motion related to demographics; abnormal if early Can be due to bony alignment, previous fracture healing, osteophytes, or other pathology such as severe arthritis, ankylosing spondylitis
Elastic	Muscle	Decreased muscle flexibility if muscle is at full length Muscle spasm due to pain or guarding
Empty	Fear responses Severe pathology Hypermobility	Protective responses prior to reaching end range (fear, symptom magnification, or other avoidance) Severe pathology resulting in joint destruction Severe hypermobility can result in empty end feel if there are no limits to motion prior to maximal stretch on other structures that cause pain

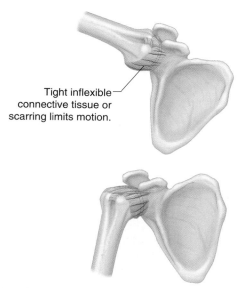

Tight inflexible connective tissue or scarring limits motion.

Fig. 4.2 Capsular restrictions during shoulder active range of motion—hypomobility.

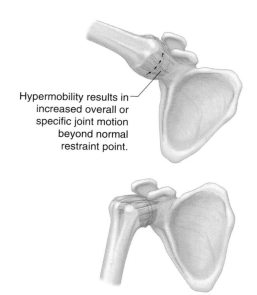

Hypermobility results in increased overall or specific joint motion beyond normal restraint point.

Fig. 4.3 Increased capsular laxity and lack of capsular restraint during shoulder active range of motion—hypermobility.

or increased with resistive isometric testing (no motion of the joint), but passive range of motion is pain-free, this points toward contractile tissue as the source of symptoms. Isotonic testing using manual muscle testing indicates relative neuromuscular strength. If RROM indicates muscle weakness in the presence of other neurological symptoms such as numbness, tingling, or cranial nerve symptoms, a full neurological screen is indicated.

The range of motion results, along with specific joint mobility tests, are compiled to determine whether there is relative joint hypomobility or hypermobility. Limited active and passive motion relative to normative values or functional requirements (with or without pain) is considered hypomobility (Videos 4.1–4.4), but the therapist will need to decide if the impairment is contributing to the primary complaints and functional deficits (Fig. 4.2). If there are mobility limitations, differentiating between joint range of motion and muscle flexibility limitations helps guide the choice between joint mobilization and muscle stretching. If the overall range of motion exceeds normal limits or the end feel is delayed, a joint is considered hypermobile (Fig. 4.3). The amount of motion is compared to the other limb or to expected ranges for patients with similar characteristics. Excessive mobility can be caused by slack or completely torn passive restraints, genetic connective tissue laxity, loss of muscle activation, impaired neuromuscular coordination, or muscle function deficits. Pain, inflammation, and edema will influence muscle function and neuromuscular coordination and can be the primary reason for activity or mobility limitations. Protective muscle guarding can mask hypermobility, and the relationship between the reported pain and movement may warrant testing after muscle guarding has been resolved. Comparing the quality and range of active, passive, and resisted motion and the point in the range of motion where pain is reproduced will help determine the impairments and guide the selection of type of exercise and exercise parameters (Clinical Example 4.3).

CLINICAL EXAMPLE 4.3   Selective Tissue Tension

Patient A

Patient A is a 68-year-old man who presents with complaints of right hip pain and difficulty putting on shoes and socks with his foot on the floor. On examination:

Test	Range of Motion	Pain Reproduction, End Feel
Hip flexion (AROM) in supine	110 degrees	Anterior hip pain 100–110 degrees
Hip flexion (PROM) in supine	110 degrees	End feel firm (capsular), reproduces anterior hip pain
Hip flexion (RROM) in supine 90 degrees	Strong 5/5	No pain
Hip extension (RROM) in supine at 90 degrees of hip flexion		
Hamstring flexibility (90/90 test)	90–20 degrees knee extension with the hip maintained at 90 degrees of hip flexion	Slight posterior tightness in the mid-portion of the hamstring muscle, does not reproduce anterior hip pain
Neural tension testing (active knee extension, ankle dorsiflexion in sitting at 90 degrees hip flexion)	90–20 degrees knee extension, full dorsiflexion	No pain, slight tightness posterior knee and calf

Evaluation

Hip flexion mobility is limited with noncontractile contributions, without hamstring flexibility or neural tension contributions. Taking into account the patient's age, the goal is set to increase hip flexion to 120 degrees of hip flexion so that the patient can tie his shoes. The goals are set based on the average range of motion to tie shoes (129 degrees +/− 9 degrees).[1]

⚡ CLINICAL EXAMPLE 4.3 Selective Tissue Tension—cont'd

Patient B

Patient B is a 48-year-old man who has right hip pain going up stairs, running up hills, and putting on shoes and socks. He is a golfer and a recreational runner. On examination:

Test	Range of Motion	Pain
Hip flexion (AROM) in supine	120 degrees	No pain
Hip flexion (PROM) in supine	120 degrees	No pain
Hip flexion (RROM) in supine 90 degrees	Strong 5/5*	No pain
Hip extension (RROM) in supine 90 degrees	Weaker than opposite side 4/5	Pain posterior hip and thigh
Knee flexion (RROM) in sitting hip at 90 degrees, knee 45 degrees flexion	Only possible against gravity 3/5	Very painful, reproduces pain in proximal hamstring area
Hamstring flexibility (90/90 test)	40 degrees knee flexion	Reproduces pain in hamstring muscle belly and insertion
Neural tension testing (active knee extension, ankle dorsiflexion in sitting at 90 degrees hip flexion)	40 degrees knee flexion, full dorsiflexion	Same symptoms as for hamstring flexibility, no additional pain with dorsiflexion
Stairs		Pain reproduced when right leg leads during upward motion
Putting on shoes and socks		Pain when hip is flexed, externally rotated and abducted

Evaluation

Contractile tissue pain (hamstring) without neural tension or joint contributions.

Comparison of Patients A and B

The major impairment for Patient A is a lack of mobility related to the hip capsule contributions, and mobility exercise will need to regain hip flexion end range. Patient B's symptoms are related to contractile structures (hamstring tendinopathy), and exercise that addresses optimal stimulus for regeneration is indicated. Progressive resistance and eccentric exercise designed to promote connective tissue replenishment and rearrangement is indicated. Patient B's exercise plan will also need to address causative factors and evaluation of movement patterns, training, and other lower extremity joints.

Reference

1. Reese NB, Bandy WD. *Joint Range of Motion and Muscle Length Testing.* 2nd ed. St. Louis, MO: Elsevier Saunders; 2010.

ALIGNMENT AND MOVEMENT OBSERVATION

Static and **dynamic** alignment along with functional movement patterns are important to evaluate during the initial examination and throughout treatment progression (Box 4.3 and Table 4.3). The information from the alignment and movement

BOX 4.3 Alignment and Movement Observation

- Static alignment assessment is useful to determine structural alignment considerations for exercise position and stress-strain relationships.
- The patient's resting posture and dynamic control affect the biomechanics of a joint.
- Prepositioning in postures that will facilitate optimal movement and recruitment during exercise is helpful to ensure pain-free, effective motion.
- If postural alignment can be corrected, regular reinforcement and feedback are necessary during or after therapeutic exercise performance.
- If position cannot be corrected by the patient, further tests and measures may be necessary to rule in or rule out impairments (mobility, pain responses, neuromuscular coordination).
- Movement analysis is used to evaluate if optimal biomechanics are being used, identify movement compensations, and assess the patient's willingness to move. This information is used to promote efficiency, distribute forces, and address causative factors.
- General guidelines for observation include observing the movement from all angles, choosing relevant movements for the functional problems, and ensuring safety.
- Movement observation includes awareness of multiple areas and observation of early or excessive motion in one area (or axis), abnormal direction or amount of motion, symmetry, and willingness to move (or avoidance).

observations impacts choice of exercise and starting positions as well as instructions and feedback. A patient's bony alignment, symmetry, curvatures and positions, and relationships between body segments can be assessed in weight-bearing or non–weight-bearing positions. **Static alignment** will influence the patient's movement strategies and the therapist's choice of exercise for the patient.[6,7] There are multiple combinations of "normal" alignment and a range of anatomical shapes and structural patterns. The underlying bony alignments may or may not contribute to accumulation of forces and tissue breakdown in repetitive strain injuries or contribute to muscle imbalances.[6,7] While postural position can be related to congenital structural alignment, habitual postures contribute to soft tissue alignment and connective tissue changes with the potential to cause repetitive strain damage. Static alignment can also be a result of compensations due to pain, lack of joint mobility, weakness, or habit.[6,7]

The information from the evaluation of static alignment is used by the therapist to explore variations in starting positions that allow the patient to assume an alignment that accommodates for his or her individual bony structure or a position where there is less likelihood of compensations due to lack of mobility or weakness (Clinical Example 4.4). If the patient is able to correct the static alignment or posture, this information is useful for instructions and feedback during exercise to help the patient to understand and practice the preferred posture. If the patient is not able to correct the position, further examination of mobility, pain, and movement coordination is needed to establish if there are impairments that can be addressed with therapeutic exercise or other interventions.

Dynamic alignment and movement should be observed in multiple planes to accurately assess components of

TABLE 4.3	Alignment and Movement Patterns to Watch for by Region	
	Alignment	**Dynamic Movement Patterns to Watch For**
Upper extremity	Upper-quarter postural position (cervicothoracic and scapular relationships) Scapular downward rotation, winging, tipping, forward shoulders Upper-extremity valgus angle	Impingement mechanics in flexion and abduction (lack of external rotation) Scapula connection, scapulohumeral relationships, early shoulder girdle elevation, or upward rotation during elevation Trunk lateral flexion to assist abduction or extension to assist flexion
Lower extremity	Leg-length discrepancy Genu valgus or varus Femoral anteversion or retroversion Knee hyperextension Excessive tibial external rotation or varus Excessive pronation or supination Weight-bearing asymmetry Pelvic rotation Movement symmetry	Dynamic internal rotation and valgus angulation Weight-bearing avoidance or asymmetry Excessive or early pronation or supination Limited pronation during stance or gait Pelvic rotation, hiking, or Trendelenburg Limited weight transfer
Spine	Anterior-posterior postural alignment (lordosis, kyphosis) Symmetry (scoliosis, height of landmarks; leg-length discrepancy, cervical midline alignment)	Axis of motion during spinal movement (early motion or excessive motion) Asymmetry of motion Deviation of motion through range Guarding or lack of motion through range Early, excessive use of global muscles Weight-bearing or range avoidance

Refer also to Figs. 4.5 through 4.20.

functional movement, including timing and coordination. The information gathered from observing dynamic alignment and movement guides choice of further examination techniques and provides information regarding willingness to move, pain behavior, and motor control patterns. Problematic functional motion should be assessed in more detail, and isolated joint range of motion and flexibility measurements are compared to the ranges observed during functional movement.[1,4,6,7] The use of video, timed tests, or repeated measurements provides further detail and allows comparison after treatment.

The physical therapist should observe the **quality** of movement as the patient actively moves through the available range of motion. Range of motion and flexibility testing is usually measured using a goniometer, but other components of the timing and patterns of movement should be documented. Movement analysis will also include detecting compensations or signs of avoidance. The information is used to choose appropriate ranges and planes of motion for exercises to limit symptom reproduction or ensure biomechanical efficiency. The therapist should continuously monitor the patient's quality of movement within available and new ranges while exercising and should attempt to correct faulty movement patterns while teaching patients how to perform the exercises (see Table 4.3).

Upper Extremity
Alignment Observation
The upper extremity depends on the muscular linkage of the scapula to the cervical and thoracic regions. As such, the trunk

and cervical posture influences the position of the scapula, muscle length–tension relationships, and overall biomechanical efficiency. Scapular motion contributes approximately one-third of the range to full shoulder elevation. The scapula rests on the thoracic cage and is connected to the thoracic spine by muscular attachments of the trapezius, serratus anterior, serratus posterior, and rhomboids. Although the acromioclavicular and sternoclavicular joints link the scapula to the clavicle and sternum, there is minimal form closure, and the position of the scapula is influenced by the slope of the rib cage. As the upper trapezius and levator scapulae attach to the cervical spine as well as to the scapulae, neck position will also influence scapular position. The anterior shoulder muscles (pectoralis major and minor, coracobrachialis, and biceps) also impact the overall position of the scapula relative to the trunk. The static postural position and the patient's ability to achieve the optimal position for upper extremity force closure helps with choice of exercise and starting positions. Observation of the scapular position in sitting or standing can provide information about the resting position that influences muscle efficiency and tension. For example, scapular downward rotation (Video 4.7), winging (Video 4.8), or tipping places passive tension on the supraspinatus tendon, rotator cuff, and/or periscapular muscles (Fig. 4.4; see Clinical Example 4.4). Forward or medially rotated shoulder positions (see Fig. 4.4) influence the length of the pectoralis muscles and the posterior scapula stabilizers or increase stress on the anterior glenohumeral capsule and biceps tendon[6,7] (see Clinical Example 4.4).

Postural positions sustained over time can result in changes in connective tissue mobility and should be considered as a potential causative factor for repetitive strain syndromes.[1,6,7]

✦ CLINICAL EXAMPLE 4.4 Postural Alignment Implications for Upper Extremity Exercise

Patient A: Downward Rotation

Patient A has a rotator cuff tear and is referred for strengthening. She has downward rotation of the left scapula noted during postural analysis (see Fig. 4.4A).

Implications for Exercise Position

Sitting with the arm supported on the plinth is chosen for rotator cuff isometrics so that the rotator cuff muscles are not working against as much gravitational force (see Exercises 10.19, 10.20, and 10.23).

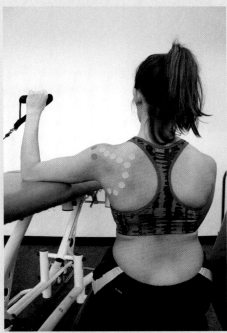

Seated position with the arm supported for shoulder isometrics in the presence of downward rotation.

Patient B: Scapular Winging

Patient B presents with anterior laxity of the right shoulder. She has a very narrow thoracic cage and winging scapula (Fig. 4.4 B).

Implications for Exercise Position and Choices

Midrange of upper extremity elevation in scaption and closed chain positions are used to teach the patient to use the serratus to rotate the scapula upward and link the scapula to the rib cage.

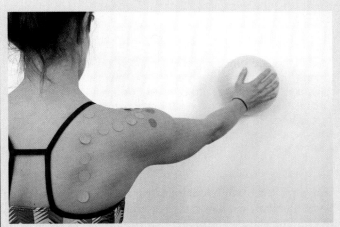

Position used to teach scapula approximation and connection in scaption with closed chain exercise.

In the scaption plane, the scapula is in a relative mid-position, and the medial border is now parallel to the spine with the scapula connected to the rib cage. The serratus, trapezius, and other periscapular muscles are in the optimum position to support the scapula and the position of the glenohumeral joint. The closed chain position also enhances proprioceptive input to promote generalized firing of all the muscles. The position in front of the body limits tension on the anterior capsule.

Patient C: Scapular Tipping

Patient C presents with bicipital tendinopathy and impingement. He has pain with active flexion from 130 to 160 degrees. In sitting, the patient has a kyphotic thoracic curve and forward head posture. He is unable to correct the kyphosis actively in sitting, and the thoracic curve does not change in supine. He has tight pectoralis minor and major muscles, and thoracic spine mobility is limited in all directions. He also presents with scapular tipping (Fig. 4.4C).

Implications for Exercise Position and Choices

In prone or four-point kneeling closed chain positions, instructing the patient to lift and maintain the head and upper body position is important to reduce the anterior pull on the scapula from the head weight (Exercises 10.25 and 11.6).

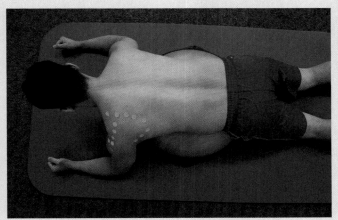

Forearm support over BOSU.

The patient's arms are slightly wider than his body to place the scapula in mid-position. The tipping is counteracted by active movement of the head and upper thoracic spine against gravity, so that the head weight does not pull the scapula forward. Once the head weight is lifted and supported, the scapula muscles can be activated in the mid-position.

Patient D: Forward Shoulders

Patient D is a 23-year-old a college student. She has anterior shoulder pain in both shoulders and presents with forward shoulders and hypermobility (see Fig. 4.4D). She can actively correct her posture, but she has difficulty maintaining a midline supported position for more than 5 minutes.

Implications for Positioning and Exercise Choices

Because the patient is able to correct the forward shoulder position, cueing and reminders to maintain the proximal position are needed rather than specific position choices, along with generalized upper-quarter muscle activation and endurance in the mid-position rather than maximal range.

BOSU, Both Sides Up Balance trainer.

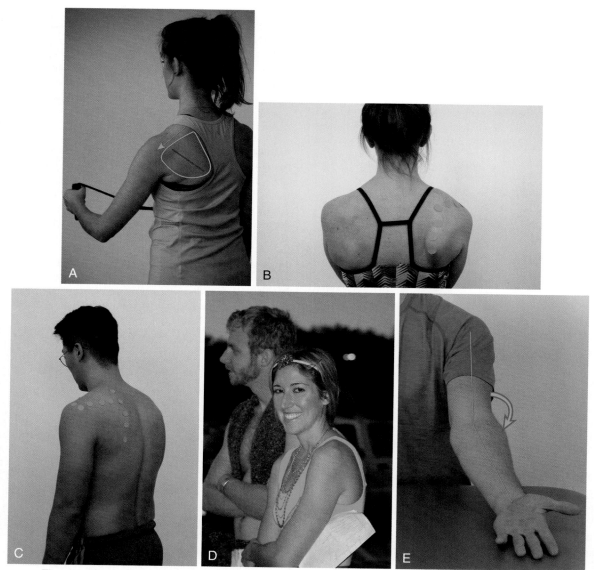

Fig. 4.4 (A) Scapular downward rotation. Scapular downward rotation occurs when the inferior angle is closer to the midline and the glenoid faces downward due to the placement of the scapula on the thoracic wall. The anterior and inferior position of the glenohumeral joint places the superior rotator cuff in a lengthened position and increases the force requirements for the rotator cuff to approximate the head of the humerus. (B) Scapular winging. Scapular winging occurs when the scapula is not approximated to or flush with the thoracic wall, the thoracic wall, often due to serratus anterior weakness or neuromuscular deficits. Scapular winging is more common with a flat thoracic spine due to the limited biomechanical advantage. (C) Scapular tipping. Scapular tipping is present when the inferior angle of the scapula separates from the rib cage or if the scapula moves superiorly to tilt the scapula forward. Tipping can be due to thoracic kyphosis, a forward head position, decreased muscle flexibility (pectoralis minor, major, upper trapezius, scalenes), or habitual stooped posture. (D) Forward shoulders. The patient's natural laxity and forward shoulder position is visible with the head of the humerus in anterior position relative to the acromion. (E) Upper extremity natural valgus angle. The natural valgus angle in the upper extremity is usually between 10 and 15 degrees. This patient's valgus angle is 19 degrees, requiring adjustment of the hand position relative to the body during closed or open chain exercise to place the arm in the natural alignment.

Bony alignment of the upper extremity (especially the natural valgus angle; see Fig. 4.4) is an important consideration for the arm position during exercise, particularly for repetitive strain injuries including lateral epicondylitis, impingement syndromes, and wrist and hand tendinopathy (Clinical Example 4.5). Some postural positions can be reversible and will be included in exercise goals, while others may need to be accepted. If the alignment cannot be adjusted easily, the exercise position and props such as pads, bolsters, balls, or pillows should be chosen to accommodate to the individual's posture (see Clinical Example 4.4).

Movement Observation and Analysis

Shoulder elevation (Fig. 4.5) includes a complex synchrony of scapular, glenohumeral, and thoracic spine motion (Videos 4.7–4.11), including:

- Scapula upward rotation (accounts for approximately one-third of total elevation; see Fig. 4.5);

- Glenohumeral flexion or abduction, depending on the plane of the movement (accounts for approximately two-thirds of total elevation; see Fig. 4.5);
- Thoracic extension or lateral flexion at the end range completes full upper extremity elevation.
- When the glenohumeral joint reaches approximately 70 degrees, glenohumeral external rotation allows the head of the humerus to clear the acromion and minimize the compression of the subacromial structures (Fig. 4.6; Video 4.10).

Impingement of the subacromial structures occurs when the space between the head of the humerus and the acromion is

---

✒ CLINICAL EXAMPLE 4.5 Bony Alignment Implications of Valgus Angle and Movement Analysis for Upper Extremity Exercise

Patient A

Patient A has pain in the forearm and lateral aspect of the elbow that developed after working with a power drill on a home project over 2 days. He has pain with active wrist and finger extension as well as resisted wrist extension. Symptoms are worse with full stretch of the wrist extensor bulk, with combined wrist flexion and pronation. He is complaining of pain with gripping and holding objects. His valgus angle is 20 degrees.

Evaluation

His valgus angle is a possible contributing factor to development of excessive stress at the extensor origin on the lateral epicondyle: normal valgus angles for males is around 10 degrees.[1,2]

Implications for Examination and Exercise Position

The overall upper extremity alignment needs to be considered during examination, exercise, and advice for functional movements. Resisted wrist, finger, and forearm motion are tested in the natural valgus alignment. As the patient improves, closed chain exercises such as push-ups or bilateral loaded exercise, need to accommodate the patient's natural position.

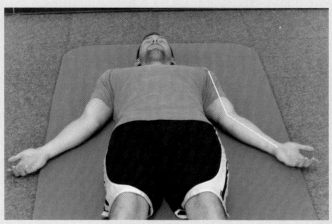

Valgus carrying angle.

Note his large carrying angle (20 degrees; *yellow lines*) and the position of his hands with respect to his body and the mat.

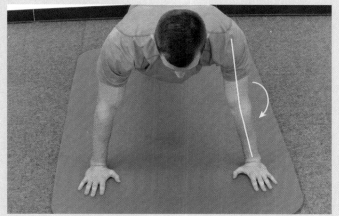

Push-up position without considering the valgus angle.

If he places his hands directly under his shoulders, the extensors are angled across the pronated forearm position (*arrow*). The shoulder is also internally rotated in this position. Even without performing a push-up there is discomfort in the lateral elbow region.

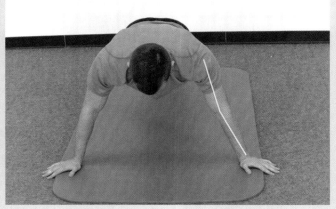

Push-up position adjusted for valgus angle.

A wider scaption position is similar to the open chain carrying angle alignment. The shoulder is also placed in neutral rotation to decrease the angulation of the muscles crossing the elbow. Changing the position relieved the discomfort. The dynamic alignment and pain responses would also be used to determine if push-ups or planks are preferred for closed chain proximal strengthening.

continued

📌 CLINICAL EXAMPLE 4.5   Bony Alignment Implications of Valgus Angle and Movement Analysis for Upper Extremity Exercise—cont'd

Patient B

Patient B is a competitive weight-lifter and has shoulder impingement symptoms. Adjustment of his weight-lifting techniques may assist with distributing forces and preventing recurrence of the repetitive strain injury.

Implications for Exercise Position

His natural valgus angle and shoulder width are considered when making recommendations for push-ups, bench press, triceps press, and biceps curls.

Adjusting the placement of the hands to a wider hand position to accommodate the natural bony angle decreases internal rotation of the shoulder and limits the amount of compressive stresses in the subacromial region. The scaption position also helps with optimal scapulothoracic and shoulder alignment. The pressure of the bar is toward the outside of the hand rather than holding the bar with the thumbs underneath the bar, which encourages shoulder internal rotation.

References

1. Neumann DA. *Kinesiology of the Musculoskeletal System: Foundations for Rehabilitation.* 2nd ed. St. Louis, MO: Mosby Elsevier; 2010.
2. Magee DJ. *Orthopedic Physical Assessment.* 6th ed. St. Louis, MO: Elsevier Saunders; 2014.

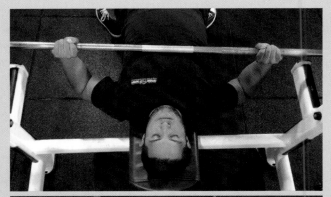
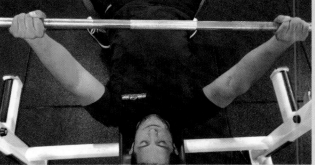

Hand position placed wide on the bar and adjusted to the natural valgus angle to prevent shoulder internal rotation and impingement stress during bench press. (Courtesy of Jonathan Castro and Brandon Wilson.)

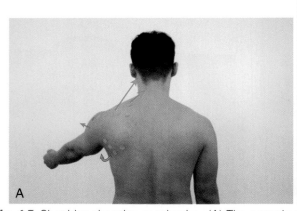
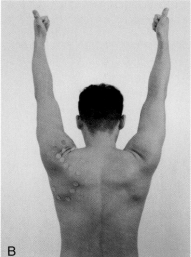

Fig. 4.5 Shoulder elevation mechanics. (A) The scapula rotates upward, with the trapezius and levator scapula acting on the spine of the scapula and superior angle of the scapula, respectively. The serratus anterior assists the upward rotation force couple with the medial border of the scapula sliding anteriorly on the rib cage toward the insertions on the first eight ribs. The motion of the scapula provides a moving base for the rotator cuff muscles that are linking the humerus to the scapula and approximating the glenohumeral joint, while the deltoid and supraspinatus also providing an upward abduction moment. (B) Full elevation into flexion. The fully elevated position requires full scapular upward rotation, full glenohumeral motion (flexion or abduction), and some thoracic motion at the end of range.

narrowed, compressing the soft tissue structures (Fig. 4.7). The supraspinatus tendon, biceps tendon, and the subacromial bursa are all potential sources of pain with the pressure or diminished circulation in the impingement positions during shoulder elevation, particularly if there is irritation, edema, or fraying of the tendons. The typical impingement range for the supraspinatus tendon is approximately 70–120 degrees of abduction or at end range flexion for the biceps tendon, and therefore it is important to watch for compensations in these ranges.[1,2] Abnormal or unconscious compensatory movements to avoid painful ranges

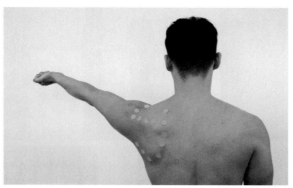

Fig. 4.6 Clearance of the acromial arch: external rotation. If the shoulder is externally rotated during the upward motion, the tuberosity clears the acromial arch. Note the relationship of the head of the humerus (pink dots) to the acromion and spine of the scapula. The glenoid is pointing forward and upward, supported by the muscle activity supported on the base provided by the scapula. The active support from the scapula position can be compared to struts supporting a shelf from underneath the shoulder, while the upward moment is provided by the superior muscle actions resisting the weight of the arm.

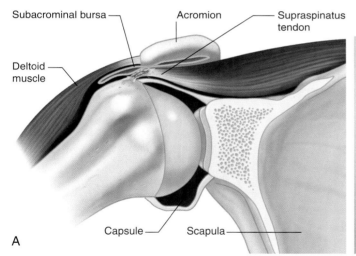

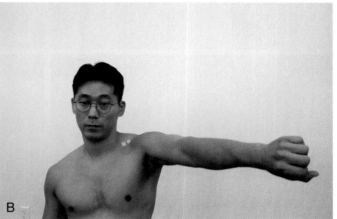

A   B

Fig. 4.7 Mechanics causing impingement. (A) Internal rotation in higher ranges of elevation. The internally rotated position places the greater tuberosity under the acromion, decreasing the subacromial space and compressing the supraspinatus tendon, subacromial bursa, and, in flexion, the bicipital tendon (at higher ranges). The "empty can" position may be a potential causative factor for impingement, and, require adjustment of the rotation during elevation and early movement reeducation strategy. All patients who have shoulder dysfunction should be assessed for impingement symptoms as impingement may be present with hypomobility or hypermobility, and any movement compensations can cause primary or secondary impingement. As a precaution, shoulder elevation exercises should be performed with early external rotation. Individuals who need internal rotation in elevated positions (throwing athletes, swimmers, laborers) may need maximal mobility of other structures to prevent early impingement or dynamic stability and coordination of the glenohumeral and scapulohumeral muscles. (B) Structural shape and subacromial impingement. The subacromial structures are compressed under the acromion as the head of the humerus migrates superiorly during elevation. The position of the supraspinatus tendon and subacromial bursa is further compromised if the shoulder is elevated while in internal rotation as the greater tuberosity is placed under the acromion. If the subacromial space is narrowed due to osteophytes under the acromion resulting from repeated stress, or when the acromion has a "hook" or "beak" shape, there is a greater likelihood of irritation and compression of the soft tissue structures passing under the acromion.

Continued

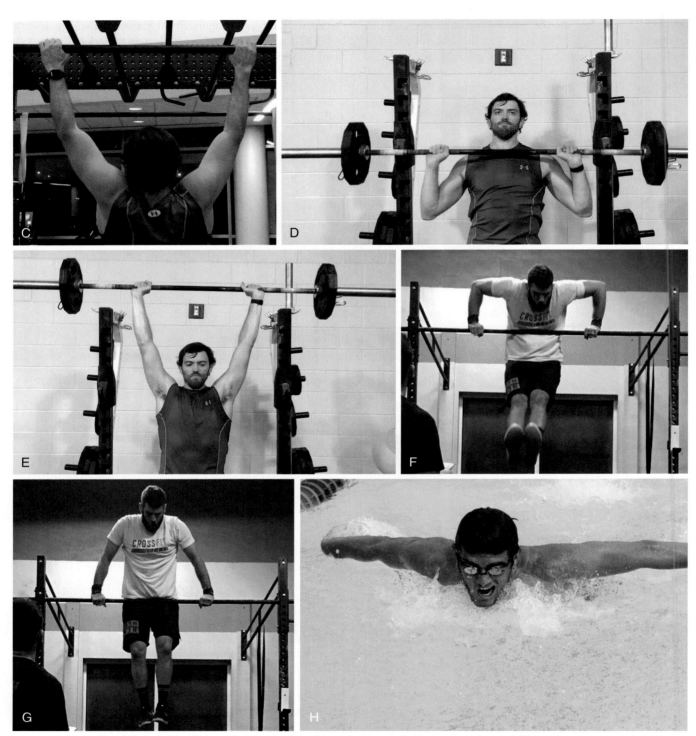

Fig. 4.7, cont'd. (C) Load in elevated positions (pull-ups). Pull-ups also place additional forces on the subacromial structures, especially during the eccentric phase. This position also places the greater tuberosity under the acromion, increasing the compressive forces on the biceps tendon and the supraspinatus tendon. (D and E) Overhead press places high compressive loads on the shoulder. (F and G) Bodyweight resistance and the dip position places the glenohumeral joint in internal rotation with superiorly directed forces. (H) Butterfly stroke involves prolonged internal rotation through the stroke cycle, increasing the risk of impingement. ([C-E] Courtesy of Brandon Wilson and Jonathan Castro; [F-H] courtesy of Carlos Gonzalez.)

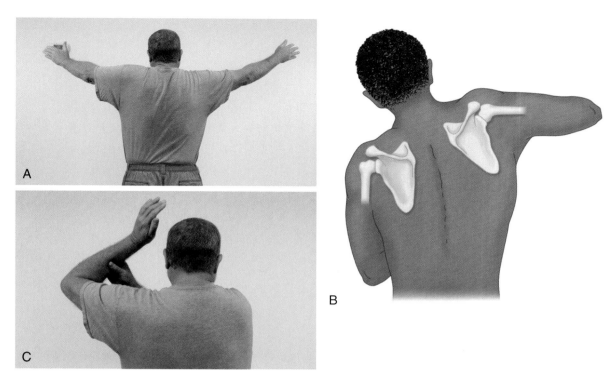

Fig. 4.8 Abnormal shoulder movement patterns (compensations for loss of mobility or neuromuscular function). (A) Early shoulder elevation (hiking). The patient is elevating his shoulder girdle early and excessively after a rotator cuff tear. (B) Trunk lateral flexion, extension, or rotation. Trunk lateral flexion is often used to compensate for lack of shoulder motion. Trunk extension is a common compensation for difficulty with flexion, and trunk rotation can be used to compensate for lack of shoulder rotation. (C) Using the opposite arm to assist the movement. The patient is unable to lift his arm and externally rotate the shoulder to place the hand behind his head due to a rotator cuff tear and uses the right arm to assist the motion.

or to accommodate for limited mobility include early scapular elevation, excessive or late scapular upward rotation (Videos 4.7 and 4.8), or trunk motion (Fig. 4.8; Video 4.9). Late external rotation of the glenohumeral joint during elevation or sustained movements with the shoulder in internal rotation is often associated with impingement (Video 4.7). Early scapular elevation, winging, or tipping will affect the timing or position of the scapula and result in increased stress on the rotator cuff during elevation[7] (see Fig. 4.8; Videos 4.7 and 4.8). The cervicothoracic position will also influence scapulothoracic relationships and relative muscle angulation (Fig. 4.9 and Clinical Example 4.4). The forearm, wrist, and hand are also influenced by excessive angulation or rotation related to bony alignment or movement patterns. The upper extremity lever arm connection to the trunk is part of functional movement analysis for these areas and should also include observing the entire upper extremity lever arm and its connection to the trunk (Clinical Examples 4.5 and 4.6).

There are simple biomechanical modifications that can help minimize shoulder impingement during elevation. During shoulder flexion or abduction into elevation, external rotation limits the amount of compression of subacromial structures (Fig. 4.10 and Clinical Example 4.7; Video 4.10). The scaption plane (between frontal and sagittal plane) places both the scapula on the rib cage and the muscles attaching to the scapula in favorable resting lengths and optimal position for form closure, while active upper-quarter spinal posture or positioning can assist with the scapulothoracic relationship during shoulder elevation (see Fig. 4.10 and Clinical Example 4.7; Video 4.11).

The functional movement analysis will also include active range of motion using isolated specific movements, physical performance measures, or simply observation of the patient performing the task (see Clinical Examples 4.6 and 4.7). Physical performance measures will be discussed at the end of this chapter and in Chapter 8.

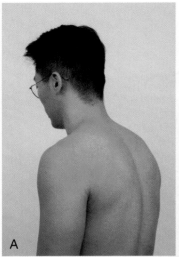
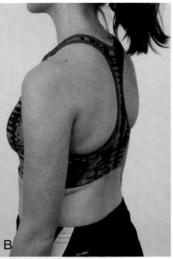
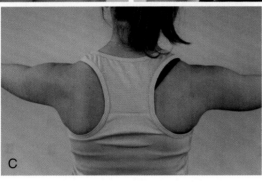

Fig. 4.9 Influence of thoracic and cervical position on relative scapula position and motion. (A) Forward head and thoracic kyphosis. A kyphotic position places the scapula in a tipped position, with additional pull from a forward head position transferred from the upper trapezius, levator scapula, and scalenes. (B) Flat thoracic spine. (C) Flat thoracic spine contributing to winging. The scapula position relative to the ribs places the serratus anterior and posterior scapula stabilizers at a mechanical disadvantage, often leading to winging or increased stress on the rotator cuff.

CLINICAL EXAMPLE 4.6   Functional Movement Analysis for Upper Extremity Diagnoses

Patient A

Patient A has adhesive capsulitis[1] with difficulty dressing and pain with shoulder movement and sleeping. Her present pain level is 4/10, but the pain goes up to 6/10 sleeping and at times wakes her up. She is an artist and is having difficulty working for more than 30 minutes on a painting. Her Quick DASH score is 45.[2]

- *Dressing:* The patient puts the affected arm into the jacket sleeve first with the jacket in front of her body. She is wearing button-up shirts and is unable to lift her arm to put on sweaters or t-shirts, but she is able to pull on loose t-shirts using her left arm.
- *Painting:* She is currently using a high stool or standing in order to paint. She also reports using smaller canvases as she is unable to use her right hand for large paintings. She is right-hand dominant but has started to use her left hand for broad brush strokes. When demonstrating how she is painting, she lifts her right arm using scapula elevation (hiking) and early upward rotation, rotates her trunk toward the direction of the movement, and uses her left hand to help her right hand. She has also rigged up a small table to support the arm.

Patient B

Patient B has been diagnosed with de Quervain tenosynovitis of the thumb extensors and abductors. She is 47 years old and works as a hotel cleaner. The pain in the hand and thumb started slowly, with progressive difficulty with her work activities: making beds, lifting her cleaning equipment, spraying cleaning fluids, wringing out cleaning cloths, washing floors, or cleaning mirrors. Her current pain level is 3/10, but the pain increases to 6/10 by the end of a shift. Her Quick DASH score is 45.[2]

- *Lifting:* Holding a bucket or lifting furniture increases pain.
- *Dressing:* She has difficulty undoing buttons with her right hand as well as closing zippers.
- *Grip activities:* Gripping the vacuum cleaner increases pain, and she uses her hand and forearm more than her legs and body. She has difficulty with

power grip (hook, fist, and cylindrical), three-fingered and lateral pinch grip, and sustained grip with objects of all sizes with pain using the thumb. She is unable to perform repeated movements.

- *Making beds:* Difficulty lifting the mattress, folding sheets, and pulling sheets
- *Cleaning:* She is right-handed and uses her right hand and wrist for washing surfaces. She has tried switching hands but discontinued using this strategy as her supervisor and peers have complained that she is taking too much time. Gripping the vacuum cleaner increases her pain to 4–5/10, while holding a bucket increases pain to 6/10.

Comparison of Patients A and B

Patient A is seeking help to obtain more range due to her limited mobility and pain, while Patient B has problems with specific repetitive movements that have contributed to overuse. In both, identifying movement compensations helps anticipate corrections needed for exercise. In both cases, exercises should match or mirror functional requirements in Phases II and III. In Phase I, functional movement reeducation is used to distribute forces and avoid pain exacerbation by limiting range for Patient A, while both patients are likely to benefit from strategies to accommodate for the painful regions. In late Phase II and Phase III, the emphasis changes to slow reintroduction of range (Patient A) and load (Patient B) prior to combining both range and load (Patient A) and load and repetition (Patient B). Distributing forces using proximal stabilization and efficient movement along, with preventing angulation and tension concentrated on the hand and thumb will be important for Patient B.

References

1. Kelley MJ, Shaffer MA, Kuhn JE, et al. Shoulder pain and mobility deficits: adhesive capsulitis. *J Orthop Sports Phys Ther.* 2013;43(5):A2–A32.
2. Mintken PE, Glynn P, Cleland JA. Psychometric properties of the shortened disabilities of the Arm, Shoulder, and Hand Questionnaire (QuickDASH) and Numeric Pain Rating Scale in patients with shoulder pain. *J Shoulder Elbow Surg.* 2009;18:920–926.

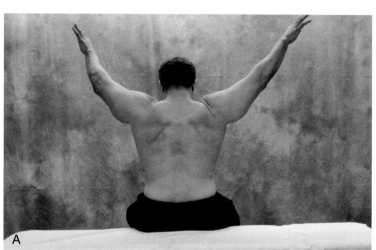
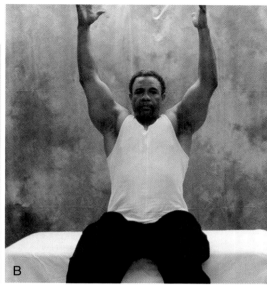

Fig. 4.10 Active range of motion with different planes and combinations: assessment for impingement. (A) Shoulder elevation. Assessing whether the patient externally rotates the shoulder to clear the greater tuberosity before the humeral head impacts the acromion, in both flexion and abduction, and identifying painful ranges helps with cueing and correction of the mechanics during exercise. The spinal posture during elevation and scapula mechanics is also important to selecting appropriate exercise positions and ranges of motion to assist with optimal mechanics. In this figure, the patient lifts his left arm without externally rotating the shoulder and reports pain at the end of the range. (B) Shoulder elevation with instructions to rotate the shoulder early. When the patient externally rotates his shoulder he is able to elevate the arm slightly further and with less pain.

CLINICAL EXAMPLE 4.7   Biomechanical Evaluation Related to Shoulder Impingement

Movement analysis is useful to assess if adjustment of movement patterns decreases impingement symptoms, particularly if the patient is continuing with his or her hobbies or activities.

The patient is an avid weight-lifter and participates in vigorous intensive work-outs. He reports pain consistent with shoulder impingement symptoms in a painful arc from 90 to 120 degrees of abduction and 100 to 135 degrees of flexion. He has minimal pain at rest, and the impingement symptoms only increase with heavy weight or intense exercise.

- *Overhead press, pull-ups, and dips against bodyweight*: The patient has been unable to perform these aggressive activities with high weight or at end range for the past 4 weeks due to pain in the extreme positions.
- *Dumbbell lateral raises*: The patient abducts the arms with the elbows straight and holding the dumbbells to the side of the body in the frontal plane. The hand position is facing toward the floor, resulting in shoulder internal rotation. The patient can perform 18 repetitions with 30 lb but his pain is reproduced on the right side.
- *Latissimus dorsi pull-downs*: The patient is holding the latissimus dorsi pull-down bar at the maximum shoulder flexion at the starting point. He pulls the bar behind the head but is unable to control the movement on the eccentric return. The behind the head action results in scapular tipping and full retraction.

The patient's work-out routine will need to be adjusted and the bar behind the neck position changed to in front of the body while he still has pain. Latissimus dorsi exercises in scaption using an angled bar can be used to limit upward compressive forces in the subacromial region. Restricting the range to below impingement symptoms, placing pressure on the outside of the palm to encourage shoulder external rotation, and proximal spinal and scapulothoracic control are preferred.

Implications for Adjustment of Weight-Lifting Program

The use of early shoulder external rotation (thumbs up toward the ceiling), choosing the scaption plane in the early phases of rehabilitation, and encouraging proximal cervicothoracic support is likely to assist with minimizing shoulder impingement biomechanics. The scapulothoracic connection and upward rotation through elevation assist the patient with optimal glenohumeral positioning and support.

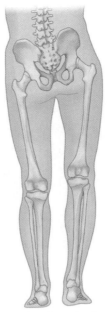

Fig. 4.11 Leg length discrepancy. A true leg length discrepancy with different femur or tibia length will result in differences in pelvic height and rotation

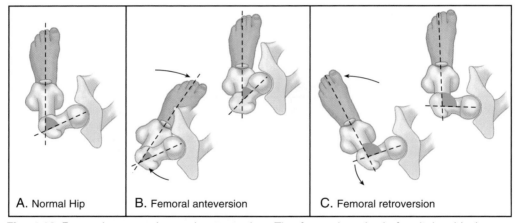

A. Normal Hip   B. Femoral anteversion   C. Femoral retroversion

Fig. 4.12 Femoral anteversion and retroversion. The femoral neck–shaft relationship impacts the "toe-in" or "toe-out" position in closed chain positions. The position of the leg is adjusted to place the femoral head within the acetabulum to create a more stable and congruent joint (A). The bony alignment cannot be adjusted and thus influences the alignment, angulation, and efficiency of muscular structures. Asking patients with femoral anteversion (B) or retroversion (C) to place the feet in the sagittal plane is likely to increase tension and angulation of soft tissue and impact the mechanics of the hip, knee, patellofemoral, and foot structures.

Lower Extremity

Alignment Observation

In the lower extremity, both the static bony alignment and dynamic muscle control are responsible for maintaining an upright lever system and the three-dimensional forces during double- and single-leg stance, gait, and other functional movements. The bony alignment influences the angulation of muscle attachments and creates a more or less efficient position for the muscles to oppose gravity and create movement in the necessary planes of motion. Static alignment is analyzed and considered during the dynamic movement. Leg length discrepancies (Fig. 4.11), genu valgus or varus (see Fig 2.35), femoral anteversion or retroversion (toeing in or out (Fig. 4.12), hyperextended knees (Fig. 4.13), excessive tibial external rotation or varus (Fig. 4.14), and altered foot position (excessive pronation or supination) (Fig. 4.15) are all examples of alignments observed during static postural analysis that might impact dynamic movement or require adjustment of exercise.

While bony alignment cannot be altered, it is possible to establish starting positions and movement planes that will place muscle–tendon complexes and joint structures in the optimal position for the patient, often the midrange of the bony alignment. Subtle changes in alignment can sometimes minimize the forces that exacerbate repetitive strain disorders[6,7] (Clinical Example 4.8). Impaired soft tissue mobility, muscle length restrictions, and compensations for inadequate dynamic muscle support can magnify the effect of extreme structural malalignment, and the distinction between contributions from bony alignment versus impairments influencing the position is an important part of the initial evaluation (Clinical Example 4.9). The static observations will be combined with those from dynamic and functional movement to identify compensations, which are important for teaching the exercises and providing feedback.

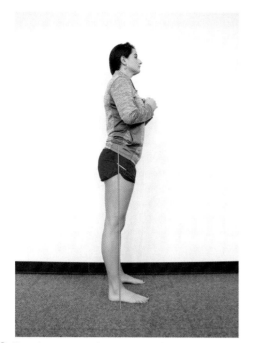

Fig. 4.13 Knee hyperextension. Hyperextending the knees in standing can result in compensatory lumbar lordosis to place the center of mass over the base. Note that the center of the knee joint falls behind the line of gravity. The posterior muscles and connective tissue are lengthened in standing when the knee is hyperextended, relying on passive constraints rather than active control. In upright standing exercises, the patient is asked to control the knee position actively rather than "hanging" on the back of the knee if a more active lower extremity position is desired to reduce stress in the lumbar spine.

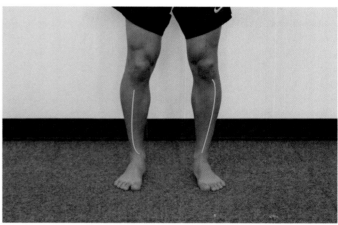

Fig. 4.14 Excessive tibial external rotation or curvature (tibial varus).

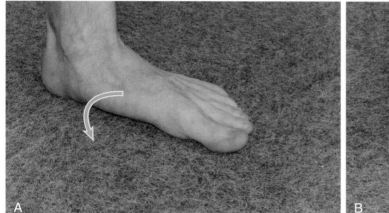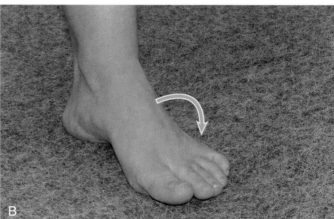

Fig. 4.15 (A) Excessive pronation. (B) Supination.

⚡ CLINICAL EXAMPLE 4.8   Bony Alignment and Dynamic Movement Implications for Starting Positions and Movement Correction

While bony alignment cannot be altered, it is possible to establish starting positions and movement planes that will place muscle–tendon complexes and joint structures in the optimal position for the patient. Subtle changes in alignment can sometimes minimize the forces that exacerbate repetitive strain disorders.

The patient is a professional Indian dance performer who has left lateral patellofemoral syndrome and patella tendinopathy. She has been unable to dance for the past 4 months. Her static bony alignment is significant for bilateral genu valgum, femoral anteversion, and tibial external torsion. She has bilateral enlarged fat pads, and the patellar tendon is painful on palpation. There is limited medial glide with tilt of the left patella and restricted mobility of the lateral iliotibial band and retinaculum. Her anteversion angle is 19 degrees (Craig's test),[1,2] and her patellofemoral angle (Q angle)[2] is 22 degrees.

Evaluation

Her bony alignment (increased anteversion, valgus, and Q angle) is contributing to the angulation of the patella tendon, and starting positions in closed chain positions will need to be adjusted to place the lower extremity in a position that minimizes angulation of the patellofemoral complex.

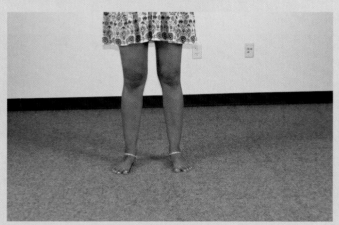

Genu valgum and tibial torsion contributing to left patella tendinopathy and lateral patellofemoral syndrome.

The patient's genu valgum and large patellar tendon angle is contributing to increased forces on a small area of the patellofemoral joint.[3] The angulation of the tendon and the fat pad enlargement are also probable pain-provoking structures.

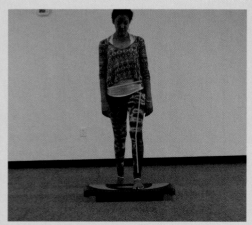

Step-up prior to adjustment of biomechanics. (Video 4.12)

The amount of force placed on the patellofemoral joint during stair-climbing is higher than walking, even with small amounts of knee flexion.[4] The tendency when stepping up a step is to place the foot perpendicular to the step. The patient places her foot toward the midline and facing straight forward, producing relative hip adduction and internal rotation, increasing the patellar tendon angulation even more than when the leg is in her natural alignment. The hip abductors and external rotators are at a relative biomechanical disadvantage to stabilize the femoro-pelvic relationship, and the rotation and angulation forces at the patellofemoral joint are increased.

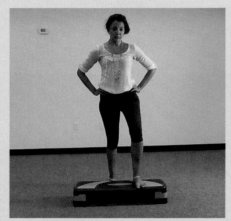

Step-up with adjustment of biomechanics (Videos 4.13 and 4.14).

The patient is asked to widen the distance between the feet to match her pelvic width (Video 4.14; see Fig. 4.7A). The natural rotation of the femur and tibia is maintained with slight external rotation in the forward step-up position (Videos 4.13 and 4.14). By allowing a neutral bony alignment, the pelvis position is more horizontal and the hip stabilizers are in mid-position to provide rotational and frontal plane control. The patellar tendon angulation is also closer to her alignment when the foot is free to move. The exercise program will need to include hip muscle activation, endurance, and strength along with neuromuscular coordination to be able to reproduce the adjusted dynamic alignment.

References

1. Magee DJ, Sueki D. *Orthopedic Physical Assessment Atlas and Video: Selected Special Tests*. St. Louis, MO: Elsevier Saunders; 2011.
2. Gelberman RH, Cohen MS, Desai SS, et al. Femoral anteversion: a clinical assessment of idiopathic in-toeing gait in children. *J Bone Joint Surg Br*. 1987;69:75–79.
3. Farrokhi S, Keyak JH, Powers CM. Individuals with patellofemoral pain exhibit greater patellofemoral joint stress: a finite element analysis study. *Osteoarthritis Cartilage*. 2011;19:287–294.
4. Goudakos IG, Konig C, Schottle PG, et al. Stair climbing results in more challenging patellofemoral contact mechanics and kinematics than walking at early knee flexion under physiologic-like quadriceps loading. *J Biomech*. 2009;42:2590–2596.

CLINICAL EXAMPLE 4.9   Dynamic Movement Abnormalities Related to Repetitive Strain Injury

The patient from Clinical Example 4.8 has a history of patellofemoral pain in the left leg. Early treatment addressed some of the soft tissue restrictions in the lateral patella region, iliotibial band, and gluteal muscles. She has enlarged fat pads and squats are painful beyond 60 degrees. A bilateral squat test is performed in neutral bony alignment and in external rotation (required for her dance positions). She is able to manage 12 repetitions in midrange, but there is pain at when straightening in the terminal range. She loses her pelvis alignment prior to the pain increasing.

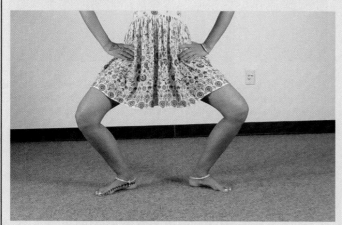

Double squat in external rotation.

Indian dance requires intricate trunk isolation and these movements are included in the movement observation by asking her to maintain a bilateral squat position in a pain-free position while performing trunk motion to challenge the alignment. This information is used to assist with exercise specificity and in evaluating the neuromuscular coordination and compensatory patterns.

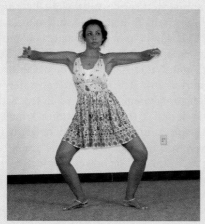

Indian dance postures and isolated movements.

The lateral trunk motion to the right challenges the stabilization of the pelvis and lower extremity relationship on the left. Note that the position of the center of mass is moved toward the opposite leg. The same actions are normally required for single-leg stance and with transitions, requiring complex coordination and control for balance and aesthetic requirements. These movements will need to be introduced slowly as part of the exercise program if they are to be specific enough for functional recovery.

At a later point in the rehabilitation she has been consistently performing bilateral isometric squats with trunk isolation as a home program without aggravating symptoms. She is able to maintain the pelvic alignment and equal weight-bearing for up to a minute, so she is asked to add upper extremity movement. Single-leg positions and postures are tested at this point, and the single-leg postures combined with upper extremity and trunk challenges result in a notable hip drop (Trendelenburg).

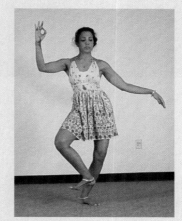

Indian dance postures and movements.

The stamping or lifting action challenges the pelvic stabilization, and the single-leg balance doubles the forces on the affected leg. The trunk isolation away from the right leg also shifts the center of mass away from the left leg, requiring opposing forces from the left hip abductors to maintain balance and weight over the left leg.

Evaluation

The progression from double- to single-leg positions is too difficult and needs to be modified. The lateral trunk motion and arm positions increase the leverage and the challenge to maintain the lower extremity alignment.

Implications for Exercise Choices

The single-leg positions are adjusted to an easier balance exercise with the opposite foot supporting 25% of the weight and only performing arm movements, rather than arm and trunk movement. This progression is included as a home program until the patient is able to control the pelvis position and balance without arm support and then progressed to single-leg balance (in external rotation) holding the opposite leg off the ground, but without arm or trunk challenge.

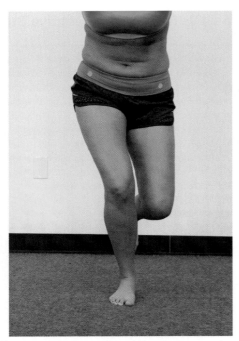

Fig. 4.16 Dynamic valgus. The patient's bony valgus angle is increased during the step-up due to a lack of muscular support from the hip stabilizers (hip abductors and adductors, external rotators). Note that the hip is lateral to the foot, and there is a relative drop of the pelvis to the opposite side (Trendelenburg position). The angulation increases the overall Q-angle and increases loading and angulation on the patellofemoral structures and the tibiofemoral joint.

Movement Observation and Analysis

Basic movement abnormalities and muscle imbalances can be observed during open chain or closed kinetic chain movement (Videos 4.12–4.16).[1,4,6] However, lower extremity closed chain movements mimic functional requirements, while upper extremity movements are often open chain. Dysfunctional movement patterns are often only apparent while observing during these activities (Videos 4.16 and 4.17). There are common movement abnormalities in the lower extremity. **Dynamic valgus** (Fig. 4.16) involves excessive generalized lower extremity medial angulation and femoral and tibial internal rotation and pronation, and can contribute to patellofemoral dysfunction (Video 4.12), knee and hip osteoarthritis (Video 4.17), shin splints, stress fractures, or plantar fasciitis (see Fig. 4.16). **Early, excessive, or prolonged pronation** or supination results in generalized rotational forces throughout

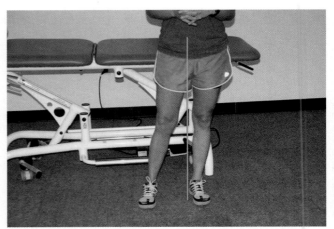

Fig. 4.17 Weight-bearing avoidance or symmetry. The patient is placing 75% of her weight on the left leg, resulting in pelvic rotation to the right. After periods of weight-bearing precautions or pain, patients may be hesitant to assume weight on the affected side or to split the weight 50/50 in bilateral stance. If this is observed in the initial evaluation, exercises using teaching techniques to help the patient self-correct the position will be part of the initial exercise prescription. Feedback using a mirror, tactile feedback using unstable surfaces or elastic resistance, or verbal cueing (see Chapter 7) will be important until the patient is able to correct the position without assistance.

the kinetic chain. **Avoidance of weight-bearing** on one leg or area of the foot (Fig. 4.17) is a common compensation for pain or other impairments, which results in further accumulation of forces on small areas (Videos 4.18 and 4.19). Limited stabilization of the pelvis can manifest as **rotation, hiking (elevation of the pelvis), or Trendelenburg gait** (pelvic drop during stance [Fig. 4.18 and Clinical Example 4.10; Video 4.20]) and can increase angulation and rotational forces assumed by soft tissue and joint structures during weight-bearing. Gait analysis (Video 4.25), stairs (Videos 4.17 and 4.20), squats (Videos 4.18 and 4.21–4.24), sit-to-stand transfers (Videos 3.4, 3.8, and 4.26), single-leg stance (Videos 2.15 and 4.27), and transitional movement (Videos 2.6 and 2.7) are all used to analyze functional movement. If the patient can safely demonstrate sports-specific movements or work-related activities, these can also be included in the examination. Dynamic movement abnormalities or compensations will need to be addressed through exercise tailored to specific muscle activation, endurance, strength, and/or power. Typically neuromuscular coordination patterns need to be altered through movement reeducation approaches as well.

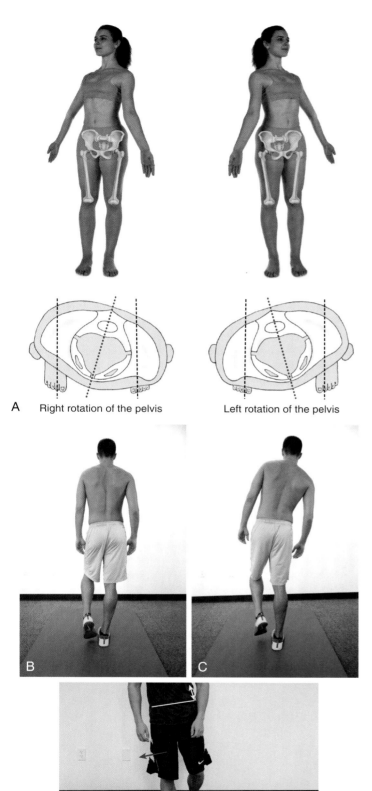

A   Right rotation of the pelvis   Left rotation of the pelvis

Fig. 4.18 (A) Pelvic rotation. Pelvis rotation creates asymmetry in the relative hip rotation in both legs, potentially contributing to other lower extremity problems. This image demonstrates the effect of trunk and pelvis rotation on fixed limbs; however, pelvis rotation can occur in one direction without the upper trunk turning, a common compensation for lumbopelvic and hip joint dysfunction. Unequal weight-bearing and hip rotator weakness will also create pelvic rotation. (From Muscolino JE. *Kinesiology: The Skeletal System and Muscle Function.* 3rd ed. St. Louis, MO: Elsevier; 2017.) (B) Trendelenburg stance. The pelvis is dropped on the left with limited stabilization from the right hip abductors. (C) Lateral trunk lean related to weak hip abductors or pain. Moving the upper trunk to the stance side is common to maintain balance over the stance leg. (D) Hip hike or lean toward the affected side. Hip hiking (lumbar side flexion) on the left and a lean toward the right is used to maintain balance and avoid stress on the lateral ankle ligaments after an ankle sprain.

CLINICAL EXAMPLE 4.10 **Movement Compensations After Femur Fracture**

The patient is 45 years old and sustained intertrochanteric and mid-shaft femur fractures 5 months ago in a motorcross accident. He is walking without crutches and has returned to work. He is self-employed as a tiler and needs to be on his knees for some jobs. He wants to add exercises that can be performed during his work day if possible.

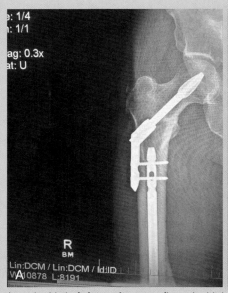
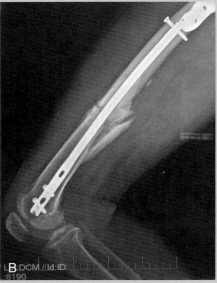

Intertrochanteric and mid-shaft femur fractures fixated with interlocking sliding screw and plate and an intramedullary rod.

As seen in the radiographs, the sliding intertrochanteric screw and plate is interlocked with the intramedullary rod, providing a very stable internal fixation. There are also two screws stabilizing the distal rod. There is extensive callus around the midshaft fracture, and the lateral view shows some displacement of a posterior fragment. The midshaft fracture has not healed completely, while the intertrochanteric fracture has healed well. There is some osteopenia in the greater trochanteric region and distal femur. The patient is able to weight-bear and progressive vertical loading, as well as muscle strengthening, is indicated to promote further bone stimulus. Precautions would include limited angulation and rotation and slow progression of loads.

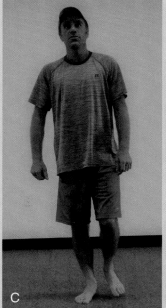
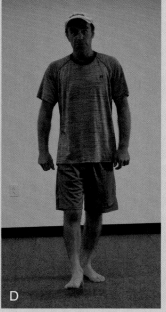

Single leg stance after right femur fractures.

In part C, the single-leg stance on the right side (fractured leg) showing a lateral trunk lean and pelvic hiking on the opposite side to accommodate for weak right hip abductors; part D shows the single-leg stance on the unaffected side.

✎ CLINICAL EXAMPLE 4.10 Movement Compensations After Femur Fracture—cont'd

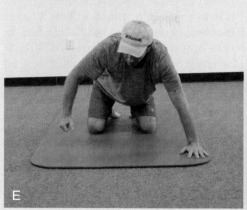 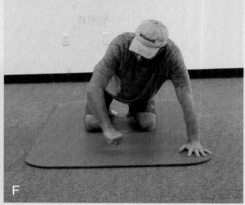

Analysis of positions and movement required for work as a tile layer.

The patient is having the most difficulty with low tasks on his knees (E and F). He is using pads underneath the knee. He is assuming the majority of his weight on the unaffected side. He does take breaks and usually stands up on the unaffected side.

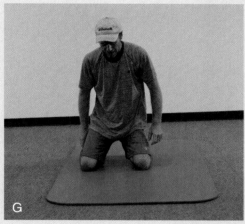

Kneeling.

The same asymmetry is noted in kneeling and when he transitions to tall kneeling (G).

Implications for Further Examination Techniques

The one-leg standing lateral shift position indicates the need to evaluate right hip abductor activation, endurance, and strength. The asymmetry noted in kneeling could be related to hip range of motion deficits, while the kneeling and high kneeling positions may be due to pain, limited muscle flexibility, knee or hip pain, or habit. The impairment results are matched to the relevant functional deficits for goals.

Implications for Exercise and Functional Activities

One-leg standing exercises can be conducted throughout the day. In addition to hip abduction strengthening in side-lying, standing on the right side with the pelvis level and moving the left leg is easy to perform throughout his work day. The transitions from kneeling to tall kneeling and the position for tiling are adjusted to encourage equal weight-bearing on both legs.

Spine

Alignment Observation

The natural curvatures in the spine (cervical lordosis, thoracic kyphosis, lumbar lordosis) result in the tendency for increased concentration of force at the transitional junction between two areas of the spine (change of direction of curvatures at the cervicothoracic, thoracolumbar, or lumbosacral junctions), which may result in relative hypermobility or instability (Fig. 4.19). Excessive curvatures (increased cervical or lumbar lordosis, thoracic kyphosis; Fig. 4.20) or reduced curvatures may result in hypomobility due to connective tissue changes or joint compression (Videos 4.28 and 4.29). Frontal plane or rotational asymmetries found in structural scoliosis or as a result of a leg-length discrepancy need to be considered when choosing starting positions for exercise and attempts to distribute forces to minimize excessive forces on joint and soft tissue. Scoliosis impacts both upper extremity and scapular alignment as well as lower extremity alignment (Fig. 4.20D and Clinical Example 4.11).

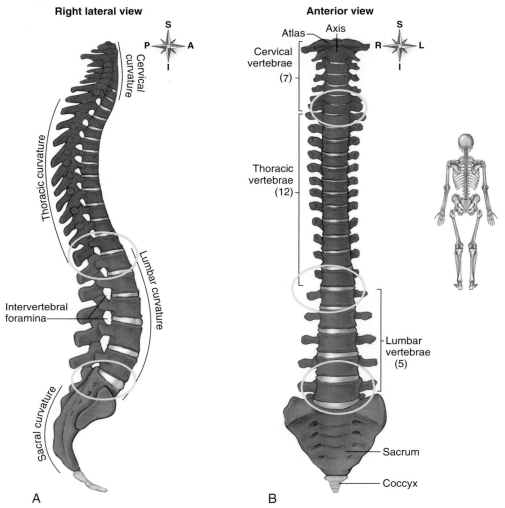

Right lateral view

Cervical curvature
Thoracic curvature
Intervertebral foramina
Lumbar curvature
Sacral curvature

S
P — A
I

Anterior view

Atlas — Axis
Cervical vertebrae (7)
Thoracic vertebrae (12)
Lumbar vertebrae (5)
Sacrum
Coccyx

S
R — L
I

A   B

Fig. 4.19 Change of direction of spinal curvatures. The junctions between curvatures (lumbosacral, thoracolumbar, cervicothoracic) are often exposed to higher translation and rotation forces. Exaggerated curvatures visible from the lateral view (A) include thoracic kyphosis, increased cervical or lumbar lordosis, and scoliosis from the anterior or posterior view (B). These areas may be vulnerable to breakdown or instability over time. Observation of the areas that move first and relatively more than other segments can be helpful to assess the axis of motion for exercise and functional movement. (From Patton K, Thibodeau G, Douglas M. *Essentials of Anatomy and Physiology.* St. Louis, MO: Mosby; 2012.)

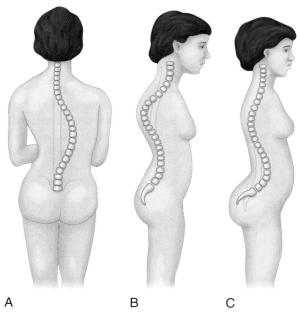

Fig. 4.20 Excessive spinal curvatures. (A) Scoliosis. (B) Kyphosis. (C) Lumbar lordosis.

⚖ CLINICAL EXAMPLE 4.11 Spinal Alignment: Scoliosis and Leg-Length Discrepancy

Scoliosis will impact exercise for all regions. Some scoliotic curves can be corrected with active muscle control, but most curvatures are established after growth has stopped. Nevertheless, active force closure can help with distribution of forces and limit accumulation of stress on those areas where the curves change. The asymmetry also influences the position of the scapula, and downward rotation, tipping, and winging differs from side to side. Spinal scoliosis also influences the pelvis alignment and muscle angles in the lower extremity.

Patient A

Patient A has a left lumbar convexity and right thoracic convexity with left scapular tipping and right scapular winging. Her center of mass is located toward the left leg, and the pelvis is rotated slightly.

connection using different strategies for each side. The asymmetry increases the complexity of exercise delivery when the therapist is choosing cues and adjusting exercise technique.

Patient B

Patient B has a 2-cm leg length discrepancy with the right leg shorter than the left and a greater valgus angle on the left. The downward rotation of her right scapula is greater in standing than in sitting, and the slope of her shoulders becomes more symmetrical. She is being evaluated for neck and shoulder pain.

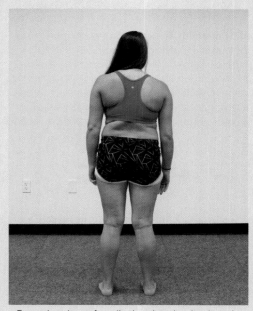

Posterior view of scoliosis related to leg length.

Posterior view of scoliosis.

Implications for Exercise Choices

Although she can work toward active support of the spine in all exercises, it is unrealistic to expect symmetry. She may have to adjust her scapulothoracic

Implications for Evaluation and Exercise Choices

Shoulder, thoracic, and cervical mobility assessment should be conducted in sitting, and sitting and supported positions would be preferred for shoulder and spinal exercise chosen to improve proximal muscle stabilization or mobility.

Movement Observation and Analysis

The large number of spinal segments allows motion to occur in some areas in response to limited motion in others (Videos 4.28–4.31). Spinal movement analysis can include observing for symmetry of motion (Videos 4.28–4.31), deviations toward one side or the other (Video 4.29), and early or excessive motion in one area, particularly at the transition between two areas of spine (movement axis) (Video 4.28; see Fig. 4.20; Clinical Example 4.12).[6,7] Repeated spinal motion testing in a particular direction can be used to assess whether pain centralizes toward the spine or is reduced, indicating that patients are likely to respond to mobility exercise in the identified direction.[8] Movement compensations or deviations can inform cueing or guidance of directions of motion during exercise (see Clinical Examples 4.12 and 4.13). Guarding, or hesitant movement, will also provide information about fear of movement or avoidance behaviors, especially in the absence of recent injury.

🔖 CLINICAL EXAMPLE 4.12   Dynamic Movement Analysis for the Spine

Neuromuscular Coordination Deficits (Lumbar Spine)

Patients with acute, subacute, or chronic low back pain with movement coordination impairments in the activation patterns and support for one or more spinal segments may present with alterations in the timing of movement, relatively more motion in specific areas, compensatory movements, or asymmetry. These patients will exhibit aberrant movement in one or more directions and often compensate to obtain the desired functional movement.[1]

Patient A

Patient A has generalized lumbar spine pain and full range of motion. On returning from full flexion, the patient uses her hands to "walk up her legs" to return to vertical, tucking her pelvis under her body and keeping her knees bent until the last few degrees of movement. If she extends without the use of the hands, the pain increases and there is increased extension through the lumbar spine. Her home exercise routine includes sit-ups. On observation, she is using the rectus abdominis and hip flexors to create lumbar flexion without transversus abdominis activation. She is also pulling her upper body up using her arms. There is also early and excessive extension and lumbar rotation with single-leg lifts in four-point kneeling.

Implications for Exercise Choices

The primary exercise focus will be teaching the patient how to activate the spinal stabilizers to protect and support the lumbar spine prior to limb motion or overall spinal movement, with an emphasis on timing, endurance, and coordination during more complex motion (Chapter 11, Section 2: Hypermobility).

Repeated Movement Testing: Centralization

For patients with acute low back pain and referred lower extremity pain or acute, subacute, or chronic low back pain with radiating pain testing with repeated movement is indicated if there is low irritability and no neurological symptoms (sensory loss or weakness). In order to be appropriate for repeated movement, the referred pain should centralize, with peripheral pain diminishing. Pain is usually increased with flexion, particularly prolonged flexion or sitting, and there may be extension mobility deficits.

Patient B

Patient B reports an acute onset of low back pain with radiating pain down the right leg. The pain is worse with sitting for more than an hour (increases from 2/10 to 4/10), but decreases with movement. Repeated extension in standing increases pain slightly in the lumbar region (3/10), but the radiating pain down the back of the leg decreases from 2/10 to 0/10. There is decreased joint mobility with posterior-anterior glides that reproduce pain in the low lumbar region, as well as decreased mobility in the thoracic spine.

Implications for Exercise Choices

Mobility exercises to the end of extension range are indicated with repeated movement (Exercise 11.10), as well as education on position reversal during work activities. Exercises can be progressed quickly for the thoracic spine to include multiple planes in sitting (Exercise 11.14).

Alignment and Axis of Motion

Patients with acute or subacute low back pain with mobility deficits will have reduced range of motion. Observing the areas of motion and the axis of motion—an area around which movement is centered—can assist with modification of movement to distribute forces. If there are regions where less movement is available, exercise can focus on reaching the end range after manual techniques in this area. If there is relative hypermobility, the goal would be to distribute motion and use multiple segments rather than allowing the forces to be concentrated in the symptomatic area. The figures here illustrate an axis of motion in the upper lumbar region with extension and right rotation, with low lumbar hypomobility and a thoracic kyphosis (Video 4.28).

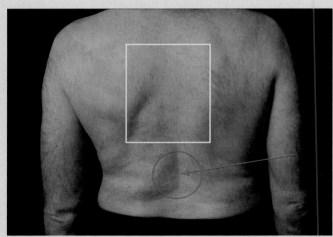

Spinal extension.

Note the axis of motion in the upper lumbar region (*arrow*) for spinal extension with range of motion concentrated in the segments above and below the axis. There is a slight curvature to the left in the lumbar region as the patient extends the spine around the axis (the region where the patient reports pain). There is limited extension in the thoracic spine (*yellow box*).

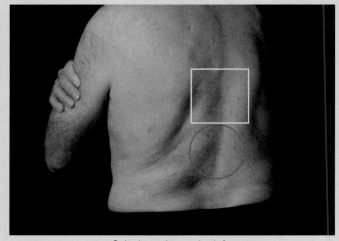

Spinal rotation to the left.

There is decreased left rotation throughout the spine and less motion than right rotation.

CLINICAL EXAMPLE 4.12 Dynamic Movement Analysis for the Spine—cont'd

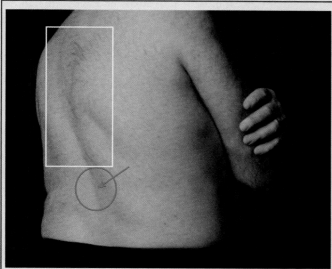

Spinal rotation to the right.

There is limited right thoracic and lumbar rotation with an axis of motion in the upper lumbar region in a similar location to the axis for the extension range of motion. Note the lean and lateral flexion deviation to the left occurring above the axis and limited movement in the low lumbar region.

Implications for Exercise Choices

Exercises to address hypomobility will need to reach end range without excessive movement at the axis. Positioning can help limit the motion to either the thoracic region when promoting thoracic extension maximize joint and soft tissue length or mobility without excessive motion at the upper lumbar axis. Exercises used to distribute forces through progressive neuromuscular coordination will also attempt to minimize early or excessive motion at the axis of motion through stabilization of the lumbothoracic region.

Reference

1. Delitto A, George SZ, van Dillen L, et al. Low back pain. Clinical practice guidelines linked to the International Classification of Functioning, Disability and Health from the Orthopaedic Section of the American Physical Therapy Association. *J Orthop Sports Phys Ther.* 2012;42(4):A1–A57.

CLINICAL EXAMPLE 4.13 Differentiating Between Bony Alignment, Mobility Impairments, and Dynamic Movement Abnormalities

The patient has a history of low back pain and has notable pelvic asymmetry in standing with the right side of the pelvis 2 cm higher than the left. The pelvis is also rotated toward the left. There are a number of possible causes of the pelvic asymmetry, each of which has implications for exercise choice and cueing:

1. Decreased weight-bearing on the left
2. Limited hip extension on the left (hip flexor tightness, limited hip joint motion)
3. Limited knee extension on the left (limited knee joint motion due to swelling, capsular restrictions, or muscle contractures)
4. Leg length discrepancy (right longer than the left)
5. Asymmetrical bony alignment with more varus or valgus on one side
6. Scoliosis

Each of the potential causes can be included or excluded by considering the results of observation of bony alignment in non–weight-bearing positions, range of motion testing, and muscle flexibility testing. There is normal joint mobility and flexibility, no difference in bony alignment or leg length, and no scoliosis (screened in sitting).

Evaluation

Weight-bearing avoidance and compensatory movement become the primary hypothesis. If the patient can correct the position with cueing, the hypothesis is confirmed.

Implications for Exercise Choices

Restoring equal distribution in standing would be an early goal. The use of motor learning concepts (Chapter 7) to teach the patient awareness of pelvic position and 50/50 distribution in bilateral standing will be important for all exercises and guides the stop point when testing exercise dosage. Bilateral exercises in closed chain positions may be progressed from supine positions (with or without equipment) where the patient can monitor the weight distribution (Exercises 9.19 and 9.21) prior to progressing to upright de-loaded squats (Exercise 9.29) and squats with tactile and visual feedback (Exercise 9.30). Weight-shifting side to side can be added to these exercises or in a lunge position (Exercise 9.22); these will be important to provide specificity for neuromuscular coordination pattern training.

SPECIFIC EXERCISE TESTING

The initial testing results in identifying the choice of type of exercise to address impairments and the specific parameters (position, range, dosage, complexity, and speed) that the patient can tolerate. Trial dosage needs to be established (resistance, repetitions, sets, time, intensity and frequency), and the exercise must be tested to set the starting point. During initial testing the patient is also taught how to perform the exercise safely without compensations. As described in Chapter 1, contraindications and precautions will override all other factors. Some tests may need to be delayed if there are healing considerations or if the SINS judgment indicates the need for caution. There

is a possibility of delayed-onset muscle soreness and joint pain after testing, so it is recommended that the therapist educate the patient that these side effects are possible after testing.

Mobility Testing (Joint Range of Motion and Muscle Flexibility)

The reader is referred to the detailed examination descriptions of measurement of joint range of motion and muscle flexibility in Reese and Bandy,[4] descriptions of evaluation concepts in Magee,[1] and the more detailed tissue related concepts in Zachazewski.[5] Expected range of motion comparisons by age and examples of some of the functional range requirements are available in Reese and Bandy.[4]

Muscle Function

Muscle function (Box 4.4) includes the ability to activate the specific motor units (including neuromuscular coordination), muscle endurance, strength, and power.[9–11] Specific testing is useful to determine if muscle function impairments are present and to establish a baseline for improvement. The testing also provides a patient-specific starting point for the exercise prescription. Quantitative measures can be used to establish goals; however, ensuring that the patient has adequate functional strength for activities of daily living is always the final goal.

Muscle Activation

Muscle activation is assessed in the clinic by asking a patient to voluntarily engage a muscle using isometric or isotonic contractions or during active movement analysis (Video 1.6). If there is no observed change in muscle tension, palpation is used to further assess if a contraction is present. If the patient is substituting other areas or muscles, the therapist can help the patient isolate the desired muscle (see Chapter 7). In addition to explanations and demonstration, repositioning or supporting the area may be necessary to decrease the load on the muscle. Muscle activation patterns are usually described qualitatively unless biofeedback or surface electromyography is used. Timing of muscle activation can also be observed and noted during exercise or functional movement (Videos 4.16, 4.17, and 4.27). A major discrepancy between active and passive range of motion is an indication that the patient may have difficulty with muscle activation, and activation in the range where control is lacking will be a goal for early exercise (Clinical Example 4.14).

📌 CLINICAL EXAMPLE 4.14 Assessment of Muscle Activation

A patient has chronic low back pain without referral into the leg. The timing of the posterior deep local stabilizers in the lumbar spine is evaluated in four-point kneeling over an exercise ball. The patient is asked to lift one leg without further instructions, and the therapist observes for the timing of muscle activation of the extensor bulk in the lumbar spine. The therapist can palpate the area if there is no visible contraction. Ideally, the spinal extensors should activate before or soon after the leg starts to extend. After a prolonged period of spinal pain, there is often delayed or absent local stabilizer activation. Absent or delayed local stabilizer activation and early use of the global movers prior to the local stabilizers indicate the need to train the neuromuscular coordination patterns to distribute forces and improve force closure. Early exercise choices involve proprioceptive, auditory and tactile cueing, and feedback, often using balance responses to activate the neuromuscular pathways that facilitate low threshold activation of the stabilizing systems (see Exercises 11.22, 11.28, and 11.35). Closed chain exercise also maximizes proprioceptive and tactile input to facilitate bilateral spinal extensor activation (Exercise 11.25), while bilateral lower (Exercises 11.24 and 11.25) or upper extremity (Exercise 11.22) exercise helps with symmetry.

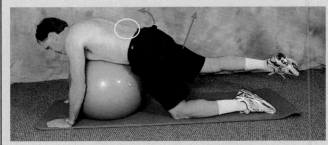

Spinal extensor activation timing.
The patient extends the right hip (*straight arrow*), allowing the pelvis to lift on the right (*curved arrow*). The primary axis of motion is at the same point in the lumbar spine as observed in the standing active spinal movement observation, indicating a pattern of concentration of movement at this point. There is limited abdominal stabilization and late spinal extensor activation.

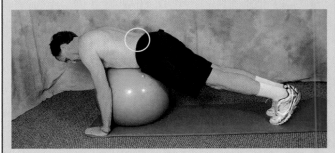

Closed chain bilateral hip extension over the ball.

Bilateral hip and knee extension with the feet remaining on the ground results in a more symmetrical position of the lumbar spine and pelvis. The patient's body weight is further over the ball, and the arms are used to assist the support. The patient is cued to lift the abdominal muscles, providing muscle support in the lumbar region, and to lift the head and focus on keeping both sides of the pelvis in contact with the ball prior to straightening the knees.

BOX 4.4 Muscle Function Testing

- Specific testing is useful to identify muscle function impairments and to establish a baseline for improvement compared to age-related normative values or in comparison to the opposite limb.
- The testing also provides a patient-specific starting point for the exercise prescription.
- Muscle activation is assessed by observing an individual muscle contraction when the patient is asked to contract voluntarily (isometric or isotonic), or during active movement analysis.
- Alternatives to assess muscle activation are biofeedback, superficial electromyography, and observing an exercise or functional movement.
- Active range of motion measurements are compared to passive range and can suggest a muscle activation problem.
- The amount of weight (body weight or external load) that the patient is able to lift is recorded, as is the number of repetitions possible, to establish a baseline measurement for strength training. Weight that allows approximately 10–15 repetitions is considered an appropriate amount for initial therapeutic strengthening, particularly for older adults or deconditioned individuals. More advanced strengthening may use weight that takes 8–12 repetitions to fatigue.
- Power testing involves maximum load within a short period and is only appropriate if the patient has sufficient strength and neuromuscular control to complete the movement.
- Power testing is conducted with a 1RM timed test using weight, body weight, or isokinetic machines.
- Muscle endurance is tested by asking the patient to perform repetitions until showing signs of fatigue. The difficulty level and resistance of exercises should allow multiple repetitions (15–30). Therapists must estimate an appropriate amount of resistance that the patient will be able to tolerate for testing, and dosage is set after trials to establish the resistance that the patient can resist prior to specific muscle fatigue.

Muscle Endurance

Muscular endurance is the ability of a muscle to repetitively or continuously contract until fatigue or loss of force is noted. Muscle endurance is measured either by recording the number of repetitions or time to failure or the maximum number of repetitions in a given time frame. Endurance exercises are performed with lower resistance. Muscle endurance goals are often among the first addressed by asking the patient to perform repetitions or isometric holds until showing signs of fatigue (Clinical Example 4.15 and 4.16; Video 4.32). If there is any indication of compromised tissue, lower loads are preferred for testing. The therapist can use this information to establish the appropriate resistance to allow at least 15–30 repetitions to challenge muscle endurance.[9] An isometric hold should last more than 10 seconds for adequate time to transition from the phosphocreatine to the glycolytic energy system (Videos 3.10 and 4.33).[11] If fatigue

---

📌 CLINICAL EXAMPLE 4.15 Muscle Endurance Testing: Isometric Holds

The patient was involved in a skiing accident 2 months ago and has residual neck pain after the fall. His pain is rated as 1/10, and the pain can increase to 3/10 with prolonged sitting (more than an hour). His goal is to be able to sit for more than 2 hours at a time in class. In the initial examination, the craniocervical flexion test using an inflatable cuff in supine is used to determine if he is able to activate the deep neck flexors sufficiently to flatten his cervical lordosis.[1,2] The cuff is inflated to 22 mm Hg before he is asked to gently flatten the front of his neck by nodding his chin to test his ability to reach and hold the 2 mm Hg incremental increases in pressure for at least 10 seconds. If the superficial muscles are used, the test is discontinued.

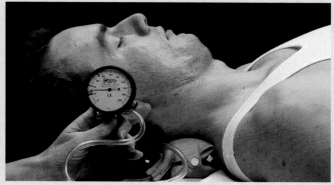

Craniocervical flexion test.

The patient is able to achieve all four levels up to 30 mm Hg and hold the position for at least 10 seconds; therefore, the supine antigravity flexor endurance test is possible.[3–5]

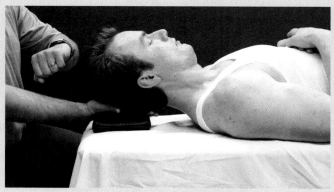

Supine antigravity flexor endurance test.

The time the patient is able to maintain his head off the table is measured to establish a baseline time. As this is more aggressive, any increase in pain is also recorded, and the test is stopped if the patient's pain increases beyond a 3/10. The patient is also asked to report pain behavior after the testing. The patient was able to maintain the antigravity position for 6 seconds prior to an increase in pain.

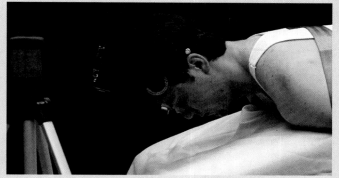

Prone neck extensor endurance test.

The patient is asked to maintain a midline cervical neutral position for as long as possible within 0.5 cm of the starting position. He is able to hold for 20 seconds before pain starts to increase.

Evaluation

The baseline measurements are used to set goals and to determine if antigravity and loaded exercise is possible. The supine antigravity position was too aggressive at this stage, and foam roller exercises are chosen to provide some challenge that does not require holding the head against gravity. The prone position goal is to hold the position for up to 30 seconds prior to increasing pain within 2 weeks.

References

1. Jull GA, O'Leary SP, Falla DL. Clinical assessment of the deep cervical flexor muscles: the craniocervical flexion test. *J Manipulative Physiol Ther.* 2008;31(7):525–533.
2. Hudswell S, von Mengersen M, Lucas N. The cranio-cervical flexion test using pressure biofeedback: a useful measure of cervical dysfunction in the clinical setting? *Int J Osteopathic Med.* 2005;8:98–105.
3. Edmondston SJ, Wallumrod ME, Macleid F, Kvamme LS, Joebges S, Brabham GC. Reliability of isometric muscle endurance tests in subjects with postural neck pain. *J Manipulative Physiol Ther.* 2008;31(5):348–354.
4. Harris KD, Heer DM, Roy TC, Santos DM, Whitman JM, Wainner RS. Reliability of a measurement of neck flexor muscle endurance. *Phys Ther.* 2005;85(12):1349–1355.
5. Shahidi B, Johnson C, Curran-Everett D, Maluf K. Reliability and group differences in quantitative cervicothoracic measures among individuals with and without chronic neck pain. *BMC Musculoskelet Disord.* 2012;13:215.

CLINICAL EXAMPLE 4.16   Muscle Endurance Testing: Repetitions to Failure

Patient A

Patient A is employed as a cargo loader for an airline company. He is recovering after rotator cuff surgery and needs to be able to lift multiple boxes or items weighing up to 25 kg. The lifting restrictions have been increased from 2 to 10 kg. Once he is capable of safely lifting 5 kg without symptoms, counting repetitions to failure would be a relevant means of testing endurance for this patient. As he progresses through rehabilitation, tracking how many times he is able to lift the weight from a table the height of the cart and then carry the weight to another table prior to fatigue establishes a baseline for training.

Evaluation

If he is able to successfully complete 30 repetitions prior to showing signs of fatigue, the amount of weight could be increased.

Patient B

Patient B is recovering after surgical debridement of his Achilles tendon. He is progressing to single-leg plantarflexion and is able to control the alignment of his lower extremity through the movement as well as maintain mid-position of the foot. The initial exercise testing for plantarflexor endurance is performed by asking the patient to perform single-leg plantarflexion with 25% support from the opposite leg for as many repetitions as possible until he fatigues or loses the alignment. He is able to perform 22 repetitions prior to local fatigue without any pain.

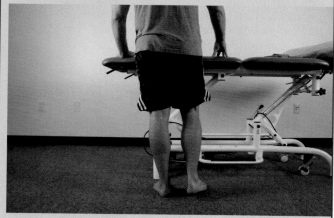

Starting point for single leg–heel lifts with 75% weight on postsurgical leg and hand support.

Evaluation

The number of repetitions before losing alignment is within the range to target muscle endurance and there was no pain. The patient will need to be able to monitor when he starts to lose the alignment in order to perform the exercise independently.

Implications for Exercise Choices

The exercise load is appropriate for muscle endurance and early tissue stress. If there is no increase in pain or swelling after the introduction of the exercise, the support from the other leg and the hands can be slowly reduced.

---

higher repetitions (>15) may be used to train muscle endurance prior to challenging the tissue with higher resistance loads.[11]

Repetitions to failure can also be used to assess endurance for functional activities (see Clinical Example 4.16). Sit-to-stand transfers , step-ups (Video 3.20), and and waist-to-overhead lifts are common examples of activities using this type of testing. Repetitions completed in a predetermined time period can be counted using body weight or equipment as resistance. Normative values for average number of repetitions for exercises such as push-ups or sit-ups are available to describe relative fitness levels.[9] These normative values are commonly used for general fitness and wellness screening but are seldom used for establishing rehabilitation goals.

Muscle Strength

Strength can be assessed using quantitative measurement devices (dynamometer or isokinetic equipment), manual muscle testing (MMT), or clinical testing using the maximum repetitions for a specific load. The dynamometer is a portable hand-held unit applied by the therapist using isometric tests. Isokinetic machines control the specific speed of movement and record forces generated by the patient throughout the range. Both dynamometry and isokinetic testing yield highly sensitive and reliable measurements but can only measure one motion at a time. Disadvantages of these methods include the cost of the equipment space, and isokinetic machines also take a significant amount of time to set up.

Manual muscle testing uses a grading system from 0 to 5 to describe the ability to move against gravity or a "break-through" for therapist-applied resistance (Table 4.4). The grading system provides a subjective comparison to the other side or to similar individuals. While the grades relying on gravity resistance provide reliable measures for individuals with severe strength deficits, the therapist-applied resistance tests may not be sufficiently sensitive without using a hand-held dynamometer.[12,13] The MMT grading system can help the therapist choose the positions for initial strengthening exercises if the individual demonstrates Grades 2 to 5. If pain is elicited during the MMT, the information is applied to the selective tissue assessment. Pain associated with a muscle contraction may indicate that the contractile tissue is involved. While MMT for any grade higher than a 2 requires the ability to move through range against gravity or resistance for assessment, resistance tests for selective tissue tension are performed with an isometric test in a neutral joint position. Maintaining the joint in a position that is unlikely to cause stress on ligament or capsule allows the physical therapist to determine whether the muscle–tendon contraction is painful.

The most common method of assessing strength for fitness purposes is the *one repetition maximum* (1RM), which is the maximum amount of weight that an individual can only lift one time.[9,10] While the 1RM may be an appropriate test for asymptomatic individuals, patients with compromised tissue may not be able to lift a maximal load without creating further damage or pain. A more conservative method used for establishing baseline resistance for therapeutic exercise is multiple repetition testing. Testing can utilize exercise equipment, free weights, body weight, or elastic resistance. This method also

---

were to occur within 10 seconds, this performance would be testing muscle strength rather than endurance because insufficient time has passed to transition from phosphocreatine to glycolytic metabolism.[11] If low loads are selected for a patient who has highly irritable symptoms or weak connective tissue,

allows the therapist to assess the specific exercises to be used in the exercise prescription. The patient is asked to exert his or her maximum effort using a specific weight, and the number of repetitions is recorded, followed by adjustment of the weight or position. The "test" load is an estimate, factoring in the patient's age, general condition, medical history, muscle bulk, and ability to move against gravity. The SINS evaluation should be used to determine if there is a need to limit the amount of weight for a patient, particularly if precautions are present. A lower starting weight is preferred, with incremental additions if the patient is able to perform multiple repetitions with ease (Video 4.34).

While loads that allow 8–12 repetitions before fatigue are recommended for strength training in healthy adults, lower weight with fatigue after 10–15 repetitions a is suitable for middle-age and older adults.[9] If the patient can lift the weight more than 15 times, the load should be increased to meet strengthening goals (Clinical Example 4.17).

There may be occasions when a patient will not be able to move against resistance in standard positions. If a patient is unable to move the limb against gravity, the limb should be supported, and at times the weight of the limb alone may provide sufficient load. Adjusting the load to allow the patient to reach the desired repetition range can be achieved by means other than increasing or decreasing the amount of weight lifted. The load can be adjusted by applying the biomechanical principles described in Chapter 2. For example changing the distance of the application of the resistance from the axis will increase or decrease the overall load and stress.

Another advantage of testing muscle strength using the multiple repetition method is the option to test the strength of a muscle in specific ranges required for function or in ranges where there is less mechanical advantage. For example, if a patient has recently had knee surgery and needs to improve quadriceps strength, knee extension in the terminal range against gravity with no additional weight may be the appropriate testing position. Multiple repetition testing can also be performed in supported positions.

TABLE 4.4 Manual Muscle Test Grades: Implications for Choice of Exercise Testing and Prescription

Grade	Description	Exercise Implications
0	No muscle activation	No neuromuscular function: indicates need to assess ability to use other muscles for functional movements
1	Trace activation	Test activation in supported positions. Activation goals with additional support for neuromuscular stimulation (electrical stimulation, overflow)
2	Able to move through range in gravity eliminated position	Strengthening dosage assessment will be started in supported gravity-eliminated positions
3	Able to move through range against gravity but no additional resistance	Strengthening dosage assessment will be started in supported gravity-resisted positions but without external resistance
4	Able to move through range against resistance but less than normal strength compared to the opposite limb and expected strength for age, gender, and other personal characteristics	Strengthening dosage assessment will be started in gravity-resisted positions with light external resistance
5	Normal strength compared to the opposite limb and expected strength for age, gender, and other personal characteristics	No strengthening impairment noted with break tests. If there are higher level functional requirements, use functional tests to assess strength for specific activities

CLINICAL EXAMPLE 4.17 Muscle Strength Testing

Patient A

Patient A is construction worker who presents with a diagnosis of lateral epicondalgia. Goals include shoulder muscle strengthening to assist the patient with developing proximal support and to distribute forces for Phase II management.

- *Initial testing:* Shoulder abduction against resistance from a pulley system with a strap above the elbow to limit forces on the lateral extensor origin:
  - He is able to perform 25 repetitions against 16 kg prior to shoulder abductor fatigue.
  - After a 2-minute rest, the weight is increased to 18 kg, and he is able to perform 15 repetitions.
  - After a 3-minute rest, the weight is increased to 20 kg, and he is able to perform 10 repetitions.

Evaluation

The weight is set at 20 kg for 2–3 sets and 8 repetitions for the initial exercise plan with the number of repetitions progressed as tolerated.

- *Strengthening goal:* The overall goal is to be able to abduct against 25 kg and hold the arm between 70 and 90 degrees of abduction to meet the functional requirements replicating the average weight of the siding and windows to be lifted to shoulder height.

Patient B

Patient B is a 72-year-old woman with a moderate rotator cuff tear who is referred for conservative management. The following active range of motion is possible:

- *In sitting:* Shoulder abduction 45 degrees
- *Supine:* Shoulder abduction 70 degrees

Strength is tested in supine with the arm on a sliding board, and the patient is asked to repeat the movement until fatigue. She is able to complete 10 repetitions to 70 degrees.

Evaluation

The supine position provides sufficient resistance for strengthening, so initial exercise dosage is set at 2 sets of 8–10 repetitions with movement on a sliding board to 70 degrees.

- *Strengthening goal:* Initial goal is to be able to abduct to 70 degrees against gravity in sitting for 8–10 repetitions.

Whether testing muscle strength or performing an exercise, the therapist should ensure that the patient is able to activate the muscle(s) of interest. Verbal guidance or careful positioning can help correct or limit compensations. Once a muscle is fatigued, a patient will typically compensate using other muscles or movement strategies. The test or the exercise is therefore no longer targeting the intended muscle(s), and the test may not reflect the results required to provide the appropriate dosage required to address the target muscles.

Muscle Power

Power is the ability to produce a rapid burst of force over a brief time period.[9,10] Athletes who are working toward returning to sport usually progress to exercises designed to improve power once other impairments have been addressed (Clinical Example 4.18). Other populations also need power for functional activities. A deconditioned patient will need to work on power if he has difficulty transferring from sit to stand quickly or efficiently (see Clinical Example 4.18). Typically power movements require use of global movers, and training for muscular power is incorporated into therapeutic exercise once other impairments have been resolved to decrease risk of injury related to high forces. The most common assessments for power are typically 1RM tests, maximum isokinetic tests, and functional power tests.

Isokinetic testing equipment allows the therapist to assess a patient's power output at specific speeds while the information is plotted across the patient's ROM. As previously mentioned, although very reliable, this type of testing restricts movement to a single joint and therefore may not translate to the need for powerful functional movement. Functional power can, however, be measured using sports-specific movements such as jumping for height or distance, hop tests, and snatch lift tests using body weight or weights.

Aerobic Capacity (Cardiorespiratory Function)

Prior to using aerobic exercise the therapist should determine if there are any contraindications or precautions for exercise intended to increase heart and respiratory rate (Box 4.5). This is particularly important for patients with risk factors such as high blood pressure, high cholesterol, smoking, diabetes, or obesity. Older adults, individuals with a history of extensive deconditioning, cardiovascular, or respiratory peripheral vascular conditions should be thoroughly screened prior to testing and exercise prescription.[14,15]

Even if there are no immediate risks identified, patients should be monitored before, during, and after exercise. Some cardiovascular conditions can mimic musculoskeletal pain, and an increase in aerobic challenge can magnify symptoms. It is therefore important to take blood pressure before and during aerobic exercise for individuals with a history of hypertension and other conditions just listed. A drop in

systolic blood pressure of more than 10 mm Hg during exercise accompanied by other signs and symptoms, or a rise in systolic blood pressure above 250 mm Hg or diastolic above 115 mm Hg immediate discontinuation of exercise, reevaluation, and referral.[9,14] Symptoms that require immediate attention include new-onset or easily provoked angina; new onset of chest, upper body, neck, or jaw pain in the presence of risk factors; dizziness; shortness of breath; nausea; or severe fatigue.[9,14–16] Clinical signs such as pallor, sweating, confusion or disorientation, inability to talk during activity,

---

⚡ CLINICAL EXAMPLE 4.18 Muscle Power and Speed Testing

Patient A

Patient A is a basketball player who is moving from Phase II to III after a medial collateral ligament injury. He has full knee range of motion and excellent strength. A squat vertical jump is used to establish the baseline height and set goals (see Table 4.5). Sprint time is also recorded prior to sports-specific training, including running and jumping drills (see Table 4.5).

Patient B

Patient B had a right posterior approach hip replacement 3 years previously and has right knee osteoarthritis. She needs to improve the use of her hip extensors to move her body weight forward over the feet and rapidly extend the hips to minimize forces on the knee joint. The 5× sit-to-stand test (timed) would be an appropriate measurement for this functional activity (see Table 4.5). After the initial test, the biomechanics are corrected and cueing is provided to encourage the patient to use her hip extensors as well as the knees for the vertical component of the movement. The verbal cueing is used to emphasize the upward motion and to perform the movement as quickly as possible. The 5× sit-to-stand test is retested at the end of the session to evaluate if the instructions have resulted in immediate improvements and is tested again at the beginning of the next session to evaluate the carryover of the movement reeducation.

The patient also underwent the 30-second sit-to-stand test. She uses her hands to provide additional support for her trunk. Her weight is toward the back of her heels, increasing the moment arm and load on the patellofemoral joint. During testing the patient is asked to perform as many repetitions as possible for the 30-second sit-to-stand or the time recorded for the 5× sit-to-stand test. Correction of the biomechanics follows the testing. If there is a need to establish baseline repeated movements for muscular endurance, the 30-second sit-to-stand is preferred.

BOX 4.5 Aerobic Capacity

- Individuals must be screened for cardiovascular risk factors before performing aerobic endurance testing.
- Aerobic testing may be necessary at different times in the rehabilitation process.
- Heart rate responses and perceived exertion are used to determine the appropriate intensity (55–90% maximal heart rate, RPE 11–13).
- Estimated maximal heart rate = 208 − (0.7 × age).[14]
- Deconditioned, older, or sedentary individuals should start with a lower intensity.
- Younger, athletic individuals should start with a higher intensity.

RPE, Rating of perceived exertion.

and vital sign abnormalities also necessitate stopping exercise, monitoring vital signs, and referring for immediate medical attention.

Improving aerobic endurance is an important goal for endurance athletes as well as for less conditioned or debilitated patients. A distance runner who has anterior knee pain may be treated initially with an emphasis on addressing the local complaints, but, further into the rehabilitative process, the focus will need to shift toward aerobic conditioning to regain his or her stamina. In some cases, aerobic exercise is used to maintain function to prevent deconditioning or improve overall mobility and postural endurance. Under these circumstances, baseline measures of aerobic function will be useful to set goals and for comparison. Aerobic testing may be indicated at different times during the rehabilitation process and could involve upper body, lower body, general, or aquatic exercise testing, depending on the precautions and impairments.

Aerobic exercise intensity for patients whose primary diagnosis is a musculoskeletal condition is usually estimated using target heart rates calculated from a formula using an age-predicted maximal heart rate $(208 - [0.7 \times age])$.[14] Exercise intensity is prescribed to reach between 55% and 90% of the maximal heart rate for individuals without cardiorespiratory diagnoses, with lower targets if the patient is deconditioned, older, or sedentary.[16] Conversely, an athlete would likely need to work at a higher target heart rate range. Heart rate responses and perceived exertion are monitored to evaluate if the patient is tolerating the intensity. These equations are often based on healthy research populations, so the predictable heart rate in those populations may not translate well to a population with comorbidities. For example if a patient is taking beta-blocker medication for hypertension, the medication influences the normal exercise-induced changes in heart rate.[9,14] Readers are referred to other sources for more detail on exercise testing and prescription for individuals with multiple medical conditions, cardiovascular disease, metabolic syndromes, kidney disease, and pulmonary diagnoses.[9]

The Borg Rating of Perceived Exertion (RPE) Scale® is a useful self-reported measure of the intensity of a specific prescribed exercise.[9,17] The ACSM guidelines for moderate-intensity exercise for most healthy adults equates to approximately RPE 11–13 on the Borg RPE Scale.[11,17] For any patients diagnosed with borderline hypertension or hypertension, the resting blood pressure should be compared to a blood pressure reading taken immediately post-exercise regardless of the perceived exertion because high arterial pressure can be asymptomatic.

Coordination and Balance

Coordination of movement requires precise, timely control of tasks while achieving the desired targets (Box 4.6). Coordination tests document successful attempts

---

BOX 4.6 Balance and Coordination Testing

- Coordination testing involves recording successful attempts for precision or movement tasks.
- Timing, order, and integration of neuromuscular activation requires observation of specific functional goals.
- Static balance is tested by timing the ability to maintain a postural position.
- Dynamic balance testing includes the ability to move from a more stable to a less stable position and regain equilibrium.

---

at complex sequences of movement. The movements can involve reaching a target, such as throwing a ball or placing items in a basket repeatedly. Other tasks may challenge precision, such as using a laser pointer, achieving a specific intensity of muscle contractions, or responding to a series of instructions or signals. Neuromuscular coordination is also used to describe the timing and order of muscle activation and the use of muscle groups designed for the appropriate task. The overuse of global movers that are activated for high-threshold, high-intensity but short-duration tasks that usually only require low threshold, low-intensity, but long-duration is inefficient and results in compensatory movements. Neuromuscular coordination testing for this type of muscle dysfunction can involve testing the ability to attain and hold a position for the length of time needed for function- or proprioceptive-type challenges, where the patient is asked to find a specific position repeatedly (Clinical Example 4.19). Functional activities, including walking around cones or in a figure-of-eight pattern, running between lines, agility drills (Video 3.15), or dodging obstacles are also examples of higher-level coordination tests or exercises. Coordination is often included in Phase III activities or once other basic impairments have been resolved.

Balance testing can include static or dynamic activities. **Static balance** requires testing the ability of a patient to achieve and maintain static positions with progressively smaller bases of support or reduced sensory input. Examples of static balance tests are the timed single-leg (Video 4.27) or the tandem stance balance tests. The ability to hold the position can be further challenged by removing sensory input by closing the eyes or by decreasing the stability of the surface, such as testing on foam. Quantitative measurement of balance is possible with force platforms that measure postural sway and the ability to maintain the center of mass within the base of support (Clinical Example 4.20).

Dynamic balance tests involve challenging the patient to move from one position to another, then reestablish a stable position (Video 4.35). A stop-and-start obstacle course and hop tests are examples of dynamic balance testing appropriate for sports-specific balance testing to determine if athletes requiring advanced balance skills are ready to return to practice (Video 3.24).

CLINICAL EXAMPLE 4.19 **Neuromuscular Coordination**

Patient A

Patient A has a history of repeated whiplash injuries and hypermobility. She has poor neuromuscular coordination, impaired proprioception, and poor position relocation. She is asked to perform precise cervical movements using a laser system mounted to a headband. The distance from the target is recorded after the patient rotates her head and is asked to find the starting position with her eyes open and closed.

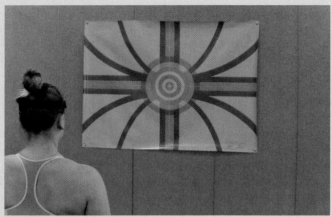

Use of a laser target for cervical coordination and position relocation training.

Patient B

Patient B is in Phase III after an anterior cruciate ligament (ACL) repair. She is asked to perform a single-leg crossover hop test (see Table 4.5) for distance as a measure of strength, power, and coordination. The result is compared to her nonsurgical leg, and she is expected to achieve at least 80% before discharge. The Illinois agility circuit test (see Table 4.5) is used to reflect her ability to change directions, speed, and coordination. The baseline test results are used to set incremental goals with a minimum of 10% improvement within 2 weeks.

CLINICAL EXAMPLE 4.20 **Balance Testing**

The Balance Master uses a force platform to provide quantitative measurement of postural sway in double- or single-leg standing positions. The baseline measurement records the distance and frequency of the sway of the line of force measured relative to the base of support. The patient is a professional dancer, and therefore both normal stance and dance positions are used during the measurement. The static balance measurements are used as a baseline to track improvement, although the visual input can be used to provide real-time feedback and incentives.

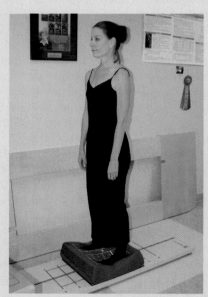

Static balance tested on an unstable surface on the Balance Master force platform.

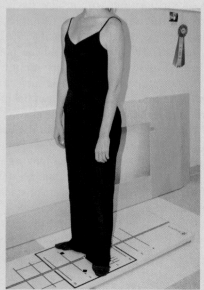

Static balance tested on the Balance Master in dance-specific positions.

CLINICAL EXAMPLE 4.20 Balance Testing—cont'd

Patient B from Clinical Example 4.19 is in Phase III after an ACL repair with microfracture surgery. She is tested on the Y balance apparatus for symmetry when reaching with the opposite leg in all directions (see Table 4.5). The average of three trials is used for comparison between sides, and results are shown in the table.

	Affected	Unaffected	Difference
Lateral reach	94 cm	102 cm	8 cm
Forward reach	39 cm	45 cm	6 cm
Posteromedial reach	84 cm	86 cm	2 cm

Evaluation
The lateral and forward reach directions will be used as part of the exercise program with the goal to achieve 90% of the reach when standing on the unaffected leg.

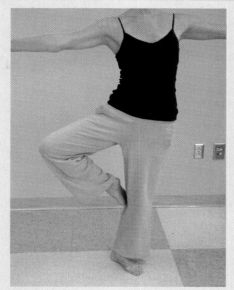

Timed single-leg stance in dance-specific positions.

FUNCTIONAL ASSESSMENT

Most patients will report functional problems when asked what their main goals are for physical therapy treatment. Self-reported, **standardized questionnaires** are helpful to determine overall functional limitations. These questionnaires can be used as **outcome measures** (see Chapter 8) as well for guiding choices of other examination procedures and establishing **goals** (Clinical Example 4.21). The information from the questionnaire can be used to select **functional performance measures** that reproduce or simulate the activity. The patient is asked to perform these activities, and the ability to perform the movement, duration, distance, or other quantitative values is recorded (see Table 4.5). Self-reported outcome measurements are also combined with the quality of movements observed to determine the match between the patient's perception of his or her ability and the observed performance. Outcome measurements are discussed further in Chapter 8.

The choice of the questionnaire is guided by evidence of psychometric properties (reliability, validity, and sensitivity). When choosing a questionnaire, the therapist should also assess if there was a particular age group or patient population used to develop the measure. Some of the measures have been tested with specific age groups or patient populations and may

CLINICAL EXAMPLE 4.21 Functional Assessment

A patient with osteoarthritis in one knee reports a score of 49/80 on the Knee Outcome Survey – Activities of Daily Living Scale (KOS-ADLS), which has good reliability and validity.[1-3] Lower scores on the scale are equivalent to greater disability. The walking item is rated as "somewhat difficult" (3/5 with 0 = unable to do, 5/5 = not difficult at all). The physical performance measures tested included a 10-m walk test (result was 16 seconds).

Evaluation
The documented gait speed (0.6 m/s) does not meet normative averages for community ambulation (1 m/s)[d]

Goals
After 4 weeks, the patient will:
1. Improve KOS-ADLS score to 58/80 (the minimal detectable difference (MDC) to exceed error is 8.4[2]; see Chapter 8 for further discussion of MDC).
2. Report minimal difficulty with walking scored as 4/5 on the KOS-ADLS instrument
3. Demonstrate adequate gait speed to meet average community ambulation speed (1 m/sec tested on the 10-m walk test)[4]

References
1. Logerstedt DS, Synder-Mackler L, Ritter RC, Axe MJ. Knee pain and mobility impairments: meniscal and articular cartilage lesions. Clinical practice guidelines linked to the International Classification of Functioning, Disability and Health from the Orthopaedic Section of the American Physical Therapy Association *J Orthop Sports Phys Ther.* 2010;40(6):A1–A35.
2. Marx RG, et al. Reliability, validity, and responsiveness of four knee outcome scales for athletic patients. *J Bone and Joint Surg (Am).* 2001;83:1459–1469.
3. Irrgang JJ, Snyder-Mackler L, Winner RS, Fu FH, Harner CD. Development of a patient-reported measure of function of the knee. *J Bone Joint Surg (Am).* 1998;80-A(8):1132–1145.
4. Fritz S, Lusardi M. White paper: "Walking speed: the sixth vital sign". *J Geriatr Phys Ther.* 2009;32:2–5.

TABLE 4.5 Functional Performance Tests[1-3,18]

TYPE OF FUNCTIONAL PERFORMANCE TEST			EXAMPLE
Balance tests (distance – symmetry or time)	Timed up-and-go Functional reach Star excursion (balance reach) Y balance Single-leg stance time	Y balance	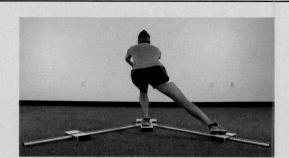
Lunge tests (maximum number of lunges or distance)	Single plane (anterior-posterior, medial-lateral) Rotational lunge	Lunge test	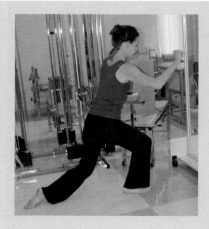
Step tests (maximum number of reciprocal steps or number of steps within a set time)	Step-up Step-down Lateral step-down Stair measure test	Step test	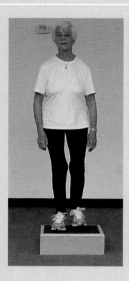
Squat tests (maximum number of squats to a specific range of motion)	Double-leg squat test Single-leg squat test	Double-leg squat test: maximum number of repetitions	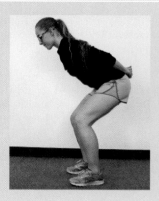

TABLE 4.5 **Functional Performance Tests**[1-3,18]—cont'd

TYPE OF FUNCTIONAL PERFORMANCE TEST			EXAMPLE
Hop tests (timed test for specific distance or maximum distance)	Single-leg hop for distance (A) Triple hop (B) Crossover hop (C) 6-m hop for time (D)	Hop test patterns[a] (single, triple, crossover, 6 m)	 A B C D
Jump tests (maximum height or distance for explosive jumps)	Bilateral or single vertical jump Drop jump Horizontal jumps	Vertical jump test for height	
Agility tests (timed tests for specific distances and directions)	Zig-zag run T-test Y-test Illinois test	Illinois agility test pattern	
Gait	6-minute walk test 10-m gait speed		
Sit-to-stand (number of repetitions within set time or time for set number of repetitions)	5× sit-to-stand 30-second sit-to-stand	30-second sit-to-stand	

[a]Image from Manske RC. *Fundamental Orthopedic Management for the Physical Therapist Assistant*. 4th ed. St. Louis, MO: Mosby Elsevier; 2016, Fig 18.16.

Further details are provided in Chapter 8.

BOX 4.7   **Criteria for Lower Extremity Functional Performance Tests[18]**

- No pain
- No effusion
- No crepitus
- Full active range of motion with good terminal knee extension control
- Good muscle strength (80% of normal or graded ⅘)

- One repetition maximum leg press >125% relative strength index
- Single-leg balance >45 seconds (eyes open and closed)
- Single-leg quarter-squat held for >45 seconds (eyes open and closed)
- Single-leg half-squat held for >45 seconds (eyes open and closed)

From Clark NC. Functional performance testing following knee ligament injury. *Phys Ther Sport*. 2001;2:101.

---

therefore have floor or ceiling effects or may not be as relevant for other patient groups. Chapter 8 discusses the use of questionnaires for outcome evaluation.

Functional Performance Measures

Functional performance measures require the patient to perform the movement with some form of objective measurement rather than just qualitative observation. These tests usually involve the entire body rather than isolated joint tests and measures. These tests usually reflect the patient's activity limitations such as gait (ability to walk a specific distance, gait speed), sit-to-stand (Clinical Example 4.18, Patient B) transfers, reaching, or combinations of movements required to return to work. The functional tests are often very similar to functional exercises, and the measures may record time taken, number of repetitions, or how accurately the task is performed (see Clinical Example 4.21). In addition, observing the movement for compensations or biomechanical elements is very important during the initial testing. These observations are used when teaching the patient how to correct movement strategies or to select methods to refine the movement patterns.

As discussed in Chapter 3, therapeutic exercise prescription should address impairments that influence a specific functional activity. Functional tests can be used as baseline measure for specific limitations in any phase, and more advanced tests are added when the patient is ready to perform the activity. The SINS and tissue healing principles (Chapter 2) will help determine if a patient is ready for this type of testing. Prerequisites for weight-bearing dynamic tests include no effusion or pain with resistance, adequate range of motion for the functional activity, and sufficient strength to support the body in gravity-resisted positions[18,19] (Box 4.7). Specific criteria have been described for progression to the next phase or next level of postsurgical or posttrauma protocols.[18,20] The tests should be chosen and performed in a logical, sequential manner.[18,19] For example, static balance is conducted before functional movements; double-leg squat tests are performed before single squats. The interpretation and use of outcome measures is discussed further in Chapter 8, and details on additional tests are available in Magee and Sueki,[2] Magee Orthopaedic Assessment,[1] Cleland and Koppenhaver,[3] and Austin.[19]

▮ SUMMARY

- Subjective information will help guide the selection of evaluation and treatment techniques.
- A more cautious objective examination is warranted if there is high severity, high irritability, or signs of acute inflammation indicating potential for aggravation. Precautions and contraindications override all other decisions related to choice of tests and measures.
- Selective tissue tension is used to determine if contractile or noncontractile structures are contributing to symptoms.
- End feel assessment assists with evaluation of range of motion and causes of limitations.
- Structural alignment (bony alignment, symmetry, curvatures, and relationship of body segments) is important to evaluate prior to movement and influences the starting position for exercise.
- The ability to correct a postural alignment provides information for the therapist to use for instructions and feedback.
- Dynamic movement observation is used to assess components of functional movement, including timing and coordination.
- Combining information gathered from assessing static and dynamic alignment and with movement analysis guides choice of further examination techniques and provides information regarding willingness to move, pain relationships, and motor control patterns.

- Muscle activation is tested by observing quality and timing or by using biofeedback equipment.
- Endurance and strength testing for therapeutic exercise purposes consists of testing using multiple repetitions against "trial" loads to determine the amount of load to be used in the initial exercise plan.
- Endurance testing involves lower loads allowing more than 15 repetitions to fatigue.
- Strength testing involves higher loads allowing between 6 and 10 repetitions prior to fatigue for normal healthy individuals or 10 to 15 repetitions for older or deconditioned individuals.
- Muscle power tests involve maximal effort over a short period and are usually functional tests for therapeutic purposes.
- Aerobic endurance testing sets a target of an age-based maximum heart rate for continuous systemic exercise or a self-reported perceived rate of exertion.
- Balance tests involve the ability to maintain a posture (static) or move from one posture to the next and return to a stable position (dynamic).
- Coordination tests involve the ability to achieve a target with precision.
- Functional assessment tests include self-reported questionnaires and tests mimicking functional tasks with repetitions, time, or accuracy recorded.

REVIEW QUESTIONS

1. Explain how the patient's subjective history, medical history, and SINS factors influence examination techniques and choice of exercise parameters.
2. Describe how selective tissue tension testing can help identify the source of impairment.
3. Describe the potential limitations with a tight, hard, elastic, and empty end feel.
4. Describe how a patient's static alignment can influence his or her dynamic alignment.
5. Discuss how information gained from movement analysis and alignment informs further testing and evaluation.
6. Differentiate among testing for muscle activation, strength, power, and endurance.
7. Provide examples of scenarios when aerobic endurance testing is indicated.
8. Provide examples of types of testing for balance and coordination.
9. Discuss the timing of functional performance tests and criteria for safe testing.

REFERENCES

1. Magee DJ. *Orthopedic Physical Assessment.* 6th ed. St. Louis, MO: Elsevier Saunders; 2014.
2. Magee DJ, Sueki D. *Orthopedic Physical Assessment Atlas and Video: Selected Special Tests and Movements.* 6th ed. St. Louis, MO: Elsevier Saunders; 2011.
3. Cleland JA, Koppenhaver S. *Netter's Orthopaedic Clinical Examination: An Evidence-Based Approach.* 2nd ed. St. Louis, MO: Elsevier Saunders; 2011.
4. Reese NB, Bandy WD. *Joint Range of Motion and Muscle Length Testing.* 2nd ed. St. Louis, MO: Elsevier Saunders; 2010.
5. Zachazewski JE. Range of motion and flexibility. In: Magee DJ, Zachazewski JE, Quillen WS, eds. *Scientific Foundations and Principles of Practice in Musculoskeletal.* St Louis, MO: Saunders Elsevier; 2007:527–556.
6. Sahrmann SA, Bloom N. Update of concepts underlying movement system syndromes. In: Sahrmann SA, ed. *Movement System Impairment Syndromes of the Extremities, Cervical and Thoracic Spine.* St. Louis, MO: Saunders Elsevier; 2011:1–34.
7. Sahrmann SA. *Diagnosis and Treatment of Movement Impairment Syndromes.* Philadelphia, PA: Mosby; 2002.
8. Delitto A, George SZ, Van Dillen L, et al. Low back pain. Clinical practice guidelines linked to the International Classification of Functioning, Disability and Health from the Orthopaedic Section of the American Physical Therapy Association. *J Orthop Sports Phys Ther.* 2012;42(4):A1–A57.
9. American College of Sports Medicine. In: Pescatello LS, Arean R, Riebe DR, Thompson PD, eds. *ACSM's Guidelines for Exercise Testing and Prescription.* 9th ed. Baltimore, MD: Wolters Kluwer Lippincott Williams & Wilkins; 2014.
10. Cipriani DJ, Falkel JE. Physiological principles of resistance training and functional integration for the injured and disabled. In: Magee DJ, Zachazewski JE, Quillen WS, eds. *Scientific Foundations and Principles of Practice in Musculoskeletal Rehabilitation.* St. Louis, MO: Saunders Elsevier; 2007:432–457.
11. Powers SK, Howley ET. *Exercise Physiology: Theory and Application to Fitness and Performance.* New York: McGraw-Hill Humanities/Social Sciences/Languages; 2011.
12. Herbison GJ, Isaac Z, et al. Strength post-spinal cord injury: myometer vs manual muscle test. *Spinal Cord.* 1996;34(9):543–548.
13. Schwartz S, Cohen ME, et al. Relationship between two measures of upper extremity strength: manual muscle test compared to hand-held myometry. *Arch Phys Med Rehab.* 1992;73(11): 1063–1068.
14. Haykowsky MJ, Hillegass EA. Integration of the cardiovascular system in assessment and interventions in musculoskeletal rehabilitation. In: Magee DJ, Zachazewski JE, Quillen WS, eds. *Scientific Foundations and Principles of Practice in Musculoskeletal Rehabilitation.* St. Louis, MO: Saunders Elsevier; 2007.
15. Boissonnault WG. Patient health history including identifying health risk factors. In: Boissonnault WG, ed. *Primary Care for the Physical Therapist.* 2nd ed. St. Louis, MO: Elsevier Saunders; 2011.
16. Smirnova IV. The cardiovascular system. In: Goodman CC, Pathology Fuller KS, eds. *Implications for the Physical Therapist.* 4th ed. St. Louis, MO: Elsevier; 2015.
17. Borg G. Borg perception. Radisvagen 124. 16573 Hasselby Sweden. http://www.borgperception.se/index.html.
18. Clark NC. Functional performance testing following knee ligament injury. *Phys Ther Sport.* 2001;2:101.
19. Austin GP. Functional testing and return to activity. In: Magee DJ, Zachazewski JE, Quillen WS, eds. *Scientific Foundations and Principles of Practice in Musculoskeletal Rehabilitation.* St. Louis, MO: Saunders Elsevier; 2007:633–664.
20. Cioppa-Mosca J, Cahill JB, Young Tucker C, eds. *Hospital for Special Surgery. Handbook of Postsurgical Rehabilitation Guidelines for the Orthopedic Clinician.* St. Louis, MO: Mosby Elsevier; 2008.

5

Exercise Prescription
Selection of Exercise Type and Parameters

Kim Dunleavy and Amy Kubo Slowik

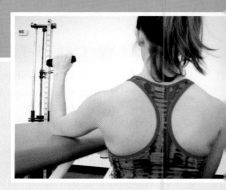

OBJECTIVES

Upon completion of this chapter, the reader will be able to:

1. Discuss the factors influencing exercise type and parameters.
2. Describe the exercise parameter categories (dosage, position, and functional requirements).
3. Discuss the types of exercise used for improving mobility, muscle function, aerobic endurance, and neuromuscular coordination.
4. List the types of exercise and suitable parameters intended to provide optimal stimulus for tissue regeneration of connective tissue (tendon, ligament, cartilage, bone) and muscle.
5. Describe how to adjust body position for support or to progressively challenge a given exercise.
6. List the types of exercise used to promote mobility and discuss how to progress the exercises.
7. List the types of exercise used to improve stability and how to progress the exercises.
8. Define and determine appropriate exercise dosage (repetitions, sets, load, duration, frequency) for selected case examples.
9. Describe how speed and complexity can be used to make exercise more or less difficult and provide examples to progress task-specific coordination.
10. Match the appropriate exercise type to goals for recovery Phases I–III.
11. Describe exercise parameters and elements to consider when establishing goals for recovery Phases I–III.

EXERCISE PRESCRIPTION: SELECTING EXERCISE TYPE AND PARAMETERS

Earlier chapters discussed some of the foundational principles involved in exercise prescription. This chapter covers the appropriate choices of **exercise type** and how to effectively manipulate the **parameters** for the best possible outcome. *Exercise type* describes the exercise, amount of assistance, use of equipment, and type of movement. *Parameters* are the factors that can be adjusted for an exercise to target goals related to the specific impairment or functional deficit. Parameters include the **position, dosage,** and requirements for function such as **complexity, speed,** and **range** of an exercise. **Dosage** is the **amount of resistance, number of repetitions, sets, intensity, time,** and **frequency** of exercise (Box 5.1).

Therapeutic exercise parameters are similar to the FITT principles (**F**requency, **I**ntensity, **T**ime, **T**ype) described by the American College of Sports Medicine (ACSM).[1] The ACSM guidelines are applicable to general fitness populations across all age ranges and for individuals with chronic diseases.[1,2] While the ACSM guidelines apply to the later phases of rehabilitation, there are some differences for therapeutic exercise to allow for tissue regeneration and to help the patient restore normal movement patterns. The phase of healing and creating an optimal stimulus for healing are important considerations when prescribing exercise for patients (Chapter 2). As an example, the ACSM guideline for **frequency** of exercise is three to five times per week for general fitness purposes. If one of the therapeutic exercise goals is to increase circulation and decrease edema, circulatory exercises should be repeated frequently (often hourly) every day until the edema is resolved. **Intensity** reflects the amount of resistance, level of effort, complexity, and speed of the exercises. The **time** component refers to both the duration of continuous exercise as well as muscle contractions. According to the ACSM guidelines, **type** refers to muscle contraction, but for therapeutic exercise, type is extended to include the amount of **assistance** required for movement and other characteristics such as **open versus closed chain exercise.** The type of exercise and the exercise parameters will change often, both within the same treatment session and over the course of treatment.

BOX 5.1 **Exercise Parameters**

- Position
- Dosage
  - Amount of resistance
  - Repetitions
  - Sets
  - Intensity
  - Time (including rest periods)
  - Frequency
- Functional requirements
  - Complexity
  - Speed
  - Range

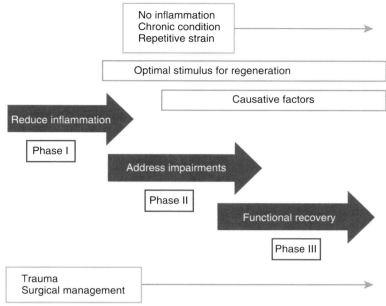

Fig. 5.1 Overlapping goals for Phases I–III.

BOX 5.2 Selection of Type of Exercise and Parameters

- Type of exercise describes the exercise, amount of assistance, use of equipment, and type of movement.
- Exercise parameters are characteristics of exercise performance that are adjusted to provide specificity for addressing impairments or recovering functional capability.
- Parameters include position, dosage, and components of movement required for functional tasks (complexity, speed, and range).
- Exercise parameters are specific to the type of tissue.
- Exercise dosage is tested and adapted to provide overload or distribution of forces for muscle function, appropriate stress and strain for mobility goals or load, and complexity, speed, and range for functional exercise.
- Selection of exercise type and parameters takes into account Severity, Irritability, Nature, Stage (SINS), injury mechanism, tissue type, and phases of healing.
- Initial assessment determines the appropriate starting point, with constant reassessment and adjustment throughout the recovery.
- Exercise prescription can be progressed within a phase and between phases.

BOX 5.3 Mobility Concepts

Range-of-motion restrictions due to	Type of exercise
Effusion or edema	Circulatory exercises in elevated positions
Capsule or connective tissue restrictions	Exercises approaching end range (prolonged hold or oscillations)
Muscle flexibility	Stretching to oppose anatomical directions of muscle

---

of forces desired for optimal stimulus for regeneration (Fig. 5.1 and Chapter 2). As the patient masters tasks and accommodates to the dosage, frequent, timely adjustments to the exercise program are indicated (Box 5.2).

PRESCRIPTION FOR MOBILITY IMPAIRMENTS

General Concepts for Mobility Exercise Prescription

Prior to including mobility exercises in the treatment plan, the therapist should determine the cause of any motion limitations (Box 5.3). As previously discussed, considerations for adding range of motion exercises also include applicable precautions for healing structures (Chapter 1 and 2) and range of motion expectations for age and functional requirements (Chapter 3).[3] The exercise parameters will differ if the limitations are due to joint or muscle structure extensibility versus effusion, pain, muscle guarding, or strength deficits. If effusion, pain, or muscle guarding is the limiting factor, the exercise parameters are based on Phase I guidelines to increase circulation and remove effusion and edema (Clinical Example 5.1). If both active and passive range of motion are restricted (see selective tissue tension Chapter 4), the exercises should approach end range of the joint capsule, connective tissue, or muscle.

Exercises should be selected to target goals by carefully considering tissue type, injury mechanism, and Severity, Irritability, Nature, Stage (SINS; see Chapter 1) Goals differ across the phases of healing but may span more than one phase (Fig. 5.1). There are a number of factors that impact selection: precautions and contraindications (Chapter 1), examination results (Chapter 4), and the influence of psychological components (Chapters 6 and 7). The patient's requirements for function (including activities of daily living, work, hobbies, and goals) will also influence the choice of exercise type. Personal characteristics and diagnosis (both primary and comorbid conditions) are critical elements to consider. Applying biomechanical principles guides the choice of starting position and the types

✈ CLINICAL EXAMPLE 5.1 Exercise Type and Parameters for Edema Resolution

Patient B from Clinical Example 4.1 is seen 3 days after a mild calcaneofibular ankle ligament sprain (Phase I). Active ankle range of motion is limited by edema as follows:

	R	L
Dorsiflexion	0 degrees (tight)	8 degrees
Plantarflexion	42 degrees (no pain)	45 degrees
Eversion	30 degrees (no pain)	30 degrees
Inversion	11 degrees (slight pulling)	20 degrees

Resisted isometric tests are all normal except for slightly less right eversion strength. There is no pain with the resisted contraction or in non–weight-bearing positions, with some pain in standing (2/10). There is mild effusion (see Clinical Examples 4.1 and 4.2).

Precautions
Avoid full tension of the injured ligament in inversion.

Goal
Increase mobility by decreasing edema.

Exercise Choices
Active range of motion to end range for plantarflexion, dorsiflexion (Exercise 9.37) is used to promote circulation as there is limited tension on the ligament in the sagittal plane and the Grade I tear does not require limitation of motion in this plane. The pumping action provides assistance with mechanical fluid motion and venous return.
- Parameters
  - *Position:* An elevated position is preferable to assist with venous return.
  - *Dosage:* Multiple repetitions and multiple sets, repeated as often as possible. There is no expectation of fatigue as the intention is to provide muscular pumping for fluid motion, and the movement is evaluated for ease of movement. As mobility improves, pain usually decreases.

The patient is taught how to perform the exercise to determine if pain in the injured area increases or if the patient needs instructions to limit the range. It is possible that range may improve even in the same session. The patient is encouraged to move as frequently as possible in a home program. Measurement of edema or active range of motion is evaluated at the end of the session.

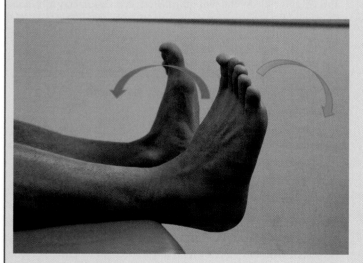

Active range of motion (AROM) dorsiflexion followed by plantarflexion (ankle pumps).

Exercise Choices
1. Isotonic exercise against elastic resistance in midrange for plantar and dorsiflexion (Exercise 9.38): Because there was minimal pain with plantar and dorsiflexion, severity is low and the Grade I tear of the lateral ligament does not require precautions to limit this plane of movement; active movements can be progressed by adding elastic resistance for this patient.
   - Parameters
     - *Dosage:* The resistance can be increased to allow multiple repetitions (>25 repetitions) with or without muscle fatigue to encourage edema removal and muscle pumping. If there is any increase in muscle pain or spasm, the amount of tension on the band and resultant resistance is decreased.
2. Isometric exercise hold against elastic resistance for inversion, eversion (exercise 9.18): Isometrics are used to promote muscle activation and assist with removal of inflammatory by-products.
   - Parameters
     - *Dosage:* In Phase I, the muscle contraction may be limited before muscle fatigue occurs, followed by a few seconds rest. As the patient progresses, the time held and the amount of resistance is increased until there is fatigue of the lateral ankle muscles. The ankle is taped to limit inversion and provide tactile sensory input.

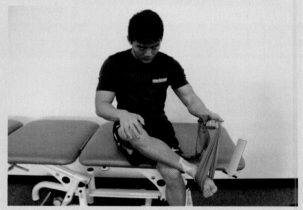

Isometric ankle eversion.

Mobility exercise is intended to increase extensibility of connective tissue and maximize soft tissue elastic and plastic properties.[4] **Elasticity** describes the ability of tissue to deform followed by returning to its initial length after the force is removed. Increased length after the forces are removed is described as **viscoelasticity**. This is more likely to occur if the tissue has a high percentage of fluid content (e.g., in cartilage or disc), but changes may not be permanent. If there is edema and effusion, early techniques to improve mobility should use "pumping" type motions to assist with increasing circulation and removing extracellular fluid, blood, or inflammatory by-products resulting from tissue damage. As improvements in mobility can be related to viscoelasticity or the removal of the excess fluid, there is therefore a need for frequent repetitive motion to keep moving the excess fluid and ultimately restoring some of the range of motion. **Creep** refers to the changes occurring from uncrimping of the wave format in collagen or the ability of the fibers to move relative to one another, often in the toe or linear regions of stress–strain curves.[4] If constant load is placed on a tissue, the tissue will adapt initially and the length will not increase further if the same load is maintained. This property is also important early after injury to keep the collagen moving, to prevent additional cross-linkages forming or the adaptation of collagen if the area is immobile or restricted due to muscle guarding and edema, while also preventing additional inflammation. All of these properties can be applied during Phase I management using exercises that do not place excessive stress or strain on the recently injured structure (Clinical Examples 5.2 and 5.3).

📌 CLINICAL EXAMPLE 5.2 Mobility Exercises: Self-Assisted Range of Motion

Mobility Parameters Week 3

A patient had an anterior cruciate ligament (ACL) reconstruction with a hamstring graft and microfracture surgery for an osteochondral defect from a previous injury. In early rehabilitation (5 weeks postop), she is performing self-assisted knee flexion in prone while still under precautions limiting active flexion due the hamstring graft.[1–3] There is some effusion in the knee, and initial flexion range is 80 degrees. After the exercise, her knee range of motion increases to 95 degrees, but the improvements are temporary and range is the same the next day.

Evaluation

Changes in mobility are most likely related to fluid motion of the effusion: **viscoelasticity.** The goal is to achieve **plastic** or permanent changes until full functional range is achieved.

Mobility Parameters Week 4

As she progresses, the effusion decreases and she is able to reach 110 degrees. During the treatment session, an additional 10 degrees of flexion is retained at the end of the treatment session.

Evaluation

Changes in mobility may be the result of **creep** or alterations in connective tissue crimping and alignment. The range is maintained by the next treatment session (plastic changes).

Mobility Parameters Week 5

After she has been inactive she complains that her knee is "tight." If she holds the self-assisted flexion position for 30–60 seconds repeatedly (up to 3 minutes), 130 degrees is possible and there is progressively less force needed to maintain the position.

Evaluation

This is an example of **stress-relaxation.** There is slight pulling pain with the prolonged stretch, and oscillations are used reaching the full end range followed by a slight release to decrease the pain responses. Changes are still possible with the oscillations using **hysteresis** principles present with oscillations, with less pain.

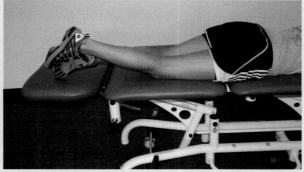

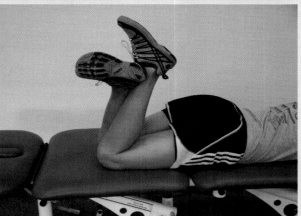

Self-assisted flexion in prone (using the opposite leg to provide passive movement to limit tension on the hamstring graft).

References

1. Wilk KE, Macrina LC, Cain EL, Dugas JR, Andrews JR. Recent advances in the rehabilitation of anterior cruciate ligament injuries. *J Orthop Sports Phys Ther.* 2012;42(3): 153–171.
2. Carofino B, Fulkerson J. Medial hamstring tendon regeneration following harvest for anterior cruciate ligament reconstruction: fact, myth, and clinical implication. *Arthroscopy.* 2005;21:1257–1265.
3. Logerstedt DS, Snyder-Mackler L, Ritter RC, Axe MJ, Godges JJ. Knee stability and movement coordination impairments: knee ligament sprain. Clinical practice guidelines linked to the International Classification of Functioning, Disability and Health from the Orthopaedic Section of the American Physical Therapy Association. *J Orthop Sports Phys Ther.* 2010;40(4):A1–A37.

CLINICAL EXAMPLE 5.3   Sustained Positions and Load for Mobility Improvements

This patient is in Phase I, 2 weeks after a Grade II right medial collateral ligament (MCL) tear after being tackled in a rugby match. There was immediate pain and swelling. He is on crutches and using a brace. There is a 1 cm difference in circumference compared to the left leg at the level of the knee joint and 5 cm above the knee, although the patient reports that the swelling has decreased. He lacks 15 degrees of extension, and there is effusion present (positive ballotment).[1] Effusion often results in the patient assuming flexed positions to avoid the full stretch of the capsule with the potential for connective tissue changes. Even a small amount of effusion also results in quadriceps inhibition,[2,3] further increasing the chance of range of motion loss due to connective tissue changes. Full extension is required for normal gait and balance and is an important reason to regain the normal range as soon as possible.

Precautions
Avoid valgus or rotational stress.

Exercise Choice
Prone knee hangs (Exercise 9.1C) and active isometric extension with a support under the ankle (Exercise 9.1B) are chosen for a home exercise program to regain full passive knee extension. The exercises do not place tension on the medial collateral ligament in the frontal plane with limited joint compression. The isometric contraction also assists with removal of the effusion.

Exercise Testing and Dosage
For the prone knee hangs, the patient is positioned with the knee joint off the edge of the table. A strap-on weight (1.5 kg) is placed on the distal tibia, and the patient is asked to report pain responses while holding as long as tolerated. The patient reports pulling and stretching pain on the posterior aspect of the knee immediately (3/10) that starts to increase after 10 seconds to 5/10. He starts to compensate by rotating his body to the left and flexing the hip. The cuff weight is decreased to 1 kg, which is less painful (1/10) and tolerable for 30 seconds prior to the stretching discomfort increasing. Dosage is set at 30 seconds and 3–5 sets twice a day. The patient is asked to report responses to the stretching (pain, effusion) during, immediately, and for 24 hours afterward.

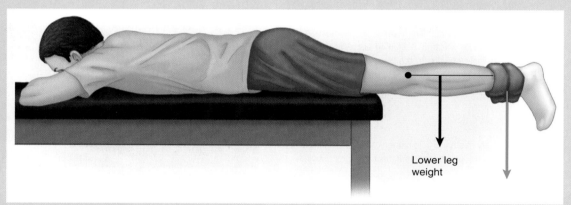

Lower leg weight

Passive knee extension (prone knee hang [Exercise 9.1C]). The unsupported weight of the lower limb and foot segment, with or without an extra weight, assists with stretch of the posterior structures. The knee is extended to the limit and the position is held for as long as possible (up to a minute is desired). The opposite leg is used to lift the leg up if the stretching becomes uncomfortable. Prolonged stretch is useful for a home program if range of motion limitations are starting to become more established or to prevent contractures. A towel underneath the femur can be used to decrease pressure on the patellofemoral region.

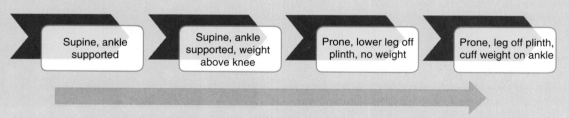

Supine, ankle supported → Supine, ankle supported, weight above knee → Prone, lower leg off plinth, no weight → Prone, leg off plinth, cuff weight on ankle

Progression of parameters to increase load to regain knee extension (prone knee hang)

References
1. Logerstedt DS, Snyder-Mackler L, Ritter RC, Axe MJ, Godges JJ. Knee stability and movement coordination impairments: knee ligament sprain. Clinical practice guidelines linked to the International Classification of Functioning, Disability and Health from the Orthopaedic Section of the American Physical Therapy Association. *J Orthop Sports Phys Ther*. 2010;40(4):A1–A37.
2. McNair PJ, Marshall RN, Maguire K. Swelling of the knee joint – effects on exercise on quadriceps muscle strength. *Arch Phys Med Rehab*. 1996;77:896–899.
3. Rice DA, McNair PJ. Quadriceps arthrogenic muscle inhibition: neural mechanisms and treatment perspectives. *Seminars Arth Rheum*. 2010;40(3):250–266.

During Phase II, the emphasis shifts to increasing the connective tissue length of restricted structures using stress or strain exceeding the yield point in the stress-strain curve (see Chapter 2). **Plasticity** occurs when there is further deformation (strain) or higher stress resulting in more permanent changes. Changes in collagen cross-links, adaptation of fiber direction, and freedom to move relative to fibers contribute to the plastic changes in tissue.[4] **Hysteresis** is another tissue property that promotes permanent improvements in mobility. Hysteresis describes changes that occur when force is applied and released repeatedly.[4] This property is particularly useful when motion is limited by muscle guarding due to pain or if there is concern that the connective tissue is weak. **Oscillations,** or exercises that move toward the end-range followed by movement away from the full tension, are a suitable option for early mobility interventions or to decrease pain.

The length (and strength) of connective tissue depends on the arrangement of collagen fibers, including the number of cross-links between the collagen fibers and the strength of the links (Fig. 5.2). If additional tissue length is required, microfailure of the cross-links, but not macrofailure of the collagen, may be needed. This involves reaching the yield point of the stress-strain curve with a slow buildup of the stress toward the end of the tissue length, but the combination of stress and strain should fall short of the critical failure point (Fig. 5.3). Typically strain (elongation) is applied with low stress in early Phase II to avoid excessive damage (see Fig. 5.3). The careful progression and selection of stress and strain can result in improvements in range of motion without causing complete tissue failure and initiating the inflammatory cycle. Too much stress or strain resulting in

inflammation triggers additional scar tissue formation and thus triggers a vicious cycle of further loss of mobility. **Stress-relaxation** properties describe a decrease in the force needed to maintain the same tissue length when the force is maintained over time.[4] This property depends on the strength of the cross-bridges between collagen fibrils. To obtain more movement, collagen fibrils need to be able to slide past each other without restriction, and longer holds with the same force can result in changes in cross bridges without damage to the collagen fibers (see Fig. 5.2 and Box 5.4). The application of low-load and longer-duration forces *or* oscillations is therefore recommended for early mobility improvements in Phase II. Once tissue has accommodated to initial stress and strain, the force can be slowly increased by increasing either of these options. Mobility exercise can also be progressed by increasing the time held in the full length using stress-relaxation properties. In order to provide sufficient force for connective tissue plasticity without excessive damage, one of these properties should be added at a time.

Body temperature will affect the physical and mechanical properties of connective tissue. Generalized aerobic exercise increases overall body temperature by a few degrees, so is useful prior to specific mobility exercises or can be included during the exercise session to promote cyclical movement to access hysteresis and prepare tissue for joint and soft tissue mobilization.[4] Superficial heating modalities can also be used to increase temperature in areas such as the hands or feet but may not influence deeper muscle and connective tissue in areas where there is more tissue bulk.[4] If the range of motion limitations are related to superficial soft tissue or joint restriction, soft tissue or joint mobilization techniques should be administered prior to exercise.

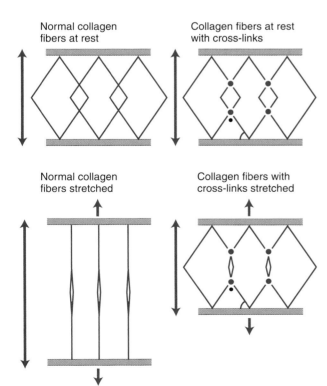

Fig. 5.2 Collagen fiber cross-links in shortened connective tissue. (From Cameron M. *Physical Agents in Rehabilitation.* 4th ed. Philadelphia: Saunders; 2013, Fig. 6.5; adapted from Woo SL, Matthews JV, Akeson WH, et al: Connective tissue response to immobility: correlative study of biomechanical measurements of normal and immobilized rabbit knees. *Arthritis Rheum.* 1975;18:262.)

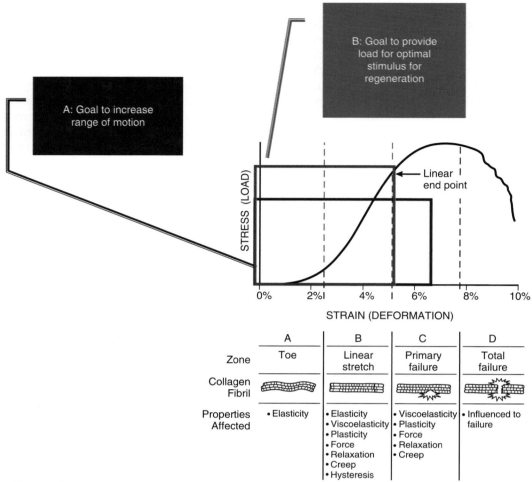

Fig. 5.3 Stress-strain curve goals for improving mobility. (From Magee DJ, Zachazewski JE, Quillen WS, eds. *Scientific Foundations and Principles of Practice in Musculoskeletal Rehabilitation.* St. Louis, MO: Saunders Elsevier; 2007; Fig. 25.11.)

BOX 5.4   Tissue Properties to Use for Increasing Mobility

- **Viscoelasticity**: Tissue deforms and some of the new length remains after the force is removed (applied with repeated movements).
- **Creep**: Holding tissue in a specific position results in changes in length of connective tissue through uncrimping of wave format and changes in cross-links over time.
- **Plasticity**: Deformation when strain or stress exceeds the yield point; results in more permanent length changes than viscoelastic responses (some changes in cross-links).
- **Hysteresis**: Force is applied and released repeatedly with some changes after the cycle of deformation and relaxation (used if there is pain, muscle guarding, or weak connective tissue; applied through repeated range of motion or oscillations).
- **Stress-relaxation**: A decrease in stress needed to maintain the same tissue length when the force is maintained over time (applied through prolonged hold stretching).

Types of Exercise Used to Promote Mobility

Exercise methods to increase range of motion include self-assisted, therapist-assisted, equipment-assisted (pulleys, buoyancy, balls), active range of motion (AROM), active-assisted range of motion (AAROM), or gravity-assisted/eliminated movement (Boxes 5.5–5.7). Mobility exercises often use gravity to assist with obtaining end range in the early phases, progressing to unsupported anti-gravity exercises to obtain functional mobility in the later phases. It may be necessary to assist the range using equipment or to stabilize the proximal area to localize the movement. Types of exercise include self-assisted, therapist-assisted, equipment-assisted, and active movement as well as passive positioning.

Self-Assisted Movement

The patient uses his or her unaffected limb (either upper extremity [Video 5.1] or lower extremity [Video 5.2]) to assist

BOX 5.5 Types of Exercise Used to Increase Mobility

- Self-assisted
- Therapist-assisted
- Equipment-assisted (buoyancy, pulleys, straps, foam rollers, exercise balls)
- Active range (with gravity assistance, elimination, or resistance)
- Positioning for prolonged stretch

BOX 5.6 Mobility Exercise Sequencing and Intensity

- Specific mobility exercises to maintain and maximize mobility gains typically follow generalized aerobic exercise and soft tissue or joint mobilization.
- Individuals with low-severity, low-irritability, chronic conditions, and strong connective tissue are likely to be able to withstand more force, longer holds, and further tension.
- Individuals with high-severity, high-irritability, acute inflammatory conditions, weaker connective tissue, and higher fear avoidance behaviors are more likely to respond to lower forces, shorter holds, and less tension during early exercise intervention.
- Oscillations can be used in the early treatment sessions to address muscle guarding, pain responses, and effusion.

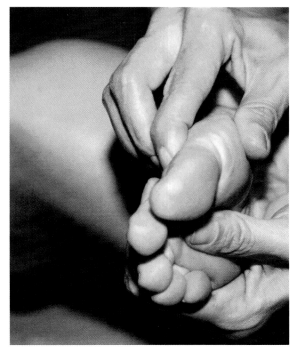

Fig. 5.4 Self-assisted range of motion of the first ray to improve forefoot mobility.

BOX 5.7 Mobility Exercise

- Circulatory exercises, done repetitively, are helpful when mobility is limited by effusion or edema.
- Oscillations (applying hysteresis properties) can be used to address range deficits without increasing pain or muscle guarding and for patients with high-severity, high-irritability, fear avoidance or catastrophizing tendencies, or weak connective tissue.
- Prolonged holds with low load are appropriate for low-severity, low-irritability, and chronic conditions (applying force-relaxation and creep properties).
- Muscle stretching takes the origin and insertion into account to place the muscle at full length. Prolonged hold, contract-relax, hold-relax, or repeated contractions reaching the end range are examples of techniques used for improving muscle flexibility. Recommendations for the amount of time for stretching vary between 15 and 30 seconds, but prolonged holds for up to 60 seconds can also be used.

the affected side to the end of range (Fig. 5.4; see Clinical Example 5.2). The patient is encouraged to increase range as tolerated and taught how to prevent compensations. Equipment such as a dowel rod, towels, belts, or straps may be used to assist the limb. Variations, such as oscillations toward the end of range, prolonged hold, or repeated motion, can be added. A disadvantage of self-assisted exercise is the tendency to compensate as soon as the end of range is reached. Self-assisted exercise is often prescribed as a home program for hypomobility or to maintain range of motion when active motion is contraindicated.

Therapist-Assisted Movement

The therapist can move the patient's limb through the available range without muscle contraction (passive movement

[Video 5.3]), and rhythmic oscillations or back-and-forward movement is a useful type of mobility intervention. Proprioceptive neuromuscular facilitation uses diagonal movement or combinations of patient active motion followed by immediate relaxation with the therapist moving the limb to the maximum range.

Passive movement. Therapist-assisted passive range of motion (PROM) is used to achieve the desired range of motion when active movement is contraindicated (e.g., post-rotator cuff repair) or to maintain range when active movement is not possible (e.g., after neurological damage such as spinal cord or a peripheral nerve injury). If the patient has permanently lost the ability to move his or her limbs, the patient or family may be taught to perform the movements as a home program.[5]

Oscillations. Therapist-assisted oscillations can be used to improve range limited by pain. Oscillations gain range without placing excessive strain on the structure. The repeated movements can decrease pain immediately and may promote intraarticular fluid motion. Oscillations or sustained holds can be combined with joint mobilization techniques through range or at the end of range (Fig. 5.5).[5] Typically, oscillations that do not reach the end of range are used to decrease pain and muscle guarding responses, decrease swelling, or promote joint gliding. Patients who have cartilage degeneration or damage may benefit from joint gliding without compression to provide the motion required to stimulate collagen formation in the superficial zones of the cartilage. Active or active-assisted exercise can also be performed using oscillations in a similar manner.

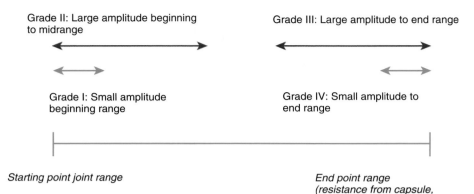

Grade II: Large amplitude beginning to midrange

Grade III: Large amplitude to end range

Grade I: Small amplitude beginning range

Grade IV: Small amplitude to end range

Starting point joint range

End point range (resistance from capsule, muscle, connective tissue)

Fig. 5.5 Maitland's grades of mobilization. (From Hengeveld E, Banks K. *Maitland's Vertebral Manipulation*, 8th ed. Edinburgh: Churchill Livingstone Elsevier; 2014.)

TABLE 5.1	**Diagonal Patterns (Proprioceptive Neuromuscular Facilitations)**	
Upper Extremity	**Shoulder**	**Forearm/Wrist**
D1 Flexion	Flexion, adduction, external rotation	Supination, wrist and finger flexion, radial deviation
D1 Extension	Extension, abduction, internal rotation	Pronation, wrist and finger extension, ulnar deviation
D2 Flexion	Flexion, abduction, external rotation	Supination, wrist and finger extension, radial deviation
D2 Extension	Extension, adduction, internal rotation	Pronation, wrist and finger extension, ulnar deviation
Lower Extremity	**Hip**	**Forearm/Wrist**
D1 Flexion	Flexion, adduction, external rotation	Dorsiflexion, inversion, toe extension
D1 Extension	Extension, abduction, internal rotation	Plantarflexion, eversion, toe flexion
D2 Flexion	Flexion, abduction, external rotation	Dorsiflexion, inversion, toe extension
D2 Extension	Extension, adduction, internal rotation	Plantarflexion, eversion, toe flexion

Data from Cameron MH, Monroe LG. *Physical Rehabilitation. Evidence-Based Examination, Evaluation and Intervention.* St. Louis, MO: Saunders Elsevier; 2007, p 415.

Proprioceptive neuromuscular facilitation techniques (PNF). Hold-relax and contract-relax techniques are forms of PNF involving contraction of antagonistic muscles (muscles opposing the desired movement). These techniques are indicated when muscle length or guarding is limiting joint movement. An isometric or isotonic contraction of the antagonist muscle is followed immediately by relaxing the muscle as much as possible. The therapist takes advantage of the relaxation of the opposing muscles to move the joint to the end range with or without holding the position. The inhibition of the opposing muscles allows the therapist to reach the maximum joint range if there are contributions to the range limitations from muscle guarding[6] (Table 5.1).

Equipment-Assisted Movement

Equipment can be set up using pulleys, exercise balls, or mechanical passive motion devices (continuous passive motion machines). Aquatic buoyancy can be used to assist movement, particularly with flotation devices.

Pulleys (Fig. 5.6A). Pulley systems can be set up to either allow the patient to use his or her unaffected limb to move through range or use the force from the weight to assist the movement (Video 5.4). Pulleys can also be used in place of or to supplement therapist assistance for contract-relax techniques. One of the advantages of using pulleys is the ability to adjust the direction of the force to assist (or resist) the desired motion easily. The pulley can be changed without moving the patient to achieve a different line of pull or resultant force.[7]

Exercise balls, foam rollers, and sliding boards (Fig 5.6B, C). Large or small balls and foam rollers can provide a moving support for a limb to reach end range (Video 5.5). Sliding boards decrease the friction between the limb and the surface. Motion is possible with the limb weight still supported on the surface without resisting gravity and friction.

Continuous passive motion (CPM) (Fig 5.6D). CPM machines are sometimes used in hospital or home settings to provide consistent motion through established ranges. The machines are usually ordered when effusion is limiting range, to provide gentle consistent motion immediately after surgery or trauma. If there is a need for intraarticular motion after surgical procedures such as microfracture, meniscus repair, or tibial plateau fracture fixation, the motion helps to shape cartilage and articular surfaces during healing. Therapists are typically responsible for adjusting the range of motion based on postsurgical protocols and patient responses (range, effusion, pain, and muscle guarding).

Aquatic buoyancy (Fig. 5.7). Aquatic therapy can be used for range of motion exercise using flotation devices and buoyancy to assist movement. There are some precautions and contraindications that preclude aquatic exercise. Patients with open wounds or any type of infectious disease are precluded from aquatic therapy. Most therapeutic pools are heated, and patients who have cardiac, vascular, or respiratory conditions will need to be screened carefully for suitability.

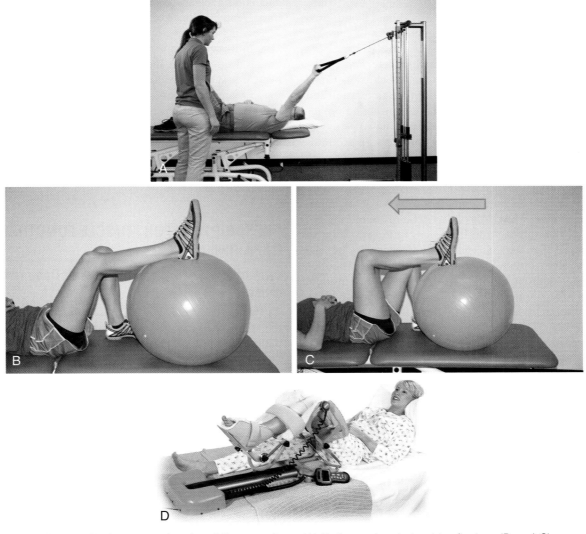

Fig. 5.6 Equipment-assisted mobility exercises. (A) Pulley-assisted shoulder flexion. (B and C) Exercise ball used to support weight of limb and concentrate active knee flexion range in mid- to inner range. (D) Continuous passive motion. (From Cameron M. *Physical Agents in Rehabilitation.* 4th ed. Philadelphia: Saunders; 2013, Fig 9.12. Courtesy of Chattanooga Corp.)

Active Movement (With Gravity Assistance, Elimination, or Resistance)

Active range of motion can be adjusted according to pain levels and ability to achieve end range. If the primary goal is mobility, the most important parameter is to reach end range, with the choice of the load, time spent in the maximal range, and speed influenced by the degree of limitation and pain responses toward the end of range.[7] Positions are selected to use gravity to assist the movement if there is major loss of strength or high pain levels (Video 5.6), while gravity-eliminated (Video 5.7) or -resisted positions (Video 4.10) also provide neuromuscular conditioning. Multiple repetitions, oscillations, or prolonged holds are all possibilities to be considered. Prolonged stretching using gravity or additional load may be used as a home program, especially if there is low irritability. Prolonged holds or sustained positions are also options to consider when there is the risk of connective tissue adaptations after surgical procedures or in the presence of effusion (see Clinical Example 5.3).

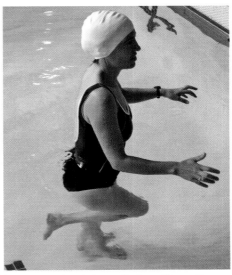

Fig. 5.7 Buoyancy-assisted knee flexion. (From Cameron, *Physical Agents in Rehabilitation.* 4th ed. Philadelphia: Saunders; 2013, Fig 17-10.)

Parameters and Dosage for Mobility

Exercises to maintain or improve mobility should be repeated frequently on a daily basis with adequate force to improve tissue length. The therapist will also need to determine the major components limiting the range when determining the dosage. If range is limited due to edema or effusion (most likely in Phase I), dosage is chosen to improve circulation and assist tissue fluid movement and edema resorption. Low loads and high repetitions using alternating "pumping" type movement with the limb elevated or using compression are indicated until the effusion is resolved. If the limitations are due to joint capsule or soft tissue restrictions, high repetitions or prolonged holds reaching the end range are important. These concepts are similar to the parameters used for joint mobilization.[5] Improving muscle flexibility requires obtaining the full length of the muscle from the origin to the insertion in the direction of the fibers. Stretching guidelines vary but the most common recommendation is to hold the full stretch for 15–30 seconds, although prolonged holds of up to a minute have also been recommended.[1,4] If muscle guarding is limiting the range, contractions followed by relaxation may be indicated (Table 5.2).

The therapist will need to consider the SINS categories, phase of healing, and the overall integrity of the connective tissue when choosing the dosage. Patients who have less severe or irritable chronic conditions are likely to tolerate longer stretching or the greater forces required for plastic changes. Under these circumstances, home programs can include exercises to retain range improvements using prolonged positioning or frequent motion reaching the end range, with the amount of load increased to reach maximum elongation (Clinical Example 5.3). In addition, bracing, splinting, and muscular activation

and endurance in the new ranges can also help retain the improvements (Box 5.6).

Patients who have lower pain tolerance or highly irritable symptoms, who demonstrate fear avoidance behaviors, or who have a diagnosis that suggests a high probability of weak connective tissue require lower forces, shorter holds, or alternating movements that assist with pain relief. The presence of high fear avoidance or catastrophizing will impact how the therapist instructs the patient and the dosage for home programs (see Chapter 6). Applying adequate force and repetitions on a daily basis is important to maintain or improve mobility; frequency is essential and home exercise programs play an important role in the prescription.

PRESCRIPTION FOR MUSCLE FUNCTION IMPAIRMENTS

Type of Exercise, Parameters, and Dosage for Muscle Activation

The first priority for restoring muscle function is to ensure that the appropriate muscles are activating in the desired range, at the right time, and at the correct intensity, essentially training the neuromuscular system initiation and sequencing (Box 5.8 and Table 5.3; Video 3.10). The type of exercise used to elicit the correct activation depends on the existing neuromuscular capabilities and patterns. While muscle activation is often a primary problem after surgical interventions, chronic postural or repetitive strain also present with movement impairments and imbalances requiring goals to change neuromuscular timing and activation.[8] Muscle activation sequencing, intensity, and synchrony are required to address the muscle imbalances often

---

TABLE 5.2 Dosage for Mobility Exercise

Goal	Type of Exercise	Range of Motion	Repetitions	Load
Improve mobility				
Decrease edema or effusion[a] Increase circulation Limit tissue stress	Isotonic: concentric isometric oscillations (pumping frequency)	Does not need to reach extreme range of motion Midrange of joint or muscle position taking into account muscle guarding Progressive increase in range as the edema or effusion decreases	Multiple repetitions >30[7]	Extremely low loads
Improve joint range of motion[b]	Isotonic: concentric oscillations	End of range	High repetitions >25,[4,7] oscillations, short hold, or sustained hold	Low loads
Improve muscle flexibility[b]	Full stretch Contract/relax Hold/relax	End of muscle range Specific direction of muscle alignment	Prolonged hold 15–30 seconds[1,4] OR repeated movement to end of range	Low loads

[a]Position is chosen to assist movement or support movement. Limit pain exacerbation in Phase I or acute trauma where there may be the potential for underlying tissue damage or protective muscle spasm. Pain should decrease with repetitions if mobility is limited by edema or effusion.
[b]Chronic conditions and established range of motion deficits with low irritability and severity, may necessitate more aggressive holds and result in stretching pain.

present with repetitive strain, chronic arthritis, and postural conditions (Clinical Example 5.4).[8]

Often the presence of joint effusion or pain results in neuromuscular inhibition.[9] Muscle inhibition may therefore be important to address for any condition that results in significant joint effusion after surgery, ligament sprains, meniscus or cartilage tears, arthritis, or fractures (see Clinical Example 5.4).[10] Under these circumstances, exercises to reduce the effusion and address pain response may be needed prior to or at the same time as muscle activation interventions. If there is limited muscle activation due to deconditioning or immobilization, the first exercise goal is to facilitate neuromuscular contraction in the desired muscle range. However, if there is any neurological or severe musculoskeletal damage, muscle activation can be more difficult and is likely to be a goal for further out in the rehabilitation time frame. Electrical stimulation, biofeedback and other forms of sensory stimuli during or in addition to exercise are indicated under these circumstances.[10,11]

Early exercise is performed in supported positions or positions that place the target muscles in the optimal position. Mid-position of a muscle commonly provides the most favorable length–tension relationship for eliciting a muscle contraction. Both isometric or small-range isotonic contractions in the desired range are useful. Enhancing sensory input with methods such as muscle facilitation techniques (tapping), hands-on gentle resistance to guide the neuromuscular contraction, or electrical stimulation can also help elicit a contraction.

BOX 5.8 Type of Exercise, Parameters, and Dosage for Muscle Activation

- Neuromuscular activation is the first priority for restoring muscle function.
- Pain and effusion results in inhibition of muscle firing.
- Exercise approaches for muscle activation can be direct (encouraging targeted muscle firing and timing) or indirect (decreasing pain responses or effusion).
- If decreased activation is related to long-term immobilization-related atrophy or nerve damage, muscle activation may be more difficult and time frames will be longer.
- Additional sensory feedback, electrical stimulation, or biofeedback might be indicated.
- Muscle imbalances and neuromuscular coordination deficits sometimes require muscle activation timing and sequencing reeducation; however these interventions are usually only used for a short time.
- Therapist-assisted, self-assisted exercise, eccentric control, or isometrics in the specific range are useful methods to promote range-specific muscle function return.
- Higher-level neuromuscular coordination exercise may require a muscle activation focus for local or global stabilizer function.

TABLE 5.3 Dosage for Muscle Function

IMPROVE STABILITY AND MUSCLE FUNCTION				
Muscle Function	**Contraction**	**Range**	**Repetitions, Load**	**Progression**
Muscle activation	Isotonic: concentric or eccentric Isometric	Protect hypermobile structures (midrange isometrics, small range isotonics in midrange) Hypomobile: isometric or isotonic to end range Range-specific activation	Start with high repetitions, low load Intensity to allow specificity of contraction	Increase sets Increase repetitions Progress to higher loads or longer holds for isometrics
Muscle endurance	Isotonic: concentric, eccentric Isometric	Any range, different loads for different muscle ranges	Low load, high repetitions, 15–30 with muscle-specific fatigue or isometric hold to fatigue >10 seconds	Increase repetitions Increase sets Increase time for isometrics Increase load to allow specific fatigue within 15–30 repetitions
Muscle strength	Isotonic: concentric, eccentric Isometric	Any, different loads for different muscle ranges	Low repetitions 6–10 repetition max (with muscle-specific fatigue) or isometric hold to fatigue	Increase sets Decrease rest time Higher loads
Muscle power	Isotonic: concentric, eccentric	Full range	Low repetitions, high loads	Increase sets Decrease rest time Higher loads Higher speeds
Neuromuscular coordination	Isotonic: concentric or eccentric Isometric control for some muscles to provide support for joints or to maintain alignment	Task-specific, throughout range or in a specific range required for function Multiple planes	Task-specificity and targets Accuracy and form are more important than resistance or repetitions Avoid compensations	Task-dependent Increase complexity Increase time or repetitions

Data from Rivard J, Grimsby O. *Science, Theory, and Clinical Application in Orthopaedic Manual Therapy. Vol I: Applied Science and Theory.* Taylorsville, UT: The Academy for Graduate Physical Therapy Inc., 2009; Riebe D, ed. Exercise prescription. In: Pescatello LS, ed. *American College of Sports Medicine. Acsm's Guidelines for Exercise Testing and Prescription.* 9th ed. Baltimore, MD: Wolters Kluwer Lippincott Williams and Wilkins; 2014:162–343.

CLINICAL EXAMPLE 5.4   Muscle Activation Deficits After Trauma

Patient A

Patient A is being seen in an inpatient acute care setting 1 day after internal fixation of greater trochanter and midshaft femur fractures (Clinical Example 4.10). The intramedullary rod was inserted through the knee and there is significant knee effusion. He reports pain levels of 5/10.

	Assisted ROM	Passive ROM
Hip flexion	30 degrees	65 degrees (pain increases to 6/10)
Hip abduction	20 degrees (assisted)	20 (pain increases to 7/10)
Knee flexion	45 degrees (limited by pain)	20–60 degrees (extension limited by a soft end feel)
		Positive patella tap or ballotment[2]

Precautions

- Touch-down weight-bearing with guarding during initial transfers and gait training
- Monitor blood pressure, pulse, and subjective responses during position changes for orthostatic hypotension
- Avoid force on the distal leg, particularly rotation and angulation
- Monitor bleeding and use universal precautions
- Slow transitions for movement of the leg and motion of the hip and knee to avoid excessive stress, limit bleeding, and allow the patient to accommodate to the new position

He is unable to achieve an active contraction of the quadriceps to straighten the knee and flexes his hip in order to move the leg laterally in the bed. He is having difficulty with bed mobility secondary to being unable to lift his right leg and needs maximal assistance to move the leg to the side of the bed for transfers.

Exercise Choices

To promote quadriceps muscle activation, isometric quadriceps contractions or quadriceps sets in a semi-reclined position with support under the knee (Exercise 9.39) are selected. The therapist places his or her hand underneath the knee joint and asks the patient to straighten the knee while watching the muscle contract. If there is still no contraction, dorsiflexing the ankle can be helpful to facilitate co-contraction and provide a posterior sling support through the gastrocnemius. Other alternatives are to provide passive assistance with terminal knee extension to the limit and gradually remove the amount of support.

- *Dosage:* If the movement is painful, short holds and adequate rest periods are used. The isometrics need to be repeated frequently to assist edema and effusion resolution and to reduce any neuromuscular inhibition.[1] At this point, the number of repetitions is less important than achieving the contraction.

Patient B

Patient B is 23 years old and plays recreational tennis. She is complaining of left hip pain and difficulty lunging for a ball. She presents with a Trendelenburg in single-leg standing, dynamic valgus, and internal rotation of the right leg going up and down steps and in lunges. Right hip abduction is weak in side-lying, and she compensates with her hip flexors to lift her leg against gravity.

Evaluation

She is having difficulty activating the posterior hip external rotators and hip abductors to stabilize the pelvis and maintain the lower extremity alignment.

- *Goal:* Improve hip abductor and external rotator activation and ability to coordinate the pelvic and lower extremity alignment during step-ups and lunges.[2]

Exercise Choices

The following exercises and instructions are chosen to improve selective timing and activation:

1. Hip abduction in supported positions (side-lying) opposing gravity (Exercise 9.26B): The patient is taught to locate and palpate the hip abductors. She is instructed to keep her leg in the natural bony alignment in line with the body rather than letting the leg drift forward into the sagittal plane, which will facilitate the hip flexors.
2. Hip external rotation in side lying using a cuff weight (clam shells [Exercise 9.26A]): The selective use of the hip external rotators is challenged in side-lying using open chain hip external rotation. The open chain exercise does not require balance responses and allows isolation and specific muscle training. The patient is taught to monitor when the body is rotating or if the anterior muscles are used in preference to the posterior gluteal musculature; she can palpate the muscles if needed to provide further feedback.

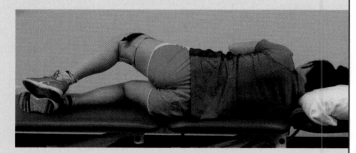

Hip external rotators in side-lying using a cuff weight (clam shells).

Gluteus medius is an external rotator when the hip is flexed and the deep rotators are important to control the lower extremity rotational alignment. In side-lying, rolling the trunk backward allows the patient to use tensor fascia latae and the hip flexors for external rotation. Asking the patient to report the areas where she is fatiguing and observing the movement of the gluteal muscles and trunk is used evaluate the timing and compensations.

Comparison of Patients A and B

Patient A has difficulty with activation of the muscles directly impacted by the trauma from the fracture, bleeding, and the surgical incisions. The activation of multiple muscle groups is important to rectify early, to assist with removal of the edema and hematoma, prevent excessive atrophy, and support the fracture sites. Patient B has isolated muscle activation deficits contributing to neuromuscular coordination deficits and accumulation of force on specific regions. Open chain, isolated exercises are used to teach the patient to activate the correct muscles with less load than required in weight-bearing positions or to activate specific muscles against gravity. For both patients, the muscle activation exercises are used early in the exercise prescription and provide the foundation to progress to muscle endurance goals.

References

1. McNair PJ, Marshall RN, Maguire K. Swelling of the knee joint – effects on exercise on quadriceps muscle strength. *Arch Phys Med Rehab.* 1996;77:896–899.
2. Crossley KM, et al. 2016 Patellofemoral pain consensus statement from the 4th International Patellofemoral Pain Research Retreat, Manchester. Part 1: terminology, definitions, clinical examination, natural history, patellofemoral osteoarthritis and patient-reported outcome measures. *Br J Sports Med.* 2016;00:1–5.

CLINICAL EXAMPLE 5.5 Range-Specific Muscle Activation

Patient A (from Clinical Example 5.4) is 2 weeks post femur fracture and internal fixation. There is still mild to moderate effusion in the right knee (2 cm difference compared to the left at the knee joint, 3 cm at 5 cm above the knee joint). The patient is ambulating with crutches and demonstrates an efficient swing-through pattern maintaining the weight-bearing precautions. His passive knee flexion range is limited to 70 degrees due to pain in the quadriceps, and he still lacks 20 degrees of extension. Active knee extension in sitting with the femur supported on a wedge is possible from 70 to 30 degrees with pain.

He has been performing isometric quadriceps (Exercise 9.39) and hamstring contractions (Exercise 9.40) at home, active heel slides in sitting for knee flexion range (Exercise 9.3), and active hip range (Exercises 9.3, 9.4, and 9.6) in semi-reclined positions. He is still having a great deal of difficulty with short arc quads and open chain knee extension (Exercise 9.43) and straight leg raises for transfers (Exercise 9.42), and he is unable to maintain his knee position in extension. When he is asked to straighten his knee (in sitting with the leg off the edge of the table), he flexes his hip and leans toward the opposite side. He has difficulty activating the quadriceps in maximum extension when the leg is resting on the table and in side-lying. When transferring from supine to sitting off the table, he lifts the leg using the hip flexors with the knee flexed throughout.

Evaluation

The patient has a quadriceps extensor lag (unable to extend throughout the range, although there is full passive range). The end range is the maximally shortened position where the length–tension relationship is the least favorable. There is still the possibility of neurogenic inhibition in the presence of pain and joint effusion.[1] He is attempting to compensate for the lack of knee extension by flexing his hip and laterally flexing his trunk away from his involved side in order to lift the lower leg higher against gravity.

Goals

The overall goal is quadriceps muscle activation to allow full active knee extension in the terminal range followed by endurance and strengthening to allow full straight leg raise for transfers. Specific goals are:
1. During the first two sessions, the patient will be able to activate the quadriceps at 10 degrees with support (isometric) and be able to control the range from 10 to 20 degrees against gravity (eccentric).
2. The patient will be able to activate the quadriceps and identify and correct compensations while performing isometric contractions.

Exercise Choice

1. Active-assisted knee extension (short arc and through available range Exercise 9.43) with assistance from the therapist, followed by self-assisted movement using a strap (Exercise 9.4) through the desired range in sitting with the leg supported. This is followed by isometrics in the available range. The patient is positioned in long sitting with the knee on a small bolster to position it at 20 degrees of flexion (see Clinical Example 3.5).

Dosage

Submaximal dosage without pain reproduction is optimal for early exercise; increased pain may cause further inhibition. The isometric contraction is possible at 20 degrees, with fatigue after 10 seconds. The time set for isometric holds is less than the maximum: 8 seconds, followed by a 10-second rest period. The exercise is continued for a total of 5 minutes. After 5 minutes, the patient is able to actively extend the knee to 10 degrees. The exercise is progressed by changing the position of the knee to 10 degrees of extension and repeated with the same parameters for another 5 minutes.

If activation is needed within a specific range, the therapist or the patient can assist the movement passively, followed by isometric exercise in the given range. The assistance is gradually removed as the patient gains control. If the individual cannot maintain the position against gravity, teaching the patient to move eccentrically with control through the range will help improve neuromuscular recruitment (Clinical Example 5.5). The exercise is progressed from activating the muscle with isometric holds, to eccentric, followed by concentric contractions. The process can be repeated to expand the patient's control through larger ranges of movements. If the patient is substituting other areas or muscles to perform the movement, further explanation or modifying the position or the load can help the patient isolate the targeted muscle or muscles. Because the pressure from edema and joint effusion can result in muscle inhibition, positioning a joint to minimize the effect of intracapsular pressure can also assist a patient with muscle recruitment.

If the activation is needed to overcome muscle imbalances or faulty movement patterns, it is most effective if the patient is positioned so that he or she can observe the muscle while learning how to localize the muscle contraction. Using mirrors for visual feedback can also help the patient to self-correct faulty movement patterns. Tactile stimuli such as props or bands, tape, or balance equipment can be used to promote automatic balance responses. While activating or isolating movements is appropriate during Phase II, the exercises will advance to integrating

BOX 5.9 Type of Exercise, Parameters, and Dosage for Muscle Endurance

- Muscle endurance follows activation parameters or can be used immediately if activation is present.
- Endurance parameters and dosage are often used in rehabilitation to slowly introduce lower loads or for muscles required for postural endurance.
- Endurance dosage involves high repetitions prior to fatigue (>15 repetitions), low loads, or long holds.
- Isometric or isotonic contractions can be used.
- The same exercise can be used to address strength or endurance by manipulating the loads and repetitions.

movement sequences into practicing more challenging and complex functional movement patterns in Phase III.

Type of Exercise, Parameters, and Dosage for Muscle Endurance

Muscle endurance usually follows muscle activation (Box 5.9). If the patient is already able to activate the target muscles, endurance parameters and dosage can be initiated immediately. Often muscle endurance parameters and dosage are used for early muscle stimulus as the loads required are lower than for strengthening and there is less likelihood of connective tissue damage.[7] Lower loads and higher repetitions are also used if a patient's symptoms are severe or highly irritable or when the nature of the problem indicates a more

---

📌 CLINICAL EXAMPLE 5.6   Muscle Endurance Exercise Type and Parameters

Patient A

Patient A has neck pain after a fall skiing (Clinical Example 4.15) with low severity and irritability (Phase II). To address local and global stabilizer endurance, gravity-resisted isometric exercises with prolonged hold are chosen. In the cervical region, the deep neck flexors are directly attached to the anterior cervical spine and counterbalanced by the deep spinal extensors (multifidi, rotatores, transversarii). However, these muscles are small, and, if the amount of load or position requires higher force to support the head weight, using the global movers that are designed to produce higher forces is a natural compensation to meet the functional need. Early exercise is conducted in supported positions to allow local stabilizer muscle activation without the need to stabilize against gravity to reestablish the neuromuscular patterns.[1–3] The patient is taught how to activate the deep stabilizers in supported positions in the early sessions. Once activation is sufficient, exercises are progressed to challenge endurance and improve ability to withstand loads.[1–4]

Exercise Choice

1. Prone forearm support over the BOSU (Exercise 11.26): The patient is observed during the exercise for loss of head and neck position below the level of the body and overuse of the sternocleidomastoid or upper cervical extensors, creating upper cervical extension. After the patient is able to perform the exercise using appropriate neuromuscular coordination, the length of time is tested for dosage. He is able to maintain the position for 30 seconds. Neck pain is monitored during the exercise, and the patient is allowed to rest if there is any increase in pain more than 3/10. The initial dosage is set at 20–30 seconds for 2 sets with a 1-minute rest period.

Progression

The initial progression is to add sets. The exercise is then progressed by decreasing the amount of body support by moving the body forward over the BOSU and challenging the position by lifting one leg at a time or both off the ground while controlling the head position (Exercise 11.27).

Patient B

Patient B had a lumbar laminectomy with residual lumbar spine and left lower extremity pain. He has progressed from lower level exercises and is able to activate his transversus abdominis and spinal extensors to maintain a neutral lumbar lordosis with alternating leg lifts (Exercise 11.21). He is also able to maintain his spinal position with leg lifts in four-point kneeling over an exercise ball (Exercise 11.28). The therapist wants to progress the patient to higher level neuromuscular training and to challenge the global stabilizers in the frontal plane. The lateral flexion endurance position was difficult to maintain due to shoulder pain and the position is adapted to provide support with a bolster under the trunk for a side plank exercise with the knees flexed for the exercise choice.[4] In the adjusted position, he is able to manage 28 seconds for the first set, 32 for the second set, and 22 with abdominal and lateral flexor fatigue.

Evaluation

The side plank (partial [Exercise 11.32]) is possible to meet muscular endurance goals in the frontal plane. The exercise is performed for as long as possible, with 30 seconds rest between sets. The initial dosage is set at 3 sets. This exercise is also used as an impairment outcome measure. If he was not able to tolerate the modified position, the side-lying quadratus lift (Exercise 11.29) is less aggressive and requires less load on the shoulder. When testing new exercises or progressions, it is useful to have more than one option to match the patient's capabilities.

References

1. O'Leary S, Falla D, Elliott J, Jull G. Muscle dysfunction in cervical spine pain: implications for assessment and management. *J Orthop Sport Phys Ther.* 2009;39(5):324–333.
2. Falla D, Jull G, Hodges PW. Feedforward activity of the cervical flexor muscles during voluntary arm movements is delayed in chronic neck pain. *Exp Brain Res.* 2004;157(1): 43–48.
3. O'Leary S, Jull G, Kim M, Vicenzino B. Cranio-cervical flexor muscle impairment at maximal, moderate and low loads is a feature of neck pain. *Man Ther.* 1997;12:34–39.
4. Magill SM, Childs A, Liebenson C. Endurance times for low back stabilization exercises: clinical targets for testing and training from a normal database. *Arch Phys Med Rehabil.* 1999;80:941–944.

---

cautious approach to exercise. Muscle endurance exercises are also important to improve control of joint position and provide postural support (Clinical Example 5.6; Video 3.9). If there is a functional need to maintain a position for prolonged periods, endurance dosage can be used throughout the rehabilitation course.

Muscle endurance parameters involve lower loads that allow higher repetitions before specific muscle fatigue occurs. Typically 15–30 repetitions are used for muscle endurance, approximately 60–75% of a one-repetition maximum[7] (Fig. 5.8). As described in Chapter 3, one-repetition maximum loads are rarely tested or used for rehabilitation purposes. Dosage is tested on the first day, and loads can be estimated from the number of repetitions to failure on the first set using the Oddvar Holten diagram[7] to estimate the approximate loads needed and to avoid having to repeat the testing multiple times if the correct load is not identified in the initial exercise testing (Fig. 5.8).[7] Individuals who have weaker connective tissue due to prolonged immobilization or bedrest and those with multiple comorbidities who are inactive or taking medications that influence connective tissue quality should be started on lower loads, and load is progressed more gradually.[1] However, the aim should still be to provide enough

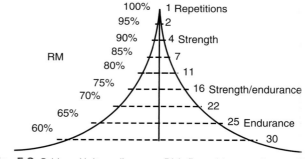

Fig. 5.8 Oddvar Holten diagram. *RM,* Repetition maximum. (From Oddvar Holten of Medical Exercise Therapy [MET].)

resistance to achieve specific muscle fatigue. The number of sets can be progressed prior to increasing load, or the time between sets can be decreased, starting with rest periods of around 2–3 minutes between sets.[7] Isometric contractions can be adjusted by increasing the amount of time that the contraction is held (Clinical Example 5.6; Videos 3.9 and 3.10). The same exercise can be used to address muscle strength or endurance by manipulating loads and repetitions (Video 5.8), and there are times when an exercise program will include some exercises with an endurance focus while others target strengthening (Box 5.10).

Type of Exercise, Parameters, and Dosage for Muscle Strength

The primary types of exercise used for strengthening are movements against body weight resistance or external loads (Boxes 5.10 and 5.11). Muscle strength parameters for rehabilitation purposes involve higher loads and lower repetitions prior to showing signs of fatigue (typically 8–12 repetitions, equivalent to approximately 75–85% of 1RM; Video 5.9).[1,7] If the patient's symptoms are severe or highly irritable or the nature of the problem suggests that a more cautious approach to exercise is indicated, using dosage to target muscle endurance is a safe

---

BOX 5.10 External Resistance Used for Strengthening and Endurance

- Body weight
- Free weights (dumbbells, cuff weights)
- Elastic resistance (bands or tubing)
- Exercise equipment (hydraulic, isokinetic, weight or spring resistance)
- Pulley systems
- Weighted balls
- Weighted bars

BOX 5.11 Type of Exercise, Parameters, and Dosage for Muscle Strength

- Muscle strength dosage involves higher loads and lower repetitions (8–12) prior to fatigue, with 10–15 repetitions for middle-aged and older adults.
- Body weight may be sufficient for strengthening purposes.
- Limb weight and leverage need to be taken into account when selecting the position of the exercise and location of external resistance.
- Specificity of exercises applies to both strength and endurance choices and should consider the range, type of muscle contraction, and requirements for function.
- Progressive increases in load are needed to promote hypertrophy.

---

starting point. The ACSM guidelines also recommend using lower weight to achieve specific muscle fatigue within 10–15 repetitions for middle-aged and older adults.[1] Dosage progression is similar to the options for endurance; the number of sets is increased prior to increasing the load or the time held for isometric contractions.

At times, the weight of the body or limbs against gravity can provide sufficient load for strengthening (see Chapter 2 "Biomechanics" and "Other Parameters Useful for Mobility, Muscle Function, and Neuromuscular Coordination Exercise Position" in this chapter). When selecting the amount of external resistance (weights, elastic bands, equipment, pulleys, balls), the patient's limb weight should also be considered. The position of the limb relative to gravity will also affect the amount of load. Likewise, the length of the patient's limbs and point where external resistance is applied on the limb will influence the length of the moment arm and therefore the overall resistance of the exercise. A patient with long legs will work against relatively greater resistance during leg lifts than a patient with shorter legs because the center of gravity of his or her leg falls further from the hip joint axis of motion. Modifying the distance from the point of application of the force to the axis of movement (the joint) will increase or decrease angular torque for overload and the forces placed on specific structures (see Chapter 2).

Exercise specificity takes the range of motion for the exercise into account because the angle of the muscle influences its capacity to produce force. Therefore, it is important to specify the desired range of motion when prescribing exercise. The starting point is often at the midrange of the muscle and at angles where the muscles is acting on the lever at optimal efficiency, progressing to inner or outer ranges (see Chapter 2). The type of muscle contraction (isometric or isotonic, concentric or eccentric) selected should reflect the patient's functional requirements and provide an optimal stimulus for tissue regeneration (Videos 5.10 and 5.11). The muscles that are responsible for weight-bearing support or movement, particularly those in the lower extremity, require more strength for functional activities than do the upper extremity muscles. In order to achieve muscle hypertrophy, progressive increases in load with one to two days between exercise sessions is recommended (Clinical Example 5.7).[1]

CLINICAL EXAMPLE 5.7 Progressive Resistance Exercise for Muscle Strengthening

Patient A

Patient A is a construction worker with a diagnosis of lateral elbow epicondylalgia. Shoulder muscle strengthening is needed to help develop proximal support and redistribute forces. His work requirements include lifting strips of vinyl siding or a window weighing up to 45 kg.

Exercise Choices

1. Scapula upward rotation and shoulder elevation in scaption against pulley resistance (Exercise 10.23): The therapist chose shoulder flexion against pulley resistance to assist the patient with distributing forces and supporting the upper extremity for holding up the siding. The resistance was determined during initial testing (Clinical Example 4.10; 20 kg, 8 repetitions, 3 sets). The elbow is kept extended with the arm in scaption and slight forearm supination

to minimize the forces on the lateral extensor muscle origins. The wrist is maintained in 20 degrees of extension, neutral deviation, and the patient is instructed to start the exercise from the shoulder rather than leading with the hand.
   - *Specific exercise strengthening goal:* To be able to perform shoulder flexion in the scaption plane against 30 kg (after 8–10 repetitions) for 2–3 sets.
2. Wrist extension strengthening using free weights (Exercise 10.32): Wrist extension is performed using free weights. The exercise is started with the arm supported and the wrist off the edge of the plinth. The weight is selected to target wrist muscle endurance (3 kg for 30 repetitions) and then progressed to a strength dosage (6 kg) with fatigue at 8 repetitions.
3. Shoulder flexion holding a free weight in front of the body: The exercise is then progressed to holding the 6-kg weight with the arm held in front of

Continueued

the body at 45 degrees of shoulder flexion, neutral pro- and supination, and 20 degrees of wrist extension. At this stage, the free weight increases the requirements for wrist and finger extensor activation to simulate the job requirements, while limiting the angulation. Three variations are used: (1) isometric shoulder endurance is challenged by holding the arm in progressive ranges of flexion for as long as possible, (2) isotonic shoulder flexion is performed through the 45- to 90-degree range, and (3) the arm is held in a stationary position in space and combined with squats. If there is any increase in the lateral elbow pain, the patient is allowed to rest for 1–2 minutes until the pain subsides. Each exercise dosage is set separately, and the weight is adjusted until muscle fatigue is experienced in either the wrist extensors or shoulder muscles with 6–10 repetitions.

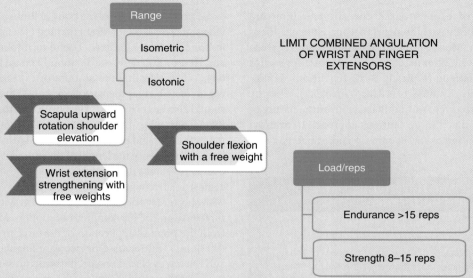

Exercise parameter progression for lateral epicondylalgia.

Patient B

Patient B is a 26-year-old man with anterior shoulder instability. He has full range of motion but reports low levels of pain in full flexion and abduction or any positions behind the frontal plane. He is a previous baseball player and has excessive external rotation and limited internal rotation. He stopped playing college-level baseball a year ago and has been weight lifting and running.

Precautions

Avoid any arm position behind the body; end range combined flexion, abduction, and external rotation; end range horizontal abduction; and end range external rotation.

Exercise Choice

Strengthening exercise parameters and dosage:

1. Shoulder internal rotation (Exercise 10.31): Shoulder internal rotation is started in mid to inner range at 45 degrees of shoulder flexion against pulley resistance. He is able to perform 12 repetitions against 15 kg prior to fatigue. The pulley stopper is set to limit the range to 10 degrees of external rotation.
2. Inner range flys (Exercise 10.24): Inner range flys are performed in sitting with the seat height set so that the shoulder is at 70 degrees of flexion. Mid to inner range is performed with the machine set to limit the range to 45 degrees in front of the frontal plane. He is able to perform 10 repetitions against 25 kg before fatigue of the pectoralis and anterior muscles of the shoulder.
3. Proprioceptive neuromuscular facilitation in standing against sports cord facing away from the attachment (Exercise 10.34): The distance is set to provide moderate tension of the cord in a limited range from 120 degrees of flexion to 50 degrees. The D2 extension, adduction, internal rotation pattern is used.

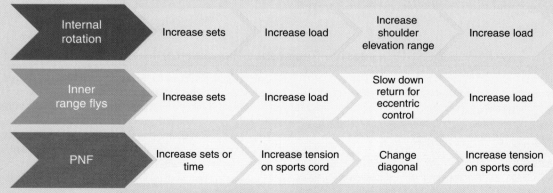

Progression for multiple strengthening exercises used for anterior instability.

Comparison of Patients A and B

Both Patient A and B are started with progressive resistance exercise; however, the precautions related to the repetitive strain injury (Patient A) and hypermobility (Patient B) drive the choices of the type of exercise. Patient A is started with exercise to distribute forces (proximal strengthening) and slow progression of stimulus of the extensor tendon origin with limitation of angulation and full loads in the fully lengthened position. Patient B needs to limit the full stretch of the anterior capsule, and strengthening loads are applied in the inner ranges of shoulder adduction and internal rotation for force closure. Exercises are progressed to include ranges and directions required for their functional requirements: lifting for construction and baseball, respectively.

Type of Exercise, Parameters, and Dosage for Muscle Power

The types of exercise used to increase power include plyometrics, high-intensity resistance equipment, and functional exercise with body weight resistance (Box 5.12). The parameters used for power are high resistance and movement within a short time frame. Power exercises involve closed chain, multi-joint movements occurring at high speed, and multi-joint motion, usually against body weight or high resistance (relative to the individual's capabilities; Video 5.12). Good balance skills, functional range of motion, and the ability to move quickly are prerequisites to this type of training (Clinical Example 5.8).

Plyometrics are a type of power exercise using full lengthening of a muscle followed by a rapid contraction to produce explosive power.[12,13] The tension created during the eccentric, or lengthening phase of the cycle, stores energy and elicits a stretch reflex, which enhances the speed and coordination for a maximal neuromuscular response. Plyometrics are only used in Phase III and once the patient can demonstrate good eccentric control throughout the full range of the movement.

The ability to control momentum or absorb shock is an essential precursor to introducing plyometric activities into a rehabilitation program. There is a risk of injury associated with plyometrics, so this type of exercise should only be introduced if this type of training is necessary to meet a patient's goals. Cipriani[12] advocates initiating plyometric-type exercise in water, which provides more support and less risk of falling. While plyometrics typically involve full-range movements suitable for sports, therapeutic exercise training in submaximal ranges, training in submaximal ranges would be appropriate when trying to mimic functional activities requiring quick changes in direction and quick responses to outside forces in smaller ranges (Videos 5.13 and 5.14).[12]

The appropriate type of muscle contraction, exercise range, and load differs according to muscle function requirements and the stage of rehabilitation. A detailed comparison of parameters and dosage for muscle activation, muscle endurance, strength, power, and neuromuscular coordination is illustrated in Table 5.2.

PRESCRIPTION FOR NEUROMUSCULAR COORDINATION

Exercise used for neuromuscular coordination involves sequencing muscle actions, often with varying goals such as stability in one area while another region is moving to achieve a target or task. Individual exercises or combined functional activities can focus on coordination with progression of planes of movement and achievement of targets or timing (Box 5.13). The progression from simple to more complex movements includes planes of movement, task orientation, changing task demands, and multiple patterns (Videos 5.12–5.17). The complexity can also be

---

BOX 5.12 Type of Exercise, Parameters, and Dosage for Muscle Strength

- Power parameters involve high-intensity exercise in a short time frame and often involve explosive movement.
- Power exercises are only appropriate for individuals who need power for sports or function and have good balance, full functional range, and sufficient strength to withstand the resistance with a slower speed.
- Power is often closed chain, rapid, and involves multiple joints, such as plyometrics.

CLINICAL EXAMPLE 5.8 Exercise Type and Parameters for Power

The patient is a basketball player in Phase III after a Grade I medial collateral ligament sprain and has full knee range of motion and excellent strength. She would like to return to basketball team practice. The power component of her exercise program consists of:

Exercise Choice	Progression
1. Squats with good eccentric control for twice as long as the upward motion, maintaining alignment. The eccentric action prepares for requirements for the landing phase	Increase speed Increase range Emphasis on the upward motion Increase repetitions Increase number of squats within a set time frame
2. Rapid motion squats holding 5-kg dumbbells in each hand above her head, emphasizing the upward motion and performing as many repetitions possible within 2 minutes	Increase repetitions within 2 minutes (speed) Increase sets Increase weight
3. Jumps on a mini-trampoline with an emphasis on the landing technique (absorbing the landing forces through movement)	Jumps on the trampoline are progressed from double-leg to single-leg jumps, then to alternating the landing on one leg, then the other.
4. Squat jumps with an emphasis on height, progressing to repeated squat jumps tracking the number of jumps reaching a height set at 75% of the maximum height in 1 minute	Increase target to maximum height in 1 minute Increase sets
5. Vertical jumps from a countermovement squat position with the emphasis on height and time	Vertical jumps are progressed to single-limb takeoff
6. Run up for 10 meters, followed by a vertical jump, with the time and height recorded	Repeated run up for 10 meters, followed by a vertical jump
7. Timed shuttle runs reaching toward the ground on each turn	Timed shuttle runs are progressed to figure-of-eight runs around cones Timed shuttle runs are combined with vertical jumps as part of the sequence

---

BOX 5.13 Exercise Prescription for Neuromuscular Coordination

- Neuromuscular coordination exercise challenges sequencing of different tasks, progression of planes of movement, grading of movement, or combinations of stability and mobility.
- Progression is from simple to complex, changing order or sequence, to more complex coordination of sequencing with distractions or achievement of targets.
- Compensations should be minimized.
- Neuromuscular coordination goals may be appropriate in any phase.

BOX 5.14 Choice of Position

- Positions can be chosen to provide more or less support and gravity resistance. These choices are important for balance and mobility versus stability focus.
  1. Gravity assistance, elimination, or resistance influences type of muscle contraction and load.
  2. Open or closed chain is used to promote muscle activation or coordination.
  3. The size of the base and position of the body relative to the base can be used to provide more support or increased challenge.
  4. Positioning can be used to maximize muscle activation against gravity or to utilize balance reactions to initiate muscle activity.

---

increased by using external distractions or targets or additional cognitive tasks. Targets for coordination can be used to record the accuracy of movement and provide feedback and goals.

A challenge to prescribing appropriate exercise dosage is the prevalence of compensations. Compensatory movements in other joints occur when a specific muscle group is unable to provide enough force to oppose the given load or torque due to pain or if habitual patterns have been reinforced due to pain or fear. There is a need for neuromuscular coordination goals in both patients with a recent history of injury (Videos 3.14 and 3.15) and those with chronic injuries to prevent adverse patterns from developing. (Videos 4.12–4.14 and 5.18).

The extent of movement alteration is also influenced by the patient's motivation and understanding of the movement. If a patient is compensating, the likelihood of reinforcing these patterns with continued repetition is high, and exercise may not meet the required overload or specificity if compensations are present. As a patient fatigues or if there is pain present, these patterns can present during an exercise. Observation and correction of the movement is therefore extremely important. The presence of pain or fear avoidance behavior plays a major role in the reinforcement of compensatory movement and impacts the choice and delivery of exercise interventions.

To ensure appropriate motion and therefore exercise dosage, the therapist must find ways to teach the patient to use the preferred patterns and not to use other muscles or momentum (Table 5.3). Clear instructions that include methods for patients to monitor their form will assist with specificity. The therapist should also ask the patient for feedback and monitor fatigue in the targeted muscle while the patient is exercising. The motor learning principles related to feedback and practice help the patient attain and retain desired movement patterns (see Chapter 7).

Neuromuscular coordination goals may be appropriate in any phase and involve teaching the patient how to use specific muscles and coordinate the contractions to achieve the required functional movement or activity. The overall control, adjustment, and timing are also important for skilled work- and sports-related goals. There are multiple methods to improve neuromuscular coordination through skilled instruction, goal setting, feedback, and practice, with consistency and efficiency as the goals for this type of exercise. The methods used for this type of goal are described in Chapter 7.

OTHER PARAMETERS USEFUL FOR MOBILITY, MUSCLE FUNCTION, AND NEUROMUSCULAR COORDINATION EXERCISE

Position

Starting positions can provide support or use gravitational forces to increase or decrease load (Box 5.14). Modifying positions can also affect the size of the base of support, increase balance challenge, or target balance reactions. Some considerations for choice of position also involve the functional requirements of the individual.

Gravity Assistance, Elimination, or Resistance

Position relative to gravity can be used to increase range of motion by using gravity to assist or resist movement. Exercises typically progress from a gravity-eliminated position to anti-gravity positions (Video 5.18). Limb or segment weight, the axis of the motion, and the lever arm all influence the overall force and torque placed on tissues with respect to gravity and external resistance (Clinical Example 5.9; see also Clinical Examples 5.4, 5.5, 5.6, and 5.8).

Open or Closed Chain

Open chain exercise is used to target specific joints or when weight-bearing is contraindicated (Videos 2.9, 2.10, 2.16, and 3.10). Closed chain exercises may be used to promote proprioceptive input from joint receptors, to enhance muscular stability around joints, and to facilitate neuromuscular responses for functional movements. Closed chain exercises are also important when there is a need to avoid the shear forces associated with open chain movement (Clinical Example 5.9; Videos 2.24 and 3.13).

Stability and Size of the Base

A large support area or base provides more stability and less challenge for the neuromuscular systems to maintain the body in equilibrium. Positions with a smaller base of support will require more frequent and rapid neuromuscular responses than those with a large base (Videos 2.5, 2.15 and 3.13). The overall size of the base and width or length of the base can be modified to either provide support, challenge stability, or facilitate mobility.

The position of the center of mass or the line of gravity with respect to the base is important when evaluating movement performance. If the line of gravity is outside the base during a stationary posture or position, muscle activity is required on the opposite side to maintain a stable position (Video 3.25). If the intention of the exercise is to promote controlled movement, the line of gravity should fall outside the base, and the movement is assisted by external moments. This concept can be used to bias and encourage the use of muscles opposing gravity and maintaining a static balance or to promote movement and use of momentum by allowing the line of gravity to fall outside the base (Clinical Example 5.10).

If the patient is compensating and using other areas or muscles to perform a desired movement, further explanation may be sufficient to correct the movement. If this is not successful, the position may need to be modified to provide more support or to isolate the movement. In the early phases of rehabilitation, more supportive positions also provide feedback and allow the patient to concentrate on activation or mobility. Compensations

---

CLINICAL EXAMPLE 5.9 Neuromuscular Coordination: Using Balance Principles and the Size of the Base of Support

Patient A

Patient A (from Clinical Example 5.5A) has neck pain after a skiing accident. He is now able to hold his cervical position for more than 60 seconds in the prone forearm support position over the BOSU.

He also has a history of chronic low back pain. In addition to his pain, he is also complaining of having difficulty with balance and carries a cane in case he needs to use it. The patient also has a high fear avoidance behavior score and activities balance confidence scale, requiring slow progression into more unstable standing positions. His exercise program is being progressed using less-stable positions.

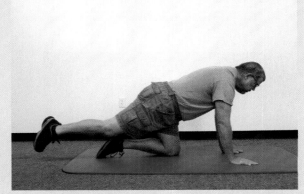

Progression to a less-stable position without the support of the ball.

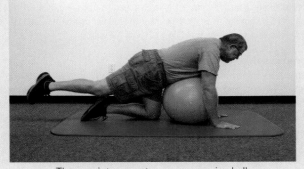

Three-point support over an exercise ball.

The timing of the proximal spinal muscle activity should occur prior to the limb motion to support the spinal structures. The local and global stabilizers will need to be recruited throughout the movement. The less stable the position, the greater the challenge to maintain position. The exercise is progressed to alternating arm and leg lifts

The exercise position requires balance responses to promote activation of the spinal stabilizers and progressively challenge balance reactions.

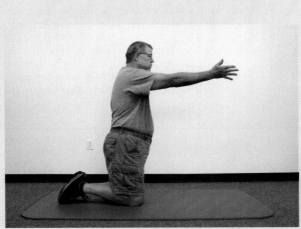
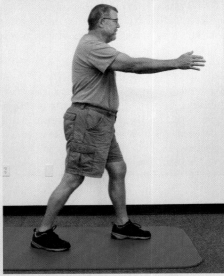

Progression from half-kneeling *(left)*. D, Stride lunge *(right)*.

Continueud

CLINICAL EXAMPLE 5.9   Neuromuscular Coordination: Using Balance Principles and the Size of the Base of Support—cont'd

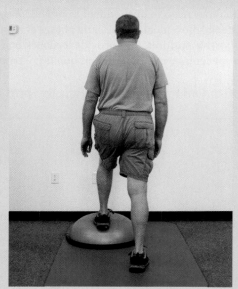

Lunge in standing with unstable base (BOSU).

An unstable base can further challenge stability by requiring muscle activation to maintain balance. Using props such as exercise balls, balance boards, rocker boards, or foam with the choice of position can provide additional challenge for balance reactions.

Patient B

Patient B is an 82-year-old woman with a history of a total knee replacement 10 years ago, cardiovascular and peripheral vascular disease, and diabetes. She has fallen six times in the past year. She has loss of sensation in a glove-and-stocking distribution on both feet up to the mid lower leg and evidence of poor venous return. There is mild effusion in the left leg around the ankle and foot and skin and nail changes consistent with poor peripheral vascular supply. She has limited dorsiflexion range with 10 degree plantarflexion contractures and bilateral hip mobility limitations with hip flexion contractures (10 degrees). She walks with a rolling walker in a forward stooped position that is reversible but results in major sway. Her base of support is very narrow, and she takes small steps following the rolling walker. She is able to stand without support, but any arm or cervical movement results in large amplitude movements and slow balance responses using hip strategies.

Precautions

The patient is at high risk of falls. Guarding during transitions, ambulation, transfers, and standing is essential. Exercises to address impairments will need to be in the most stable position possible. Cardiovascular precautions must include monitoring vital signs and careful observation during exercise for adverse signs and symptoms. Precautions related to diabetes and sensory loss include checking with the patient on her dietary intake, medication use, and symptoms. The loss of sensation requires teaching the patient to use vision and spatial awareness rather than sensory input for lower extremity movement. Visual inspection of the skin and peripheral circulation will be needed at each visit.

Evaluation

The patient has significant balance impairments with multiple contributing factors including loss of sensation in the feet and ankles, generalized limited lower extremity strength and reaction times (particularly foot and ankle neuromuscular function), decreased ankle dorsiflexion and hip extension, and gait patterns and postural positions placing the center of mass outside a small base. Limited overall activity and cardiovascular disease is also leading to generalized inactivity and deconditioning. The multiple cardiovascular and metabolic comorbidities have a negative impact on the overall prognosis and require consistent monitoring. The patient is at a high risk of falls.

Exercise Choice

The exercise program includes strategies to increase the size of her base in standing to provide more stability. Exercises chosen to address some of the contributing impairments (ankle mobility, hip and knee mobility, general lower extremity strength) are performed in stable positions (supine, four-point kneeling, sitting, side-lying) to limit the risk of falling. Functional strengthening and training will also use a wider or more stable base rather than starting with less-stable positions. The patient is encouraged to use the walker to provide some security but not to allow the walker to lead her gait pattern and to keep her feet apart during sit-to-stand and gait with the walker.

Comparison of Patients A and B

Exercises chosen for Patient A are performed in positions to encourage recruitment of the local and global stabilizer muscles to oppose gravity and provide muscle support for the spinal segments. The progression uses different bases of support to challenge the spinal stabilizers in different planes of movement and directions. The progression is also used as a form of graded exercise exposure to build confidence, improve balance confidence, and reduce fear avoidance behavior. Patient B has significant balance deficits, multiple contributing impairments, and is at high risk of falling. Exercise choices need to be in positions where there is limited fall risk, while functional reeducation also involves **increasing** the base of support to reduce the risk of falling. She has permanent loss of peripheral sensory stimuli and will need to learn how to use information from other areas and senses to improve static and dynamic balance.

References

1. Childs JD, et al. Neck pain: Clinical practice guidelines linked to the International Classification of Functioning, Disability, and Health from the Orthopedic Section of the American Physical Therapy Association. *J Orthop Sports Phys Ther.* 2008;38(9):A1–A34.
2. Delitto A, George SZ, van Dillen L, Whitman JM, Sowa G, Shekelle P, Denninger TR, Godges JJ. Low back pain. Clinical practice guidelines linked to the International Classification of Functioning, Disability and Health from the Orthopaedic Section of the American Physical Therapy Association. *J Orthop Sports Phys Ther.* 2012;42(4):A1–A57.

Patient A

Patient A had an anterior cruciate ligament (ACL) reconstruction (hamstring tendon) and microfracture procedure for an articular cartilage lesion of the lateral femoral condyle 6 weeks ago.

Precautions

The microfracture surgery precautions include non–weight-bearing ambulation until 8 weeks. The postsurgical protocol is more conservative than for an isolated ACL tear.[1] Introduction of hamstring exercise has been delayed until 6 weeks.[1,2]

Exercise Choice

Gradual introduction of weight-bearing and range of motion is important to promote healing of the cartilage and bone matrix.[1] Early stimulus of the hamstring muscles using isometrics in mid range is also a goal at this stage.[1,2] The therapist chooses closed chain isometrics in supine at 90 degrees of knee flexion against an exercise ball on the wall to promote muscle activation while adhering to the range and weight-bearing precautions. Between 50 to 100 degrees of flexion limits the amount of load placed on the ACL graft.[1,3] Flexion to 90 degrees also places less compression on the femoral subchondral bone and allows slow progression of intermittent compression and decompression, which is recommended to promote articular cartilage repair.[1,4]

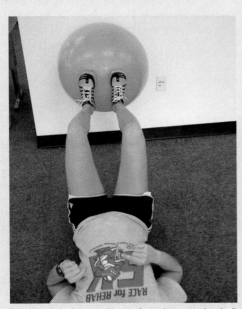

Closed chain isometrics against the exercise ball.

The end point of the lower extremity kinetic chain is in contact with the ball and any motion at one joint results in joint motion higher in the chain. The patient is working to hold the ball still against the wall, so while this is an example of a closed chain exercise, no motion will occur at any joints. This exercise increases the general proprioceptive input, which in turn results in co-contractions of the quadriceps and hamstrings in a flexed position. The unstable base also provides challenge for frontal plane stability at the hip and ankle joints in addition to the knee.

Patient B

Patient B is a college student who fell on an outstretched arm while roller blading. There were no fractures, but she did sustain a ligamentous sprain of the midcarpal region with the possibility of subluxation of the lunate. She has used a wrist splint for the past 6 weeks and is able to start active range of motion of the wrist. Her pain level at rest is 0/10 with mild pain with wrist extension and moderate pain (6/10) with weight-bearing such as pushing off a chair. She has difficulty with heavy household chores (mild), carrying bags (moderate), and is unable to participate in yoga. Her quickdash score is 25. Compared to her right side, she lacks 23 degrees of ulnar deviation, 12 degrees of radial deviation, 6 degrees of flexion, 35 degrees of extension. Her average grip strength of 3 trials is 15 kg whereas the right side is 24 kg.

Precautions

No weight-bearing, cautious increase in force with resistance exercise, limit motion to one plane, avoid functional activities placing excessive force or angulation on the wrist and requiring extreme range. Avoid weight-bearing positions and limit combined extremes of stress and strain.

Evaluation

The patient's primary impairments are limited mobility and decreased grip strength. Severity and irritability of symptoms are relatively mild, but the nature of the problem (palmar wrist ligament sprain with the possibility of lunate subluxation, with 6 weeks of immobilization and need to protect the healing ligaments from excessive stress and strain) and stage (6 weeks post injury, incomplete healing, starting point for restoration of mobility) indicate slow progression within pain tolerance and adherence to precautions.

Exercise Choice

Open chain exercise is indicated due to the amount of wrist extension range and need to limit load with full strain of the palmar ligaments. Exercises to address wrist mobility will reach end range in open chain positions without excessive force or prolonged hold initially. Exercises to address grip strength and upper extremity function will require pain-free wrist range, with a functional position of the wrist (15–20 degrees of extension) to maximize grip but without radial or ulnar deviation. Because she has sufficient wrist extension for the functional grip position, open chain exercise holding a handle can be used to target proximal shoulder endurance and strength for functional tasks.

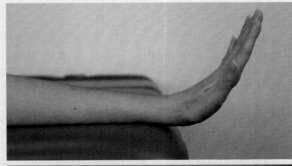

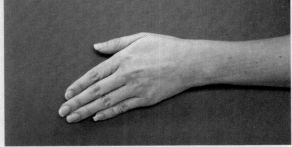

Active wrist movement.

Continued

CLINICAL EXAMPLE 5.10   Use of Open or Closed Chain Parameters—cont'd

Active wrist extension, radial and ulnar deviation is performed to the end range. The goal is to reach end range without holds and to perform multiple repetitions in each plane separately. There is no expectation of fatigue and only mild pain is acceptable.

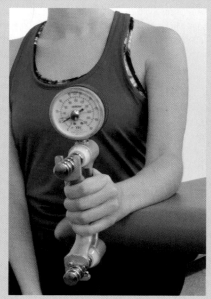

Grip dynamometer.

Active isometric grip is performed with forearm support in a neutral forearm position at 20 degrees of wrist extension. Her initial maximal grip strength was 15 kg (average of 3 repetitions). Dosage is set at 60% of 1 RM: 9 kg for 15 repetitions and 3 sets.

Comparison of Patients A and B

Closed chain exercise offers the advantage of promoting force closure and isometric activation of the quadriceps, hamstrings, and hip stabilizers without excessive strain or shear force on the ACL reconstruction for Patient A.[1,2] The flexed position also limits the amount of direct compression on the microfracture region on the lateral femoral condyle but still allows the pressure on the ball and co-contraction of the muscles to provide low levels of intermittent compression and decompression without body weight. Weight-bearing closed chain exercises, such as squats, leg press, steps and step downs, and lunges performed in greater angles of knee flexion have been advocated for isolated ACL reconstruction to promote general lower extremity muscle function recruitment and are the preferred method to train functional alignment and proprioception.[1,3] However, the microfracture weight-bearing restrictions are most important in the early recovery, and bone or articular cartilage precautions override impairment or functional recovery requirements to promote healing of these structures.[1,4] Open chain knee extension (non–weight-bearing) resistance in ranges between 0 and 30 has been found to result in greater tensile load placed on the ACL.[1,3]

In comparison, Patient B's wrist mobility is limited, and closed chain positions for the upper extremity require at least 45 degrees of wrist extension. The palmar wrist ligaments also need to be protected from full strain to avoid healing in lengthened positions.

In both cases, the primary choice was impacted by precautions and healing requirements for the injured tissue, with the degree of the mobility impairment also influencing choices for Patient B.

References

1. Wilk KE, Macrina LC, Cain EL, Dugas JR, Andrews JR. Recent advances in the rehabilitation of anterior cruciate ligament injuries. *J Orthop Sports Phys Ther.* 2012;42(3): 153–171.
2. Carofino B, Fulkerson J. Medial hamstring tendon regeneration following harvest for anterior cruciate ligament reconstruction: fact, myth, and clinical implication. *Arthroscopy.* 2005;21:1257–1265.
3. Escamilla RF, Macleod TD, Wilk KE, Paulos L, Andrews JR. Anterior cruciate ligament strain and tensile forces for weight-bearing and non-weight-bearing exercises: a guide to exercise selection. *J Orthop Sports Phys Ther.* 2012;42:208–220.
4. Buckwalter JA. Articular cartilage: injuries and potential for healing. *J Orthop Sports Phys Ther.* 1998;28:192–202.

can also be due to too much load, and a more supported position or lower load may be required until muscle function has improved. As edema and joint effusion can result in muscle inhibition, positioning a joint to minimize the effect of intracapsular pressure can assist a patient with muscle recruitment. The mid-position of a muscle provides a more favorable length–tension relationship to allow contraction, and other methods of enhancing sensory input such as muscle facilitation techniques (tapping), hands-on gentle resistance to guide the neuromuscular contraction, or electrical stimulation can be used to obtain a contraction. As patients progress, positions are changed to less stable and more challenging ones, with eventual progression into functional positions.

Speed

Exercises performed at slower speeds are typically easier if the movement is simple or in a supported position. However, controlling the speed of movement against gravity can also impact the difficulty of the exercise and also influence the type of muscle contraction that may or may not be desired for optimal stimulus. Slower, controlled eccentric contractions can be used to provide overload or optimal stimulus for connective tissue and muscle (especially for tendon) regeneration. Faster speeds during more complex movements can result in compensations, so slowing down motion may be necessary to target stabilizing muscles or to ensure proper alignment. Adjusting the speed of exercise is also used to target optimal stimulus for regeneration, neuromuscular coordination, or return to function requiring higher speed in Phase III (Table 5.3).

PRIORITIES AND PROGRESSION RELATED TO TYPE OF EXERCISE, DOSAGE, AND FUNCTIONAL REQUIREMENTS

As discussed in Chapter 1 and illustrated in this chapter's Clinical Examples, precautions override impairment or return to function goals in order to prevent further damage and allow time for tissue healing. The next priority is to provide a slow progression of the appropriate type of load (Table 5.4) to promote

TABLE 5.4   Types of Exercise and Parameters to Provide Optimal Stimulus for Tissue

Target Tissue	Type of Exercise	Range of Motion	Repetitions	Load
Connective tissue: tendon	Isotonic-isometrics or concentric without increasing pain during exercise, progressing to eccentric	Start short to mid-range (of muscle–tendon complex) Progress to full range Length and direction dependent	Multiple repetitions in one plane Start with movements in planes other than the plane of the injured tissue Progress to plane of tissue	Start with low loads Evaluate and minimize strain in Phases I and II by adjusting the lever arm, amount and angle of force Increase higher loads in midrange before providing loads in full functional range
Connective tissue: ligament	Isometric, isotonic	Start in planes other than injured ligament Avoid full tension early in Phases I, II Progress to plane of ligament and increase range	Multiple repetitions	Start with low loads Progress to loads adequate to meet functional requirements
Cartilage	Isotonic Gliding Intermittent compression/decompression	Gliding of joint without weight-bearing Progress from non–weight-bearing to partial weight-bearing (intermittent) to increasing time in full weight-bearing Advance to progressive weight-bearing Distribute forces by ensuring proper muscle support of proximal joints Equalize weight-bearing between both limbs Promote central alignment around joint axis	Multiple repetitions	Low loads Compression/decompression requires alternating contractions Rest periods if necessary
Bone	Vertical loads Muscle attachment tension (isometric–isotonic)	Depends on type of fracture Progress based on stability and angulation		Cancellous bone tolerates lower loads than cortical bone
Muscle • Local stabilizers (postural)	Isotonic or isometric (tonic) Oscillations Maintaining alignment or position	Neutral joint range (mid-range or isometrics throughout range)	Multiple repetitions prior to fatigue (15–30) Multiple sets (can use different exercises with same focus)	Low loads Increase to longer holds
• Global stabilizers	Isotonic or isometric Eccentric contractions are important in end range Maintaining alignment or position Controlling or stopping movement	Neutral joint range to end ranges	Multiple repetitions progressing to less repetitions (10–15)	Larger loads and challenge Multiple joints Complex movement
• Global movers	Isotonic (phasic) Increase speed Propulsion Power Fine-tuned specific movement Eccentric for shock absorption Plyometrics	Throughout functional range if available	Low repetitions (6–10) Increased speed Complex movements Short bursts	Higher loads Direction-specific Increased speed Complex movement

tissue stimulus and recovery without excessive stress and strain (see discussion of stress-strain relationships in Chapter 2). Table 5.5 summarizes the parameters for impairments. There are also relative priorities of impairments that depend on the diagnosis, primary impairments (Chapters 3 and 4), injury mechanism (Chapter 2), and requirements for function (personal factors; Chapter 3).

The implications of hypomobility or hypermobility impairments and injury mechanism are discussed in Chapter 6.

Muscle function parameters will start with muscle activation and build to muscle endurance and finally to strength or power parameters if needed (Fig. 5.9). As the patient moves through the phases of rehabilitation, progression for impairments may be different, and the therapist will need to evaluate the relative contributions of the impairments to functional problems (Clinical Example 5.11). Examples of progression through phases as well as examples of starting exercise at different levels are provided at the end of each section in Chapters 9–11.

TABLE 5.5   Exercise Parameters

Goal	Type of Exercise	Range of Motion	Repetitions	Load
Improve Mobility				
Decrease edema Increase circulation Limit tissue stress	Isotonic: concentric Isometric	Avoid extremes Midrange of joint or muscle position taking into account muscle guarding	Multiple repetitions >30	Extremely low loads
Improve joint range of motion	Passive Assisted Isotonic: concentric	End of range	High repetitions >25, OR sustained hold end of range	Low loads
Improve muscle flexibility	Full stretch	End of range	Prolonged hold 15–30 seconds OR repeated movement to end of range	Low loads
Improve Stability and Muscle Function				
Promote muscle activation	Isotonic: concentric, eccentric Isometric	Protect hypermobile structures (midrange motion) Hypomobile through range	Start high repetitions	Low loads, Isometrics - long holds
Muscle endurance	Isotonic, isometric, concentric, eccentric	Any, different loads for different muscle ranges	High repetitions >15 with muscle-specific fatigue or isometric hold	Low
Muscle strength	Isotonic, isometric, concentric, eccentric	Any, different loads for different muscle ranges	Low repetitions (6–10) with muscle-specific fatigue or isometric hold	Higher than for endurance
Muscle power	Isotonic, concentric, eccentric	Full range	Low reps	Higher than for endurance or strength, high speed
Increase neuromuscular coordination	Isotonic	Task-specific, throughout range, multiple planes	High with task-specificity and targets Goal-dependent accuracy and form more important, avoid compensations	Task-dependent usually low or body weight for function

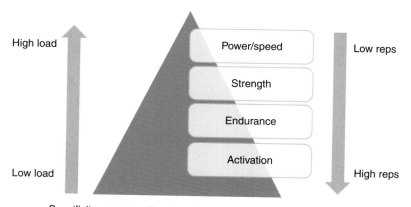

Fig. 5.9 Muscle function progression and priorities.

A patient is referred for management of patellofemoral syndrome and patella tendinopathy. He reports a history of intermittent right knee pain for approximately a year and increasing frequency of symptoms. He has pain in terminal extension and in closed chain squats starting at 45 degrees. There is pain and effusion around the patella tendon with an enlarged fat pad. There is pain and restriction of the lateral retinaculum, iliotibial band, and quadriceps, along with limited gastrocnemius flexibility and bony alignment contributions (tibial varus and torsion, pronation). He has decreased hip muscle activation and endurance contributing to dynamic valgus when squatting, going up and down steps, and jumping.

Evaluation

The patient is in Phase I and SINS is moderate (pain increases to 6/10 going down stairs, running after 15 minutes, or landing from jumps).

Precautions

Limit angulation and rotation in closed chain weight-bearing positions. Limit load in weight-bearing with slow progression of load with knee flexion beyond 30 degrees. Slow progression of combined load and compressive forces (the patella starts to rest within the femoral groove around 20–30 degrees, with greater compressive contact forces as the knee flexes). Avoid full knee extension due to fat pad enlargement.[1–4]

Exercise Choice

Muscle function exercise must progress across phases.

Phase I

Exercise focuses on proximal hip activation and endurance without excessive forces on the patellofemoral complex.[1–3] Open chain hip extension, abduction using the multihip machine (Exercise 9.20), open chain hip external rotation (Exercise 9.26A), and side-lying hip abduction (Exercise 9.26B) are used to teach hip muscle activation and timing, followed by testing for the amount of load the patient can resist for between 15 and 20 repetitions (muscle endurance). As there is no increase in his knee pain, isometric lower extremity activation, endurance, and early load for the patellofemoral complex is introduced using isometric holds on the leg press at 30 degrees of knee flexion. The position is held for 45 seconds against 40 kg. The leg press is advanced by performing two more sets at 45 degrees and 60 degrees prior to starting single-leg exercises on the equipment.

After 2 weeks, his pain has decreased. He has full range in open chain positions with minimal pain in full terminal extension from 5 degrees flexion to 5 degrees hyperextension. His single leg quarter-squat R is painful (4/10, loss of midline

position, dynamic valgus). Line of gravity is maintained behind the knee throughout movement. He is only able to complete 5 repetitions (increased pain to 6/10).

Phase II

The emphasis moves to addressing knee muscle function, progressive weight-bearing activities, and the introduction of specific load on the patellofemoral region. After the patient is able to perform isometrics on the leg press in double-leg positions against loads up to 75% of his body weight in ranges up to 70 degrees, closed chain double leg isotonic motion (70–10 degrees) is started. Elastic resistance is used around the upper thighs to encourage hip external rotator activation to maintain the lower extremity alignment. The weight is decreased by 50% for the single-leg version of the exercise. Double-leg mini-squats (Exercise 9.30) are started with isometrics at 45 degrees with elastic resistance around the upper thigh to maintain hip external rotator activation to limit dynamic valgus and an exercise ball behind his back to provide feedback for alignment with the center of mass over the feet. The isometrics are progressed by increasing range before starting isotonics. The exercise is then progressed by shifting more weight to the symptomatic leg in increments, maintaining the pelvis alignment. When single-leg squats are introduced, parallel bars are used to provide some support and the same sequence is repeated: isometrics starting at 30 degrees, progressing range, then adding isotonics.

Phase III

Exercise is progressed to address the remaining impairments, increase load, progress functional training, and prepare the patient to return to playing basketball.

A greater emphasis and time during treatment sessions is allocated to functional improvement with progressive speed, complexity, and directional challenge. To progress to jumping, he needs to be able to perform single-leg leg press or similar exercises against approximately 150% of body weight for 8–10 repetitions without increasing pain during or after the exercise (within 24 hours), as well as performing single-leg squats without difficulty.[4,5] Similar to the progression in Phase I and II, jumping is started on equipment to decrease the amount of load on the knee. He begins with double-leg jumps on a shuttle, with the range limited to 60 degrees of knee flexion, followed by single-leg jumps. The range of lowering is progressively increased as well as resistance. Jumps are then started on a mini-trampoline (double, then single) prior to starting squat jumps (Exercise 9.51).[5,6] Running and agility drills (Exercise 9.52) are added to drills as the final component of preparation to return to basketball (see Clinical Example 5.8).

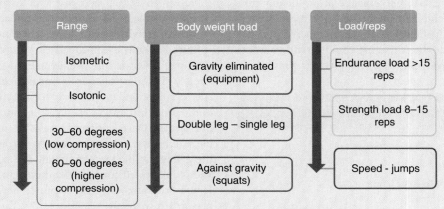

Adjusting parameters over Phases II and III for patellofemoral dysfunction.

References

1. Dolak KL, Silkman C, Medina McKeon J, et al. Hip strengthening prior to functional exercises reduces pain sooner than quadriceps strengthening in females with patellofemoral pain syndrome: a randomized clinical trial. *J Orthop Sports Phys Ther.* 2011;41:560–570.
2. Khayambashi K, Mohammadkhani Z, Ghaznavi K, et al. The effects of isolated hip abductor and external rotator muscle strengthening on pain, health status, and hip strength in females with patellofemoral pain: a randomized controlled trial. *J Orthop Sports Phys Ther.* 2012;42:22–39.
3. Crossley KM, et al. 2016 Patellofemoral pain consensus statement from the 4th International Patellofemoral Pain Research Retreat, Manchester. Part 1: terminology, definitions, clinical examination, natural history, patellofemoral osteoarthritis and patient-reported outcome measures. *Br J Sports Med.* 2016;00:1–5.
4. Willy RW, Davis IS. The effect of a hip-strengthening program on mechanics during running and during a single-leg squat. *J Orthop Sports Phys Ther.* 2011;41:625–632.
5. Silva RS, Ferreira ALG, Nakagawa TH, Santos JEM, Serrao FV. Rehabilitation of patellar tendinopathy using hip extensor strengthening and landing-strategy modification: case report with 6-month follow-up. *J Orthop Sports Phys Ther.* 2015;45(11):899–909.
6. Janssen I, et al. Predicting the patella tendon force generated when landing from a jump. *Med Sci Sports Exerc.* 2013;45:927–934.

Phase I: Exercise Type and Goals (Initial Healing and Resolution of Inflammation)

There are also typical priorities for each phase of rehabilitation. During Phase I, the primary goals are to (1) assist with resolving inflammatory by-products, (2) facilitate healing through increasing circulation to the area while protecting the injured structures from excess force, and (3) minimize the effects of immobility and facilitate muscle activation, if appropriate (Box 5.15; see Table 5.1)

Removing inflammatory by-products and improving circulation require high repetitions with low loads to facilitate generalized circulatory responses and muscle "pumping" to improve vascular return. Positions should support the area, limit stress on the injured region, and, if necessary, provide elevation to assist with removal of edema and effusion. If effusion and edema are present, reducing the localized fluid accumulation is an early priority to improve mobility and decrease pain. The sooner the effusion and edema are resorbed, the quicker the improvements. Precautions to limit stress or strain on the injured structure are a priority, but motion in planes other than the injured structures using active low-intensity isotonic exercise with alternating contractions in relatively pain-free positions or isometric contractions can be used to achieve these goals (Table 5.6).

Deciding which exercises should be included in a home exercise program and when to start exercising without supervision is always individualized to the patient. Assessing the patient's personality and likelihood of doing too much is important in determining the number and difficulty level of exercises. The precautions are addressed first with the patient, particularly for postsurgical or macrotrauma healing precautions. In Phase I, the goals to reduce inflammatory by-products and increase circulation require exercises to be performed frequently as a home program. In addition to pumping or alternating contractions, using compression and elevating the limb are helpful.

Home exercise choices take into consideration the environment, available equipment, and preferences for type of exercise. For example, if the patient has a gym membership or has a stationary bike at home, the therapist could provide a home program utilizing the available equipment versus prescribing simple home exercises using limb weight or elastic resistance. Home program instruction should also include instructions for modifying exercises if pain is elicited or for how to adjust activities of daily living so that there is less stress on injured tissues. Home programs can play a key role in the patient's rehabilitation, especially if there are financial or insurance restrictions on the number of clinical visits. In these cases, the therapist should start planning how to include a home program for the patient very early in the treatment process (see Table 5.4).

Phase II: Exercise Type and Goals (Tissue Repair and Early Regeneration)

Not all patients will start in Phase I; patients with a chronic musculoskeletal condition, a recurrence, or a repetitive strain disorder may start in Phase II. Others will progress from Phase I to Phase II once inflammation has resolved. Goals in Phase II are to (1) address impairments, (2) provide optimal stimulus for tissue recovery, and (3) progress toward return to functional activity (see Table 5.5). The relative contributions of impairments contributing to functional deficits and causative factors are included in the exercise prescription decision-making process.

1. **Impairments** (decreased joint range of motion, muscle flexibility, strength, endurance, aerobic endurance) that influence functional problems are addressed with supervised exercise and supplemented with a home program. The extent of the impairments and the length of time expected for changes to occur will influence which goals are addressed first.

2. During this phase, the amount of load and the force direction are important considerations for providing an **optimal stimulus for tissue regeneration.** The emphasis in Phase II moves from completely avoiding the specific forces that could cause further tissue damage to slowly progressing the forces in the planes of injured tissue. The amount of force and complexity are increased more rapidly for the uninvolved areas that can assist with force distribution.

3. Exercises that incorporate or simulate components of **functional activities** with lower than normal loads are introduced as early as appropriate for the degree of tissue healing.

Home programs are usually needed to provide sufficient frequency of exercise to address impairments, promote optimal tissue regeneration, and reintroduce functional activity. Typically, home programs are necessary for maintaining the range gained during therapy sessions and should be initiated as early as possible. Exercises for endurance and strengthening are included once the patient is able to demonstrate the exercise using good form and is able to self-monitor the dosage to meet the desired goals. Home programs can help reinforce new movement patterns if performed correctly (see Chapter 7). The home program should include parameters such as the desired range, position, load, frequency, and repetitions. The patient must be able to perform multiple repetitions without compensations and with correct form in order to effectively reinforce the desired movement. If patients are taking an active role in their own recovery, they are also more likely to work toward return to their functional activities, and home programs can promote self-efficacy. However, the "no-pain no-gain" attitude does indicate some caution with overall intensity and progression of the home program (Table 5.7).

BOX 5.15 General Goals of Exercise for Phases I to III

Phase I
- Remove by-products of inflammation
- Protect injured structures
- Minimize effects of inactivity and immobility

Phase II
- Address impairments contributing to functional problems (range of motion, flexibility, muscle strength or endurance, cardiovascular endurance, pain)
- Provide optimal stimulus for tissue regeneration
- Promote functional recovery

Phase III
- Address remaining impairments
- Progress load for optimal tissue strength and functional length
- Promote return to functional and sports activity

TABLE 5.6   Goals and Choice of Type Of Exercise During Phase I

Goals	Exercise Choices	Parameters	Elements to Consider	Examples
Increase circulatory supply to region Assist with removal of edema and effusion	Active, low-intensity exercise of other joints around the injured region Alternating active muscle contraction within available and relatively pain-free or low pain-producing range Isometric muscle contraction for short durations followed by relaxation Generalized movement of the affected limb or trunk while adhering to precautions	High repetitions, or as tolerated with larger number of sets (fatigue is not necessary, but movements may be limited by pain) Low loads Complete rest periods Positioning or support for injured area Low complexity Speed as tolerated As tolerated in unaffected areas	Distal joint activity will assist with venous return, particularly if the limb is elevated (e.g., ankle pumps) Only used if likelihood of bleeding is small Active contractions are likely to provide mechanical "pumping" actions for circulation as well as promote movement of extracellular edema or intra-articular effusion Motion of proximal or distal joint or other areas of the body can increase overall circulatory flow and challenge	Straight leg raises without motion of the ankle for a patient after ankle surgery stabilized in a cast boot Ankle pumps Isometric quadriceps and hamstring contractions Bike for patients who are unable to load the lower extremity but are allowed to move the joints
Protect injured structures (precautions)	Avoid placing excessive load on injured tissue or reaching length at which microfailure or macrofailure is likely to occur (see stress-strain curve in Chapter 2) Additional protection may be provided by use of assistive devices, bracing, or taping		Motion without excessive load may be possible in planes other than the anatomical plane in which the injured tissue is located	Ankle pumps (plantar and dorsiflexion in the sagittal plane) may be used to increase circulation and assist with removal of effusion 3 days after an ankle sprain, while the injured lateral ligaments are placed in a mid position using an Aircast brace that limits inversion and eversion
Minimize effects of lack of activity or immobilization (deconditioning)	Generalized activity for other limbs or trunk Specific movements in affected limb, adhering to precautions and guidelines		Mechanisms to minimize muscle atrophy and cardiovascular effects of immobility for the uninvolved regions and general body systems Adhere to precautions and allow healing of the affected structure	Bike, aquatic therapy, or upper extremity ergometer conditioning may be used for lower extremity injuries when weight-bearing is not allowed
Maintain or increase range of motion (ROM) related to swelling, pain	ROM may improve as swelling or pain diminishes, however, there are times when exercises are specifically intended to maintain ROM in order to prevent the consequences of immobility		Passive ROM may be used to maintain ROM while precautions limit active motion due to stress on muscle or ligament	After a rotator cuff tear passive movement is allowed to prevent loss of shoulder ROM, but active use of the rotator cuff is not allowed
Facilitate muscle activation	Specific muscle activation around the injured area may be required to maintain neuromuscular responses		Avoid compensation with other preferred or stronger muscles	Isometric quadriceps contraction is important to provide force closure while a femur fracture heals, but it is very easy to compensate using the hip flexors when performing straight leg raises
Maintain ROM and strength for unaffected areas			Mechanisms to allow movement in other regions and joints include equipment or support	Aquatic therapy, upper body ergometry, upper body and trunk, or uninvolved resistance exercise if the lower extremity is healing or multi-hip strengthening for a knee or ankle injury

TABLE 5.7 Goals of Exercise Phase II

Goals	Exercise Choices	Parameters	Elements to Consider
Address impairments contributing to functional problems			
• Improve range of motion	Active exercises reaching end range Passive positioning or stretch at end range	Position for gravity-assistance/gravity-resistance, if no compensations Reach end range of restricted tissue with short holds, progress to holding at end range or oscillations at end of range	Reproduction of pain response may result in muscle guarding Prolonged stretch or assisted range of motion (AROM) exercise can be progressed by increasing the range or the time held at end range Using oscillations prior to or after the prolonged hold can decrease immediate pain responses Monitor for compensations (shifting alignment or using other joints) when approaching end range and full stretch Stabilizing neighboring joints can assist with isolating desired movements
• Improve muscle flexibility	Muscle stretching reaching end range	End range Prolonged hold, 20–30 seconds	Techniques to inhibit muscle guarding such as hold-relax, contract-relax proprioceptive neuromuscular facilitation Ensure full length of two-joint muscles Isolated stretching of a muscle takes into account the angle of muscle attachments and stabilization of the proximal attachment area Progress range to move toward plastic range
• Facilitate muscle activation	Specific exercises that promote target muscle activation by using anti-gravity positioning, anatomical alignment, or feedback	Specific activation of the muscle High repetitions Low load Appropriate timing of contractions	Address compensations using motor learning principles, visual input, feedback, and isolating the joint or area (as opposed to more complex coordination exercises) Balance activities can be used to promote intrinsic feedback Can use extrinsic feedback with tactile input or props such as elastic resistance, and balls can be used to promote muscle activation
• Improve or maintain muscle endurance	Progressive resistive exercise, active exercise against external or body weight resistance Active exercise against resistance	Load that will allow repeated muscle contraction to fatigue >15 repetitions for isotonic contractions Load sufficient to fatigue for isometric contractions >10 seconds Increase number of sets	Target muscles should fatigue and need to be monitored using self-report and observation of movement patterns (specificity) Monitor for compensations (shifting alignment or using other muscles, particularly larger global movers) when starting to fatigue Progress by increasing repetitions or time held before increasing load
• Improve muscle strength	Progressive resistive exercise, active exercise against external or body weight resistance	Load or resistance to challenge muscle to fatigue for 6–10 repetitions or isometric contractions for <10 seconds Progress load	Starting point and progression of resistance depends on tissue status Monitor for soreness and delayed-onset muscle soreness to assess resistance levels Progress resistance to meet overload principles
• Improve or maintain cardiovascular endurance	General exercise requiring increase in cardiac or respiratory responses	Cardiovascular targets including moderate intensity for 20–30 minutes	Cardiovascular target responses (60–80% age adjusted pulse, progress from mild to moderate perceived exertion)
• Address neuromuscular coordination patterns	Targeted active exercise to promote efficient movement	Motor control concepts (see Chapter 7)	Address compensations due to pain, altered sensory input from connective tissue restrictions, early mechanoreceptor input, habitual patterns, or individual perceptions of desired goal for movement Once desired muscle pattern is achieved, encourage repetition and practice with feedback Progress by removing feedback

TABLE 5.7 Goals of Exercise Phase II—cont'd

Goals	Exercise Choices	Parameters	Elements to Consider
Provide optimal stimulus for tissue regeneration • Provide slow increase in stimulus to injured tissue for regeneration (within tissue capability)	See Table 5.6	Careful positioning is important to promote desired force direction Amount of load will be slowly increased	Slower progression in the anatomical plane of the injured tissue Avoid placing excessive load on injured tissue or reaching length at which micro or macrofailure point is likely to occur (see stress-strain curve) Movements in specific directions may be contraindicated depending on extent of damage and repair Monitor for signs of inability to withstand force: edema, effusion, pain
Promote functional recovery • Promote restoration and improvement of efficient neuromuscular patterns for functional recovery	Simple to complex progressions Single- to multiple-plane progressions Balance and reaction time Functional and sports specific tasks (part to whole)	Smooth, coordinated movement Accuracy is more important than repetitions Practice with feedback, followed by self-monitoring	Motor control concepts (Chapter 7) Practice Use of proprioceptive, visual, auditory feedback Feedback to ensure that desired movement is accurate, without compensations

Phase III: Exercise Type and Goals (Tissue Maturation and Remodeling, Functional Recovery)

Phase II and III often overlap, but the primary focus of Phase III exercises is functional recovery. Any remaining or contributing impairments are addressed, and the exercises should be designed to continue to apply adequate forces to stimulate tissue regeneration. Training should emphasize neuromuscular coordination, advanced strengthening in functional positions and ranges, and muscle and aerobic endurance as needed. If the patient's goals involve higher-level work or recreational activities, this phase may be extended, but some postsurgical protocols include a separate phase for this type of advanced training (Table 5.8).

Some postsurgical protocols subdivide the timelines within Phase II or III and specify prerequisite range of motion or strength achievements for advancing to the next level. In this text, Phase III will cover the criteria for returning to both basic functional activities and advanced sport or physically demanding job duties. However, most patients will be discharged once they have achieved their basic functional goals.

During Phase III, the patient should be returning to his or her pre-injury functional activities, so the frequency of exercise is adjusted if the patient is integrating functional strengthening or sports training into daily activities. Some exercises will need to be discontinued or used less frequently if the goals have been achieved. If more complex or challenging exercises include the subcomponents of Phase II exercises, the earlier exercises can be discontinued. Home exercises may be discontinued if functional activities are providing sufficient challenge, or exercises are advanced to address the range of motion or strength needed for elite performance. The home exercise program should be reassessed at this point, taking into account the personal and environmental considerations described in the ICF model. It is important to ensure that the program is realistic for the patient's lifestyle and motivational level. The patient may be more motivated to continue exercise in a group format or with friends and may need guidance and referrals to appropriate classes or programs in the community. Discharge planning might also include prevention or fitness recommendations.

Chapter 6 expands the information provided in this chapter by comparing and contrasting the choices for general categories for extremes of mobility (hypomobility and hypermobility) and mechanisms of injury (repetitive strain or trauma), as well as discussing the overlapping influence of psychological impairments. These categories are provided to assist with decision-making and establishing priorities for exercise prescription. Additional examples of exercise prescription are provided in the workbook.

TABLE 5.8   Phase III Goals of Exercise

Goals	Exercise Choices	Parameters	Elements to Consider
Continue to address remaining impairments contributing to functional problems or potential factors for injury			
• Improve joint and connective tissue range of motion (ROM) and muscle flexibility	Same as for Phase II	Prolonged hold Range requirements for all functional activities	May not be needed if hypermobility is present, no causative factors or full ROM is achieved ROM should be within functional limits at this stage; however, causative factors may require continuation of this goal into Phase III, particularly for athletes or those performing high-level functional activities to prevent further injury
• Facilitate neuromuscular coordination	Simple to complex progressions Single to multiple plane progressions Balance and reaction response activities	Speed Achieving specific targets	Motor control concepts (see Chapter 7) Practice Use of proprioceptive, visual, auditory feedback Equal weight-bearing and limited compensations should be present prior to more complex multi-planar closed chain movement Monitor for compensations when more complex movements are added to the program
• Improve or maintain muscle endurance	Same as for Phase II	Progress ability to maintain isometric holds Or increase number of repetitions Increased load Increased complexity of movement	Monitor for compensations as functional endurance requirements are advanced
• Improve muscle strength and/or power	Progression to functional strengthening or power Body weight or external resistance Open or closed chain	Progress load to 6–10 repetitions with specific fatigue or power dosage with high speed Progress to functional strengthening	Functional strength or power exercises require full range of motion and ability to perform the movements with less load Equal weight-bearing and limited compensations should be present prior to more complex multi-planar closed chain movement
• Improve or maintain aerobic endurance	Same as for Phase II	Progress duration of activity (time) Increase difficulty or exertion level	
Promote functional activity or sports specific return			
• Improve ability to perform requirements for function or sport	Functional and sports-specific tasks Plyometrics Contact or non-contact activities	Complex coordination and task achievement goals Full ROM Sports- or work-related strength, mobility, endurance-specific activities Increase speed or repetition	Drills Sports-specific practice Use functional tests to establish goals Blocked-to-random practice (see Chapter 7)
Continue to promote optimal stimulus for regeneration			
• Provide optimal stimulus for tissue regeneration (within tissue capability)	See Table 5.6	Increased load Multidirectional and planes	Continue to progress load and direction of forces required for functional movement at higher level

SUMMARY

- Type of exercise describes the exercise, amount of assistance, use of equipment, and type of movement.
- Parameters are those factors that can be adjusted for an exercise to target goals related to the specific impairment or functional deficit. Parameters include the position, dosage, and requirements for function such as complexity, speed, and range of an exercise.
- Dosage is the amount of resistance, number of repetitions, sets, intensity, time, and frequency of exercise.
- Mobility exercise increases the extensibility of connective tissue and maximizes soft tissue's elastic and plastic properties using oscillations or isotonic movement (high repetitions, low load) or flexibility (low load and longer duration of force) reaching the end range. If the major limitation is due to edema or effusion, multiple repetitions using pumping oscillations with very low loads and high repetitions are used without necessarily holding the end of range.
- Dosage for muscle function is different for muscle activation, endurance, strength, and power, with low loads and higher repetitions used for activation and endurance and higher load and lower repetitions used for strength or power.
- Neuromuscular coordination requires task specificity to achieve targets in smooth and controlled movements.

- In Phase I, the primary goals are to remove edema and effusion using low intensity around the injured region, alternating active muscle contractions, isometrics, or generalized motion of the limb or trunk while protecting injured structures and minimizing effects of deconditioning.
- In Phase II, the goals switch to addressing impairments—range of motion, muscle function deficits, cardiovascular endurance, and neuromuscular coordination—along with providing tissue-specific stimuli for regeneration and facilitation of functional recovery.
- In Phase III, exercise is progressed further to address the remaining impairments and provide tissue-specific stimuli while addressing functional goals. The emphasis of this phase is functional training, including practice and refinement of performance.
- Exercise parameters are also aligned with the type of tissue, with isotonic concentric and eccentric exercise used for tendon and connective tissue recovery, gliding and intermittent compression and decompression used for cartilage, and vertical loads and pull from muscle tension used to stimulate bone growth. Muscle stimulus is specific to the muscle's function as a stabilizer or mover.

REVIEW QUESTIONS

1. Differentiate between the types of exercise used for hypermobility and hypomobility. What parameters would be used for each category?
2. Describe exercise parameters appropriate for a patient with postural syndromes.
3. What are the primary considerations when choosing type of exercise and parameters for a patient postsurgery?
4. List the parameters used for goals of exercise for Phases I–III.
5. Differentiate between open and closed kinetic chain exercise and provide examples for when each type of exercise is contraindicated.

REFERENCES

1. Riebe D. Exercise prescription. In: Pescatello LS, Arena R, Riebe D, eds. *ACSM's Guidelines for Exercise Testing and Prescription.* 9th ed. Baltimore, MD: Wolters Kluwer Lippincott Williams & Wilkins; 2014:162–343.
2. Garber CE, Blissmer B, Deschenes MR, et al. American College of Sports Medicine Position Stand. The quantity and quality of exercise for developing and maintaining cardiorespiratory, musculoskeletal, and neuromotor fitness in apparently healthy adults: guidance for prescribing exercise. *Med Sci Sports Exerc.* 2011;43(7):1259–1334.
3. Reese NB, Bandy WD. *Joint Range of Motion and Muscle Length Testing.* 2nd ed. St. Louis, MO: Elsevier Saunders; 2010.
4. Zachazewski JE. Range of motion and flexibility. In: Magee DJ, Zachazewski JE, Quillen WS, eds. *Scientific Foundations and Principles of Practice in Musculoskeletal Rehabilitation.* St. Louis, MO: Saunders Elsevier; 2007:527–556.
5. Maffey LL. Arthrokinematics and mobilization of musculoskeletal tissue: the principles. In: Magee DJ, Zachazewski JE, Quillen WS, eds. *Pathology and Intervention in Musculoskeletal Rehabilitation.* St. Louis, MO: Elsevier Saunders; 2009:487–526.
6. Cameron MH, Monroe LG. *Physical Rehabilitation. Evidence-Based Examination, Evaluation and Intervention.* St. Louis, MO: Saunders Elsevier; 2007.
7. Rivard J, Grimsby O. Science, theory, and clinical application in orthopaedic manual therapy. In: *Applied Science and Theory. Vol. I.* Taylorsville, UT: The Academy for Graduate Physical Therapy Inc.; 2009.
8. Sahrmann SA, Bloom N. Update of concepts underlying movement system syndromes. In: Sahrmann SA, ed. *Movement System Impairment Syndromes of the Extremities, Cervical and Thoracic Spines.* St. Louis, MO: Mosby Elsevier; 2011:1–34.
9. Rice DA, Mcnair PJ. Quadriceps arthrogenic muscle inhibition: neural mechanisms and treatment perspectives. *Semin Arthritis Rheum.* 2010;40(3):250–266.
10. Adams D, Logerstedt D, Hunter-Giordano A, Axe MJ, Snyder-Mackler L. Current concepts for anterior cruciate ligament reconstruction: a criterion-based rehabilitation progression. *J Orthop Sports Phys Ther.* 2012;42(7):601–614.
11. Kim KM, Croy T, Hertel J, Saliba S. Effects of neuromuscular electrical stimulation after anterior cruciate ligament reconstruction on quadriceps strength, function, and patient-oriented outcomes: a systematic review. *J Orthop Sports Phys Ther.* 2010;40:383–391.

12. Cipriani DJ, Falkel JE. Physiological principles of resistance training and functional integration for the injured and disabled. In: Magee DJ, Zachazewski JE, Quillen WS, eds. *Scientific Foundations and Principles of Practice in Musculoskeletal Rehabilitation.* St. Louis, MO: Saunders Elsevier; 2007:432–457.

13. Chmielewski TL, Hewett TE, Hurd WJ, Snyder-Mackler L. Principles of neuromuscular control for injury prevention and rehabilitation. In: Magee DJ, Zachazewski JE, Quillen WS, eds. *Scientific Foundations and Principles of Practice in Musculoskeletal Rehabilitation.* St. Louis, MO: Saunders Elsevier; 2007:375–387.

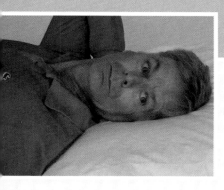

Mobility, Trauma, and Psychologically Informed Concepts for Exercise Choice, Parameters, and Progression

Kim Dunleavy

OBJECTIVES

Upon completion of this chapter, the reader will be able to:
1. Compare and contrast the types of exercise used for hypomobility or hypermobility.
2. Compare and contrast the management of repetitive strain versus traumatic conditions.
3. Discuss exercise choices when applying psychologically informed practice.

4. Use concepts applicable for each category to identify goals and select exercises and parameters.
5. Discuss progression within and across phases of rehabilitation for the exercise categories.
6. Discuss the overlap between categories.

CONCEPTS TO ASSIST WITH CHOICE OF TYPE OF EXERCISE AND PARAMETERS

The guidelines for prescribing exercise in the three phases of healing were discussed in previous chapters. The SINS categories (Severity, Irritability, Nature, and Stage) will also influence decisions about establishing an appropriate intensity for initial exercise testing and for anticipating how rapidly subsequent exercises should be progressed. Building on these concepts discussed in earlier chapters, this chapter will discuss concepts related to extremes of mobility impairments, type of trauma, and circumstances when psychologically informed practice can assist clinical decision-making for exercise choices and approaches (Table 6.1 and Box 6.1). Choices related to impairments on either end of the mobility spectrum leading to dysfunction will be described for *hypomobility* (range of motion or flexibility is less than required for function; mobility deficits)[1] and *hypermobility* (excessive joint and connective tissue mobility or loss of passive restraint systems requiring reliance on neuromuscular coordination[1]; see Fig. 6.1 and discussion in Chapter 3). The *mechanism of injury* will also influence the contributing factors, extent of damage, and need to protect and promote healing for the injured structures. The concepts for choices of exercises to address *repetitive strain disorders* (including postural or alignment contributions from microtrauma)[2-4] and *postsurgical or posttrauma management* (related to macrotrauma)[5,6] will be presented. (See also discussion in Chapter 2.)

An additional concept, *psychologically informed exercise delivery*, is used when psychosocial components (presence of fear avoidance, catastrophizing behaviors, anxiety or depression manifestations) have a major impact on activity and participation limitations (see Chapter 3).

The type of mobility deficit is distinguished using information gleaned from the subjective and objective evaluation, especially selective tissue tension and range of motion tests (see Chapter 4).[1] The mechanism of injury is determined from the history and onset of symptoms. [2-4] The therapist uses observation of patient behavior, subjective pain reports, and self-report instruments to decide if a psychologically informed approach is needed.

These conceptual categories can be used to assist with clinical reasoning and choosing appropriate exercises. Combinations of categories frequently exist simultaneously for different structures and regions.[2,3] For example, a patient with primary hypomobility in the cervical region may have a relative hypermobility at the cervicothoracic junction. A patient with knee instability may present with limited gastrocnemius flexibility. The microtrauma and macrotrauma categories can present with hypomobility or hypermobility depending on the stage of healing. For example, a patient who has an anterior cruciate ligament tear is likely to present with joint hypermobility as a primary category, but, after surgery, effusion limits range of motion and early goals are to restore functional range of motion as soon as possible. Once full range of motion has been achieved, the need to protect the ligament reconstruction during healing becomes a priority, and hypermobility concepts will apply. A patient who has been treated conservatively with a cast and ankle boot for 8 weeks after a fracture is likely to present with ankle hypomobility due to immobilization, and early exercise management to restore range is the main priority along with stimulus for bone healing. In the *Clinical Practice Guidelines* provided by the American Physical Therapy Association Orthopaedic section, diagnoses are now described using movement system labels as the first part of any category, emphasizing the importance of movement considerations.[5–6,7–15] Hypomobility is consistent with mobility deficit classifications in the guidelines, and hypermobility is consistent with loss of force closure requiring improvement in neuromuscular coordination. Not all classification systems use the same terminology, but the concepts can be used to assist with choices.

Psychological factors coexist with the mobility or trauma categories (Fig. 6.2). People with high fear avoidance behaviors or catastrophizing (pessimistic and ruminating thinking) will present with characteristics of any of the four groupings.[16–21] One of the critiques of traditional attempts to classify patient presentations or responses to treatment is not addressing the psychosocial elements of care.[22,23] Exercise selection, parameters, and progression will differ under these circumstances, and the delivery of exercise integrates educational and behavioral modification methods as well as motivational and psychological support.

The main impairments or contributing factors are prioritized after the initial evaluation, and, as patients improve, the reasoning process will continue. The therapist should make frequent adjustments to the type and parameters of exercises selected for their patients. The phases of healing are applied across each of these categories with some commonalities in the type of progression across phase for each category. Other concepts discussed earlier in the text are also applied, such as providing optimal stimulus for regeneration, adjusting biomechanics to distribute forces (see Chapter 2), specificity (see Chapter 5), and linking impairments and function (see Chapter 3). Examples of exercises are included in this chapter, with additional exercises provided in the workbook using the same categories. Though many exercises may be acceptable for a given patient, following these general concepts can guide goals, initial exercise selection and parameters, and progression to provide the most appropriate challenge for each individual (Table 6.1).

HYPOMOBILITY

The presence of **hypomobility** (Box 6.2) or **hypermobility** as a main priority for exercise goals is determined using selective tissue tension and assessing active range of motion and passive physiological and accessory joint motion, as well as performing special tests.[24,25] If the therapist's findings indicate that the primary issue is related to hypomobility, exercises target improvement of range of motion of the affected areas. The primary contributions to the loss of mobility need to be determined in the initial assessment as each area will need slightly different

TABLE 6.1 Categories to Guide Reasoning for Exercise Prescription

Musculoskeletal Condition Category	Description
Hypomobility	Range of motion or flexibility is less than functional requirements
Hypermobility	Excessive joint and connective tissue mobility or loss of passive restraint systems
Repetitive strain/postural syndromes (microtrauma)	Microtrauma: repetitive strain conditions and postural or alignment contributions
Trauma/post surgery (macrotrauma)	Macrotrauma with tissue disruption including postsurgical

BOX 6.1 Categories to Guide Reasoning for Exercise Prescription

- Categories can be used to compare and contrast the concepts used for extremes of mobility and extent of force from trauma.
- Concepts used for extremes of mobility can be compared for hypomobility and hypermobility.
- Concepts can be compared for forces resulting in injury related to microtrauma resulting from repetitive strain and/or postural syndromes and macrotrauma resulting from major trauma and/or surgery.
- Psychological influences can overlap any of the categories.
- Categories are not mutually exclusive for an individual.
- Hypomobility and hypermobility can occur simultaneously within the same individual.
- Repetitive strain injuries often include combinations of hypomobility and hypermobility.
- Traumatic or postsurgical injuries can include hypermobility if there is a loss of ligamentous support, fractures, or meniscal damage, or hypomobility if there is swelling or adhesions resulting from inflammatory responses and immobilization.

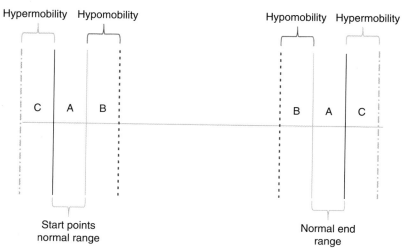

Fig. 6.1 Extremes of mobility impairments: hypomobility and hypermobility concepts. *A*, Normal end feel and joint range; *B*, hypomobility; *C*, hypermobility.

parameters, although all exercises need to progressively reach the end of the available range of motion, with the ultimate goal of improving the range to the functional requirements (Fig. 6.3).

In Phase I, the presence of edema and effusion requires a different emphasis. If edema or effusion is present, the emphasis of the exercise is to provide circulatory stimulus and use muscle activity to provide alternating compression and relaxation to facilitate fluid motion. The use of the "pumping" motion created by active isotonic motion (e.g., pumps), generalized limb motion (e.g., using a bike through range), or isometric contractions with

a short hold, all help with resolution and absorption of fluid that is interfering with normal joint mobility (see Clinical Example 6.1). Mobility exercise involves large- or small-amplitude motion reaching the limits of range with the expectation that (1) moving past the available range is possible and (2) if the effusion and edema are influenced by progressive movement, further range will be possible, even within the same session (Fig. 6.3). Similar to concepts used for joint mobilization, small- or large-range

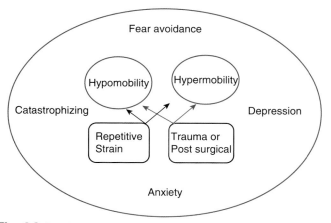

Fig. 6.2 Psychological factors overlapping mobility and trauma categories.

> ### BOX 6.2 Goals, Exercise Selection, Parameters, Sequencing, and Progressions for Hypomobility
>
> - Exercise goals for mobility deficits are to increase range of motion and flexibility to meet functional requirements.
> - Exercise choices include passive, active-assisted, active, self-joint mobilization, and muscle stretching.
> - Manual therapy and aerobic warm-up exercises before mobility exercise are useful to maximize connective elasticity and plasticity.
> - Once mobility has improved, active exercise to retain the newly acquired range is important.
> - Parameters include reaching end range using oscillations or holds at the end of range.
> - Amount of stress and strain is adjusted based on connective tissue status.
> - Early mobility exercises address edema, effusion, and pain with oscillations; Phase II mobility exercises address connective tissue plasticity.
> - Progression of range, hold, sets, and stress is based on responses during and between sessions.

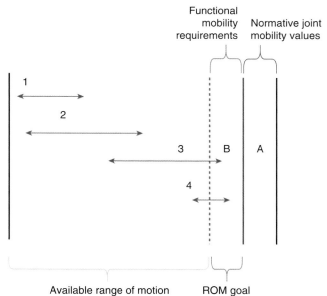

Fig. 6.3 Use of oscillations for hypomobility and mobility goals. Goals for range of motion are set based on functional requirements (B) and take into account age and other personal characteristics, such as body type and muscle bulk. These goals might not be to reach full age-related normative values (A) if the range is not necessary for the patient's functional requirements. Oscillations can be used to address pain responses and guarding in the beginning of range (small oscillations, Grade I; larger oscillations without reaching end range, Grade 2), or reaching the end of the available range (large oscillations, Grade 3; small oscillations Grade 4). If the primary limitation is muscle guarding, the range of motion barrier will change during treatment with progressive mobility toward the functional goal. If the limitation is due to connective tissue limitations, and severity and irritability are low, prolonged stretch or holds are possible.

A 16-year-old female soccer player had anterior cruciate ligament (ACL) reconstruction and meniscus debridement 5 days ago.

Precautions

She is wearing a protective knee brace and is non—weight-bearing on crutches due to the meniscus tear.

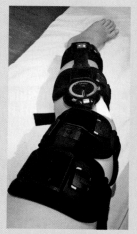

Knee brace to protect the knee from rotation and angulation stresses.

She has a moderate effusion around the knee and edema in the lower leg, with ecchymosis (bruising). Her passive knee range of motion is limited by a soft end feel (15–60 degrees). The edema and blood products move toward the ankle over time.

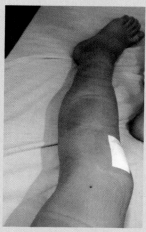

Effusion, edema, and ecchymosis in the lower compartment on day 5.

Evaluation

The patient's mobility limitations are due to the effusion and edema. Phase I goals are to assist with removal of the postsurgical fluid and blood products to prevent permanent connective tissue adaptations and the potential for deep vein thrombosis.

Exercise Choices

Active-assisted and active exercises are used to regain as much range as possible. The mobility exercises are performed in supported positions to limit stress on the knee. Knee extension is performed with the ankle supported on a towel, and the patient provides pressure on the femur. She also assists knee flexion in the same position. Circulatory exercises (ankle pumps) and isometric quadriceps contractions are performed in supine to promote absorption of the extracellular fluids and blood products.

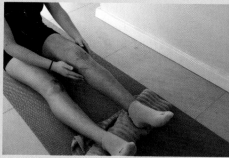

Starting position for self-assisted knee extension range on day 8.

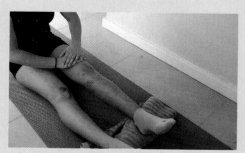

Self-assisted knee extension range on day 8.

The patient places pressure on the femur to obtain a gentle stretch into extension, releases the stretch, and repeats multiple times. Because she tolerates the pressure and there is limited muscle spasm, the stretch is held for longer, working up to a 30-second hold. The ankle placement on a towel provides some gravity assistance. An alternative is to place a light strap-on weight above the knee.

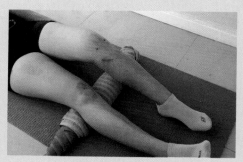

Isometric hamstring contractions at 45 degrees.

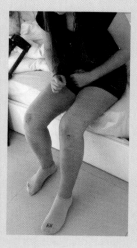

Heel slides (Exercise 9.3) on a tiled surface with multiple repetitions, followed by progressive holds reaching end range.

Reference

1. Wilk KE, Macrina LC, Cain EL, Dugas JR, Andrews JR. Recent advances in the rehabilitation of anterior cruciate ligament injuries. *J Orthop Sports Phys Ther.* 2012;42(3):153–171.

✦ CLINICAL EXAMPLE 6.2 Restoring Mobility: Connective Tissue Restrictions

An 80-year-old woman with knee osteoarthritis and a history of a hip replacement 2 years ago lacks 15 degrees of knee extension. The knee extension limitations are related to joint effusion (Figure 2.7), connective tissue adaptations, and possible bony changes. Her impairments are influencing her functional activities; she has difficulty going up and down stairs and walking and standing for long periods (see Clinical Example 3.1).

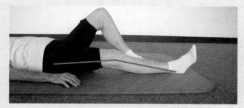

Limited knee extension in supine.

Exercise Choices

To improve knee extension mobility: A non–weight-bearing position is chosen to limit vertical load on the knee. The foam roller decreases friction between the heel and the surface and allows repeated motion without excessive forces. Multiple repetitions of low-load knee and hip flexion and extension (with the emphasis on extension) is used with the intention of providing joint gliding and removal of effusion (Video 2.23). While other equipment options such as using an exercise ball (Exercise 9.4B; Video 2.23) or using a strap to assist extension (Exercise 9.4A) are also good choices, the foam roller allows full knee extension with gravity assistance. The emphasis of the action is on the extension and performing 2 to 3 sets of end range motion.

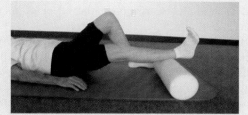

Self-assisted knee extension using a foam roller.

This is followed by passive knee extension with a cuff weight above the knee (Exercise 9.1A), then isometric quadriceps contractions to reach maximal extension and hold for 20 to 30 seconds (Exercise 9.1B) to address the connective tissue restrictions. Other options include a warm-up on a bike with the seat height set to achieve maximal knee extension (Exercise 9.7) and use of joint mobilization techniques in extension before the exercise. Prone knee hangs could also be used as a home program (Exercise 9.1C).

Comparison of Patients in Clinical Examples 6.1 and 6.2

Both patients have some limitation in knee extension mobility due to intraarticular joint effusion related to trauma (Clinical Example 6.1) and repetitive strain (Clinical Example 6.2). The intraarticular fluid volume increases tension on the capsule, and both patients are likely to assume a flexed position to relieve the pressure. Goals to restore full knee extension are therefore important to prevent contractures and further connective tissue changes for both patients, with a more favorable prognosis for achieving full knee extension for the younger patient who had full knee extension before her injury. Both patients have cartilage damage requiring precautions to limit vertical upright weight bearing, although the precautions for the postsurgical recovery after the ACL surgery and meniscus repair require non–weight-bearing for 6 weeks. The patient with osteoarthritis is ambulating without an assistive device, and progression to closed-chain weight-bearing exercises is possible; however, the major priority for mobility exercise is to obtain as much extension as possible, and the supine position uses gravity assistance to encourage full range. The postsurgical swelling and bleeding is also extraarticular and descends into the lower leg with time. The exercises to address overall venous return and removal of the blood products will also include ankle pumps and isometrics in elevated positions. Ankle pumps are not indicated for the patient with osteoarthritis. Active quadriceps contractions (isometrics or isotonics) are indicated for both patients to access any knee extension improvements and to restore activation in the terminal range, an important goal for ambulation.

---

oscillations can also be used to target pain relief and related muscle guarding without reaching the end of available range (Fig. 6.3). Oscillations will take advantage of hysteresis properties, while prolonged holds toward the end of an available or a new range promote connective tissue changes through creep (see Chapter 2). Although edema and effusion related to immediate trauma or surgery are usually addressed in Phase I, if there is articular cartilage damage related to trauma or arthritic changes (osteoarthritis or inflammatory systemic arthritic conditions such as rheumatoid arthritis), intermittent effusion is possible. The presence of intraarticular effusion causes a "balloon" effect, with capsular stretch causing pain and the fluid limiting full joint excursion. With persistent effusion, joint compression or shear forces should be limited (see Clinical Example 6.1).

Many injuries or diagnoses that involve prolonged positioning, protective muscle spasms, or immobilization cause hypomobility. Loss of joint range of motion can be due to prolonged functional positions, pain, or compensations producing capsular tightness or soft tissue shortening. Connective tissue adapts to the direction and amount of stress. If there is repetitive use of a structure in a specific range, the collagen linkages and alignment can become limited over time. Restricted range of motion causes further stress on structures, and a cycle of pain, swelling, and avoidance of motion frequently occurs with joint restrictions.

In Phase II or III, increasing range of motion involves improving the extensibility of muscle, joint capsule, and other connective tissue if these structures are restricted. Exercises used to improve mobility need to reach the end of the available range with some load to achieve permanent length changes (plasticity) (see Chapter 2 for stress-strain concepts). The amount of stress is adjusted based on the individual's personal factors such as age, connective tissue strength, history of disease, and medications, but the emphasis is to obtain maximum length of the tissue (strain) with lower loads to avoid damage and further inflammation. Exercises should reach end range using oscillations (Video 2.23) and progress to prolonged holds (Videos 6.1 and 6.2; see Chapter 5).[25,26] The more established the connective tissue adaptations are, the less change is expected in one session (see Fig. 6.3 and Clinical Example 6.2). As the patient's mobility improves, higher repetition, longer holds, and slow progression of load are indicated to allow adaptations to the stress applied to the tissue.

TABLE 6.2   Type of Exercise for Hypomobility Exercise, Rationale, and Indications

Type of Exercise for Hypomobility	Description	Rationale	Indications
Active-assisted mobility exercises	Gravity-assisted	Gravity provides passive motion without muscular contraction	When active muscle contraction is contraindicated or muscle spasm is limiting movement
	Self-assisted	The opposite limb, straps, or other equipment assist with movement through range	Home programs to increase or maintain mobility
	Pulley-assisted	Pulley systems provide smooth assistance through range	Promote or maintain mobility
	Therapist-assisted	Therapist provides additional assistance at the end of range	Used when active mobility is possible but additional range is required
Active mobility	Gravity-resisted agonist contractions	Active muscle contractions through range against gravity	Regain active mobility through functional range
	Antagonist muscle contraction Hold/relax	Active isometric muscle contraction of muscle opposing direction of limited mobility followed by relaxation and passive motion toward limitations	Used when muscle spasm or loss of flexibility of the antagonist is limiting mobility
	Contract/relax	Active isotonic muscle contraction of muscle opposing direction of limited mobility followed by relaxation and passive motion toward limitations	Used when muscle spasm or loss of flexibility of the antagonist is limiting mobility and there is a need to strengthen the antagonist muscle through range
	Generalized aerobic mobility	Active aerobic exercise (with repeated movement through range using equipment) for generalized mobility	Used for warm-up and/or generalized motion
Self-joint mobilization		Positions or movements to increase joint mobility	Home programs to maintain or increase mobility
Muscle stretching (self-stretch)		Positions or movements to obtain maximal muscle length with prolonged (20–30 second) holds	Home programs to maintain or increase muscle flexibility

Types of exercise used to improve mobility include passive range of motion (Video 4.3) and active-assisted mobility exercises (Videos 1.3 and 1.4), active exercise using gravity (Video 4.3), self-assistance from other limbs (Videos 6.4 and 6.5), or pulleys (Video 5.3) (Table 6.2). In some cases, passive, prolonged stretching or positioning using load is appropriate to address extensive connective tissue or muscle restrictions. Depending on which structures are limiting the motion, range of motion and/or muscle stretching exercises will be indicated. Both require reaching the end of the structural range, with or without holding the position. The direction of the stretch or movement needed to obtain the full length is matched to the anatomical angles and directions of the connective tissue or muscle (Videos 6.6–6.8). If the major limitation to motion is muscle flexibility (or spasm), techniques that involve maximum contraction using isometrics (hold/relax) or isotonics (contract/relax) are used to facilitate the maximum relaxation of the opposing muscle, followed by holding the fully stretched position.

Manual techniques, such as soft tissue (Video 6.6) and joint mobilization, neural mobilization, and joint manipulation are useful before mobility exercises for diminishing pain and improving connective tissue length and mobility. The combination of manual therapy and exercise has been shown to be more effective than manual therapy or exercise therapy alone for mobility deficits in the cervical and lumbar regions.[9,10,27–29] Mobility exercises are usually implemented immediately following therapist-delivered manual techniques or prolonged static stretch to help maintain any newly gained motion. The exception is generalized aerobic activity, which is useful before specific exercise. An overall increase in tissue temperature and generalized cyclical activity is thought to enhance connective tissue viscoelasticity to maximize the effect of manual and stretching techniques.[26]

To retain any gains in tissue extensibility or improved range, it is important to regain active muscular control (with specific emphasis in the newly acquired range). Active range of motion exercises, self-joint mobilization with movement (Video 6.10), and muscle stretching (self-stretch or therapist-assisted stretching) will all address mobility impairments and can all be performed as part of a home program (Videos 4.5, 6.2-6.5, 6.8, and 6.11–6.13). Typically, mobility limitations require home programs to supplement individualized supervised exercise in the clinical setting as repeated movement shapes the connective tissue and helps with resolution of edema. The additional exercise at home is needed to provide sufficient and consistent slow remodeling of connective tissue and improvement in muscle orientation and length (see Clinical Example 6.2). If there is a loss of neuromuscular function, especially with complete damage of neural structures, the likelihood of permanent contractures is high, and consistent passive or active-assisted motion will be important to prevent loss of range[30] (see Clinical Example 6.3). It is important that home exercises are chosen and adapted to reinforce range of motion gains from mobilization and exercise interventions in the clinic. As range of motion increases, exercise goals may also include muscle activation, endurance, and strengthening in the new range. In order to ensure that the targeted tissue is stretched during exercise, the therapist should diligently observe the patient for compensations during exercises and may need to limit motion at proximal structures. Props or positioning may be utilized to localize the stretch, maintain alignment, or assist the patient's kinesthetic awareness of proper end-range stretching of the structure.

CLINICAL EXAMPLE 6.3 Shoulder Hypomobility: Peripheral Nerve Damage

A 44-year-old man was involved in a motor vehicle accident 8 weeks before being referred for physical therapy treatment. He sustained major lacerations in the anterolateral aspect of the cervical region that have healed, but he is unable to move his shoulder actively. On initial evaluation, he is using a sling and is not using his left arm for any functional activities except eating with his arm in a supported position. Initial examination included differential diagnosis of C5–C6 nerve root or upper trunk brachial plexus injury; suprascapular, dorsal scapular, and long thoracic nerve injury; and rotator cuff injury, as well as evaluation of mobility, muscle function, and functional impairments. The patient is referred for further tests to determine the extent and prognosis of the nerve injury. He has significant pain (average 5/10 goes up to 7–8/10) and is unable to sleep through the night. If he takes his arm out of the sling, the pain increases by 2/10 immediately.

Precautions

No long lever stretching or aggressive neural stretching before further workup to establish the extent of nerve damage. Limit stress and strain to within elastic limits.

Evaluation

The patient's impairments include mobility deficits of the left shoulder and cervical region related to posttrauma immobilization and lack of active muscle control, decreased sensation in the left upper arm, and severely decreased muscle activation of the left shoulder (abduction, external rotation, internal rotation, scapula upward rotation and protraction). He has major functional deficits with lifting objects including his baby, dressing, bathing, and household and work activities. Despite the timeframe since his original injury, the patient is in Phase I as there are still signs of acute inflammation, muscle guarding, and severe pain. His symptoms are moderately irritable and the nature of the problem—the traumatic wound and nerve injury—requires further diagnostic workup to determine the extent of the nerve injury and the potential for surgical repair. The lack of neuromuscular function and immobilization have resulted in secondary shoulder mobility deficits.

Exercise and Initial Intervention Choices

1. Manual therapy to improve integumentary and muscle extensibility in the cervical region
2. Manual therapy for the left shoulder (inferior glides, distraction, posterior rotator cuff stretching)
3. Passive and active-assisted exercise choices: (1) Passive and active-assisted flexion, abduction in scaption, and rotation in neutral provided by the therapist (Exercise 10.32). (2) Active-assisted (self-assisted) movement using a pole (Exercise 10.4), pulleys (Exercise 10.5), and self-assisted rotation with the arm supported on a table on a sliding board.

Parameters

- Range is determined by end feel and stopped before guarding or severe increases in pain
- Oscillations to address pain responses
- If there is significant guarding or increased pain, passive physiological motion or accessory glides can be used between sets to relieve pain

Example of Passive Movement

Pendular exercises are performed in the sling (Exercise 10.50). The patient is standing in a forward lean position with the opposite arm supported on a table. He is taught how to create a passive pendular motion by using his legs and trunk to start and continue motion of the shoulder in the sling. The home exercise goal is to provide gentle motion for pain relief and to prevent further loss of range.

Parameters

- Range is determined by patient within pain limits
- Frequent sets throughout the day are used rather than prolonged stretch in one session
- Gentle motion using flexion and circumduction

Evaluation

The patient is observed for compensations (shoulder hiking or elevation and cervical or thoracic motion, as well as monitoring pain responses during and after exercise.

Progression (second visit)

- Gravity-assisted shoulder flexion (prone on plinth; Exercise 10.2)
- Range of the self-assisted flexion is progressed using T bar in scaption (Exercise 10.4)
- Active-assisted flexion in sitting position using latissimus pull-down bar to end range (Exercise 10.32; modification for range assistance)

Reference

1. Wadsworth MK, Mills JT, Michener LA. Diagnosing suprascapular neuropathy in patients with shoulder dysfunction: a report of 5 cases. *Phys Ther.* 2014;84(4):359–372.

Passive movement	Active-assisted movement
Therapist-assisted physiological movement	Supine self-assisted flexion, abduction (wooden pole)
Joint mobilization—accessory and physiological movement with Grade II oscillations	Self-assisted rotation in neutral
Pendular exercises	Pulley-assisted flexion
Prone gravity-assisted flexion, circumduction	Pulley-assisted rotation

Passive and active-assisted movement to address mobility deficits after nerve damage.

As described in Chapter 5, choices regarding positioning for prolonged holds or oscillations are based on pain responses, connective tissue strength, and tolerance to stretching. When using mobility exercise there is always a risk of placing excessive strain beyond the tissue's capability to withstand it and initiating

> ## BOX 6.3   Goals, Exercise Selection, Parameters, and Progression for Hypermobility
>
> - Exercise goals for hypermobility are to improve neuromuscular control (including muscle function and proprioception) to limit excessive range, to promote force closure, and to distribute forces.
> - Exercise type: Closed-chain exercise using isometric and isotonic exercises
> - Exercise parameters: Midrange isometric and small- or specific-range isotonic exercise to address muscle activation, endurance, and strength
> - Isometrics may include alternating contractions, prolonged hold, or maintaining a position with outside challenges.
> - Balance responses, oscillations, and perturbations assist with muscular initiation to maintain a position.
> - Proprioceptive and sensory feedback are important for promoting timely neuromuscular coordination using closed-chain exercises, taping or other tactile input, as well as alternate sensory input from visual and auditory sources.
> - Initial emphasis is to promote activation of local stabilizers for controlling joint position.
> - Functional positions and movements will require loading the global stabilizer muscles and developing control through the range.
> - As patients progress, sequencing the local and global stabilizers before the global movers is needed for functional activities requiring higher loads or speed.
> - Parameters include positioning or active control in midrange, muscle activation, and endurance dosage initially, followed by strengthening and power with appropriate sequencing.
> - Progressing range, hold, sets, and stress is based on responses during and between sessions.

the inflammatory cycle; therefore, it is important to slowly progress the amount of load or tissue length. Major pain exacerbation that lasts after the exercise ends is a negative response, and the intensity or range of the stretch should be decreased. If severity and irritability is low, some stretching discomfort might be acceptable. For patients with higher irritability, techniques are adjusted to limit increasing pain responses. During Phase I, range of motion corresponding to the amount of edema, effusion, or pain is monitored. In Phase II, the emphasis moves to impairment-based exercise, and specific and functional range of motion is measured. Because the ability of the tissue to withstand force is lower in the fully lengthened position, care should be exercised with applying high forces to obtain additional range. (See discussion of the stress-strain curve in Chapter 2.) Mobility exercises are adjusted to further increase or maintain any range improvements while taking into account that connective tissue length changes need some time to become permanent. The rate of progression and amount of force used to gain new ranges should always take the patient's connective tissue status and SINS factors into account (see Clinical Examples 6.1–6.3).

HYPERMOBILITY

Types of Hypermobility

Hypermobility (Box 6.3) or excessive range (Fig. 6.4) is related to impaired form closure due to structural abnormalities, connective tissue laxity, traumatic damage, or growth-related changes.[31–32] Degenerative joint changes can present with hypermobility due to narrowing of cartilage or disc spaces and hypermobility.[33] Approximately 10% of the population have been described as having generalized hypermobility associated with weaker or less elastic connective tissue.[34] Inadequate neuromuscular support can also contribute to hypermobility. During and after pregnancy, one in three pregnant women complain of back pain (Videos 6.14 and 6.15),[35] and increased mobility of peripheral joints related to

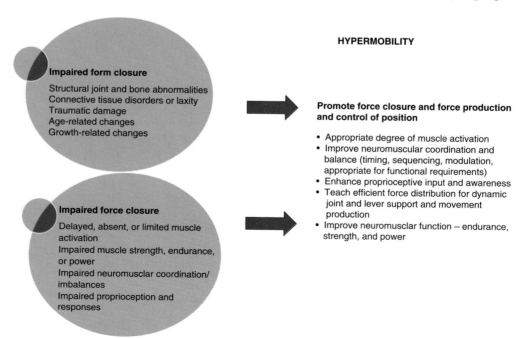

Fig. 6.4 Hypermobility (form and force closure) and exercise approaches.

hormonal changes is present throughout and after pregnancy[35,36] (see Clinical Example 6.4). Hypermobility can be generalized in the presence of congenital laxity or connective tissue disorders such as Ehlers-Danlos syndrome[37] (Clinical Example 6.5), or specific, such as previous ligament and capsule damage (e.g., anterior shoulder instability; see Clinical Example 6.6).[38] Structural abnormalities such as hip dysplasia will also present with increased mobility and breakdown of stabilizing connective tissue or joint structures from altered biomechanics.[39] Under these circumstances, information from the medical history will assist with early hypotheses.

History and Presentation

The typical history for a patient who has hypermobility is a slow progression of symptoms without a specific incident. Others are able to identify previous trauma resulting in ligament or connective tissue damage. Hypermobility due to microtrauma or microtrauma requires testing for ligament and capsule integrity.

Hypermobility may present with aberrant (uncoordinated) movements or movement compensations.[9,10,40] If the passive or inert restraint system is lax or missing, excessive joint motion occurs beyond the normal range. If the individual is able to control the area using the active systems, this may not be symptomatic.[41-43] Typically, hypermobility is problematic if there is insufficient neuromuscular control and forces are transmitted to joint structures,[1] with the subsequent risk of micro- or macro-injury when forces are applied to a local area.[32,44-46] Not all individuals who present with hypermobility are symptomatic, but the presence of hypermobility can be problematic over time.[47] Joint

---

CLINICAL EXAMPLE 6.4 Hypermobility: Pregnancy

A 30-year-old woman is 6 months pregnant and is complaining of low back pain. Her pain is worse with prolonged standing, going up and down stairs, and moving from sitting to standing (Video 6.15).

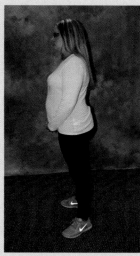

Standing posture during pregnancy.

The patient will need to be educated on the optimum balanced position and to take frequent breaks, rather than placing stress on the structures for prolonged periods.

Precautions

Exercise management should take into account the increased connective tissue laxity related to increasing hormonal levels during pregnancy. Toward the last trimester, all ligaments and tissue become more extensible, and the weight and position of the baby increases the stress on the lumbar spine. The baby starts to drop into the pelvis, and the sacroiliac relationships adjust to provide space for the baby. Stretching of muscles attaching to the pelvis and lumbar spine is discontinued. Exercise is also limited to sitting, standing, or side lying as lying supine for prolonged periods is contraindicated. As the biomechanical and hormonal influences are time-limited, exercises are intended to maintain support to the end of term.

Implications of Pregnancy for Exercise Choices and Education

The baby's weight pulls the lumbar spine into an increased lumbar lordosis. There is also limited support from the stretched abdominal muscles working in the end range and with additional resistance and pressure from the baby's weight. The stress on the posterior lumbar spine stretches the iliolumbar and sacroiliac joint ligaments that are more extensible due to the increasing hormonal levels in the last trimester. Active muscle support from the abdominal, gluteal, and

pelvic floor muscles becomes more important for force closure of the sacroiliac and lumbar spine joints. The ability to maintain the isometric support for longer periods becomes progressively more difficult with the changing dynamics, and therefore exercise is aimed at maintaining support and building the ability to provide active support for short periods.

Exercise Choices

Exercise focuses on activation of the abdominals and pelvic floor to support the spinal and lumbopelvic structures (Video 6.16). Double-leg, closed-chain positions with bilateral isometric activation and overall core stability are preferred to single-leg exercises. Single-leg lower extremity movements toward end of range in open- or closed-chain positions are more likely to result in transfer of stress to lumbopelvic structures. Exercise focus is on distributing forces through active muscle control and avoiding extreme ranges as much as possible to limit additional tension on the stretched structures.

Movement Reeducation

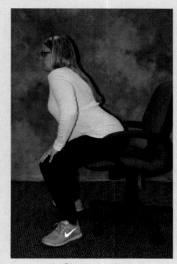

Sit to stand.

Movement reeducation for transferring from sit to stand is provided to decrease the axis of motion in the lumbar spine as she stands up (Video 6.15). Note the increased lordosis as the patient moves her body forward. The hips are externally rotated to accommodate the baby's position. She is using her hands to assist with the momentum and vertical movement, relying primarily on the hip musculature to lift her body weight. She is instructed to move her body weight as far forward on the edge of the chair as possible and to engage the abdominal and pelvic floor muscles before initiating the movement using her hips and knees.

CLINICAL EXAMPLE 6.5 Generalized Laxity: Ehlers-Danlos Syndrome

A 30-year-old patient presents with intermittent low back and knee pain. During the initial examination, he reports that he is very flexible. He has a Beighton scale score of 8/10, and excessive laxity of his skin and joints. There are no other positive special tests except for excessive range of motion and muscle flexibility. He has no history of trauma. General exercise prescription would follow guidelines for the hypermobility category (Table 6.3; Type of Exercise, Table 6.4 Exercise Parameters).

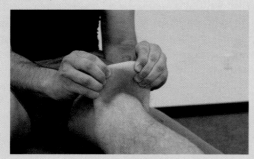

Excessive skin laxity.

Beighton Scale[1,2]
Test positive score (+1)
1. Passive extension 5th finger: Greater than or equal to 90 degrees

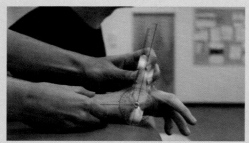

Passive extension.

2. Passive hyperextension elbow: Greater than or equal to 10 degrees

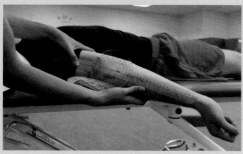

Passive hyperextension elbow.

3. Passive hyperextension knee: Greater than or equal to 10 degrees

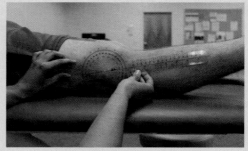

Passive hyperextension knee.

4. Opposition of the thumb to the forearm: Full contact to forearm

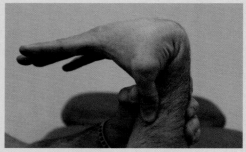

Thumb opposition.

5. Trunk flexion in standing: Palms to floor

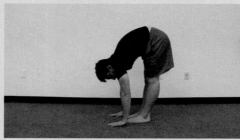

Trunk flexion to floor.

Items 1–4 are measured bilaterally; item 5 contributes 1 point for a total score out of 9. Scores of 0–2 indicate no generalized hypermobility, 3–4 mild hypermobility, 5–9 major hypermobility.

References
1. Magee DJ, Sueki D. *Orthopedic Physical Assessment Atlas and Video: Selected Special Tests and Movements.* 6th ed. St. Louis, MO: Elsevier Saunders; 2011.
2. Van der Giessen LJ, Liekens D, Rutgers KJ, Hartman A, Mulder PG, Oranje AP. Validation of Beighton score and prevalence of connective tissue signs in 773 Dutch children. *J Rheumatol.* 2001;28(12):2726–2730.

degeneration can be a long-term consequence of hypermobility, especially when there is limited structural support, such as with hip dysplasia[48] or after traumatic joint damage.[5] Evaluation of the possibility of generalized or specific hypermobility is part of the full objective examination and includes the Beighton score[47] (Clinical Example 6.5), comparison of active and passive range to normative values, end feel, and specific special tests.[24,25,49,50]

Hypermobility can also be relative to other areas of hypomobility, with stress on the segments that move first or most.[3] Often the hypomobility in other areas contributes to increased stress in these areas of vulnerability, resulting in a cycle of dysfunctional mechanics and concentration of forces in the hypermobile region. Specific laxity is also a possibility if there is overuse in extreme ranges of motion, a situation often related to sports or work activities (see Clinical Example 6.6). If there is an acute traumatic onset with partial loss of some of the supporting structures, precautions will be necessary to keep the structures in a mid- to shortened position during healing (see Clinical Example 6.7).

CLINICAL EXAMPLE 6.6   Anterior Laxity of the Glenohumeral Joint Related to Overuse

A 28-year-old woman has generalized shoulder pain with a slow increase of symptoms over the past 6 months. She works out using a home exercise video and at the gym. She was a gymnast until 16 years old. She has excessive shoulder flexion and external rotation in higher level ranges. There is no pain with the movement but she reports low levels of pain the day after weight lifting. Her weight-lifting program involving the shoulders includes bench press with dumbbells, push-ups, burpees, chest press in sitting, biceps and triceps exercise with free weights, lateral raises, latissimus dorsi pulldowns, and punches with free weights. Her passive flexion is excessive compared to the left side in supine, and external rotation exceeds the left shoulder by 20 degrees (110 degrees). Joint play is greater for the right shoulder with mild apprehension and muscle guarding with horizontal abduction, external rotation. She has extremely good strength.

Evaluation

The patient has hypermobility of the right shoulder with greater anterior laxity.

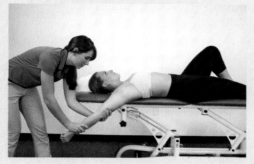

Specific hypermobility related to training (previous gymnastics). Passive flexion range in supine is excessive on the right.

Exercise Choices

For anterior instability: Closed-chain exercises are used to promote proprioceptive training along with strengthening parameters in the mid- or inner range. As she is working out regularly, her program is started at a higher level than someone who is not as active. Balance and unstable positions are also used to train scapulothoracic and glenohumeral muscle coordination with an emphasis on muscle endurance and maintaining force closure. The initial exercise tolerance is evaluated using progressively more challenging positions.

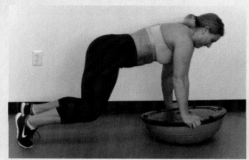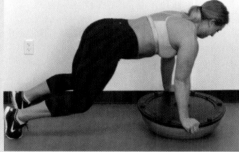

Plank with unstable surface. She is able to hold the position for up to 25 seconds.

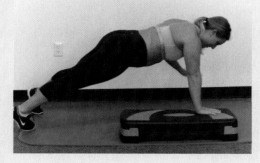

Plank with one-hand lift off a step.

Evaluation

The additional challenge with one-arm support on a step is more difficult, and she is unable to maintain her scapula connection and head position with the arm lift. If she is unable to correct the position with cueing, the same exercise is attempted without a step. If she is still unable to maintain the position with good scapulothoracic connection, the full plank using the BOSU is used with multiple sets as the primary exercise and progressed to weight shifting and motion of the BOSU to challenge neuromuscular coordination and endurance.

CLINICAL EXAMPLE 6.7 Hypermobility: Anterior Shoulder Dislocation

A 25-year-old man sustains an acute anterior shoulder dislocation while playing ice hockey. He slammed his shoulder into the boards, and the shoulder immediately dislocated. His shoulder was relocated in the emergency department, and he is presently using a bolster sling to protect the shoulder. He is referred for isometric stabilization and assisted range of motion 2 weeks after the injury.

Precautions
No horizontal abduction, especially with external rotation (recreating the anterior dislocation position). Midrange isometric and small-range isotonic exercise with low loads.

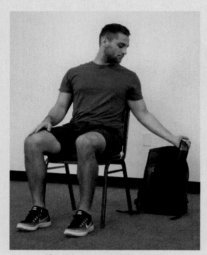

Positions to be avoided.

The opposite arm is used to demonstrate the positions to avoid during dressing and with functional movements. Lifting a backpack off the ground behind the body, dressing with the injured arm behind the body, and using the arm behind the back are all positions that will place excessive strain on the anterior shoulder.

Exercise Choices
Initial Choices: Isometrics With Alternating Rhythmic Stabilization
The patient is taught to use self-assisted motion to place the arm on a foam pad at 50 degrees of flexion in front of the body to limit stresses on the anterior shoulder. With the arm supported, a slow buildup of resistance in multiple directions provides stimulus for muscle activation. This exercise is progressed to holding for as long as possible with challenge in multiple directions or in one direction with a timed hold.

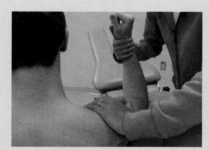

Isometrics: alternating rhythmic stabilization.

The therapist stabilizes the shoulder while providing a gentle build-up of resistance, asking the patient to keep the shoulder in the same position

("Don't let me move you"). The therapist applies resistance for internal and external rotation (alternating the directions) with a slow buildup and release, then progressively increases the rate of alternating the direction of force. The proximal hand is placed over the shoulder to limit motion and compensations.

Progression
Isometrics are progressed to small-range isotonics against elastic or pulley resistance in a supported position. The position and starting tension of the pulley system is set to stop the arm from returning past the neutral point to avoid stretching the anterior structures.

Four Weeks After the Injury: Isometric Midrange Resistance Exercise
Two weeks later, the patient is able to progress to isometric endurance and strengthening against resistance. His pain levels have decreased to 2/10, and he is able to activate the rotator cuff and scapula stabilizers and hold against moderate self-resistance in one direction for up to 20 seconds.

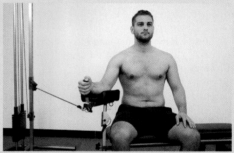

Isometric endurance progressing to strengthening dosage against pulley resistance.

The pulley system and patient starting position are set to challenge the shoulder internal rotators and adductors without allowing the shoulder to move into external rotation or horizontal abduction to protect the anterior structures. The forearm support decreases the load required to hold the arm up against gravity and allows specificity of resistance for the pectoralis major, anterior deltoid, and subscapularis.

Six Weeks After the Injury: Closed Chain Exercise
The patient is able to progress to closed-chain exercise in four-point kneeling over an exercise ball and with a balance board (Exercise 10.25). His pain levels have decreased to 2/10, and he is able to activate the rotator cuff and scapula stabilizers and hold against moderate self-resistance in one direction for up to 20 seconds.

Scapular stabilization and isometric shoulder activity are enhanced by the need to maintain the position of the unstable equipment. The patient is asked to establish a stable position requiring scapular protraction and connection to the thoracic wall, followed by small movements of the balance equipment to facilitate further muscle activation in multiple directions around a centralized axis of motion.

Progression
Exercise is progressed from closed-chain stabilization to open-chain oscillations using the body blade (Exercise 10.22) and open-chain isotonics in protected ranges with progressive resistance concentrating on the scapula stabilizers (Exercise 10.24) and anterior shoulder muscles. Inner range strengthening is progressed in sitting using machine resistance (Exercise 10.33) and in side-lying controlling the movement eccentrically (Exercise 10. 24A).

CLINICAL EXAMPLE 6.7 Hypermobility: Anterior Shoulder Dislocation—cont'd

Midrange isometrics

Closed-chain isometrics

Open-chain rhythmic oscillations protected range

Open-chain isotonics protected range

Progression of exercise.

Comparison of Exercise Choices for Different Types of Hypermobility in Clinical Examples 6.5, 6.6, and 6.7

While the patients in Clinical Examples 6.5, 6.6, and 6.7 will all require midrange exercise and avoid full range of motion, the patient in Clinical Example 6.7 will

need to be monitored more carefully to prevent excessive motion after the acute trauma. The extent of trauma for the hockey player was much greater than for the female patient with anterior shoulder laxity. Both the patient with anterior laxity and the patient after the anterior dislocation require limitation of a specific direction, avoiding positions with the arm behind the body especially in horizontal abduction and with external rotation. The patient who has generalized laxity will need to avoid the end range in all directions. The stage of rehabilitation and acuity also influences the amount of load and the use of open- versus closed-chain exercises. In Phase I after the acute dislocation, isometrics using rhythmic stabilization are preferred to weight-bearing exercise, while the patient with anterior laxity is in Phase II and has low intensity and irritability allowing more aggressive closed-chain exercise during the first visit.

Exercise Concepts for Hypermobility: Neuromuscular Coordination and Force Closure From Local and Global Stabilizers

Exercise to address hypermobility should emphasize improving the ability to control midrange or limit movement beyond the normal functional limits with *dynamic stabilization and neuromuscular coordination training* (Table 6.3; Videos 6.16–6.24). Panjabi was one of the first researchers to describe the need for active support in the neutral zone and the importance of active support to prevent buckling or instability.[51, 52] In cases of increased local joint movement or generalized connective tissue laxity, support or force closure from the local stabilizing muscles closest to the joint controls the mid-position of the joint in the neutral zone; therefore, these muscles are the emphasis in early rehabilitation (Phase I or II [Videos 6.16–6.18 and 6.20–6.21]).[40] As the forces and complexity of movement increase during Phase II or III, the global stabilizers (see Chapter 2) become more important to control joint structures against higher forces through the range (Videos 6.22–6.24). The function of the local stabilizing muscles is to control the joint position, while the global stabilizers can absorb and distribute larger forces, particularly when speed increases or toward the end-point of motion. If the stabilizing muscles are recruited at the appropriate time and threshold, the global movers can then be used to improve efficient movement without excess force being absorbed by the connective tissue and joint structures. While hypermobility indicates the need for neuromuscular coordination approaches, the use of these exercises may also be appropriate for neuromuscular support for patients who have hypomobility once further range of motion has been achieved. Hypermobility, on the other hand, does not progress to stretching or mobility approaches unless the goals are to address areas where hypomobile structures are influencing the force attenuation.

Stability Concepts: Centralized Axis of Motion and Force Distribution

Force closure provided by local and global stabilizing muscles can help to maintain support with a centralized axis of motion (Video 6.25). Active neuromuscular coordination involves multiple areas and muscles to distribute forces for dynamic and flexible support rather than stiffening the area completely.[53] Distribution of forces over multiple joints and through the neuromuscular system decreases excessive absorption of force by any one structure.

It is important to develop appropriate sequencing of the types of muscle activity, degree of appropriate muscle support and function, and neuromuscular training mechanisms. Using the local stabilizing muscles before larger global muscles supports joint structures and distributes forces to enable efficient lever systems. The fine-tuning of the timing, coordination of contractions, and the ability to control or counterbalance forces are all important elements of the neural and motor pattern training.

Stability Concepts: Anticipatory Neuromuscular Timing

The ability to initiate local stabilizer function in the trunk muscles early or before movement of limbs (**anticipatory muscle activity**) is often impaired when pain is present.[54] Anticipatory muscle activity refers to muscle activity, usually in a proximal region, that occurs fractionally before movement of a limb (Videos 6.17, 6.18, and 6.21). Limb motion without proximal or "core" stability can result in the forces being absorbed by the mobile joint structures in the spine. Delayed motor programming can be accompanied by generalized overactivation or lack of coactivation of muscles during movement. These patterns can last even after pain has resolved, with compensatory movements becoming the normal practiced pattern. Patients with chronic or repeated episodes of pain should be evaluated for appropriate neuromuscular coordination patterns and appropriate "grading" of muscle activity for the task. Motor control approaches used to teach the appropriate timing and recruitment have been found to achieve appropriate neuromuscular activation and coordination that is retained [55–57] (see Chapter 7).

Stability Concepts: Parameters

In addition to adjusting or fine-tuning the timing and sequencing of the contractions, muscle endurance is needed to maintain positions to protect joint structures and distribute forces for sustained postures and movements.[53,57–60] Lower loads and low-intensity contractions repeated multiple times or isometric holds are therefore appropriate for this type of exercise. As the patient progresses, endurance parameters are progressed, followed by increasing movement challenges in different directions and with more complex movements. Strength training is added once adequate neuromuscular control is possible. As with all patient populations, the patient's personal characteristics (age, fitness levels, occupation, hobbies) will also drive the types of movement requirements and the need for higher-intensity strengthening progression. There are varied results from the research

TABLE 6.3 Type of Exercise for Hypermobility

Type of Exercise and Parameters Used for Hypermobility		Description	Rationale	Indications
Stabilization, neuromuscular coordination, and promotion of force closure	Isometrics or small-range isotonics	Muscle activation, endurance, or strength challenge to maintain joint in midrange	Promotes control of the joint and distribution of forces through contractile structures	Used in Phase I for muscle activation; resistance is added in Phase II to challenge endurance or strength
	Rhythmic stabilization	Therapist provides external resistance in multiple directions or alternating directions with the patient resisting the forces to maintain the position	Responses to external forces initiate muscle activation while maintaining the joint in a stable position	Teaching muscle activation
	Oscillations	Rapid motion in small ranges	Promotes local stabilizer activation around the joint and increased sensory input	Postural muscle activation or pain control. Can be used for muscle endurance with resistance or higher speed of oscillations
	Closed-chain	End point of the lever system is in contact with a surface and does not move	Joint compression increases sensory input from the capsule and promotes postural muscle control; neuromuscular coordination is enhanced by multijoint motion, which occurs naturally with closed-chain motion	Phase II stabilization if weight bearing is tolerated
	Midrange	Varies based on total joint range of motion and joint structure	Midrange is used to limit stresses at the end of range related to lack of adequate inert stability	Indicated in Phases I and II
Neuromuscular coordination	Unstable base or balance reactions	Use of an unstable base or dynamic balance reactions to promote postural reactions	Balance reactions are the fastest and most automatic responses to activate postural muscle support	Can be used in all Phases. Phase I, muscle activation; Phase II with additional challenge can be used to improve reaction speed; Phase III can be used if needed for functional activities
	Increased sensory input	External tactile, visual, or auditory input to increase proprioception	Use other types of sensation or alternate areas to enhance input and awareness of proprioception	Usually used in Phases I or II; taping or bracing may be used in Phase III
	Slow reversals	Muscle contraction is followed by contraction of the antagonists against resistance (small ranges)	Strengthen muscles surrounding the hypermobile joint	Requires external resistance (therapist or machines). Indicated after sufficient activation and control is present in midrange
	Reaction responses	Challenges to react to task-specific requirements	Reactions to external forces or the ability to stop, change direction, or absorb forces are necessary for functional movements	Phases II or III
	Perturbations	External challenges while the patient tries to maintain the position	External challenges are provided by the therapist to challenge response time	Indicated after activation and sufficient endurance, strength, and control are present
	Eccentric control	Lengthening contraction to control speed and range of motion	Required to limit movement toward or past the end of range	Phase II. Indicated for improving proprioceptive responses. Late Phase II or Phase III. Requires activation, endurance, and sufficient strength. The introduction of eccentric movement starts in midrange and progresses toward end range control. Props, verbal, visual, or tactile feedback may be needed to ensure the movement stays within a safe range

comparing the use of low-load motor control exercises to higher-load or generalized strength training; as researchers strive to recruit samples with similar characteristics and presentations, studies may help inform future directions for overall treatment efficacy.[5–10,23,55,61–62] Detailed description of all the types of classification systems for spinal pain is beyond the scope of this text.

The initial choice of an acceptable range will be determined by the type of hypermobility. For example, if there is generalized hypermobility, the midrange is desired and extremes in all directions would be avoided (Video 6.25 and 6.26). On the other hand, if there is specific hypermobility (as in the case of anterior glenohumeral instability or an incomplete ligament tear), specific directions of motion should be limited and exercises are progressed first in planes of movement that are the most stable or do not stress healing structures.

Props can be placed to position joints in midrange, thereby limiting the length of the surrounding passive joint restraints. Tactile feedback from taping or bracing can provide additional cues to help with neuromuscular responses to limit strain on elongated or painful tissues. Small balls or resistance bands can be used to provide additional sensory feedback to promote muscle activation around a joint during movement (Videos 6.25 and 2.21). Hands-on, tactile input using techniques such as proprioceptive neuromuscular facilitation (rhythmic stabilization (Video 2.20) or approximation) are helpful to promote the correct muscle activation or teach desired patterns. These techniques are typically followed with independent, active exercises without the assistance in order to teach patients how to perform the exercise in a realistic context. Visual input using mirrors or targets can also provide feedback.

Stability Concepts: Need for Proprioceptive and Sensory Input

Hypermobility is also characterized by delayed sensory receptor input from the lax ligaments, capsule, or tendon and the timing and grading of neuromuscular responses is influenced by the disruption of the sensory mechanisms (see Table 6.3). The neuromuscular coordination system is reliant on incoming sensory information about position (proprioception). When joint hypermobility is present, proprioception is often impaired due to delayed responses from stretch receptors in the slack tissue. Using sensory information from other sources (e.g., tactile input from elastic resistance, taping, equipment, or positioning or visual/auditory input) should therefore be used to assist with feedback while learning how to perform or refine exercises. Closed-chain exercise is beneficial to further enhance feedback.

Stability Concepts: Type of Exercise

Isometric contractions, small midrange isotonic contractions, oscillations, rhythmic stabilization, or **agonist/antagonist reversals** are all appropriate methods for enhancing muscle support within midrange (see Table 6.3). **Closed-chain** positions provide joint compressive forces that result in sensory feedback, which, in turn assists with postural muscle activation and support (Videos 2.24, 6.16, and 6.18).[63] Coordinated muscle activation around the joint creates a centralized axis of motion and increases stability of the lever system. Closed-chain exercise involves movement at multiple joints, and motion at the proximal or distal joints can be used to help distribute forces. If motion is distributed to surrounding joints, the forces on the injured or hypermobile area are reduced and there is less chance of reaching the extreme ranges where the tissues are most vulnerable to combinations of stress and strain. Exercising in the midrange and avoiding the end range decreases the excessive shear forces and motion allowed by slack or absent support from the inert structures. Therefore, it is important to include goals to improve range-specific muscle activation, endurance, and strength. Balance activities trigger vestibular and ocular reflexes that automatically stimulate the balance and equilibrium reactions that involve postural muscle activity to bring the body back to a midposition (Videos 6.21 and 6.26). Therefore, using balance responses is one of the quickest and most automatic methods for promoting postural muscle stability. Oscillations or perturbations challenge alternating muscles and also create the same effect (Videos 6.21 and 6.25).[64,65] A comparison of the types of exercise and parameters used for hypomobility and hypermobility impairments is illustrated in Fig. 6.5 and found in Table 6.4.

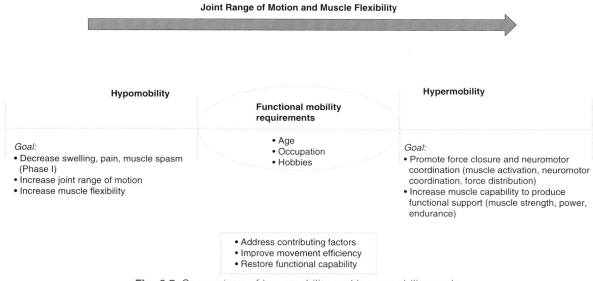

Fig. 6.5 Comparison of hypomobility and hypermobility goals.

TABLE 6.4 Comparison of Hypomobility and Hypermobility

Type of Exercise and Parameters		Hypomobility	Hypermobility
Goals		Improve range of motion or pain-free range of motion Use available range of motion during functional activities Maintain improvements in range of motion or maintain available range of motion	Limit excessive forces, particularly at end ranges Improve force closure to distribute forces Facilitate neuromuscular activation Improve muscle endurance and strength to limit forces on inert structures Improve neuromuscular coordination Improve proprioceptive awareness
Type of exercise		Usually open-chain (progression into closed-chain if required for function in Phase III) Active-assisted, gravity-assisted, therapist-assisted, or pulley-assisted Passive positioning Passive or active-assisted prolonged stretching Active isotonic Followed by isometric or isotonic contractions to maintain range	Closed-chain Active isometric or small-range isotonic followed by isotonic through midranges Controlled movement through end range (not excessive or beyond normal limits)
Precautions		Avoid excessive stress or strain (especially combined) resulting in connective tissue critical failure and inflammation	Avoid extreme range Avoid prolonged holds or positions toward end range
Parameters	Position	End range (joint or muscle) Use gravity, pulleys, or active muscle contractions to assist full range or stretch Progress to positions requiring anti-gravity motion	Midrange (joint and muscle) Supported, progressing to unsupported Progress to positions challenging control through range Closed-chain to promote centralized axis of motion
	Dosage	Progress from low loads in the extreme ranges with high repetitions to low loads with sustained holds Oscillations to reach end range without excessive strain or to address pain Maximal length of affected tissue Progress time of hold or load Allow some time to accommodate to new lengths before progressing load	Progress from low loads, high repetitions (activation) focusing on correct timing, sequencing, and targets to low loads, high repetitions *OR* prolonged isometric holds with low loads (endurance). Progress to higher loads, lower repetitions in midrange (strength) Oscillations to promote alternating muscle activation in midrange (neuromuscular activation) Mid- or shortened range of affected tissue Ability to maintain position is a priority before progressing load Progressing range is the last priority
	Functional requirements	Progress toward functional range requirements	Progress toward performing functional activities without exceeding joint or muscle extremes of range
Priorities		Increase or maintain range of motion Avoid compensations at other joints or areas to isolate the affected area Ensure that hypomobility is related to restricted soft tissue and not due to muscle spasm that is masking hypermobility	Maintain midrange or avoid reaching extreme ranges Avoid early or excessive motion at hypermobile region Address neuromuscular coordination with progressive muscle challenge: muscle activation (anticipatory), recruitment of local stabilizing muscles before global stabilizing muscles, followed by global movers Ability to monitor and adapt movement strategies Proprioceptive awareness Postural muscle endurance
Evaluation and monitoring		Pain responses during and after exercise (delayed-onset muscle soreness) Range of motion End feel (especially for muscle guarding)	Pain responses after exercise (delayed-onset muscle soreness) Specific muscle function capabilities Neuromuscular coordination; support and stability around hypermobile area before distal movement
Tips		Avoid excessive pain; use oscillations or short hold if pain responses are causing muscle guarding	Use motor learning principles to facilitate muscle activation and change motor patterns Practice new patterns with feedback, then fade feedback as retention improves External feedback (taping, props, equipment, visual input, auditory input) can be used to augment sensory input
Other interventions		Joint mobilization or manipulation	Taping

---

BOX 6.4 Goals, Exercise Selection, Priorities, and Progression for Repetitive Strain Disorders

1. Exercise management of repetitive strain injuries includes:
   - Adjusting contributing factors that cause excessive load on the tissue
   - Progressively introducing tissue-specific stimuli (optimal stimulus for regeneration)
   - Correcting movement and alignment abnormalities
   - Addressing training factors or other contributing factors such as nutrition, footwear
2. Goals and related exercise choices are selected to address or adjust for contributing factors including:
   - Components that cannot be adjusted but need to be considered, such as static bony alignment
   - Flexibility and joint range of motion restrictions
   - Muscle imbalances or lack of force closure
   - Inefficient movement patterns or patterns that result in accumulation of forces
   - Training factors
3. Priorities during Phases I and II include:
   - Precautions to avoid combinations of forces resulting in microfailure (avoiding directions or type of forces, ranges, or specific movements or adjusting biomechanical factors)
   - Exercises designed to distribute forces and reeducate movement in areas distant from the area of the injured tissue
   - Exercises intended to address contributing factor impairments

4. Progression during Phases II and III includes consideration of:
   - Slow introduction of specific forces for the tissue
     - Tendinopathy: Isometric or concentric exercise followed by eccentric exercise without angulation or compression of the tendon
     - Stress fractures: Slow vertical loading forces without rotation or high-impact forces
     - Cartilage: Intermittent compression and decompression and gliding with reduced weight-bearing loads
5. Reeducating dynamic alignment is crucial to distribute forces and prevent recurrence of injury. Training to:
     - Use proximal joints
     - Use muscles designed to provide the appropriate forces
     - Adjust moment arms for efficiency
     - Avoid movement compensations
     - Address muscle imbalances
     - Reinforce new movement patterns and prevent further injury through repetition and practice
6. Phase III addresses return to functional activities, including training and movement patterns, progression, and higher level neuromuscular coordination
7. Goals overlap, and treatment is often started in Phase II

REPETITIVE STRAIN DISORDERS

Repetitive strain disorders (Box 6.4) develop over time, and it is important to address the distal factors that are contributing to the accumulation of forces at the primary injury site and facilitate the recovery of the injured tissues. While both traumatic and repetitive strain mechanisms require consideration of extent of tissue damage, tissue healing times, and phases of healing, management of repetitive strain injuries includes addressing all elements that could have contributed to a long process of microtrauma. Patients with repetitive strain injuries (e.g., shoulder impingement syndrome) or postural syndromes (e.g., mechanical neck pain) report a slow onset of symptoms without a specific incident. Tissue breaks down when stress and/or strain is greater than tissue capacity, with microtrauma causing small amounts of damage. If the forces are continually applied without sufficient time to recover, microdamage occurs. If the inflammatory cycle is initiated, pain and dysfunction follow, with the patient avoiding using the area, and then secondary muscle atrophy. As the tissue structure changes, less force causes damage. The avoidance and compensatory patterns become ingrained, often causing further concentration of force on the injured tissue. Eventually the tissue becomes weak and connective tissue is disorganized, leading to a chronic cycle of pain, disuse, further damage, and movement dysfunction.[66–68]

Repetitive movements or sustained postures that place structures in consistent extreme lengths result in tissue adaptation to the lines of force (see Chapter 2). These adaptations can cause tight and shortened tissue or tissue degeneration. The imbalances and asymmetries increase the tendency to move earlier or more at selected points. The progressive concentration of forces results in more mobility at these junction points and a cycle of hypermobility and tissue breakdown causing pain. Extreme postural alignments or repeated movement can thus result in

muscle imbalances including relative stiffness or loss of flexibility and limited muscle activation and endurance to counterbalance the resulting passive tension.

While individual joint or regional hypomobility or hypermobility does occur, the presence of both mobility impairments in the same patient is very common. The entire kinetic chain needs to be considered when evaluating and treating patients with repetitive strain injuries, and postural habits are likely to result in imbalances of tight versus lengthened structures and areas where forces accumulate. The combination of joint restrictions and areas of excessive motion concentrates forces on the hypermobile regions with the body moving in the "path of least resistance."[3] Sahrmann and associates[3] describe the patterns for different regions and have named these movement system *impairment syndromes*. Sahrmann[3] also suggests that hypermobility is more likely to result in pain and dysfunction when both hypermobility and hypomobility are present. As such, the hypermobile area should be regarded as the priority for treatment and principles for stability and neuromuscular control applied to the symptomatic area. In situations where hypomobility is present, relative hypermobility in specific segments or regions becomes the major problem. A refined approach is needed to adjust and teach the most efficient movement patterns and alignment in order to distribute the forces, promote increased mobility in the restricted areas, and improve muscle function to support the hypermobile regions. The relationships among patterns of movement, habitual postures and movements, muscle imbalances, and other biomechanical influences are discussed in more detail by Sahrmann.[3]

Treating repetitive strain injuries will include goals to address contributing factors causing excessive load on the tissue. In addition to training patterns (Video 6.27), movement and alignment patterns are addressed to distribute forces (Clinical Example 6.8; Videos 4.11, 4.12–4.14, 4.21, and 4.22).

CLINICAL EXAMPLE 6.8   **Repetitive Strain: Adjusting Functional Activities to Decrease Force Accumulation**

Patient A

Patient A is a 25-year-old athlete who developed pain in his left shoulder after rigorous pull-ups and rope climbing 2 weeks ago and has been diagnosed with bicipital tendinopathy. The pain is not limiting his activities of daily living, but he wants to return to exercising. He is experiencing pain with any exercise (loaded) in the higher ranges. He has tight pectoralis, latissimus dorsi trapezius muscles along with a forward head position and tipping. The postural alignment is exacerbated with higher level shoulder exercises or when he fatigues.

Adjustments of Weightlifting Parameters

One of the first interventions is to work with the patient to adjust his overhead strengthening to limit the compressive forces.[1,2] Teaching the patient to support the upper quarter with active proximal posture during higher level shoulder movements will be the first component of any of the prescribed exercises. Exercise is limited to ranges below 120 degrees of flexion to avoid the ranges where the biceps tendon is compressed. Loads are decreased, particularly in higher ranges. Pull-ups and overhead weights such as triceps extension with full shoulder extension and shoulder press are discontinued. Olympic lifting is limited to lifting weights to waist height but not overhead, and push-ups are done in a limited range.

Patient B

Patient B is a female volleyball player who has been diagnosed with patella tendinopathy.

Jumping Modifications and Program

Jump landing modifications are included in the exercise program using motor control approaches (see Chapter 7) to teach the patient to land softly to assist with dissipation and distribution of forces away from the patella tendon. She is trained to maintain her lower extremity alignment without allowing her knees to collapse medially (dynamic valgus) and encouraged to maintain a forward trunk inclination with squat progressions to decrease the moment arm and resultant forces on the patellofemoral joint. Her strengthening program consists of hip external rotator, abductor, and extensor exercises with progressive resistance to challenge specific muscle activation, then endurance and finally strength parameters.[3-5] Jumps are started with body weight support in supine on a reformer (progression from Exercise 9.19), followed by jumping on the trampoline (Exercise 9.51), and progressed to hop training (Exercise 9.50). Jumps from the ground to a box are added, followed by drop jumps, then countermovement jumps and finally progressed to a drop jump off a step followed by a maximum vertical jump. At the end of 12 weeks, the patient is able to return to full participation in competitive volleyball.

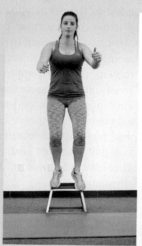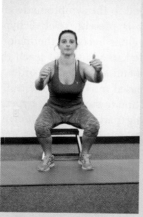
Drop jump with forward trunk lean and hip flexion.

Patient C

Patient C is a 30-year-old woman who is complaining of shoulder and chronic mechanical back pain that increases with lifting her child or laundry. She has a flat thoracic spine and scapula winging and tipping. In Phase II, she has progressed through spinal and shoulder activation and endurance exercises.

Lifting Reeducation and Training

Techniques using the legs and a stable spinal unit during lifting are introduced. Concepts related to adjusting leverage by bringing objects as close as possible to the base of support and using the legs to create the movement once the trunk position has been established are taught and practiced with small loads.[6] The patient is instructed in different forms of lifting. A golfer's lift may be appropriate for lifting groceries out of a car, while a double-leg squat lift would be more appropriate for lifting a laundry basket (Exercises 11.43–45). Integrating core muscle activation before the lift and using the legs is integrated into other exercises to supplement the lifting training, such as squats and lunges, while progressing scapulothoracic, shoulder, abdominal, and spinal extensor strengthening.

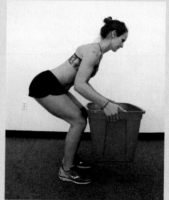
Double-leg squat lift without scapulothoracic connection.

Her scapula is tipping anteriorly, thus decreasing the connection to her thoracic spine and trunk and increasing the reliance on the rotator cuff muscles. Practicing lifting techniques without teaching her how to connect the scapula to the thoracic spine before the lift would only reinforce this pattern.

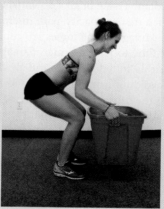
Double-leg squat lift with scapulothoracic connection.

Once the patient is able to link the scapula to the ribs, weight is added to the crate. The instructions on how to achieve this pattern are provided in closed-chain positions or in supine. The patient is taught how to approximate the scapula to the ribcage, maintaining the position when the arms reach forward and when she lifts the object. The isometric stabilization of the lumbar spine neutral position is also achieved before the lift rather than after the object is already off the ground (anticipatory timing).

CLINICAL EXAMPLE 6.8   Repetitive Strain: Adjusting Functional Activities to Decrease Force Accumulation—cont'd

Comparison of Patients A, B, and C

Part of the treatment plan for all three patients is to distribute forces from the symptomatic area. For Patient A, the avoidance of upward compressive forces with load in higher ranges of shoulder flexion is used to decrease stress and allow the biceps tendon to recover in Phases I and II. Patient B has progressed through early muscle activation exercises, and progressive muscle endurance and strengthening are used along with movement reeducation for jumping techniques in Phase III. Patient C's exercises are matched to the activities of daily living that are causing problems and the movement patterns changed to avoid localization of stress. Activities are adjusted to deload the symptomatic tissue in Phase I and early Phase II (Patient A), and movements are slowly reintroduced in Phase II and III to allow progressive return to function (Patients B and C).

References

1. Lewis J, Mccreesh K, Roy JS, Ginn K. Rotator cuff tendinopathy: navigating the diagnosis – management conundrum. *J Orthop Sports Phys Ther.* 2015;45(11):923–937.
2. Wilk KE, Hooks TR. The painful long head of the biceps brachii. *Clin Sports Med.* 2016;35(1):75–92.
3. Janssen I, Steele JR, Munro BJ, Brown NA. Predicting the patella tendon force generated when landing from a jump. *Med Sci Sports Exerc.* 2013;45:927–934.
4. Zhang SN, Bates BT, Dufek JS. Contributions of lower extremity joints to energy dissipation during landings. *Med Sci Sports Exerc.* 2000;32:812–819.
5. Silva RS, Ferreira ALG, Nakagawa TH, Santos JEM, Serrao FV. Rehabilitation of patellar tendinopathy using hip extensor strengthening and landing-strategy modification: case report with 6-month follow-up. *J Orthop Sports Phys Ther.* 2015;45(11):899–909.
6. Haddas R, Yang J, Lieberman I. Effects of volitional spine stabilization on lifting task in recurrent low back pain population. *Eur Spine J.* 2016;25(9):2833–2841.

CLINICAL EXAMPLE 6.9   Repetitive Strain Injury: Mobility Exercise to Distribute and Limit Forces on the Lumbar Spine

The patient presented in Clinical Example 4.11B has low back pain with radiating pain down the right leg. The pain is worse with sitting for more than an hour (increases from 2/10 to 4/10), but decreases with movement. Repeated extension in standing increases pain slightly in the lumbar region (3/10), but the radiating pain down the back of the leg decreases from 2/10 to 0/10. There is decreased joint mobility with posterior-anterior glides that reproduces pain in the low lumbar region, as well as decreased mobility in the thoracic spine.

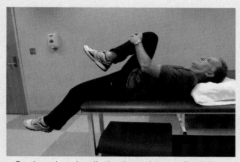

Supine showing limited quadriceps flexibility.

Contributing Factors

Tng factors include (1) thoracic kyphosis with decreased active extension, lateral flexion, and rotation; and (2) decreased hip flexor flexibility limiting the hip to 0 degrees in the supine Thomas test position along with quadriceps tightness. His lumbar lordosis is slightly increased with a specific axis of motion in the mid-lumbar spine with extension, rotation, and lateral flexion.

In supine the patient is able to achieve 0 degrees of extension but the hip tends to abduct and the knee flexion is limited to 45 degrees (positive Ely's test). When the patient is positioned at the edge of the table, his hip extension remains at 0 degrees (Video 6.8).

Exercise Choices to Address Contributing Factors

Reversal of upper thoracic kyphosis and pectoralis major stretch in sitting, leaning against a gym ball with the knees flexed.

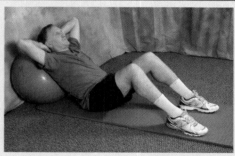

Reversal of upper thoracic kyphosis and pectoralis major stretching against an exercise ball without stress on lumbar spine.

The position leaning against the ball allows the patient to open the chest and extend the upper thoracic spine while the pelvis is in a slight posterior pelvic tilt to limit extending at the typical axis of the motion. The position also limits any stress on the lumbar spine from the hip flexor restrictions (Video 6.2).

- Hip flexor and quadriceps stretching in prone

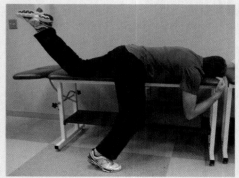

Stretching hip flexors and quadriceps in prone to avoid stress on the lumbar spine.

The supported position with the pelvis stabilized on the plinth limits compensations when reaching the end range of the hip flexion and knee flexion. The patient is performing the knee flexion actively, followed by releasing the contraction. He is also shown how to use a strap to assist the stretch (Video 6.12).

📌 CLINICAL EXAMPLE 6.10   **Repetitive Strain Injury: Addressing Contributing Impairments**

Progressive Endurance of the Proximal Scapulothoracic Region for Bicipital Tendinopathy

Patient A from Clinical Example 6.5A has multiple contributing factors leading to development of subacromial stress on the biceps tendon. His workout program involves high loads while the tendon is compressed, and his flexibility and mobility limitations contribute to his forward head and tipped scapula with subacromial compression earlier in the flexion range.

Precautions
Avoid higher range elevation with loads, particularly in upward direction. Address upper body position and scapula support to limit compression of the tendon under the acromion.[1,2]

Exercise Choices to Address Contributing Factors
1. Flexibility exercises for the pectoralis (Exercises 10.8 and 10.9), latissimus dorsi (Exercise 10.11), trapezius, scalene, and levator scapulae (Exercises 11.16, 11.17, and 11.18) muscles.
2. Mobility exercises to increase upper thoracic spine extension and rotation (Exercises 11.14 and 11.15) with the shoulder below 120 degrees to distribute the forces.
3. Proximal upper-quarter support and thoracic mobility are addressed using the Airdyne bike (Exercise 10.27) and rowing machine. The Airdyne bike focus is on thoracic mobility with the cervical spine vertical alignment maintained to challenge postural endurance. The rowing machine range is performed with a mirror to monitor excessive tipping or forward head position during dynamic motion.
4. Scapulothoracic and cervicothoracic endurance is addressed using closed-chain exercises. A forearm support plank starting from the BOSU is progressed by moving more body weight onto the shoulders followed by walkouts on the ball. In all of the upper body closed-chain exercises, higher levels of flexion are avoided to limit stress on the biceps tendon.

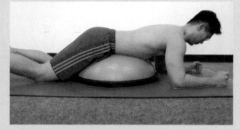

Progressive positions against gravity for scapulothoracic and spinal muscle endurance. Prone on elbows starting from BOSU.

The patient is instructed to move his ribcage and head up slightly, away from the ground, to obtain the closed-chain scapular protraction with neutral cervical and thoracic alignment. Note that he does need to change his gaze toward the floor in front of the BOSU to use the trapezius and cervical extensors to limit scapula tipping.

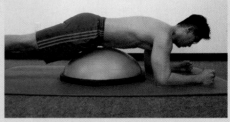

Forearm support over BOSU to challenge endurance of the cervical region and for scapulothoracic connections.

Further load is added to the exercise by straightening the knees, requiring a plank position.

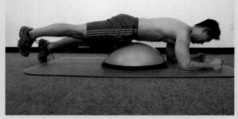

Progression by decreasing the base of support.

The exercise is progressed by shifting his weight to one leg and lifting the opposite leg.

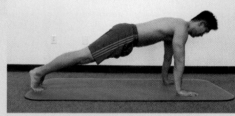

Full plank progression, increasing load by decreasing the size of the arm support and leverage by raising the body further against gravity.

Biomechanical Alignment Adjustments
In a full plank position, the upper extremity starting position is established to accommodate the natural valgus angle of the upper extremity with a wider starting position of the arms with respect to midline.

Both the scapulothoracic and proximal cervicothoracic positions are also adjusted before the plank and observed for loss of position during the exercise.

References
1. Lewis J, Mccreesh K, Roy JS, Ginn K. Rotator cuff tendinopathy: navigating the diagnosis – management conundrum. *J Orthop Sports Phys Ther.* 2015;45(11):923–937.
2. Wilk KE, Hooks TR. The painful long head of the biceps brachii. *Clin Sports Med.* 2016;35(1):75–92.

Correcting the movement and alignment abnormalities are critical to repetitive strain injury management. Specific impairments may be in the area of the pain and dysfunction or in other body regions, and impairments can range from limited muscle endurance, strength, and neuromuscular coordination to mobility impairments described for hypomobility and hypermobility (see Clinical Examples 6.9 and 6.10). In Phase I, relative rest or distribution of force away from the injured region is important to decrease inflammation and allow the healing process to occur. As the injured tissue is unable to withstand as much stress or strain compared to before the injury, the analysis of how to limit forces is important. Addressing the contributing factors can start in Phase I, and these exercises are progressed throughout rehabilitation. The reintroduction of tissue-specific stimuli (optimal stimulus for regeneration; see Chapter 2) is added slowly in Phase II

CLINICAL EXAMPLE 6.11   Introducing Forces for Optimal Regeneration for Achilles Tendinopathy

A 45-year-old runner is in Phase II after surgical debridement of his left Achilles tendon (Clinical Example 4.16). He has a prolonged history of Achilles tendinopathy related to running. Progressive resistive exercise is introduced to begin reloading the Achilles tendon.[1–4]

Exercise Choices to Introduce Specific Forces for Regeneration

1. Body weight support bilateral exercise: Double heel raises (supported weight bearing on leg press or reformer) to neutral dorsiflexion in natural bony alignment, maintaining equal weight bearing
2. Progression to vertical weight bearing: Double heel raises standing on floor
3. Eccentric lowering (to the floor then standing on a step)
4. Single heel raises

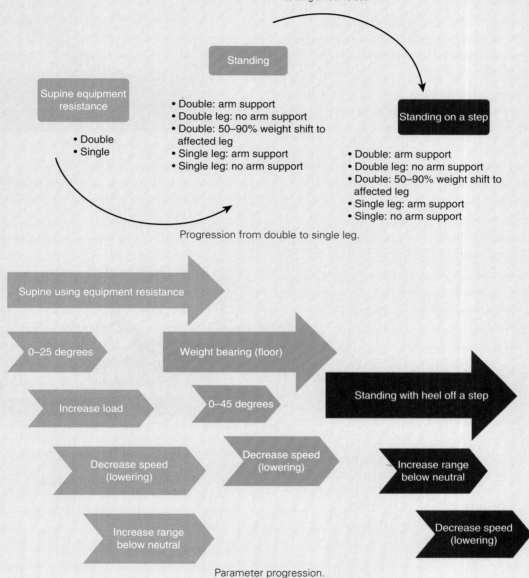

Progression from double to single leg.

Parameter progression.

References

1. Silbernagel KG, Crossley KM. A proposed return-to-sport program for patients with mid-portion Achilles tendinopathy: rationale and implementation. *J Ortho Sports Phys Ther.* 2015;45(11):876–886.
2. Silbernagel KG, Thomee' R, Erikssson Bi, Karlsson J. Continued sports activity, using a pain-monitoring model, during rehabilitation in patients with Achilles tendinopathy: a randomized controlled study. *Am J Sports Med.* 2007;35:897–906.
3. Komi PV, Fukashior S, Jarvinen M. Biomechanical loading of Achilles tendon during normal locomotion. *Clin Sports Med.* 1992;11:521–531.
4. Couppe' C, Svemssom RB, Silbernagel KG, Langberg H, Manusson SP. Eccentric or concentric exercises for the treatment of tendinopathies? *J Ortho Sports Phys Ther.* 2015;45(11):853–863.

CLINICAL EXAMPLE 6.12   **Introducing Forces for Optimal Regeneration Hamstring Tendinopathy**

The patient is a 25-year-old man referred for management of proximal hamstring tendinopathy with a diagnosis of hamstring tendinopathy. He started to experience pain at the right hamstring tendon insertion 3 months ago while running. He has been running for a year, typically 4 to 5 km at a time. He also participates in competitive soccer and ultimate Frisbee and works out at the gym. His pain levels are around 3/10, but the pain can go up to 8/10 after driving. Sitting is also painful, and he experiences moderate pain (6/10) after sitting for 10 minutes. Activity decreases the pain, and he has no pain standing or walking. One of the goals is to introduce forces to the hamstring tendon without reaching the combination of maximal stress and strain for the two joint muscle. He wants to be able to sit for lecture requirements (sometimes up to 2 hours) and drive without pain. He is still playing all his sports and running. He has tried to perform hamstring curls in sitting with 25 to 30 kg but experiences sharp pain. He continued to perform the exercises by leaning to the opposite side and was able to perform 10 repetitions at a time. He is also doing bridging at home (double- and single-leg).

On examination, he has full hip and knee range of motion with the exception of decreased active hip extension in prone (3 degrees). Manual muscle tests are equivalent bilaterally and do not reproduce his pain. Hamstring flexibility is decreased, although no pain is experienced (90–52 degrees in the 90/90 position).

Evaluation

The patient has moderate irritability exacerbated by sitting (direct pressure) on the tendon. His symptoms are consistent with hamstring insertion tendinopathy with contributions from restricted hamstring flexibility and neural mobility. Range of motion and manual testing did not reproduce symptoms, and exercise testing is used to establish comparable symptoms and dosage. Full tension of the two joint hamstring muscle is at 90 degrees of hip flexion and 52 degrees of knee flexion. The initial choices to apply load will need to avoid this extreme position to avoid application of full stress and strain simultaneously.

Exercise Choices to Introduce Force to the Hamstrings
Bridging (Exercise 9.21)

Double-leg isometric and isotonic bridging was possible without any pain and exceeded the amount of time and repetitions for strengthening effect (>30 seconds for isometric, >30 repetitions for isotonic). Placing resistance balls under the feet increased the challenge to the hamstrings, and he reported fatigue after 20 seconds. The double-leg position with the feet on the resistance balls was chosen to work on specific muscle endurance. The unstable position requires more hamstring muscle activation compared to placement of the feet on the ground. He is asked to hold the position for as long as possible.

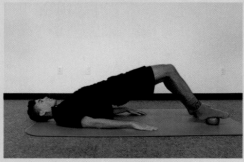

Bridging on an unstable surface.

He was able to perform single-leg bridges (without the unstable surface) with some fatigue in the left hamstrings after 8 repetitions and a slight increase in pain (2/10). He was able to continue with the exercise until 12 repetitions, and the pain increased to 3/10. Single-leg bridging is chosen for strengthening and optimal stimulus by providing an overload without full stretch of the hamstrings at the hip.

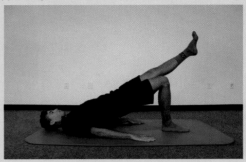

Single-leg bridging.

Hamstring Curls (Exercise 9.44)

Isometric hamstring curl in prone against pulley resistance was started at 8 kg. The patient was compensating by flexing his hip. After correcting the action by keeping his pelvis in contact with the mat, he was only able to maintain 5 kg and hold the position for 20 seconds before fatigue. The exercise dosage was set at 5 kg and held to fatigue for 2 sets. He had no pain during the exercise.

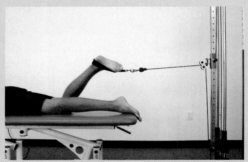

The load is slowly progressed to allow the tendon to respond.

Parameters, Dosage, and Progression for Hamstring Curls

1. The amount of time the patient is able to hold the position is increased slowly until he is able to maintain the position for 30 seconds.
2. The sets are increased up to 5 sets.
3. The weight is increased by 1 kg, and the patient is able to hold the position for 20 seconds for 3 sets.
4. The range for each set is adjusted, and one set each is performed at 60 degrees, 45 degrees, and 25 degrees of knee flexion.
5. The weight is increased again, and the dosage tested for eccentric isotonic contractions from 60 degrees to 25 degrees. The weight he is able to control for 15 repetitions is 8 kg. The dosage is set at 3 sets with a 60-second rest.
6. Once the patient can perform 18 repetitions and the pain decreases during the exercise to 1/10, the dosage is increased again to 10 kg. He is able to perform 12 repetitions for a strengthening effect

Reference
1. Goom T, Malliaris P, Reiman M, Purdam C. Proximal hamstring tendinopathy: clinical aspects of assessment and management. *J Orthop Sports Phys Ther*. 2016;46(6):483–493.

CLINICAL EXAMPLE 6.13 Introducing Forces for Optimal Regeneration: Stress Fractures

A 22-year-old woman was training for a 5K run by running 45 to 50 miles per week on roads, trails, and a track. She developed pain in the outside of the foot about 3 weeks before the race. The pain increased progressively, and, while running, she stepped on an uneven surface and felt a crack. Radiographs revealed a 5th metatarsal fracture. She was immobilized in a rocker boot for 8 weeks. At 8 weeks, she is allowed to walk without the boot and to start increasing her aerobic capacity using a stationary bike without load on her foot.

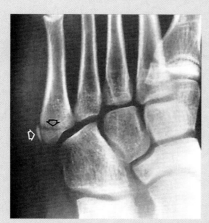

Fracture of the 5th metatarsal. (From Eisenberg RL, Johnson NM. *Comprehensive Radiographic Pathology*. 6th ed. St. Louis, MO: Elsevier; 2016, Fig 4.108.)

Precautions up to Week 8
Reduce vertical loads, avoid rotation, and institute relative rest of the area

Exercise Choices
Cardiovascular endurance can be maintained with non–weight-bearing exercise (cycling, swimming, aquatic running, core and lower extremity strengthening in open chain or non–weight-bearing positions).

At 8 weeks, she is able to start non–weight-bearing stretching of the hip and knee regions and strengthening of the lower extremity without weight on the midfoot. Open-chain multihip strengthening (Exercise 9.20) is possible along with reformer-based lower extremity strengthening with the heel on the bar (Exercise 9.19). Ambulation is allowed, with pain responses limiting the distance.[1,2] The strengthening exercises are progressed to weight-bearing activities including squats, single-leg balance with and without unstable surfaces, and transitions from foot to foot. At 12 weeks, the weight-bearing precautions are lifted, and she is allowed to start running. She is still walking with slight avoidance of the area and limited stance time. Interval fast-pace walking is started on a soft flat surface until her gait pattern is symmetrical.

Reintroducing Running
The absence of local point tenderness, the ability to stand independently on the affected leg, and the ability to walk without pain allow progression to running. Running is started on a shock-absorbing track with walk/run intervals using supportive shock-absorbing shoes. The distance and volume are slowly reintroduced, monitoring pain responses before and after running provides indicators of tolerance to the program. Frequency and the ratio of walking to running is progressed slowly, starting with 4 minutes of walking, with 1 minute of jogging for 10 minutes every second day. If there is no increase in pain, the following week the ratio is increased to 1 minute walking, 1 minute jogging every second day. In the third week, the patient is able to run for 10 minutes every second day, and, by the fourth week, the time is increased to 15 minute. The time is increased by 5 minutes every week. Distance limits are set at no more than 30% of the preinjury training program for up to 12 weeks after the injury and progressed by no more than 10% each week.[1,2] Movement observation on the treadmill is performed using video analysis. Goals are to achieve equal weight bearing, an increased cadence, and decreased stride length with a slight overall body lean rather than sending the legs out in front of the body. The placement of the legs under the trunk weight decreases the angulation and absorption of forces on the lateral aspect of the foot at impact and decreases the time with loads on the area. Changes in her pattern take time, and the sessions are scheduled with time to adjust her mechanics.

References
1. Warden SJ, Davis IS, Fredrickson M. Management and prevention of bone stress fractures in long-distance runners. *J Orthop Phys Ther*. 2014;44(1):749–765.
2. Willy RW, Davis IS. The effect of a hip-strengthening program on mechanics during running and during a single-leg squat. *J Orthop Sports Phys Ther*. 2011;41:625–632.

while the contributing factors are being addressed (see Clinical Examples 6.11, 6.12, and 6.13).

Contributing Factors

There are usually multiple contributing factors that cause localization of forces and microtrauma (see Boxes 6.4 and 6.5, Table 6.5). Most of the issues can be addressed with exercises designed to distribute forces and movement reeducation to allow the injured area to recover. The approaches to treatment may include strategies to address mobility deficits in areas other than the painful region[9,69] and to improve neuromuscular coordination for local movement impairments.[9] General movement inefficiencies and patterns that may have been a contributing factor or a result of a long history of movement compensations are addressed through movement reeducation. The causative factors are sometimes distant from the area of the injured tissue and can often be addressed during Phases I or II using exercises that do not recreate forces similar to those creating the dysfunctional patterns. Alignment and movement patterns can be corrected and new patterns trained as a primary goal while tissue recovers. While some alignment characteristics limit prognosis, the goal is nonetheless to minimize and distribute forces in order to allow healing (see Chapter 2). Some factors such as bony alignment cannot be adjusted, but positioning choices can be used to accommodate the patient's natural bony alignment. If postural alignment is related to habit, muscle imbalances, or soft tissue restrictions, the related postural impairment may be reversible. Slowly building the complexity and degree of difficulty of exercises using the adjusted movement patterns will culminate in functional training during Phase III. A comparison of contributing factors for development of Achilles tendinopathy, lateral elbow tendinopathy, tibial stress fracture, and hamstring tendinopathy is available in Table 6.6.[70–78] The type of exercise and parameters used for a repetitive strain injury compared to the choices after macrotrauma or surgery is presented in Table 6.7.

BOX 6.5 Contributing Factors for Repetitive Strain and Postural Disorders

- Movement patterns or prolonged positions that localize forces
- General overuse without sufficient time for recovery
- Bony and postural malalignment
- Range of motion deficits
- Poor force closure (muscular activation, support or endurance)
- Muscle imbalances and inefficient neuromuscular coordination patterns resulting in localization of forces

---

TABLE 6.5 Contributing Factors for Repetitive Strain Disorders

Contributing Factors	Intervention	Goals and Prognostic Factors	Intervention Timeframe
Bony alignment	Adjust static or dynamic alignment to patient's natural bony alignment, midrange of joint Choose exercises that promote natural alignment	Prognosis influenced by degree Requires higher level of motor control/strength with more extreme bony malalignments	Motor control adjustment proportional to static alignment degree
Flexibility/joint restrictions	Stretching, soft tissue and joint mobilization	Sports or activity-specific requirements Influenced by repetitive stresses	Flexibility and joint restrictions are addressed early as functional improvements may take 4 to 6 weeks of consistent stretching and mobilization. Functional changes are dependent on need for functional range of motion requirements Requires ongoing flexibility support
Muscle function (activation, endurance, and strengthening) Neuromuscular coordination	Muscle initiation for local stabilizers (low load, sequencing, supported positions), followed by global stabilizers (higher load, speed, mid- to end range) before global movers (high load, speed, phasic high coordination and movement goals) Progress to endurance focus: high repetition with motor control principles	Cognitive understanding; practice once appropriate initiation is achieved (breaking down reinforced movement patterns) Requires minimal pain, no active inflammation	1 to 2 sessions to learn how to activate the appropriate local stabilizer or global stabilizers Activation exercises are usually started in supported positions 4 to 6 sessions to aim to achieve the appropriate neuromuscular coordination in gravity-resisted/upright positions Progress to endurance in stationary positions, Integrate into functional movements; this is variable depending on understanding and the extent that previous patterns were reinforced Endurance activities take consistent practice for functional activities
Motor patterns/learning	Teach optimal positioning, efficient movement patterns Improve proprioceptive awareness Reinforce patterns	Prognosis influenced by length and repetition of mechanics influencing forces Psychological components can influence desire to change patterns (e.g., "No pain no gain") Internal competition to lift heavy weights, fear avoidance patterns, kinesiophobia	Dependent on understanding of desired patterns, the ability to achieve new patterns, body awareness, and practice
Sports and activities of daily living preferred patterns/ required skills	Functional progression and simulated skill patterns Movement reeducation, drills Depends on skill level, motor coordination, and learning styles	Managing alignment, muscle initiation, flexibility Outside influences: coaches, training schedule, motivation	Skill level, motor coordination, and learning capabilities

TABLE 6.6 Comparison of Contributing Factors for Achilles Tendinopathy, Lateral Elbow Tendinopathy, Tibial Stress Fracture, and Hamstring Tendinopathy

	Bony and Postural Alignment	Range of Motion Impairments	Muscle Function Impairments	Neuromuscular Coordination and Movement Pattern Impairments	Tissue Force Considerations
Achilles tendinopathy [70–71]	Rearfoot varus, tibial varus, genu valgum	Tight gastrocnemius-soleus, hip extension, and ankle range of motion limitations	Limited hip abduction and external rotation activation and endurance, decreased endurance and strength gastrocnemius complex	Lower extremity angulation and rotation in standing, walking, and running (early pronation, overstriding, narrow base of support, upright posture)	Need to withstand elongation and forces from contraction
Lateral elbow tendinopathy [72–74]	Increased upper extremity valgus Scapular tipping, forward head, thoracic kyphosis	Tight pectoralis major, minor, trapezius, limited neural mobility, decreased pronation	Limited proximal support from upper quarter and scapulothoracic connection; decreased spinal extensor endurance, scapulothoracic connection, serratus anterior activation and endurance, decreased extensor carpi radialis brevis endurance	Midline activity requiring shoulder internal rotation, forearm pronation, and radial deviation Overuse; holding heavy weights for household repairs	Need to withstand elongation and forces from contraction
Low back pain [2,3,9]	Mild scoliosis, thoracic kyphosis, lumbar lordosis	Tight pectoralis major, minor; trapezius; limited neural mobility; limited hip extension; tight hip flexors and quadriceps	Decreased spinal extensor, hip abductor activation and endurance, abdominal muscle activation and sequencing	Prolonged sitting for occupation Home exercise program is not addressing impairments	Need for force distribution to alter concentration of forces in mid-lumbar regions
Tibial stress fracture [75]	Pes cavus (supination), tibial varus	Tight gastrocnemius/soleus, hip flexors, iliotibial band, gluteal muscles	Decreased hip extension endurance and strength	Limited shock absorption Heel strike pattern with rapid transfer in stance phase	Need to distribute vertical loading and shock absorption
Hamstring tendinopathy [76–78]	Moderate scoliosis Increased lumbar lordosis Right hip anteversion	Tight hamstrings Decreased neural flexibility		Upright running inclination Decreased hip extension Trunk rotation asymmetry	Need to withstand elongation and forces from contraction

POSTSURGICAL MANAGEMENT

Postsurgical or trauma management (e.g., rotator cuff tears or rotator cuff repair) involve both stability and mobility training (Box 6.6). Goals are prioritized and informed by the approximate healing timelines and postsurgical protocols. Precautions and contraindications are related to healing of the surgical incisions, damaged structures, and altered anatomical structural alignment and take precedent when selecting exercises and parameters. Some postsurgical limitations include avoiding certain planes of movement, ranges of motion, and types of exercises during the earlier phases of healing. Both the repaired structure and the structures that have been incised and sutured need to be protected during healing, and exercise selection is based on the surgical protocols and the surgeon's orders (Clinical Example 6.14). As the tissue healing progresses, resolving impairments becomes more important (Clinical Example 6.15). Exercises directed at preventing range of motion deficits and minimizing muscle atrophy may be indicated after immobilization, deconditioning, or weight-bearing precautions.

There are a multitude of surgical procedures,[79] with new innovations emerging constantly. Physical therapists and physical therapist assistants should have working knowledge of the more common surgical procedures and their relevant precautions. Procedures can include repairing (e.g., rotator cuff repair) or replacing (e.g., total knee replacement) damaged structures. There are also procedures designed to stimulate healing, such as stem cell implantation or stimulation of bone bleeding to replace irregular defects. Other procedures aim to improve the biomechanical alignment or smooth joint surfaces to slow down arthritic damage. Intraarticular loose bodies or excessive scar tissue may be removed. Internal or external fixation devices can be used to support a fracture site until sufficient bone healing has taken place. Tissue type and approximate healing times are therefore vital considerations following trauma or surgery, and protocols to guide recovery are based on approximate timeframes for tissue healing (Clinical Example 6.16). Some protocols outline specific milestones required to advance to the next phase. Even if postsurgical protocols are available, the therapist will need to understand the surgical procedure, particularly when structural changes result. As surgical procedures evolve, changes in the rehabilitation process are required, and it is the therapist's responsibility to understand the new requirements.

TABLE 6.7   Comparison of Repetitive Strain and Postural Conditions (Microtrauma) to Postsurgical or Trauma (Macrotrauma)

Type of Exercise and Parameters		Repetitive Strain and Postural Alignment (Microtrauma)	Postsurgery or Macrotrauma
Goals		Distribute forces to avoid excessive forces on inflamed or irritated structures Address causative factors increasing forces on the structures and impairments resulting from compensations Adjust dynamic biomechanical alignment if possible Promote tissue healing and optimal regeneration Promote functional recovery	Protect surgically incised and repaired structures until sufficient tissue strength is present to withstand functional forces Address impairments resulting from surgery, immobilization, or weight-bearing precautions Promote tissue healing and optimal regeneration Promote functional recovery
Type of exercise		Dependent on phase, type of tissue, correct pathomechanics	Dependent on phase, type of tissue, protocols
Precautions		Use care or avoid ranges, planes of motion, and types of movement that place stress on symptomatic structures (e.g., impingement) Dependent on injured tissue, extent of microtrauma, and damage	Use care or avoid ranges, planes of motion, and types of movement that place stress on damaged structures or surgical sites Dependent on injured tissue, extent of traumatic injury, surgical incision, and surgical technique
Parameters	Position	Dependent on precautions, phase, impairments, biomechanical alignment, optimal stimulus for tissue Initially supported to avoid stress on damaged tissue; later, progress toward movements contributing to localized stress once the patient is able to correct the biomechanics	Dependent on precautions, phase, impairments, optimal stimulus for tissue regeneration Slower progression in planes and directions of motion placing stress on healing structures
	Dosage	Phases I and II: Low weight, high reps until activation and dynamic alignment are corrected Progressive endurance with increasing challenge for regions surrounding injured tissue to distribute forces before focus on injured tissue Address causative factors with appropriate dosage for mobility impairments and muscle function Phases II and III: Progress load in plane of tissue before multiple directions of stress Precision of movement with feedback followed by practice once self-monitoring is accurate	Phase I: Circulation and edema, restoration of functional mobility and muscle function, prevention of deconditioning Phase II: Dosage for impairments with slower progression for surgically incised tissues Phase III: Continued progression of loads for injured tissue to provide optimal stimulus
	Functional requirements	Phase II exercises prepare for return to functional movements Phase III: Return to sport, work, or activities of daily living components with movement reeducation and adjustment Include attention to movement reeducation and resolution of contributing factors Address training and preparation for required intensity and duration	Progress toward functional activities while adhering to healing timeframes and surgical protocols Timelines to enter Phase III will differ based on healing status of surgically incised or healing tissue
Priorities		Consider alignment, biomechanics; avoid excessive forces, promote distribution Address causative factors while protecting symptomatic area Areas of hypermobility take precedence over hypomobility Local stabilizers, global stabilizers, and global movers recruited in order Adjust training and movement patterns to promote efficient movement Improve muscular and cardiovascular endurance	Dependent on healing timeframes, resolution of impairments Adhere to postsurgical precautions and protocols Prevent loss of range of motion and minimize atrophy during weight-bearing or movement restrictions Provide optimal stimulus for regeneration, progressive forces for resolution of impairments
Evaluation and monitoring		Impairment-based measures Self-reported outcome measures Movement observation and functional performance measures	Same as for repetitive strain but depends on postsurgical precautions and benchmarks for healing time frames
Tips		Motor learning concepts focus on learning new patterns to distribute forces, learn mechanisms to avoid localization of forces	Surgical protocols or healing time frames can help guide progression
Other interventions		Dependent on specific impairments	

CLINICAL EXAMPLE 6.14 Management After Periacetabular Osteotomy

A 26-year-old female ballet dancer has a history of hip pain since she was 16 years old. She started experiencing popping and clicking when in higher-range ballet positions, followed by increasing pain in the groin. At 20 years old, her hip pain started to increase, with intermittent lateral hip, low back, and lateral thigh pain. She also had episodes during which she felt that her hip would "give way" with higher intensity activity. At 26 years, she was having problems with lateral thigh pain and quadriceps spasm on a daily basis. She was seen by an orthopedic surgeon and diagnosed with bilateral hip dysplasia, femoroacetabular impingement, and degenerative osteoarthritis (see Clinical Example 2.8 for radiographs). She was scheduled for a periacetabular osteotomy to realign the ilium and ischium to reorientate the direction of the acetabular coverage.[1]

Preoperative Exercise Choices

Before the surgery, exercise focused on increasing muscle activity to improve force closure around the hip with decreased load on the superior acetabulum and femoral head using deloaded positions. Extremes of range were avoided, and muscle function, endurance, and strengthening activities were performed before surgical correction of the biomechanical alignment.[2]

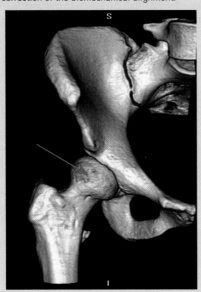

A three-dimensional computed tomography (CT) scan. Note the abrasion and femoral head arthritis, the shallow acetabular angle, and the lack of femoral head coverage.

Postoperative Precautions

After surgery, postoperative time frames are guided by bony healing of the osteotomy site[1] and band muscle healing related to the surgical technique. Weight-bearing restrictions are maintained until 8 weeks with slow progression of single-leg weight bearing. Precautions prohibiting resisted hip flexion or knee extension were in effect for the same time frame because of the ilioinguinal incision and the rectus femoris detachment during surgery.

Postoperative Exercise Choice

- *Phase I (0–8 weeks):* Continuous passive movement (CPM) machine daily for 2 weeks, passive hip flexion, external rotation (500×/day), circulatory exercises (ankle pumps, gluteal sets) (Exercises 9.37, 9.41)
- *Phase II (8–12 weeks):* Muscle activation; range of motion progressive weight bearing; active hip flexion, extension, rotation, and abduction standing open-chain; prone hip extension on BOSU (open-chain; Exercise 11.27); bridging (with legs supported on an exercise ball; combination of Exercise 11.9 with neutral spine bridging action similar to Exercise 9.21); hip external rotation; abduction in side-lying against resistance bands (Exercise 9.26); core stability exercises (Exercises 11.20, 11.21, 11.23, and 11.29); hip flexor stretch (Exercise 9.8); Thomas' stretch; and prone knee flexion stretches (Exercise 9.8).
- *Phase III (12–16 weeks):* Functional progression. Elliptical (Exercise 11.41), single-leg balance on unstable surfaces (Exercise 9.24), progressing to single-leg balance with UE motion, bilateral and unilateral squats (Exercise 9.30), lunges on BOSU (sagittal, frontal planes; Exercise 9.49), ladder drills (Exercise 9.52), Pilates reformer classes.[2,3]

References

1. Matheney T, Kim YJ, Zurakowski D, Matero C, Millis M. Intermediate to long-term results following the Bernese periacetabular osteotomy and predictors of clinical outcome. *J Bone Joint Surg Am.* 2009;91(9):2113–2123.
2. Billingsley R, Dunleavy K. Rehabilitation post periacetabular osteotomy. Rehabilitation of a 27 year old ballet dancer post periacetabular osteotomy: A case study. *J Orthop Sports Phys Ther.* 2012;42. February (1):A60–A113. OPO1195.
3. Sucato DJ, Tulchin K, Shrader MW, DeLaRocha A, Gist T, Sheu G. Gait, hip strength and functional outcomes after a Ganz periacetabular osteotomy for adolescent hip dysplasia. *J Pediatr Orthop.* 2010;30(4):344–350.

CLINICAL EXAMPLE 6.15   Management After Rotator Cuff Repair

Patient A

Patient A is a 45-year-old man who underwent an arthroscopic rotator cuff repair (supraspinatus). He wants to return to his job as a cargo loader for an airline company (Clinical Example 4.14). He sustained a moderate tear of the rotator cuff (infraspinatus and supraspinatus) after trying to catch a box that fell off the conveyor belt. After the surgery, he was immobilized in a sling for 2 weeks, followed by slow progression of passive range of motion from weeks 2 to 6.[1,2]

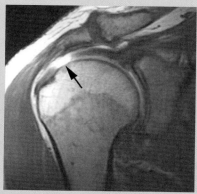

From Rynders SD, Hart JA. Orthopaedics for Physicians Assistants. Philadelphia: Saunders; 2013, Fig 2.13.

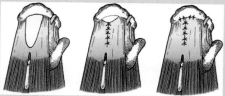

From Rynders SD, Hart JA. Orthopaedics for Physicians Assistants. Philadelphia: Saunders; 2013, Fig 2.15.

Precautions

- *For up to 6 weeks:* protected passive range up to 90 degrees, only up to 30 degrees external rotation in front of the body.[1,2] No resisted shoulder abduction or external rotation until early healing.
- *For week 6 to week 12:* slow progression of resisted movement for abduction and internal and external rotation. Avoid high stress toward end of available range.

Exercise Choice

- *For up to 6 weeks:* passive range of motion (therapist) (Exercise 10.52), pendular exercises (Exercise 10.50), self-assisted flexion (Exercise 10.4).
- *At week 6:* Active range of motion was introduced with progression of load at week 8 as the patient's pain levels have decreased to 2/10 on a numeric pain rating scale (approximate time for tissue healing).[1,2]
- *At week 8:*
  1. Therapist- and self-resisted isometric internal rotation in neutral, in scaption at 45 degrees and 70 degrees with the arm supported on a table (Exercises 10.19 and 10.20).[1,2]
  2. Pulley-assisted flexion, resisted extension to neutral against pulley resistance (scaption; Exercise 10.30).
  3. Elbow flexion arm supported on a table with different ranges of elevation (Exercise 10.38).

4. Elbow extension arm supported on a table with different ranges of elevation (Exercise 10.39).
5. Active flexion without weight.
6. Rows from 70 degrees of flexion using bilateral pulleys and a reclined bench (Exercise 10.44).
7. Scapula stabilization in four-point kneeling with the body weight supported on an exercise ball (Exercise 10.25).

Patient B

Patient B is a 72-year-old woman who has a moderate rotator cuff tear and a reverse total shoulder replacement.

Precautions

For the first 6 weeks, no extension beyond neutral, no internal rotation, no abduction in the frontal plane. Abduction pillow is used constantly. No active range of motion.[3]

Exercise Choices

- *Up to week 3:* Her initial protocol included passive range of motion, active elbow, wrist and hand activity (with the arm supported). Range is slowly increased without stress at the end of range to a maximum of 90 degrees flexion. External rotation up to 30 degrees is performed in the scapular plane.[3] Submaximal isometrics (abduction, flexion, horizontal flexion, horizontal extension, scapula stabilization) are performed for the rotator cuff and deltoid and scapula stabilizers in supported positions with the arm in scaption.[3]
- *From week 3 to week 6:* Passive flexion in scaption is increased to up to 120 degrees, with external rotation progressed to 30 degrees, respecting muscle guarding and end feel.
- *At week 6:* Active assisted range of motion and active range of motion is started with gentle strengthening in small ranges of motion and without external load. Length of time for the submaximal isometrics is increased.
- *At week 8:* Internal and external rotation submaximal isometrics are performed in supported positions.

Dosage Example

She is only able to abduct her shoulder to 45 degrees in the scapula plane in sitting with 120 degrees of passive movement possible in supine. Dosage for shoulder abduction is tested in supine using a sliding board and a roller. She is able to abduct her shoulder from 0 to 70 degrees on the sliding board 17 times. The supine position provides sufficient resistance for an early muscle endurance effect; initial exercise dosage is set at 2 sets of 15 repetitions.

Shoulder abduction is performed in supine on a sliding board to support the arm weight, with dosage set at two sets of 15 repetitions, from 45 to 70 degrees.

- Progression
  1. Increase number of sets.
  2. Progression to shoulder abduction in sitting once the patient is able to perform 3 sets of 20 repetitions without specific fatigue. The exercise in a seated position starts with the arm supported in 40 degrees abduction on the plinth. The elbow is flexed to 90 degrees to decrease the lever arm. Initially, the patient is asked to perform isometric contractions at multiple angles throughout the available range with the arm resting on the table, which is raised in increments.
  3. The exercise is progressed by attempting to lift the arm off the plinth and holding the contraction until fatigue.

CLINICAL EXAMPLE 6.15   Rotator Cuff Tear—cont'd

Comparison of Patients A and B

The arthroscopic repair for Patient A does not disrupt the capsule as much and does not require extensive range of motion restrictions. While both patients had moderate tears (between 1 and 3 cm), Patient A is younger and physically active, with the potential for return to work. Prognosis is higher due to the rate of healing and the connective tissue strength, along with presurgical activity and muscle function.[3] Muscle activation and endurance exercise can therefore be started at a higher intensity and progressed more rapidly. The postsurgical precautions after a total shoulder replacement are more restrictive due to the open anterior deltopectoral incision and the alteration of the biomechanics from the joint replacement. The reverse shoulder arthroplasty is indicated for individuals with major osteoarthritic changes along with humeral head instability related to a rotator cuff tear.[4] The prosthesis design increases the deltoid tension and moment arm to compensate for the rotator cuff, but often the active range of motion expectations are significantly less than age-related norms.[4] Patient B's age suggests that her connective tissue and muscle capability to withstand stress or strain is lower: slow

progression using low loads will be safer. As Patient B is unable to perform abduction against gravity past 45 degrees, using gravity-eliminated positions provides enough resistance for early muscle conditioning.

References

1. Maschi RA, Fives G. Rotator cuff repair: arthroscopic and open. In: Cioppa-Mosca J, Cahill JB, Cavanaugh JT, Corradi-Scalise D, Rudnick H, Wolff A, eds. *Handbook of Post-Surgical Rehabilitation Guidelines for the Orthopaedic Clinician.* St. Louis, MO: Mosby Elsevier; 2008:383–392.
2. Thigpen CA, Shaffer MA, Gaunt BW, Leggin BG, Williams GR, Wilcox RB. The American Society of Shoulder and Elbow Therapist's consensus statement on rehabilitation following arthroscopic rotator cuff repair. *J Sh Elb Surg.* 2016;25(4):521–553.
3. Fermont A, Wolterbeek N, Wessel R, Baeyens J, De Bie R. Prognostic factors for successful recovery after arthroscopic rotator cuff repair: a systematic literature review. *J Orthop Sports Phys Ther.* 2014;44(3):153–163.
4. Boudreau S, Boudrea E, Higgins LD, Wilcox RB. Rehabilitation following reverse total shoulder arthroplasty. *J Orthop Sports Phys Ther.* 2007;37(12):734–743.

CLINICAL EXAMPLE 6.16   Considerations for Timelines and Precautions After Anterior Cruciate Ligament (ACL) Repair

Differences between patients with different types of ACL reconstructions or comorbidities at the same stage after surgery (6 weeks)[1]:

Post ACL Reconstruction With Patella Tendon Graft

Patella compression forces and load on the patella tendon increases with greater ranges of flexion. Range of isometric closed-chain squats is limited and progressed slowly, while the patient is observed for valgus forces, "hanging" back on her heels, and biomechanics of the squat that may increase patellofemoral forces

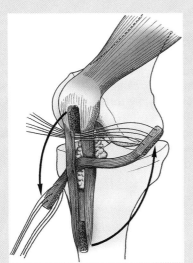

Patella tendon graft. (From Rynders SD, Hart JA. Orthopaedics for Physicians Assistants. Philadelphia: Saunders; 2013, Fig 11.94.)

Post ACL Reconstruction With Hamstring Graft

No isolated hamstring strengthening until 8 weeks, slow progression of load and hamstring stretching.

Post ACL Reconstruction With Allograft and Meniscus Repair

Slower progression of weight bearing to single leg, only active knee flexion against gravity (no resistance) until 8 weeks to avoid pull on the meniscus. Avoid any angulation or rotation in weight bearing; ensure equal weight bearing with squats or sit-to-stand

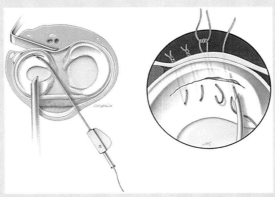

Meniscus repair. (From Rynders SD, Hart JA. Orthopaedics for Physicians Assistants. Philadelphia: Saunders; 2013, Fig 7.28.)

Post ACL Reconstruction With Patella Tendon Graft and MCL Tear

More aggressive range of motion restoration due to the potential for adhesions, especially in extension. Knee brace to limit valgus angulation during weight-bearing exercises and open-chain hip exercises.

Reference

1. Wilk KE, Macrina LC, Cain EL, Dugas JR, Andrews JR. Recent advances in the rehabilitation of anterior cruciate ligament injuries. *J Orthop Sports Phys Ther.* 2012;42(3):153–171.

BOX 6.7   Exercise Approaches in the Presence of Psychological Impairments

- Affective and cognitive elements related to fear avoidance, fear catastrophizing, or anxiety states can complicate exercise choices and progression.
- Cognitive-behavioral, motivational, and self-efficacy approaches may be a higher priority than optimal stimulus for regeneration or impairment-based dosage and type of exercise for individuals with psychological contributions to functional deficits.
- The two approaches for individuals with fear avoidance or catastrophizing are graded exercise and graded exposure.
- Graded exercise sets the amount of activity and exercise with a focus on quota attainment (*not pain abatement*).
- Graded exposure uses a fear-provoking activity to challenge avoidance behaviors with slow reintroduction of the movement or load with easier versions used initially to develop patient confidence in abilities.
- Communication strategies for psychologically informed exercise delivery are important and involve motivational techniques, education and explanations, and setting patient expectations.
- Cognitive strategies include explaining the reasoning behind exercise choices and shaping patient beliefs, education about maladaptive pain responses, addressing concerns, and goal setting.
- Behavioral techniques include reinforcement of positive responses, reward systems, distraction, and extinction of negative responses.
- Motivational techniques include motivational interviewing, goal setting, reward systems, reminders of positive responses and encouragement, and addressing patient expectations as well as a positive patient–therapist relationship.
- Promotion of self-efficacy includes movement reeducation and control, reintroduction of functional activity, and progressive steps toward functional goals.
- Fear avoidance may occur at any point in recovery and for patients with low- or high-level functional activities.

EXERCISE APPROACHES IN THE PRESENCE OF PSYCHOLOGICAL IMPAIRMENTS

Psychological state should be considered when selecting exercise as a treatment modality (Box 6.7). While pain is normally associated with protective responses to avoid further injury, there are occasions when avoidance behaviors influence exercise performance.[80] Even healthy individuals will respond with heightened pain responses to stretching or other stimuli if they have higher fear or catastrophizing traits.[16] Affective and cognitive elements related to fear avoidance, fear catastrophizing, or anxiety states can complicate exercise choices and progression and call for different approaches to teaching exercise.[18,81,82] While operant conditioning theories have been used for some time by psychologists to assist patients with addressing negative pain behaviors, integrating cognitive-behavioral, motivational, and self-efficacy approaches into therapeutic exercise approaches is a more recent focus for patients with chronic pain behavior.[83–87] These psychologically informed communication and coaching strategies may override the choices of exercise parameters or even type of exercise when negative pain behaviors are impacting function. Under these circumstances, using objective tests for exercise and functional performance provides a more appropriate baseline and ongoing reflection of the patient's status than self-reported pain or disability.

If a patient presents with a long history of high pain severity and irritability and reports minimal changes in symptoms regardless of position or movement, evaluating the psychological contributions to the patient's disability is advised. High values on the Fear Avoidance Behavior questionnaire, Tampa Kinesiophobia questionnaire, or high-risk categorization on the Start Back tool are indicators that the psychological elements are a major priority. Psychologically informed exercise and communication strategies would then be the primary approach (see Tables 6.8 and 6.9) while still taking mobility and trauma concepts into account.

Activity, Exercise Dosage, and Progression Using Psychologically Informed Approaches

There are two major approaches to prescribing and progressing exercise for patients with significant fear of pain or catastrophizing: *graded exercise* and *graded exposure*.[81,82] Graded exercise is a quota-based approach using preplanned exercise and activity dosage based on pain tolerance. The amount of activity and exercise is established at baseline, with the focus on quota attainment and not pain abatement. In this mode, activity and exercise progression can be increased without waiting for pain to decrease. By working through a preplanned sequence without adjusting for pain intensity, patients learn that progressive movement and exercise is possible even when experiencing pain (see Clinical Example 6.17).

With graded exposure, the goal is to slowly introduce a fear-provoking activity to challenge avoidance behaviors.[81,82] Exposure is started with a task or movement that is normally avoided or elicits a fear response, then modified to make it less challenging. The patient is persuaded to practice the movement using an easier version of the exercise to develop confidence in his or her abilities without the risk of flaring up a high-pain experience.[21] The progression is based on the lessening of fear/anxiety responses rather than dosage for mobility, neuromuscular function, or aerobic endurance as discussed in Chapter 5. If the patient's exacerbating activity

TABLE 6.8   Communication and Interaction During Exercise for Individuals With Fear of Movement or Pain

Techniques	
Cognitive	Explanation of the purpose of exercise, expected outcomes, and any potential responses Patient education to modify dysfunctional beliefs about maladaptive pain responses Addressing the patient's concerns about outcomes and promote positive expectations Goal setting
Behavioral	Positive reinforcement Establishing reward systems Distraction or extinction techniques to limit rewards and focus for maladaptive pain behavior
Motivational	Motivational interviewing Goal setting Reward systems Reminders of positive experiences Encouragement Positive patient–therapist relationships Addressing patient expectations
Promoting self-efficacy	Include functional activity modification or methods to improve biomechanics early in the treatment course Promote control of movement and provide movement reeducation Encourage small steps toward returning to basic functional activities

TABLE 6.9   Exercise Approaches in the Presence of Psychological Impairments: Graded Exercise Compared to Graded Exposure

Graded Exercise	Graded Exposure
• Initial quota is conservative based on the dosage of the activity or exercise that the patient is not able to tolerate due to pain (dosage is set at the patient's pain tolerance point). Principles of progression are based on pain behaviors or identified impairments rather than on pain abatement • Dosage is increased when the preset quotas are attained as well as following the progression concepts discussed in Chapter 5 • Does not require decreased pain responses to progress • Exercise monitoring is objective • Compensatory movements should be avoided and corrected • Goals are to progressively increase the patient's tolerance for increased intensity of activity or exercise • Motivational encouragement is used when a quota is attained; if a quota is not attained, the therapist persuades the patient to attempt more, rather than less, movement	• The patient is asked to develop a hierarchy of the most feared or painful movements • Exercise starts using the least-feared movements and progresses toward the most feared • The prescribed exercise or movement incorporates the activity or motion that the patient is avoiding • The activity may be modified or parameters set at a low dosage to slowly introduce the patient to the stimulus • Progression and dosage can be further modified until the therapist is satisfied that the patient's confidence and tolerance are increasing • The parameters that are least likely to increase fear/anxiety are the first to be progressed but may not provide an optimal stimulus for regeneration until the patient is more comfortable with the movement • Exercise monitoring is objective but additional information about confidence in performing the activity is helpful • Compensatory movements should be corrected • Motivational encouragement is used during the exercise to allay fears and persuade the patient to attempt more, rather than less movement
Example: A patient who exhibits fear avoidance behaviors while recovering after shoulder surgery for fixation of a humeral fracture is asked to perform as many repetitions of resisted shoulder flexion as possible using a 3-lb weight. The fracture is completely healed, and there are no precautions. He is only able to perform 8 repetitions before complaining of increased pain (5/10). The weight is lowered to 2 lb and he can perform 15 repetitions before the pain increasing. The dosage is set at 2 lb and 15 repetitions for 2–3 sets, but he is encouraged to perform as many repetitions as possible. Once the patient is able to perform 25 repetitions before pain onset, the weight is increased to 3 lb and, as the patient is able to complete 14 repetitions before pain increasing, the dosage is progressed.	**Example:** If a patient is fearful of bending forward, hip hinging without lumbar flexion in a pain-free range can be taught as an exercise with the goal of improving biomechanics and decreasing the fear of the movement. Initial dosage would include ranges without exacerbation, monitoring for loss of spinal stability, and setting the repetitions based on an established number of exercises rather than based on symptoms or fatigue. The exercise would be progressed by increasing the number of repetitions in smaller ranges followed by increasing the degree of bending until the patient is able to fully bend over to tie his shoes.

⚷ CLINICAL EXAMPLE 6.17 **Graded Exercise and Graded Exposure Exercise Approaches**

A patient presents with high fear avoidance behaviors and kinesiophobia after a motor vehicle accident resulting in back and neck pain. The therapist decides to use a graded exercise approach for exercise delivery. The initial exercises are chosen to match impairments (decreased spinal muscle activation, endurance, and strength; decreased aerobic endurance; movement compensations and impaired neuromuscular coordination for simple and complex movements). Her general pain levels are reportedly moderately high (4–6/10) all the time with exacerbations to 8/10. Her NDI and Oswestry scores show moderate to high disability.

Exercise Choices

- *Week 1*: Exercises to address local spinal muscle activation are performed in supine on a foam roller (Exercises 11.19 and 11.22), supine (Exercises 11.20, 11.21, 11.23, and 11.24), four-point kneeling (Exercise 11.28), and side-lying (Exercises 11.29 and 11.30). During the exercise assessment the patient is asked to perform as many repetitions as possible for each exercise before fatigue or an increase in pain above 6/10. Dosage is set at 60% of the maximum number possible with 2 sets performed. Feedback and cueing is provided during the exercise. Aerobic endurance is targeted with 5 minutes on the UBE and 5 minutes on a bike before the spinal stabilization and neuromuscular activation exercises. The patient is educated on the mechanisms of chronic pain, and achievement of the target is rewarded by acknowledging the patient's performance (form and quotas). The expectations are also set that the pain levels may not decrease but that the goal is for the patient to be able to perform more sets or more repetitions, along with functional activity goals.
- *Week 2*: After a week of performing the exercise program, the number of repetitions is increased to 80% of the maximum, and the number of sets increased to 3 sets of each exercise. Feedback is slowly reduced once she is able to perform the exercise without compensations in appropriate alignment and with anticipatory muscle sequencing. The aerobic endurance exercise is increased to 14 minutes. Light weights are added to selected exercises (Exercises 11.22 and 11.30), and lower extremity exercise is added on the leg press (Exercise 9.19). The exercise tolerance is tested and exercise stopped if the pain increases beyond 6/10, with the load adapted to provide muscular endurance. The dosage is set at 60% of the maximum for the new exercises. The

patient is informed of the possibility of some exercise-related soreness after adding the new exercises and reassured that this does not indicate damage or reinjury. The frequency of her home program is increased from 15 minutes every second day to every day.

- *Week 3*: Exercises are continued, with some of the supported exercises only performed as a home program. The loads are increased by 0.5 kg for the arm weights, and single-leg leg press actions are included at half the resistance. Vertical positions are added to the exercise program with mini-squats performed with light arm support on a table. Side-lying leg lifts and clam shells (Exercise 9.26) and single-leg balance activities (Exercise 9.24) are added. The time for her exercise program is increased to 20 minutes daily and walking for 10 minutes at a moderate intensity.
- *Week 4*: In week 4, a graded exposure approach is added to the exercise program for specific functional movements. In her initial Oswestry and NDI disability index, she reported only being able to lift very light weights. She also reported being fearful of lifting any objects at work or at home as she thinks the activity increases her pain. To prepare her for lifting tasks, a modified hinge position (Exercise 11.37) is practiced with arm movement to challenge maintaining the position for short periods, and, after teaching her positions and methods to decrease leverage, lifting light objects from a high surface to another high surface is added to the program. The activity is started with only a few repetitions, and the number of repetitions is increased slowly as she regains some confidence and her fear decreases. The load is only increased once she reports minimal fear related to the movement and is able to repeat the movement multiple times. The earlier exercises are progressed to more vertical upright positions and seated postures (Exercises 11.39 and 11.35), initially with resistance from arm movement and with small free weights or light pulleys.

References

1. George Zepperi, George SZ, Wittmer VT, Fillingim RB, Robinson ME. Comparison of graded exercise and graded exposure clinical outcomes for patients with chronic low back pain. *J Orthop Sports Phys Ther.* 2010;40(11):694–704.
2. George SZ, Zeppieri G. Physical therapy utilization of graded exposure for patients with low back pain. *J Orthop Sports Phys Ther.* 2009;89:969–979.
3. Forster B, Bishop M, Dunleavy K. "Back in action" – a streamlined patient-centered approach to teach movement strategies. *Int J Student Sch in Phys Ther.* 2016;2:1–15.

---

is an everyday occurrence, performing limited versions under clinical supervision is likely to be of minimal benefit due to inevitable repetition of the activity outside the clinical setting. The patient will therefore need to practice modified versions during work or activities of daily living as much as possible (see Clinical Example 6.11).

Communication Strategies During Psychologically Informed Exercise Delivery

Cognitive-behavioral strategies, positive encouragement and reinforcement, enhancing self-efficacy, motivational strategies, distraction, graded motor imagery, and reducing fear of movement can be included as part of the exercise delivery and interactions with therapists.[83,84] Cognitive approaches involve explaining how the maladaptive pain responses are not reflective of a major threat or damage and shaping expectations for exercise. As fear-avoidance behaviors are often linked to specific pain-provoking movements, the therapist can use the exercise to explain mechanisms of pain and the need to address pain beliefs as well as encourage positive coping approaches to return to normal activities.

Patient expectations are likely to play a role in the outcomes, and the therapist's ability to communicate with the patient is critical.[85–87] The therapist should clearly and carefully explain each exercise, choosing words that resonate with the patient. The therapist should also respond to the patient's concerns in a positive but realistic manner (see Chapter 7). Cognitive strategies are used to explain expectations and shape the patient's beliefs while developing positive attitudes toward improving functional ability. Specific, realistic goals are part of the "contract" to direct attention toward the future and are established in conjunction with the patient. Behavioral concepts use operant conditioning principles to reinforce positive behavior and achievements with rewards and encouragement and to extinguish negative responses (including avoidance). Avoidance behaviors are consistently pointed out to the patient, and the patient is provided with alternatives. If at all possible, exercises and activities that the patient enjoys are used because the patient needs to associate exercise with positive experience.

If patients are demonstrating elevated fear avoidance behaviors, exercise choices can be modified to limit stresses, with slow and deliberate progressions in areas least likely to trigger fear. The pain- or fear-provoking activity is eventually reintroduced. Progressing dosage to provide optimal stimulus for regeneration may be less important until the fear avoidance behaviors have decreased. Biomechanical adjustments can help decrease the overall forces and moment arms. Improving neuromuscular coordination can increase confidence once movement is easier and more efficient. For some highly fearful patients, the thought of exercise, without any actual activity or movement, can trigger a sympathetic response and increase pain perception.[80] These patients will require more education about their pain experience and why they need to exercise or maintain activity levels. Patients who demonstrate high anxiety levels may need extensive assurance that the exercise is suitable and will not result in negative consequences. This will apply regardless of whether the therapist uses a graded exercise approach or a graded exposure tactic.

In some patients, fear avoidance or lack of confidence only arises later in the treatment progression, particularly when weight-bearing activities or a return to the same type of movement involved in their injury is required. Athletes who are starting to return to higher-level activities cannot afford to be wary of full weight-bearing or moving in a particular direction. In fact, avoiding the feared movement can lead to injury-causing compensations. While the extent of fear avoidance is not always the same as that in chronic pain patients, confidence in all required movements and activities is a vital component returning patients to their preinjury function and participation.

USE OF THE CONCEPTUAL CATEGORIES

Five conceptual categories of dysfunction to assist with selecting and progressing exercises and parameters were introduced in this chapter (Box 6.8). Extremes of mobility (hypomobility and hypermobility), types of trauma (microtrauma, including repetitive strain and postural syndromes; macrotrauma, including traumatic damage and postsurgery), and psychological impairments (fear of pain or reinjury, catastrophizing, depression and anxiety) overlap and can exist simultaneously for different structures and regions.

The categories presented in this chapter are not exclusive for an individual, and, as the patient progresses, the area of emphasis may shift for specific exercises or for the overall approach. The concepts provided in this text are useful as a general guide for the clinical reasoning processes and are not meant to function as a "recipe" for exercise prescription. It is common for areas of hypomobility and hypermobility to be present simultaneously in patients with repetitive strain injuries. If ligament or capsule damage is the result of major trauma, hypermobility is present in the macrotrauma category. If the healing precautions after surgery involve immobilization or avoidance of movement, hypomobility is a possible primary impairment once the precautions are lifted, although major damage also results in laxity, and hypermobility might also be the most important impairment in Phases II and III. Some

surgical procedures, such as subacromial decompression for shoulder impingement syndromes or articular debridement for patellofemoral dysfunction, are meant to address contributing factors to repetitive strain injuries. The selection of exercises and parameters will therefore require careful and frequent evaluation, and priorities may change as the patient progresses.

Psychological elements can coexist with any of the mobility or trauma categories. The degree of fear avoidance or catastrophizing behaviors will determine if graded exposure or graded exercise parameters are indicated. These types of interventions should be considered if a patient refuses to exercise or complains of extreme pain during testing or at their next visit.

Multiple classification systems have been proposed to address different presentations for specific anatomical regions, particularly for spinal pain. Spinal disorder classification systems for low back pain, including the movement impairment approach,[2,3,88] treatment-based,[9,69] mechanical diagnosis,[89] and pathoanatomic[90] classifications and a system described by O'Sullivan,[91] have areas of consistency and overlap and other areas where there is discordance. A full discussion of these systems is beyond the scope of this text. The information in this chapter is intended to help with the clinical reasoning approach required to deliver focused exercise prescription at different points in the continuum.

BOX 6.8 Major Priorities for Categories

1. Hypomobility: Type of exercise is chosen to assist reaching end range using oscillations or prolonged holds. Dosage includes multiple repetitions or prolonged hold at end range.
2. Hypermobility: Exercises are selected to assist force closure, improve neuromuscular coordination and muscle function, and improve proprioception. Exercise targets local postural stabilizers and global stabilizers to support joint structures. Closed-chain exercise is preferred for initial exercise prescription. Positions include midrange for elongated or hypermobile structures. Additional sensory feedback and balance activities are used to promote neuromuscular timing and sequencing.
3. Repetitive strain and postural syndromes: Exercises are chosen to address contributing factors, muscle imbalances, and neuromuscular coordination. Correcting faulty movements and applying biomechanical concepts are used to redistribute forces. Optimal stimulus for regeneration is important during Phases II and III, with exercises targeting the injured tissue progressing more slowly than those directed at the contributing factors. Phase III exercise includes functional movement reeducation using improved movement patterns and motor learning concepts.
4. Precautions related to tissue healing are the primary consideration for posttraumatic and surgical cases and often follow posttrauma and surgical guidelines for progression. Progression and optimal stimulus for regeneration are determined by extent of initial damage, the surgical procedure, and the type and condition of the damaged or incised structures.
5. Types of exercise appropriate for patients with overriding psychological influences on treatment include graded exercise and graded exposure. Additional relevant approaches include cognitive-behavioral approaches, motivational techniques, and coaching to improve self-efficacy.

SUMMARY

- Five conceptual categories include two impairment-based categories, hypomobility and hypermobility, two categories based on type of trauma, repetitive strain and trauma/post-surgical, and psychological contributions.
- Categories overlap and priorities differ depending on the phase of healing as the patient progresses and the extent of impairments.
- Categories can be used to guide clinical reasoning for the type of exercise, exercise parameters, and precautions.
- Categories are determined from subjective and objective examinations, history, and interpretation of the pattern of patient problems.
- Hypomobility and hypermobility are determined from selective tissue tension, overall range of motion, and joint evaluation.
- Hypomobility treatment requires different types of exercise and parameters if there is edema or effusion. Circulatory exercise using pumping actions, limited resistance, and oscillations or repeated motion helps with removal of fluid limiting motion. Once effusion or edema has resolved, other impairments (hypomobility/hypermobility and muscle function) will require program adjustments.
- Hypomobility related to muscle flexibility or capsule/connective tissue restrictions requires reaching the end range on a continuum from short hold and repeated movement to prolonged hold and load. The amount of load and degree of strain depend on personal factors and determination of SINS, particularly related to tissue status and presence of inflammation.
- Hypomobility exercises include passive or active-assisted exercise using gravity or limbs other than the one injured, pulleys, or additional assistance from the therapist.
- Muscle stretching may include contractions prior to full stretch, but tissue alignment is considered during the elongation.
- Mobility exercise usually follows manual interventions and/or aerobic warm-up.
- Generalized or specific hypermobility exercise is performed in midrange, with a progression of muscle function exercises and an emphasis on dynamic stabilization and neuromuscular coordination to address compensations or protect the hypermobile structures from reaching full length.
- Neuromuscular coordination exercise for hypermobility progresses from an emphasis on the local stabilizers to the global stabilizers prior to functional progression and strengthening of the global movers.

- Stability requires a central axis of motion and appropriate timing and degree of neuromuscular activity with anticipatory stabilization of postural and proximal muscles.
- Early activation of the stabilizing muscles is enhanced by additional sensory input using closed chain proprioceptive input and additional visual, tactile, or auditory input, as well as exercises using balance or postural responses.
- Other parameters for stabilization include oscillations, rapid alternating movement of limbs, or alternating resistance stimulus. Balance exercises use an unstable base of support or targets for maintaining postural position within the base of support.
- A history of repetitive strain injury requires identifying contributing factors and including a multidimensional program to address any potential impairments resulting in overuse or concentration of forces. The emphasis of early exercise is to distribute forces to allow the injured tissue to heal.
- Movement and alignment patterns, training patterns, muscle function, mobility, and coordination impairments may be progressed at the same time or sequentially through exercise prescription.
- After surgery or trauma, exercise choices and progression are impacted by the extent of tissue damage and guidelines for tissue healing time frames. Impairments will vary across recovery time, but healing precautions take precedent. Some exercise goals will be geared toward preventing mobility or limiting muscle function deterioration while adhering to weight-bearing or immobilization precautions.
- Exercise in the presence of psychological impairments requires different teaching approaches and dosage parameters, with communication and coaching strategies to assist with progressive return to function.
- Exercise approaches in the presence of significant fear of pain, catastrophizing, avoidance, or kinesiophobia include graded exercise and graded exposure.
- Graded exercise involves preplanned progression and activity dosage designed to attain quotas without pain abatement or requiring decreased pain intensity.
- Graded exposure introduces fear-provoking activity to challenge avoidance behaviors with slow progression of intensity.
- Both graded exercise and graded exposure use cognitive-behavioral strategies, motivational techniques that include reinforcement and enhancement of self-efficacy, graded motor imagery, and progressive education to decrease maladaptive pain and fear responses.

REVIEW QUESTIONS

1. Differentiate between exercise goals for hypermobility and hypomobility.
2. Discuss how the mechanism of injury (repetitive strain vs. trauma/surgery) influence the priorities for exercise selection.

3. Discuss two exercise approaches for individuals with overriding psychological contributions to symptoms.
4. Compare and contrast the difference between types of exercise and exercise parameters used for primary hypomobility compared to hypermobility.

5. Discuss the priorities to manage contributing factors for repetitive strain injuries.
6. Provide examples of how contributing factors related to hypomobility can influence outcomes for a patient with repetitive strain injuries.
7. Discuss how introduction of optimal forces and movement reeducation is important during exercise progression.
8. Discuss how the healing timeframes influence progression of exercise for patients who are recovering from a major traumatic injury or surgery.
9. Describe how the categories discussed in this chapter can overlap or present to different degrees in the same patient.

REFERENCES

1. Magee DJ, Zachazewski JE. Principles of stabilization training. In: Magee DJ, Zachazewski JE, Quillen WS, eds. *Scientific Foundations and Principles of Practice in Musculoskeletal Rehabilitation.* St. Louis MO: Saunders Elsevier; 2007:388–413.
2. Sahrmann SA. *Diagnosis and Treatment of Movement Impairment Syndromes. Movement System Impairment Syndromes of the Extremities, Cervical and Thoracic Spine.* Philadelphia, PA: Mosby; 2002.
3. Sahrmann SA, Bloom N. Update of concepts underlying movement system syndromes. In: Sahrmann SA, ed. *Movement System Impairment Syndromes of the Extremities, Cervical and Thoracic Spines.* St. Louis MO: Mosby Elsevier; 2011:1–34.
4. Carcia CR, Martin RL, Houck J, Wukich. Achilles pain, stiffness, and muscle power deficits: achilles tendinitis. Clinical practice guidelines linked to the International Classification of Functioning, Disability and Health from the Orthopaedic Section of the American Physical Therapy Association. *J Orthop Sports Phys Ther.* 2010;40(9):A1–A26.
5. Logerstedt DS, Snyder-Mackler L, Ritter RC, Axe MJ, Godges JJ. Knee stability and movement coordination impairments: knee ligament sprain. Clinical practice guidelines linked to the International Classification of Functioning, Disability and Health from the Orthopaedic Section of the American Physical Therapy Association. *J Orthop Sports Phys Ther.* 2010;40(4):A1–A37.
6. Logerstedt DS, Snyder-Mackler L, Ritter RC, Axe MJ. Knee pain and mobility impairments: meniscal and articular cartilage lesions. Clinical practice guidelines linked to the International Classification of Functioning, Disability and Health from the Orthopaedic Section of the American Physical Therapy Association. *J Orthop Sports Phys Ther.* 2010;40(6):A1–A35.
7. Ludewig PM, Lawrence RL, Braman JP. What's in a name? Using movement system diagnoses versus pathoanatomic diagnoses. *J Orthop Sports Phys Ther.* 2013;43(5):280–283.
8. Godges JJ, Irrgang JJ. ICF-based practice guidelines for common musculoskeletal conditions. *J Orthop Sports Phys Ther.* 2008;38(4):167–168.
9. Delitto A, George SZ, Van Dillen L, et al. Low back pain. Clinical practice guidelines linked to the International Classification of Functioning, Disability and Health from the Orthopaedic Section of the American Physical Therapy Association. *J Orthop Sports Phys Ther.* 2012;42(4):A1–A57.
10. Childs JD, Cleland JA, Elliot JM, et al. Neck pain: Clinical practice guidelines linked to the International Classification of Functioning, Disability, and Health, from the Orthopedic Section of the American Physical Therapy Association. *J Orthop Sports Phys Ther.* 2008;38(9):A1–A34.
11. Cibulka MT, White DM, Woehrle J, et al. Hip pain and mobility deficits–hip osteoarthritis: clinical practice guidelines linked to the international classification of functioning, disability, and health from the orthopaedic section of the American Physical Therapy Association. *J Orthop Sports Phys Ther.* 2009;39(4):A1–A25.
12. Enseki K, Harris-Hayes M, White DM, et al. Nonarthritic hip pain. Clinical practice guidelines linked to the International Classification of Functioning, Disability and Health from the Orthopaedic Section of the American Physical Therapy Association. *J Orthop Sports Phys Ther.* 2014;44(6):A1–A32.
13. Kelley MJ, Shaffer MA, Kuhn JE, et al. Shoulder pain and mobility impairments: Adhesive capsulitis. Clinical practice guidelines linked to the International Classification of Functioning, Disability and Health from the Orthopaedic Section of the American Physical Therapy Association. *J Orthop Sports Phys Ther.* 2013;43(5):A1–A31.
14. Martin RL, Davenport TE, Paulseth S, Wukich DK, Godges JJ. Ankle stability and movement coordination impairments: ankle ligament sprains. Clinical practice guidelines linked to the International Classification of Functioning, Disability and Health from the Orthopaedic Section of the American Physical Therapy Association. *J Orthop Sports Phys Ther.* 2013;43(9):A1–A40.
15. Martin RL, Davenport TE, Reischl SF, et al. Heel pain – plantar fasciitis; revision 2014. Clinical practice guidelines linked to the International Classification of Functioning, Disability and Health from the Orthopaedic Section of the American Physical Therapy Association. *J Orthop Sports Phys Ther.* 2014;44(11):A1–A23.
16. Beneciuk JM, Bishop M, George SZ. Pain catastrophizing predicts pain intensity during a neurodynamic test for the median nerve in healthy participants. *Manual Therapy.* 2010;15(4):370–375.
17. Beneciuk JM, Robinson ME, George SZ. Low back pain subgroups using fear-avoidance model measures: results of a cluster analysis. *Clin J Pain.* 2012;28(8):658–666.
18. George SZ, Stryker SE. Fear-avoidance beliefs and clinical outcomes for patients seeking outpatient physical therapy for musculoskeletal pain conditions. *J Orthop Sports Phys Ther.* 2011;41(4):249–259.
19. Hirsh AT, George SZ, Bialosky JE, Robinson ME. Fear of pain, pain catastrophizing, and acute pain perception: relative prediction and timing of assessment. *J Pain.* 2008;9(9):806–812.
20. Leeuw M, Goossens ME, Linton SJ, Crombez G, Boersma K, Vlaeyen JW. The fear-avoidance model of musculoskeletal pain: current state of scientific evidence. *J Behav Med.* 2007;30:77–94.
21. Vlaeyen JW, De Jong J, Geilen M, Heuts PH, Van Breukelen G. The fear of movement/(re)injury in chronic low back pain: further evidence on the effectiveness of exposure in vivo. *Clin J Pain.* 2002;18:251–261.

22. Karayannis NV, Jull GA, Hodges PW. Physiotherapy movement based classification approaches to low back pain: comparison of subgroups through review and developer/expert survey. *BMC Musculoskelet Disord*. 2012;20:13–24.

23. Hodges P. Motor control and pain. In: Sluka K, ed. *Mechanisms and Management of Pain for the Physical Therapist*. 2nd ed. Philadelphia, PA: IASP Wolters Kluwer; 2016:67–81.

24. Magee DJ. *Orthopedic Physical Assessment. St. Louis MO*. 6th ed. Elsevier Saunders; 2014.

25. Maffey LL. Arthrokinematics and mobilization of musculoskeletal tissue: the principles. In: Magee DJ, Zachazewski JE, Quillen WS, eds. *Pathology and Intervention in Musculoskeletal Rehabilitation*. St. Louis, MO: Elsevier Saunders; 2009:487–526.

26. Zachazewski JE. Range of motion and flexibility. In: Magee DJ, Zachazewski JE, Quillen WS, eds. *Scientific Foundations and Principles of Practice in Musculoskeletal Rehabilitation*. St. Louis, MO: Saunders Elsevier; 2007:527–556.

27. Kelley MJ, Shaffer MA, Kuhn JE, et al. Shoulder pain and mobility deficits: adhesive capsulitis. Clinical practice guidelines linked to the International Classification of Functioning, Disability and Health from the Orthopaedic Section of the American Physical Therapy Association. *J Orthop Sports Phys Ther*. 2013;34(5):A1–A31.

28. Gross AR, Goldsmith C, Hoving JL, et al. Conservative management of mechanical neck disorders: a systematic review. *J Rheumatol*. 2007;34:1083–1102.

29. Gross AR, Hoving JL, Haines TA, et al. A Cochrane review for manipulation and mobilization for mechanical neck disorders. *Spine*. 2004;29:1541–1548.

30. Wadsworth MK, Mills JT, Michener LA. Diagnosing suprascapular neuropathy in patients with shoulder dysfunction: a report of 5 cases. *Phys Ther*. 2014;84(4):359–372.

31. Rombaut L, Malfait F, De Wandele I, et al. Muscle mass, muscle strength, functional performance, and physical impairment in women with the hypermobility type of Ehlers-Danlos syndrome. *Arthritis Care Res (Hoboken)*. 2012;64(10):1584–1592.

32. Jansson A, Saartok T, Werner S, Renström P. Evaluation of general joint laxity, shoulder laxity and mobility in competitive swimmers during growth and in normal controls. *Scand J Med Sci Sport*. 2005;15(3):169–176.

33. Deane KA, McGregor AH. Current and future perspectives on lumbar degenerative disc disease: a UK survey exploring specialist multidisciplinary clinical opinion. *BMJ Open*. 2016;15(6):e011075. https://doi.org/1136/bmjopen-2016-011075.

34. Remvig L, Jensen DV, Ward RC. Epidemiology of general joint hypermobility and basis for proposed criteria for benign joint hypermobility syndrome: review of the literature. *J Rheumatol*. 2007;34(4):804–809.

35. Lindgren A, Kristiansson P. Finger joint laxity, number of previous pregnancies and pregnancy induced back pain in a cohort study. *BMC Pregnancy Childbirth*. 2014;14:61.

36. Marnach ML, Ramin KD, Ramsey PS, Song SW, Stensland JJ, An KN. Characterization of the relationship between joint laxity and maternal hormones in pregnancy. *Obstet Gynecol*. 2003;10(2):331–335.

37. De Paepe A, Malfait F. The Ehlers-Danlos syndrome, a disorder with many faces. *Clin Genet*. 2012;82(1):1–11.

38. Magee DJ, Mattison R, Reid DC. Shoulder instability and impingement syndrome. In: Magee DJ, Zachazewski JE, Quillen WS, eds. *Pathology and Intervention in Musculoskeletal Rehabilitation*. St. Louis, MO: Saunders Elsevier; 2009:125–160.

39. Smith CD, Masouros S, Hill AM, Amis AA, Bull AM. A biomechanical basis for tears of the human acetabular labrum. *Br J Sports Med*. 2009;43(8):574–578.

40. Meadows J, Armijo-Olivio SL, Magee DJ. Cervical spine. In: Magee DJ, Zachazeweski JE, Quillen WS, eds. *Pathology and Intervention in Musculoskeletal Rehabilitation*. St. Louis MO: Saunders Elsevier; 2009:17–64.

41. Nadler SF, Wu KD, Galski T, Feinberg JH. Low back pain in college athletes. A prospective study correlating lower extremity overuse or acquired ligamentous laxity with low back pain. *Spine (Phila Pa 1976)*. 1998;23(7):828–833.

42. Kim HJ, Yeom JS, Lee DB, Kang KT, Chang BS, Lee CK. Association of benign joint hypermobility with spinal segmental motion and its clinical implication in active young males. *Spine (Phila Pa 1976)*. 2013;38(16):E1013–E1019.

43. Baeza-Velasco C, Gely-Nargeot MC, Pailhez G, Vilarrasa AB. Joint hypermobility and sport: a review of advantages and disadvantages. *Curr Sports Med Rep*. 2013;12(5):291–295.

44. Konopinski MD, Jones GJ, Johnson MI. The effect of hypermobility on the incidence of injuries in elite-level professional soccer players: a cohort study. *Am J Sports Med*. 2012;40(4):763–769.

45. Pacey V, Nicholson LL, Adams RD, Munn J, Munns CF. Generalized joint hypermobility and risk of lower limb joint injury during sport: a systematic review with meta-analysis. *Am J Sports Med*. 2010;38(7):1487–1497.

46. Smith R, Damodaran AK, Swaminathan S, Campbell R, Barnsley L. Hypermobility and sports injuries in junior netball players. *Br J Sports Med*. 2005;39(9):628–631.

47. Fujii M, Nakashima Y, Yamamoto T, et al. Acetabular retroversion in developmental dysplasias of the hip. *J Bone Jnt Surg*. 2010;92(4):895–903.

48. Van der Giessen LJ, Liekens D, Rutgers KJ, Hartman A, Mulder PG, Oranje AP. Validation of beighton score and prevalence of connective tissue signs in 773 Dutch children. *J Rheumatol*. 2001;28(12):2726–2730.

49. Magee DJ, Sueki D. *Orthopedic Physical Assessment Atlas and Video: Selected Special Tests and Movements*. 6th ed. St. Louis, MO: Elsevier Saunders; 2011.

50. Cleland JA, Koppenhaver S. *Netter's Orthopaedic Clinical Examination: An Evidence-Based Approach*. 2nd ed. St. Louis MO: Elsevier Saunders; 2011.

51. Panjabi MM. The stabilizing system of the spine: Part II. Neutral zone and instability hypothesis. *J Spinal Disord*. 1991;5(4):390–396.

52. Panjabi MM, Cholewicki J, Nibu K, Grauer J, Babat LB, Dvorak J. Critical load of the human cervical spine: an in vitro experimental study. *Clin Biomech*. 1998;13(1):11–17.

53. Hodges PW, Ferreira PH, Ferreira ML. Lumbar spine: treatment of instability and disorders of motor control. In: Magee DJ, Zachazeweski JE, Quillen WS, eds. *Pathology and Intervention in Musculoskeletal Rehabilitation*. St. Louis MO: Saunders Elsevier; 2009:389–425.

54. Masse'-Alarie H, Flamand VH, Moffet H, Schneider C. Corticomotor control of deep abdominal muscles in chronic low back pain and anticipatory postural adjustments. *Exp Brain Res*. 2012;218(1):99–109.

55. O'Sullivan P. Diagnosis and classification of chronic low back pain disorders: maladaptive movement and motor control impairments as underlying mechanism. *Man Ther*. 2005;10:242–255.

56. Tsao H, Hodges PW. Persistence of improvements in postural strategies following motor control training in people with recurrent back pain. *J Electromyogr Kinesiol*. 2008;18:559–567.

57. Richardson C, Hodges P, Hides J. *Therapeutic Exercise for Lumbopelvic Stabilization: A Motor Control Approach for the Treatment and Prevention of Low Back Pain.* 2nd ed. Edinburgh, UK: Churchill Livingstone; 2004.

58. Falla D, Bilenkij G, Jull G. Patients with chronic neck pain demonstrate altered patterns of muscle activation during performance of a functional upper limb task. *Spine.* 2004;29(13):1436–1440.

59. O'Leary S, Falla D, Elliott J, Jull G. Muscle dysfunction in cervical spine pain: implications for assessment and management. *J Orthop Sport Phys Ther.* 2009;39(5):324–333.

60. O'Leary S, Jull G, Kim M, Vincenzino B. Craniocervical flexor muscle impairment at maximal, moderate and low loads is a feature of neck pain. *Man Ther.* 2007;12:34–39.

61. Aasa B, Berglund L, Michaelson P, Aasa U. Individualized low-load motor control exercises and education versus a high-load lifting exercise and education to improve activity, pain intensity and physical performance in patients with low back pain: a randomized controlled trial. *J Orthop Sports Phys Ther.* 2015;45(2):77–85.

62. Fersum KV, Dankaerts W, O'Sullivan PB, et al. Integration of subclassification strategies in randomized controlled trials evaluating manual therapy treatment and exercise therapy for non-specific chronic low back pain: a systematic review. *Br J Sports Med.* 2010;44:1054–1062.

63. Kibler WB, Livingston B. Closed-chain rehabilitation for upper and lower extremities. *J Am Acad Orthop Surg.* 2001;9:412–421.

64. Chmielewski TL, Rudolph KS, Snyder-Mackler L. Development of dynamic knee stability after acute ACL injury. *J Electromyogr Kinesiol.* 2002;12(4):267–274.

65. Chmielewski TL, Hurd WJ, Rudolph KS, Axe MJ, Snyder-Mackler L. Perturbation training improves knee kinematics and reduces muscle co-contraction after complete unilateral anterior cruciate ligament rupture. *Phys Ther.* 2005;85(8):740–749; discussion 750–754.

66. Morrissey D. Guidelines and pathways for clinical practice in tendinopathy: their role and development. *J Orthop Sports Phys Ther.* 2015;45(11):819–822.

67. Gross MT. Chronic tendinitis: pathomechanics of injury, factors affecting healing response, and treatment. *J Orthop Sports Phys Ther.* 1992;16(6):248–261.

68. Scott A, Backman LJ, Speed C. Tendinopathy: update on pathophysiology. *J Orthop Sports Phys Ther.* 2015;45(11):833–841s.

69. Delitto A, Erhard RE, Bowling RW, DeRosa CP, Greathouse DG. A treatment based classification approach to low back syndrome: identifying and staging patients for conservative treatment. *Phys Ther.* 1995;75:470–489.

70. Silbernagel KG, Crossley KM. A proposed return-to-sport program for patients with midportion Achilles tendinopathy: rationale and implementation. *J Ortho Sports Phys Ther.* 2015;45(11):876–886.

71. Silbernagel KG, Thomeé R, Bi Erikssson, Karlsson J. Continued sports activity, using a pain-monitoring model, during rehabilitation in patients with Achilles tendinopathy: a randomized controlled study. *Am J Sports Med.* 2007;35:897–906.

72. Coombes BK, Bisset L, Vicenzino B. Management of lateral elbow tendinopathy: one size does not fit all. *J Orthop Sports Phys Ther.* 2015;45(11):938–949.

73. Alizadehkhaiyat O, Fisher AC, Kemp GJ, Vishwanathan K, Frostick SP. Assessment of functional recovery in tennis elbow. *J Electromyogr Kinesiol.* 2009;19:631–638.

74. Alizadehkhaiyat O, Fisher AC, Kemp GJ, Vishwanathan K, Frostick SP. Upper limb muscle imbalance in tennis elbow: a functional and electromyographic assessment. *J Orthop Res.* 2007;25:1651–1657.

75. Chen TL, An W, Chan ZYS, Au IPH, Zhang ZH, Cheung RTH. Immediate effects of modified landing pattern on a probabilistic tibial stress fracture model in runners. *Clin Biomech.* 2016;33:49–54.

76. Goom T, Malliaris P, Reiman M, Purdam C. Proximal hamstring tendinopathy: clinical aspects of assessment and management. *J Orthop Sports Phys Ther.* 2016;46(6):483–493.

77. Plinsinga ML, Brink MS, Vicenzino B, Van Wilgen P. Evidence of nervous system sensitization in commonly presenting and persistent painful tendinopathies: a systematic review. *J Orthop Sports Phys Ther.* 2015;45(11):864–875.

78. Michenor L, Kulig K. Not all tendons are created equal: implications for differing treatment approaches. *J Ortho Sports Phys Ther.* 2015;45(11):829–832.

79. Cioppa-Mosca J, Cahill JB, Young Tucker C, eds. *Hospital for Special Surgery. Handbook of Postsurgical Rehabilitation Guidelines for the Orthopedic Clinician.* St. Louis, MO: Mosby Elsevier; 2008.

80. Sueki DG, Dunleavy K, Puentedura EJ, Spielholz NI, Cheng MS. The role of associative learning and fear in the development of chronic pain – a comparison of chronic pain and post-traumatic stress disorder. *Phys Ther Reviews.* 2014;19(5):352–266.

81. George SZ, Wittmer VT, Fillingim RB, Robinson ME. Comparison of graded exercise and graded exposure clinical outcomes for patients with chronic low back pain. *J Orthop Sports Phys Ther.* 2010;40(11):694–704.

82. George SZ, Zeppieri G. Physical therapy utilization of graded exposure for patients with low back pain. *J Orthop Sports Phys Ther.* 2009;89:969–979.

83. Monticone M, Ambrosini E, Rocca B, et al. Group-based multimodal exercises integrated with cognitive-behavioral therapy improve disability, pain and quality of life of subjects with chronic neck pain: a randomized controlled trial with a one year follow-up. *Clin Rehab.* 2016:1–11. https://doi.org/10.1177/0269215516651979. Online ahead of print.

84. Dunleavy K, Kubo Slowik A. Emergence of delayed posttraumatic stress disorder symptoms related to sexual trauma: patient-centered and trauma-cognizant management by physical therapists. *Phys Ther.* 2012;92(2):339–351.

85. Bialosky JE, Bishop MD, Cleland JA. Individual expectation: an overlooked, but pertinent, factor in the treatment of individuals experiencing musculoskeletal pain. *Phys Ther.* 2010;90(9):1345–1355.

86. Bishop MD, Bialosky JE, Cleland JA. Patient expectations of benefit from common interventions for low back pain and effects on outcome: secondary analysis of a clinical trial of manual therapy interventions. *J Man Manip Ther.* 2011;19(1):20–25.

87. Bishop MD, Mintken PE, Bialosky JE, Cleland JA. Patient expectations of benefit from interventions for neck pain and resulting influence on outcomes. *J Orthop Sports Phys Ther.* 2013;43(7):457–465.

88. Karayannis NV, Jull GA, Hodges PW. Movement-based subgrouping in low back pain: synergy and divergence in approaches. *Physiother.* 2016;102(2):159–169.

89. Hefford C. McKenzie classification of mechanical spinal pain: profile of syndromes and directions of preference. *Man Ther.* 2008;13:75–81.

90. Petersen T, Laslett M, Thorsen H, Manniche C, Ekdahl C, Jacobsen S. Diagnostic classification of non-specific low back pain. A new system integrating patho-anatomic and clinical categories. *Physiother Theory Pract.* 2003;19:213–237.

91. O'Sullivan PB. Lumbar segmental 'instability': clinical presentation and specific stabilizing exercise management. *Man Ther.* 2000;5:2–12.

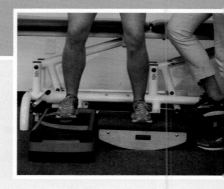

7

Teaching and Learning Concepts for Exercise

Kim Dunleavy and Amy Kubo Slowik

OBJECTIVES

Upon completion of this chapter, the reader will be able to:

1. Describe how incoming sensory information, central processing, and motor output influence teaching and learning motor tasks and specific exercises.
2. List the factors that influence motor learning and motor skill development.
3. Describe elements that should be considered when first explaining and instructing an exercise.
4. Analyze and adjust instructions and explanations based on a patient's preferred learning style and personal factors including motivation.
5. Differentiate between internal and external focus.

6. Describe and apply the stages of motor skill acquisition to exercise progression.
7. Apply feedback and feedforward mechanisms to exercise delivery, choice of feedback, and additional support for performance.
8. Apply feedback, sequencing, practice, and context concepts to exercise progression.
9. Use motivational skills to facilitate patient buy-in and follow-through.
10. Discuss teaching and learning implications for home program planning and education.

TEACHING AND LEARNING CONCEPTS FOR EXERCISE INSTRUCTION

Therapeutic exercise influences physiological tissue adaptation, but neuromuscular coordination and efficiency are just as important. Changing neuromuscular coordination requires two-way communication and an understanding of the patient's personality and learning styles (Table 7.1). Learning how to perform an exercise and developing effective movement patterns involves changing and reinforcing patterns that are influenced by habit, training, pain experiences, and individual goals. Skilled therapeutic exercise instruction and feedback are therefore dependent on the ability of the therapist to explain the desired movement and coach the patient using a variety of individualized techniques (Box 7.1). This chapter covers teaching and learning concepts with an emphasis on learning how to perform, monitor, and adjust exercise and movement strategies.

It is becoming increasingly important for therapists to teach and reinforce movement patterns quickly due to the time restrictions for treatment. Teaching the patient how to perform the exercises safely with the correct form and self-monitoring is therefore very important prior to the patient being able to continue the exercises at home. While patient motivation and consistency are important for a successful outcome, the therapist's ability to teach and convey the message in a manner that resonates with the patient is possibly one of the most important skills for any therapist to cultivate. After

TABLE 7.1	Learning Styles and Explanations
Preferred Learning Style	**Methods of Explaining Exercises or Providing Feedback**
Visual	Physical demonstration Mirrors Video Pictures Demonstration of directions Use of props for direction or targets: poles, bands, tape on the floor Imagery with visual images
Tactile	Passive movement followed by active or active-assisted movement Proprioceptive neuromuscular facilitation Manual resistance Movement guidance or blocking Props (balls, pads) Taping
Auditory	Verbal instructions Use of neurolinguistics Music or metronomes to provide rhythm or speed Imagery and words using auditory cues
Kinesthetic	Allow patient to experience movement before offering visual demonstration or use minimal verbal instructions Use equipment to assist motion Passive movement followed by active movement Proprioceptive neuromuscular facilitation

BOX 7.1 Teaching and Learning Concepts

- Improving neuromuscular coordination requires two-way communication and understanding the patient.
- Learning how to perform an exercise and developing effective movement patterns involves changing and reinforcing patterns that are influenced by habit, training, pain experiences, and goals.
- Instructions and explanations are individualized based on the patient's background and individual characteristics.
- Teaching the patient how to perform the exercises safely with the correct form and self-monitoring is important prior to the patient being able to continue the exercises at home.
- Providing a list of exercises with pre-set instructions does not address variations in patient needs and understanding.
- Teaching, motor learning, and skill acquisition concepts should be applied to the introduction, reinforcement, and modifications of exercise and functional activities.

selecting the appropriate exercises, the therapist is responsible for selecting appropriate instructions and images to teach the patient how to move in the desired sequence, intensity, and pattern. The choice of words, images, and methods of instruction should be different for each individual and at different stages. It is essential that patients understand how to perform the exercise, and simply providing a list of exercises with pre-set instructions does not address variations in patient needs and understanding. Once the patient understands the exercise or movement, fine-tuning and reinforcement of new or adapted movement patterns takes place throughout treatment as the patient progresses.

The skill to effectively teach a patient involves strong communication strategies and professional interaction skills that, in turn, can assist with motivation and patient confidence. Teaching patients how to move efficiently is a skill that is learned and practiced in the clinical setting, and often therapists will need to try multiple approaches with a patient before finding the most effective teaching method suited to each patient's needs. This chapter provides an overview of teaching methods for different learning styles and patient characteristics, as well as motor learning concepts that can be applied during **introduction, reinforcement,** and **modification of exercise and functional activities**.

MOTOR CONTROL CONCEPTS

Motor control is defined by Shumway-Cook[1] as the "ability to regulate or direct the mechanisms essential to movement."[1] Movement requires a complex integration and processing of incoming sensory input, coordination, and control of movement through neurological pathways and motor output from neurological and muscle systems.[1] Deficits in any one element of the motor control system may require emphasis on another element during exercise, or restoration of function may require maximizing all aspects of the systems (Clinical Example 7.1). Unconscious and subconscious cognitive processes such as attention, planning, and problem-solving influence the acquisition of skills,[1] and memory systems are used to shape or change patterns.[2]

Motor learning is defined as the process of acquiring or adapting patterns through practice of movement or tasks, resulting in permanent changes in performance ability.[3,4] There is enormous potential to learn new patterns at all ages, a characteristic described as **neural plasticity**. The integration of neural connections can be shaped and improved through learning and practice, and each element of motor control—sensory input, central neural processing and integration, and motor output—has implications for the use of exercise as an intervention (Fig. 7.1). Learning how to move in a different manner is a process; short-term working memory involves new neural connections and efficiency, and repetition and reinforcement result in patterns being stored in long-term memory storage areas of the brain.[1] Each component of motor control is important to consider when patients are attempting to learn, relearn, or change functional movement patterns to recover after an injury or to prevent injury.[3] If sensory input has been impacted by injury or other medical diagnoses, using different forms of sensory input will be needed to learn how to change movement (Videos 2.4, 2.24, and 3.16–3.19). If motor function is impaired, using additional sensory input can be helpful to promote neuromuscular recovery in early phases and is also used to provide feedback. Throughout the learning process, central processing is involved in the immediate coordination of movement and in converting short-term to long-term memories of skill acquisition patterns.

Patient A

Patient A is 8 weeks after a revision of a previous ACL reconstruction (3 years ago) with a hamstring graft. She also had microfracture surgery on the lateral femoral condyle to address osteoarthritic changes. She has difficulty with accepting full weight on the affected side after 6 weeks of non–weight-bearing and 2 weeks of partial weight bearing. In order to improve proprioception and to restore symmetrical weight bearing,[1] she is asked to perform isometric squats with additional visual feedback using a mirror to monitor weight-bearing distribution and elastic resistance around the thighs to enhance hip muscle activation (Video 2.24). She has some pain in the anterior knee region related to an enlarged fat pad, and patellofemoral pain and taping is used to provide additional sensory input and pain relief.

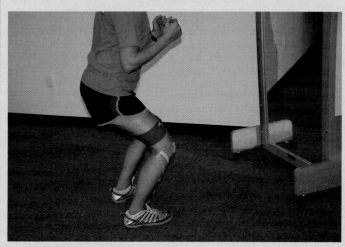

Focus on visual and tactile input to improve weight bearing distribution after ACL injury.

Additional sensory input from other regions might be used to promote awareness of weight-bearing distribution in Phase II,[2] such as enhanced visual feedback from the mirror, tactile input from elastic resistance around the legs to minimize dynamic valgus through the movement, and patellofemoral taping after anterior cruciate ligament reconstruction. The patient is instructed to "Keep equal tension on the band as you lower toward the floor," or "Imagine your kneecaps are the headlights on your car and keep the lights facing down the road."

Once equal weight bearing is possible, squats using an exercise ball against the wall are used to provide additional tactile input to promote a forward trunk lead while holding a deeper squat position.

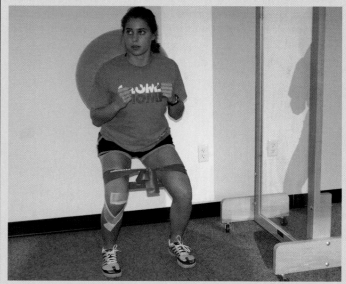

Additional intrinsic feedback (tactile input) from exercise ball for body position.

Additional intrinsic feedback is provided by the exercise ball behind the back. The hinged hip and trunk angle requires hip extensor control as well as hamstring and quadriceps activation, while the range minimizes excessive anterior translation stress on the ACL. The elastic resistance is used to promote feedback to activate and use the hip external rotators and abductors to maintain dynamic femoral alignment in the frontal plane during the squat, thus preventing excessive dynamic valgus or lower extremity rotation to limit unnecessary stress on the patellofemoral structures.

Patient B

Patient B (from Clinical Example 3.1) has limited control of the relationship between the femur and the pelvis in the frontal and transverse planes related to a total hip replacement 2 years previously and right knee osteoarthritis. She has difficulty with sit-to-stand (Video 4.26), stairs (Videos 4.17 and 4.20), and step-ups/-downs (Video 4.16). Exercise testing for sagittal plane movement is conducted using open-chain movement due to the knee pain in weight-bearing positions.[3] Supine knee and hip extension against elastic resistance is used to train sagittal plane movement and proprioception. Initially, the right leg drifts toward the midline.

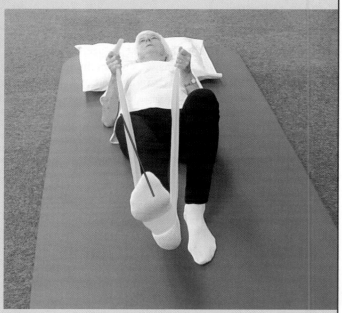

Supine knee and hip extension against elastic resistance. In the initial exercise testing, the patient allows the right leg to drift toward the midline.

After correction and education, she is able to maintain a midline position. The non–weight-bearing position has the advantage of lower joint compression forces while providing visual input and feedback on alignment. The elastic resistance provides some tactile input and additional visual input to guide the position of the leg. After cueing to keep the leg in line with the hip joint, the exercise is meeting the goal of providing resistance for hip and knee muscle strengthening as well as hip rotation activation and training (neuromuscular coordination) to correct the hip alignment. Although the exercise needs to be progressed to vertical positions to match the functional requirements, this is an early exercise starting point. Specific open-chain exercises to increase hip extension, abduction, and external rotation strength in non–weight-bearing positions (Exercise 9.26A and B) are also included in the early prescription, with progression to weight-bearing positions with additional feedback (Exercises 9.30 and 9.31).

continued

📌 CLINICAL EXAMPLE 7.1 Use of Visual and Tactile Input to Guide Neuromuscular Coordination Training—cont'd

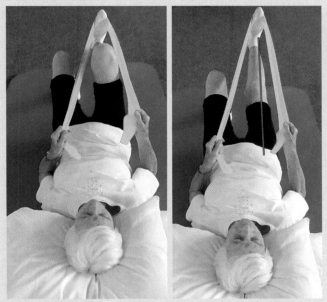

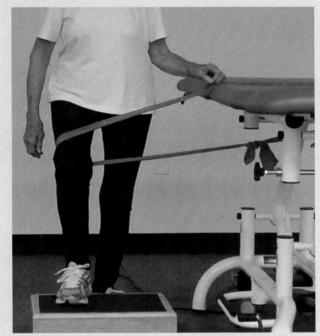

Hip and knee flexion and extension against elastic resistance with concentration on maintaining the lower extremity in line with the hip to train hip control.

Angulation and placement of the foot toward the midline is also observed while ambulating or stair climbing. Preparation for step-up position with elastic resistance to provide feedback for alignment (modification of Exercise 9.31).

Comparison of Patients A and B

In both patients, additional tactile and verbal input are used to accommodate for sensory impairments to adjust neuromuscular patterns and dynamic alignment. The use of the resistance bands provides input to enhance hip muscle activation to enhance hip muscle activation to control the tendency for dynamic valgus and medial drift of the leg. While both patients need to work on maintaining weight distribution between legs and limiting angulation, the choice of closed-chain exercise for Patient A enhances generalized muscle activation around the knee in the midranges after the ligament reconstruction, whereas, for Patient B, non–weight-bearing positions are chosen for the majority of the exercises to limit compressive stress on the osteoarthritic knee.

References

1. Relph N, Herrington L, Tyson S. The effect of ACL injury on knee proprioception: a meta analysis. *Physiotherapy.* 2014;100(3):187–195.
2. Benjaminse A, Gokeler A, Dowling AV, et al. Optimization of the anterior cruciate ligament injury prevention paradigm: novel feedback techniques to enhance motor learning and reduce injury risk. *J Orthop Sports Phys Ther.* 2015;45(4):170–182.
3. Chang A, Lee S, Ren Y, Zhang L. Impaired varus-valgus proprioception and neuromuscular stabilization in medial knee osteoarthritis. *J Biomech.* 2014;47(2):360–366.

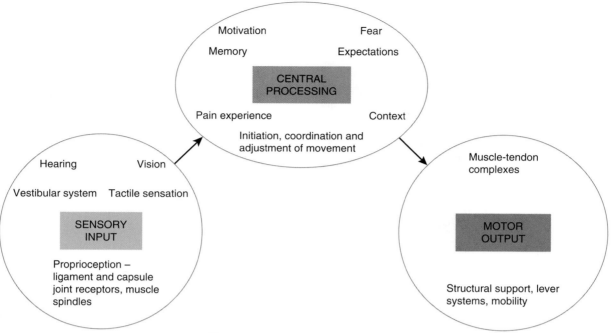

Fig. 7.1 Motor control components.

INITIAL EXPLANATIONS AND GOAL SETTING

The first step in the teaching process and exercise instruction is explaining the **what**, **why,** and **how** of the exercise to the patient (Boxes 7.2 and 7.3). This is also the opportunity to establish rapport and buy-in from the patient. The exercise name, position, and goals are a good starting point to introduce the exercise (**what**). The **why** component can involve explanations about the diagnosis and injury, anatomy, physiology, and expected timeframes. The why element might also involve explanations of why the exercise was chosen, a particularly important component when psychological elements are involved (see Chapter 6). The expectations for recovery or prognosis and a treatment plan can assist with setting realistic goals and are informed by a thorough evaluation. The "why" also includes the goals of treatment and exercise, expectations for how long it will take to see improvement, intended outcome, and how the exercise is linked to the patient's personal goals. The why question also provides an opportunity for the therapist to initiate two-way open communication and establish a foundation for trust.[5,6] A strong relationship and rapport with the patient (**therapeutic alliance**) sets the stage for the best outcome possible.[5,6] The initial discussion of what the patient expects to achieve during treatment and outcomes and his or her experience with exercise can help with tailoring explanations and further education. This is also an ideal time to establish rapport and buy-in from the patient. The therapist's ability to listen and receive verbal and nonverbal communication from the patient is especially important if there are fear avoidance behaviors.

The **how** involves instructions on the movement and direction as well as explanations of the sequence, duration, repetitions, or other parameters. These integrated components will be adjusted throughout the treatment progression and for different exercises. Therapists will develop their own repertoire of explanations, images, and words to use for instructions and feedback, and level, language, and methods are adjusted to

the individual's cognitive understanding and learning style (see Table 7.1).

Goals establish the guidelines and expectations and provide further explanations of what the patient needs to achieve. A patient-centric approach to goal setting is imperative for creating meaningful goals and for avoiding patient dissatisfaction. Goals should be relevant and have a direct relationship to activities that interest the patient. Compliance and motivation are likely to suffer if the goals are not patient-centric. Goal-setting

S: Specific
M: Measurable
A: Achievable
R: Relevant
T: Time

CLINICAL EXAMPLE 7.2   Setting Goals for a Patient With Shinsplints

A runner with shin splints has 5 degrees of ankle dorsiflexion. He is only able to tolerate running on a treadmill for 15 minutes before pain in the anterior shin is reproduced.

Short-term goal:
• Within 2 weeks, the patient will:
  • Demonstrate 10 degrees of ankle dorsiflexion using the standing lunge technique

Long-term goal:
• Within 6 weeks the patient will:
  • Demonstrate 20 degrees of ankle dorsiflexion during the stance phase of running on the treadmill (using videotaping)[1]
  • Be able to run for 30 minutes without increasing pain levels at a perceived exertion level of 11 in order to return to running for cardiovascular fitness.

Reference
1. Simoneau GG. Kinesiology of walking. In: Neumann DA, ed. *Kinesiology of the Musculoskeletal System.* St. Louis, MO: Mosby Elsevier; 2010:627–681.

---

is activity-based and impairment-driven using the SMART goal-writing technique. SMART goals are **S**pecific, **M**easurable, **A**chievable, **R**elevant, and have a **T**ime set in which to achieve the goals. **Specific** goals refer to both the activity and the key impairments and match the patient's expectations for therapy. Making goals **measurable** and setting a threshold for goal achievement removes subjective expectations from the outcomes, such as "I think that I am better." Measurable goals are also valued by insurance providers to determine if the patient is progressing in order to approve reimbursement (Box 7.4). The use of objective and validated tests and measures is useful to create measurable goals (see Chapter 8).

Achievable goals are important for both the patient and clinician. Goals that are too ambitious or too easy to reach will result in failure or premature discharge from therapy. **Relevance** refers to matching the goals with patient expectations but also using clinical reasoning to determine the most appropriate goals for the patient's personal and environmental context. **Time**-dependent goal-setting ensures that all parties are held to task but is an area that newer practitioners may find particularly challenging. Time-dependent yet reasonable goals are created using a combination of prognostic factors, soft tissue healing times (see Chapter 2), and clinician experience. Limited experience shifts the decision-making to the first two components. Therapists will need to constantly reevaluate and adjust goals as patients improve (Clinical Example 7.2).

SMART goals can be established for short-term impairment-based goals and long-term goals. The linkages between improvements in the impairment and activity are included in the goals. Both short- and long-term goals are specific and measurable using identified thresholds for success and are achievable and time-dependent. Explaining the timeframes and how the impairment (e.g., limited dorsiflexion) is linked to running participation is likely to be relevant to the patient and therefore more likely to provide motivation to perform the stretching as prescribed than it would be without explanations.

The specific goal for each exercise is established during the initial testing for exercise dosage, but it is helpful to explain to the patient that goals change during the course of treatment. The general goals should change between phases, but the therapist also needs to adjust the specific exercise goals by adjusting the exercise parameters regularly. For example, if a patient meets the initial goal of performing an exercise with appropriate muscle activation patterns, the dosage will change to meet muscle endurance goals and again once the patient's goals are adjusted to start to address muscle strength. If the patient improves more quickly than expected or additional impairments or functional goals are identified, individual exercise goals will also change. As these goals and the related parameters need to change frequently, not all individual exercise goals are documented in detail for each exercise, but the therapist will need to keep adjusting exercise goals and dosage to achieve more general short- and long-term goals.

The **how** element also involves teaching the patient to perform the exercise. How an exercise is taught and performed will vary based on **individual characteristics** including **age, learning styles**, **motivation**, and **intellectual capability**. The methods used to demonstrate and teach exercise will differ based on the patient's motor task familiarity and skill. The ability to effectively learn movements can also be challenged by a patient's protective patterns caused by injury or pain, such as fear avoidance behavior (see Chapter 6).[2] The patient's literacy and education levels, as well as language will also influence how to instruct the patient. For example, a patient who speaks English as a second language may require very short, simple verbal instructions with more demonstration, and the therapist will need to take more time to ensure that the patient understands the message. Age, background, and socioeconomic elements also influence the choice of exercises for home programs and for images and analogies based on relevance. For example, if an older adult is receiving home therapy, it is easier to identify where to exercise, what position is the safest, and what equipment is available. If the older adult used to skate as a hobby, using the image of a skating-type action with the hip for standing abduction might be an appropriate image. If the patient's vision is impaired, demonstrating the exercise in a position where the patient is able to see the therapist and speaking clearly and slowly is imperative. Socioeconomic elements usually influence the type of equipment available and home and community resources.

The initial explanations can be adjusted according to the patient's familiarity with a specific exercise, preferred learning style, personality, and other personal characteristics, such as occupation or age (Fig. 7.2 and Clinical Example 7.3). If a patient has a strong preferred learning style, care should be taken to ensure that the information is conveyed using the preferred learning medium (see Table 7.1). In some cases, explanations will be adjusted based on the diagnosis, comorbidities, or impairments. For example, if the patient has sensory limitations such as hearing, vision, proprioception, or tactile sensation impairments, these are important to take into account when choosing

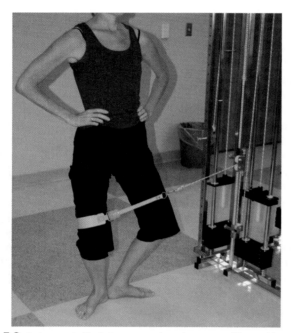

Fig. 7.2 A dancer is likely to respond to dance-specific positions and terms when explaining the exercise and positions. "First position demiplié" is readily understood and immediately relevant to return to her preferred exercise. In addition, the specificity of the exercise increases carryover and preparation for function.

appropriate explanations, feedback on performance, and props. For example, visual demonstration is appropriate for a patient with hearing loss, and standing in front of the patient so that this patient can lip read is vital to deliver instructions. If the patient is blind, auditory instructions with clear and descriptive explanations or using passive movement may be useful. Individuals with loss of sensation are likely to need increased sensory information from other areas or visual input to maximize the receptive components needed to perform the exercises.

ACQUISITION OF MOTOR TASKS

Internal Versus External Focus

If a patient is concentrating on a specific body part or a muscle action in isolation when learning or practicing a movement, this is defined as an **internal focus**. In contrast, **external focus** involves concentrating on achieving a goal or a target external to the body.[3,4,7] The patient's focus is influenced by the therapist's instructions and what the patient is asked to think about (see Box 7.4). For example, asking a patient to focus on contracting the quadriceps muscle after knee surgery would be considered internal focus, while instructions to throw a weighted ball at a target emphasizes an external focus. Internal focus is suited for tasks when isolated muscle activation, endurance, or strengthening is desired (often in Phase I or early Phase II), while external focus is faster and results in the coordination of multiple systems and areas. External focus is therefore appropriate for concentration on complex tasks requiring high levels of complexity, fast speeds, and reaction times (late Phase II or III; Video 7.1) and is used for functional endurance, strengthening, power, or mobility exercise or functional movement training.[3,4] External focus is also very

---

CLINICAL EXAMPLE 7.3 **Individualized Instructions, Explanations, and Exercise Choices**

Patient A

Patient A is a concert pianist who has cervical pain. The therapist is explaining how she can maintain her seated postural position with upper extremity challenges to work on her cervical endurance (Exercise 11.35). The patient is anxious and has a tendency to recruit the global movers (trapezius, sternocleidomastoid, biceps, deltoid, and pectoralis) creating a fast, stiff movement. If the larger muscles are recruited at a high intensity, she is unlikely to be able to support the cervical spine while she is practicing. In order to decrease the intensity of the contraction and recruit the local stabilizers at a lower intensity, the therapist needs to use instructions that are customized to her personal characteristics. Her preferred learning style is auditory, and her background as a concert pianist can be used to provide analogies using musical terms to achieve the desired intensity such as: "Imagine that you are playing a soft, lyrical song rather than using staccato or crescendo-type intensity." The amount of weight used should be light to avoid increasing the challenge for high-threshold muscle activation. In addition, if the therapist speaks softly and lyrically when providing cues, the movement is more likely to encourage low-intensity muscle activity.

Patient B

Patient B is an engineer who also has cervical pain. He is taught the same exercise (Exercise 11.35, seated postural endurance with upper extremity weights) to work on seated endurance for his work-related activities. He analyzes and processes information in a sequential and concrete fashion and is likely to respond

to clear instructions in a logical sequence. He might also respond to explanations using forces, directions of forces, and efficiency.

Patient C

Patient C is an ophthalmologist and has cervical pain. He is likely to respond quickly and accurately to instructions using anatomical terminology as opposed to the typical lay terminology. While Exercise 11.35 is useful, the position that he uses for his examinations is a forward lean position looking into the patient's eyes. Exercise 11.37 can be used to challenge the forward lean position in sitting or in standing. The exercises can be adjusted to challenge this position with additional weight applied to the cervical region to simulate another occupation task requirement—to be able to resist the weight of the magnifying glasses worn for at least 20% of his time at work.

Comparison of Patients A, B, and C

Each patient's occupation and personality characteristics are unique and require adjustments for the exercise instructions, cues, corrections, and exercise alternatives. For Patient A, the instructions, analogies, and imagery as well as the voice intensity is used to match the patient's musical ability, while for Patient B the sequencing of instructions as well as examples using visualization of forces is more likely to match his educational background and occupation. Patient C's exercise choices are matched to his job requirements—a factor that is also more likely to result in improvements in the required muscle function along with providing relevance.

CLINICAL EXAMPLE 7.4 Internal and External Focus for a Patient Post Femur Fracture

Patient A

Patient A sustained a right femur fracture after a motorcycle accident (see Clinical Example 4.10) is evaluated 6 weeks after the surgery. He has major wasting and atrophy of the quadriceps, hamstrings, and gluteal muscles, and there is still some effusion in the knee joint. There are scars on the distal lateral femur where the screws for the intramedullary rods were inserted, a scar distal to the patella where the rod was inserted through the knee joint, and a long scar in the superior lateral femur where the sliding screw was inserted for an intertrochanteric fracture. The patient is employed as a construction worker and is extremely motivated to return to work because he has no other source of income.

One of the major goals during the first treatment is to teach the patient to be able to activate the quadriceps to address the quadriceps lag demonstrated when trying to lift his leg. The patient is positioned in supine with a small ball under the knee. He is asked to push the back of the knee down into the ball to stabilize the femur and avoid compensating by lifting the leg with the hip flexors. He is then asked to place his hands on the muscle and focus on straightening his knee by contracting his quadriceps. The therapist assists the movement by lifting the foot to demonstrate the desired movement. Concentrating on the muscle is an example of **internal focus.**

As the patient progresses to weight-bearing activities and demonstrates good quadriceps control, exercises are selected to address the next goal of being able to transfer weight onto the injured limb. The parallel bars are used to support some of his body weight, and the patient is able to practice shifting weight onto the injured leg. Once he tolerates weight bearing without excessive compensations, other challenges can be added such as kicking a ball with the opposite leg. This encourages coordination and requires multiple adjustments for balance and coordination. Concentrating on the accuracy and speed of the ball is an example of **external focus.** The external focus also has the advantage of distracting any fear of weight bearing and increases confidence in being able to take weight fully on the injured leg. At this point, if the therapist asked the patient to concentrate on keeping the quadriceps active, the instructions may distract the patient from the coordination required to respond to the outside stimulus.

Patient B

Patient B is a runner who has iliotibial band syndrome. The use of internal or external focus changes as the patient progresses through phases of rehabilitation.

In Phase II, addressing hip external rotator endurance to distribute forces and control dynamic valgus during running might include clam shells (Exercise 9.26A) in side lying. The exercise is taught with the patient palpating and concentrating on the activation by having her palpate the muscle during the movement and concentrate on achieving specific muscle fatigue (**internal focus**).

However, asking the patient to concentrate on keeping her kneecap facing forward toward a target during step-ups and step-downs (Exercise 9.31) and using a laser pointer strapped to her leg to guide the alignment is useful to address the closed-chain functional sequence. This would be indicated after she is aware of how to activate the muscles and her endurance is improving.

When she returns to running, using a metronome to increase the cadence can help decrease stride length (**external focus**) without her thinking too hard about changing her running mechanics. She can also be directed to listen to the sound of her landing with the aim of improving shock absorption. The patient needs to coordinate all areas using complex systems for the running, and concentrating on muscle activation of one muscle may lead to constraining movement.

---

important for adjusting complex motion when compensatory patterns have contributed to injury or for prevention of injury. A number of studies have shown that external focus is effective in improving jumping, throwing, racquet sport actions, and golf performance.[4,7] While the majority of research in this area has been conducted on healthy athletes, there is also research showing improved biomechanics using external focus for patients after anterior cruciate ligament (ACL) reconstruction,[3] adjusting running biomechanics to prevent accumulation of forces known to contribute to repetitive strain injuries,[8] and improving jumping biomechanics.[9,10] There is also some evidence that directing too much attention using internal focus can interfere with complex movement coordination, and therefore the therapist will need to pay attention to what the patient is concentrating on and the type instructions used for functional movement strategies or complex movements in Phases II and III[4,9] (Clinical Example 7.4).

Stages of Motor Learning

Fitts and Posner[11] classified the process of learning motor skills into 3 stages: cognitive (conscious control), associative and autonomous (automatic) stages (Box 7.5).[1,3] Goals progress from understanding the desired movement to being able to perform the movement without concentrating on the activity (Fig. 7.3).

Cognitive Phase: Conscious Control and Understanding the Desired Movement

When the patient is learning a new task or adjusting and replacing a maladaptive pattern, the first priority for the therapist is to ensure that the patient understands the exercise position and

BOX 7.5 Acquisition of Motor Tasks

- **Internal focus** is concentration on a specific body part or a muscle action, often in isolation, and is appropriate in Phases I or II to address specific impairments (muscle function or mobility).
- **External focus** is related to concentration on achieving a goal or a target external to the body and is useful during Phases II or III to address neuromuscular coordination, functional endurance, strengthening, power exercise, or functional movement training.
- **Stages of learning** progress from **conscious cognitive** control to a more automatic or **autonomous stage.**
- The first step in learning a new exercise is **understanding** the desired exercise structure, position, and movement.
- The second step involves **fine-tuning and correcting** the performance with **feedback** and **error detection.**
- Once the movement performance is optimal, **practice** is needed to reinforce and change patterns.
- After the patient is able to perform the movement without significant concentration in a more autonomous manner, the exercise complexity, speed, and timing can be progressed for **functional movement training.**

movement and how to perform the movement before being expected to perform the exercise without feedback. During this stage, the patient will need to think about the movement and concentrate on achieving the desired movement or skill. Errors and compensations are common, and patients are not always aware of how they need to improve.[12] However, concentration on learning the movement or exercise can also result in the patient trying so hard that the movement is highly variable or stiff and inefficient.[7] Under these circumstances, the therapist may need to adjust the

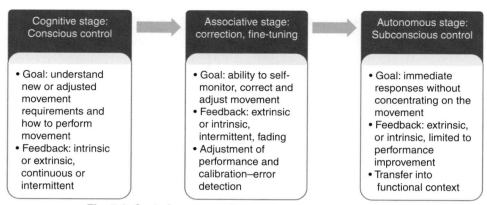

Fig. 7.3 Goals for stages of motor learning during recovery.

instructions or use another exercise that the patient has mastered and return to the more difficult task at a later point.

If the patient is unable to demonstrate the exercise successfully, it is the therapist's responsibility to explain, demonstrate, and instruct the desired movement to the patient in familiar terms until the activity is performed correctly. It is very easy to assume that the patient is not compliant with an exercise program rather than assessing what the therapist needs to adjust in order for the patient to understand the what, why, and how and to provide opportunities for the patient to demonstrate his or her understanding. The patient's preferred learning style and personal factors are used to provide one or more explanations using a variety of methods including visual demonstration, tactile guidance (Videos 7.2–7.4), verbal instructions, or other forms of explanation such as videotaping (Clinical Example 7.4). The patient's perception of what the desired pattern is can be influenced by previous training or ingrained patterns or thoughts (Clinical Example 7.5). A useful teaching method is to ask the patient to explain what he or she understood from the initial instructions to check whether the message needs to be clarified. This "repeat back" method also provides further information about the patient's preferred learning methods or vocabulary, and the patient's words or analogies can be used to provide feedback at a later point.

Although a step-by-step process is often used to teach movement or exercise, breaking down movement into minute steps or providing excess information is not always needed and can inhibit fluid complex motion.[3] Too much detail or the incorrect instructions can distract the patient's attention, inhibit learning, and be very frustrating for the patient.[4,7] There is also some thought that allowing patients to self-identify errors (as long as they know what the error is and the movement is safe) can speed up the process of skill acquisition.[12] Not allowing the patient to identify his own movement errors can often be problematic for novice therapists and even for some experienced clinicians.

Any negative thoughts or beliefs interfering with optimal movement, such as fear of pain, further injury, or falling, will impact learning. Under these circumstances, ensuring that the patient feels safe and that the exercise is unlikely to harm them will be important. The ability to understand what an exercise looks like, perform the exercise correctly, and adjust the movement requires attention and the desire to change. Often patients will require time and repetition to understand what they are being asked to do,

and, therefore, the movement may need to be slow and deliberate at first. If the patient is impatient about returning to work or sport, this would potentially impede a gradual progression without increasing inflammation, just as fear or lack of motivation to try the movements will not address the desired goals. During this stage of learning, clear instructions of what to do and choosing how much information to provide are important. Motivation and encouragement and/or education about the intent, future progressions, and reasons for the intensity or type of exercise may be needed. The therapist needs to provide sufficient information for the patient to understand the movement while at the same time avoiding overwhelming the patient with information.

Associative Stage: Correction, Fine-Tuning, and Practice

Once the patient understands the format of an exercise, the next stage involves **fine-tuning** and **practicing** a task using the correct movement patterns.[8,12] Rarely will a patient be able to perform an exercise perfectly on the first attempt. Movements should become more consistent and efficient with practice,[13] and the amount of feedback from the therapist is slowly faded. Correct performance may require adjusting alignment (Videos 5.12 and 7.5), percentage weight bearing (Video 7.6), timing of movement (Videos 7.7 and 7.8), and range or intensity, and limiting compensations (Videos 7.2 and 7.6–7.7). Often compensatory patterns have been reinforced for some time, and the therapist might need to explain, demonstrate, or adjust the exercise multiple times using different methods of instruction before correct performance is achieved. Only after the correct form is demonstrated should the patient be asked to repeat the movement, particularly without supervision as a home program. Error detection is therefore critical (see later discussion). Practicing with correct form will solidify the neural memory. If the exercise is performed with compensations, practice will only serve to reinforce the incorrect movement pattern. Therefore, the therapist should take ample time to ensure that the desired movement is understood and achieved. During this phase, practice depends on successful performance using a variety of exercises in environments similar to those required for function while allowing error detection and correction (Videos 5.12, 7.8, and 7.9).[3] The "association" with a previous or new environment is thought to reinforce the pattern, while movement in a different context is not necessarily transferred to functional requirements.

📌 CLINICAL EXAMPLE 7.5 Adjusting Ingrained Patterns

A patient is in Phase II after an ACL reconstruction and has a natural bony valgus alignment.

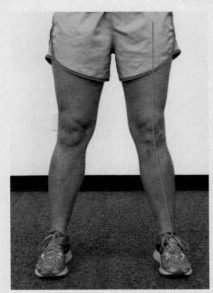

Valgus bony alignment.

When she is performing bilateral squats (Exercise 9.30), she adopts a wide stance, further increasing the valgus forces on the knee. During the exercise, the patient is hanging backward, with her line of gravity behind her heels. She has been complaining of anterior knee pain. This movement pattern increases load on the patellofemoral joint and could be related to pain avoidance, habit, or the patient may be thinking about "keeping the knees from moving over the toes." This is a common misperception, and the therapist will need to clarify if the patient is performing the exercise to avoid knee pain, to increase her overall stability, or if this is her habitual alignment related to prior training. If this is the case, her thought pattern and the ineffective movement pattern need to be replaced to correct the pattern. This could involve multiple strategies including demonstrating the position, instructing the patient to set up the position with the feet slightly closer together, and using a mirror to observe the actual compared to the desired pattern. While a smaller base is desired, dynamic valgus is not, and an external focus such as asking her to point her knees toward cones or a line in front of her or asking her to hold a pole and keep it parallel to the ground and in front of her body, may be useful to promote alignment without multiple complicated instructions.[1]

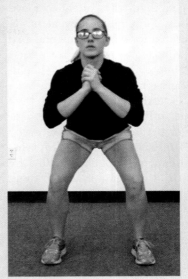

Squat with wide base and slightly asymmetrical weight distribution.

The patient's weight distribution is slightly toward the right side. Note that the overall muscle bulk and activation is greater on the right leg compared with the left leg.

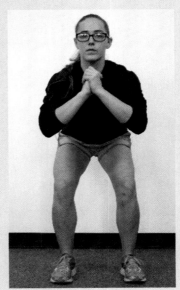

Squat with smaller base and improved weight-bearing distribution.

Smaller base of support with the feet underneath the hips and improved distribution of weight results in more symmetrical muscle activation and decreases the valgus forces on the knee.

Reference

1. Benjaminse A, Gokeler A, Dowling AV, et al. Optimization of the anterior cruciate ligament injury prevention paradigm: novel feedback techniques to enhance motor learning and reduce injury risk. *J Orthop Sports Phys Ther.* 2015;45(4):170–182.

Autonomous Stage: Automatic Control with Progressing Complexity

The eventual goal is for the patient to move toward **automatic responses**. Functional movement, particularly for sports, requires reinforced fundamental patterns to allow attention to be directed toward play or more skilled activity. As the patient improves, movements should become more fluid, accurate, and efficient and be processed more automatically without excessive concentration.[3] Usually this phase is only achieved in Phase III, but if the patient is a highly skilled athlete or performer, this stage may be accelerated. Skilled instructions matching the patient's specific needs and external focus of attention can help with achieving the level of coordination and integration needed to get to this point and shorten the first stages of motor learning. There are strategies to facilitate the progression from conscious control to more automated but still efficient patterns. Balance and equilibrium strategies often provide the fastest and most efficient response system, with multiple sensory systems providing input into this complex system. As one of the most

critical systems for human function, balance and equilibrium responses operate at an unconscious level, and a patient is required to maintain or regain balance if challenged even if he or she is not able to consciously create the same movements at high speed. Exercise choices that include using unstable surfaces, a small base of support, or challenges to maintain balance (perturbations or external challenges) can all be used to promote these responses with guarding and appropriate care to ensure patient safety.

When automatic control is achieved, the task is progressed by altering a number of variables: progression of speed, timing, coordination (**progressing the complexity of the movement** [Videos 3.22, 3.23, and 7.1]). At this point feedback from the therapist should be minimal, and the patient will need to self-monitor and correct errors independently. Error correction progresses from immediate feedback **during** the performance to feedback **after** the exercise (knowledge of results; see later discussion). As patients progress to functional movements in Phase II and III, practice is varied and embedded in the context of functional skills or tasks (Clinical Example 7.6).

📌 CLINICAL EXAMPLE 7.6   Progressing From Conscious Control to Associative Stage (ACL Repair)

One of the major goals for patients after ligament reconstruction is to improve neuromuscular control to provide timely responses to help stabilize the joint during dynamic motion. This requires progressive challenge to train neuromuscular responses to be able to execute movement with unconscious control. The overall awareness of position (proprioceptive training) and the timing and coordination of movement will be a major priority to return to function and prevent further injury while developing adequate neuromuscular endurance, strength, and, finally, power.

Precautions After ACL Repair

During early recovery, precautions need to be followed to protect the healing areas. Weight-bearing closed-chain exercises such as squats, leg press, step-ups and step-downs, and lunges performed in greater angles of knee flexion have been advocated for isolated ACL reconstruction to promote general lower extremity muscle function recruitment and are the preferred method to train functional alignment and proprioception.[1,2] However, bone or articular cartilage precautions override impairment or functional recovery requirements to promote healing of these structures.[1] Open-chain knee extension (non–weight-bearing) resistance in ranges between 0 and 45 has been found to result in greater tensile load placed on the ACL.[1,2]

Conscious Control (Phase I or early Phase II)

The closed-chain isometric squat for Patient A in Clinical Example 7.1 offers the advantage of promoting force closure and isometric activation of the quadriceps, hamstrings, and hip stabilizers without excessive strain or shear force on the ACL reconstruction. The use of closed-chain exercise offers the advantage of promoting force closure and isometric activation of the quadriceps, hamstrings, and hip stabilizers without excessive strain or shear force on the ACL reconstruction. This position limits stress on the graft by using active force closure between 45 and 90 degrees and uses closed-chain exercise to limit anterior translation.[1] The patient is instructed to "keep the ball still while pushing toward the wall."

Associative Stage (Late Phase II, Phase III)

As the patient progresses through Phase II, and with sufficient time for healing, precautions are lifted and the patient is allowed to exercise through range. Closed-chain bilateral squats are used to promote proprioceptive input, force closure,

and muscle endurance with the aim to progress through the pain-free range. The patient is asked to react to outside stimuli and respond without using conscious control. This is especially important for complex movements or to train reaction time. Techniques such as using external focus to keep a bar horizontal while balancing on an unstable surface or maintaining alignment with a line on the floor or cones to guide the sagittal plane movement can be used to help with developing unconscious control of lower extremity alignment; however, there is a greater reliance on integrating responses rather than breaking down the movements.

As the patient progresses, an unstable surface is used to further challenge proprioception.

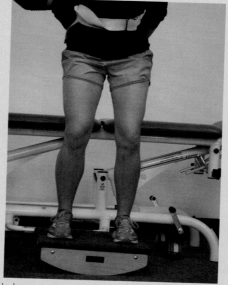

Double-leg squats with an unstable base (balance board).

The most unstable direction of the balance board is used in the frontal plane to challenge equal weight-bearing distribution. If the patient moves toward the unaffected leg, the loss of balance is an immediate source of feedback.[2–4] The patient is instructed to "keep the balance board still."

continued

📌 CLINICAL EXAMPLE 7.6 Progressing From Conscious Control to Associative Stage (ACL Repair)—cont'd

As the patient progresses, pertubations are used to challenge balance responses without the patient anticipating the movement or directions to respond to. The need to respond quickly and accurately to maintain balance helps train the neuromuscular response time and overall proprioceptive awareness.[3,4]

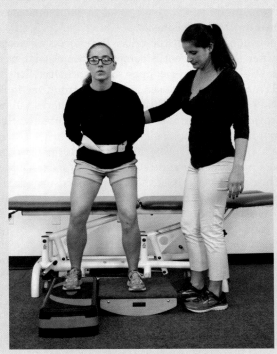

Unstable surface for surgical side.

The patient is challenged to maintain the stable position by external motion of the balance board created by the therapist. The patient is instructed to "keep the balance boards still while I challenge your position."

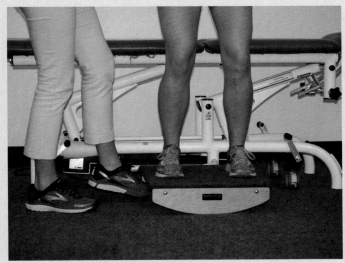

Pertubations.

Autonomous or Automatic Phase

As the patient progresses to dynamic movement and masters slower drills, the complexity is increased with fine tuning and practice. Drills are performed in a semi-squat starting position running between cones, with changes of direction around cones and responding to sport-specific requirements such as another player running toward the patient or requiring the patient to dribble a soccer ball and avoid players. The patient is required to adapt and use the acquired dynamic balance and neuromuscular coordination responses before returning to contact sports.

The action is translated into the context in which the patient needs to be able to reproduce the movements, such as running sideways on a soccer field. The uneven surface challenges responses and is a familiar environment. The movement is started slowly, allowing the patient to develop confidence, with progressive speed and range of motion. The exercise is progressed to different angles and directions (starting slowly and picking up speed before varying direction).

References

1. Adams D, Logerstedt D, Hunter-Giordano A, Axe MJ, Snyder-Mackler L. Current concepts for anterior cruciate ligament reconstruction: a criterion-based rehabilitation progression. *J Orthop Sports Phys Ther.* 2012;42(7):601–614.
2. Wilk KE, Macrina LC, Lyle Cain E, Dugas JR, Andrews JR. Recent advances in the rehabilitation of anterior cruciate ligament injuries. *J Orthop Sports Phys Ther.* 2012;42(3):153–171.
3. Chmielewski TL, Hurd WJ, Rudolph KS, Axe MJ, Snyder-Mackler L. Perturbation training improves knee kinematics and reduces muscle co-contraction after complete unilateral anterior cruciate ligament rupture. *Physical Ther.* 2005;85(8):740–749.
4. Chmielewski TL, Hewett TE, Hurd WJ, Snyder-Mackler L. Principles of neuromuscular control for injury prevention and rehabilitation. In: Magee DJ, Zachazewski JE, Quillen WS, eds. *Scientific Foundations and Principles of Practice in Musculoskeletal Rehabilitation.* St. Louis, MO: Saunders Elsevier; 2007:375–387.

ERROR DETECTION AND FEEDBACK/ FEEDFORWARD MECHANISMS FOR MOTOR PERFORMANCE

Error detection uses stored memories of successful versus unsuccessful attempts at movement, allowing for adjustment of planning and processing tasks (Box 7.6). Error detection is often affected by injury or reinforced patterns related to pain or fear avoidance. Sensory receptor activation is reduced or late after ligament injuries and in the presence of hypermobility, resulting in impairments in proprioception, response time, and neuromuscular coordination. Maladaptive patterns result from the combination of sensory impairments, fear avoidance, pain, or muscle function impairments. As a patient regains muscle function and movement, the restoration of patterns relies on regaining **accurate** error detection to promote efficient functional movement patterns. Slower, controlled movement allows sensory information processing during the movement and makes error detection possible. If a movement is faster, processing sensory feedback is more difficult, particularly if sensory systems are affected by injury. In the early stages of exercise introduction and fine-tuning, slower exercise with focus on correcting error may be easier, while in the later stages, higher speed is necessary to test neuromuscular coordination (Clinical Example 7.7).

Correcting movement will involve either feedback or feedforward systems. If the analysis or processing occurs after the movement, **feedback** mechanisms are used to **detect** error and adjust future performance. In contrast, **feedforward** mechanisms occur when repeated practice allows anticipation of the required motor performance, they are faster, and they **prevent error**. Most functional movement is performed using feedforward mechanisms in individuals with normal function. Faster movement or more complex tasks may rely on memory of the requirements for the task and only allow error detection after the movement. Feedforward mechanisms are also needed for anticipatory adjustments required for postural tasks (Clinical Example 7.8).

BOX 7.6   Error Detection, Feedback, and Feedforward Systems

- **Error detection** integrates stored memories of successful versus unsuccessful attempts at movement, allowing for adjustment of planning and processing tasks.
- Slower, controlled movement is used early in the learning process while more rapid movement is used once neuromuscular control is achieved.
- If error detection mechanisms are impaired or need to be reestablished, feedback and feedforward processing loops assist with movement correction and control.
- **Feedback** mechanisms occur after the movement and are used to *detect* error and adjust future performance.
- **Feedforward** mechanisms occur when repeated practice allows anticipation of the required motor performance, are faster, and **prevent error.**
- Feedback and feedforward loops can be facilitated using visual, auditory, or tactile information provided by equipment, the therapist, or the patient.
- Balance responses provide rapid sensory information and can be used to facilitate moving from conscious to unconscious control.

Knowledge of performance is the perception or awareness of movement patterns using **concurrent feedback** while moving.[1] Feedback can also be provided using videotaping, peer evaluation, achievement of a specific target, auditory tones such as a metronome, or a computerized program such as the Wii or Balance Master. Visual, auditory, and tactile sensory input, along with balance responses, allow the patient to adjust position, stop movement, or correct alignment, thus providing **intrinsic or implicit feedback**.

Knowledge of results describes the process of using feedback **after** the movement is completed. Knowledge of results informs the patient whether he or she has achieved the goal and correct movement and is used to develop error detection methods and to fine-tune or adjust movement patterns.[1] Therapists can provide knowledge of results using both corrective feedback for improvement or motivational feedback when a patient performs a movement correctly, but the goal is for the patient to be able to self-monitor and detect errors for maximal learning. Feedback about performance success depends on an accurate understanding of the desired result.

There is some evidence that therapists and coaches should allow patients time to analyze and process the success of the movement (error detection) on their own before offering verbal **explicit** feedback. The frequency of feedback is important as constant feedback has been found to slow down learning motor skills and diminish long-term retention.[4,13,14] Often intrinsic or implicit feedback is being processed by the patient at the unconscious level, and frequent or detailed explicit feedback interferes with the integration of information or results in the patient becoming dependent on the therapist for approval.[4] Ideally, concurrent explicit feedback during and after the movement is **faded** or offered only as needed as the patient improves. Typically, less feedback is required once the patient has reached Phase III or before discharge. Each exercise will be different, however, and new exercises may require additional correction at first.

Highly skilled individuals, with well-developed neuromuscular coordination, body awareness, and error detection capabilities do not require as much correction from the therapist. For these patients, feedback frequency, timing, and word choice should be carefully considered so that there is limited interference with the individual's error detection mechanisms.[1] The therapist may interfere with the unconscious automated motor control processes when using unfamiliar terms, excessive instructions, or poorly chosen corrections.

The eventual goal of practice for all patients is to be able to utilize the unconscious feedforward mechanisms that can be translated into activities of daily living. *Dyad training* is a method where two peers alternate in the performance and feedback roles.[13–15] The combination of practice and opportunities to observe and evaluate someone else's performance can result in more effective learning and higher retention than either one of these options alone.[13–15] Alternating practice and observation trials also provides some physical rest and relief from high concentration that may be beneficial for individuals who are "overthinking" or trying too hard[4] (see Clinical Examples 7.10 and 7.11).

Patient A

Patient A has chronic low back pain with hypermobility. The initial goals are to promote neuromuscular coordination and activation of the local stabilizers to provide force closure and force distribution. Exercises are performed in supported positions. Spinal stabilization muscle activation techniques are performed in supine with a blood pressure cuff placed under the lumbar lordosis to provide a visual feedback system related to intensity of a transversus abdominus contraction to support a neutral spine position without excessive pelvic tilting (Exercise 11.20). Timing of the instructions helps with anticipatory sequencing for the transverse abdominus contraction to facilitate feedforward training before leg lifts off an exercise ball (Exercise 11.21; Video 6.17). The anticipatory timing is facilitated by the timing of the verbal instructions to:

- "Prepare your body to keep it still before you lift your leg." (Anticipatory timing)
- "Keep the center of your pelvis on the table/floor and try to keep it from tipping back and forward or side to side as you lift your leg." (External focus)
- "Watch the gauge of the blood pressure cuff and keep the pressure still while you lift the leg" (External focus and error detection)

Although external focus is often faster and more effective for coordinated movements, internal focus can be useful in the early stages when muscle activation is required and tactile feedback allows error detection. Alternate instructions using an internal focus are:

- "Place your index finger on the front of your pelvis and your thumbs on your ribs. Imagine that you have suspenders between your fingers. Try to keep the space the same. Monitor the position and, if the space changes or pelvis starts to move, increase the amount of muscle contraction you are using (Video 6.17)." (Internal focus and tactile error detection)

Once the patient is able to engage the abdominal muscles, lying on a foam roller provides rapid sensory feedback (tactile and balance responses) to maintain midline position (intrinsic feedback; see Exercise 11.21).

Patient B

Patient B has a history of whiplash 6 months previously with complaints of cervical pain and headaches making it difficult for her to sit for more than 30 minutes. She has problems with computer work and driving. During the initial evaluation the therapist determines that she is having difficulty with cervical endurance against gravity, and she has difficulty with accurate repositioning after moving her cervical spine. Exercises are selected to address both the endurance and coordination deficits. The patient was able to hold the positions required for the deep cervical flexor test against gravity, but fatigued very quickly (after 5 seconds) and pain levels increased with the anti-gravity flexor endurance test (see Clinical Example 4.15).

Exericse Choices

Exercise 1: Unstable support from a partially deflated ball encourages the patient to utilize the postural stabilizing muscles while performing upper extremity exercise. If the cervical muscles are not controlling the midposition, the patient will be able to feel the movement of the ball. After stabilizing the cervical region, she is asked to keep her cervical spine stable while she challenges the position by lifting one leg to a 90-degree position. The exercise is progressed using the foam roller for anterior cervical stabilization (Exercise 11.22) as the relatively unstable position provides feedback if there is movement of the roller but does not involve holding the head up against gravity.

Upper extremity movement is added to further challenge endurance and activation. The patient is asked to monitor the position of the foam roller, and fatigue or pain in the cervical region is the limiting factor for the dosage (Video 6.21).

Exercise 2: Cervical endurance against gravity (Exercise 11.26). The head and neck position is more difficult to control and to monitor in prone as the patient cannot use tactile input to detect position or the desired target. The therapist places a wooden rod above the patient's head for the patient to reach and monitor when she achieves the position. Video taping can be used to point out the coordination patterns and alignment desired if the patient only uses the upper cervical extensors rather than a counterbalanced force couple of the deep cervical flexors with the upper and lower cervical extensors and the upper cervicothoracic extensors.

Exercise 3: After she has developed sufficient awareness and control of the head position, fine-tuning the dynamic coordination is indicated to improve the consistency of repositioning accuracy. A laser device attached to a head strap is used to provide feedback related to cervical positioning and to train neuromuscular coordination by tracking shapes on the target or by following instructions to reach the target points. Variation in the directions, distances, and response time is built into the training (Clinical Example 4.19).

The laser is used to train neuromuscular coordination and improve the accuracy of returning to a midline position along with fine-tuned tracking using external focus and feedback systems. The visual target provides concurrent feedback to train the coordination systems.

Patient C

Patient C is in Phase II after a hip resurfacing procedure. She needs to be able to monitor her weight-bearing symmetry throughout the squat range. A force platform and visual display (Balance Master) provides concurrent feedback for immediate adjustments when she shifts toward her nonsurgical limb.

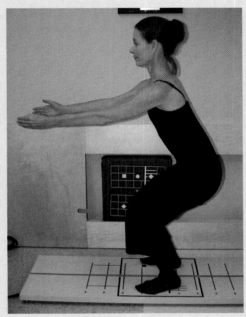

Balance Master.

Concurrent feedback of weight-bearing symmetry is measured on the force platform and is visible on the computer monitor during squats, which allows adjustment while moving through range.

As she progresses, balance reactions on an unstable surface (mini-trampoline) are used to promote hip muscle activation on the standing leg by facilitating automatic postural and balance responses. Movement of the opposite leg requires adjustments of intensity, direction, and coordination from the stabilizing muscles.

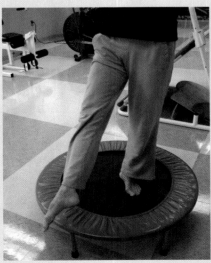

Use of balance responses on mini trampoline.

⚑ CLINICAL EXAMPLE 7.8 Feedback

A patient is recovering after a hip labral tear pain and wants to be able to return to basketball. In her initial Phase II exercise program she was addressing her hip stability in a single-leg squat. In order to monitor her hip position, single-leg squats are performed in front of a mirror with markers placed on the anterior superior iliac spines of her pelvis. The pelvis position (see Fig. 4.18) shows the "hip drop" or Trendelenburg position, with the unsupported side of the pelvis dropping below the supporting side. The limited support from the hip abductors increases the overall passive stress placed on the lateral soft tissues of the right leg and increases the compressive forces on the hip joint.

She is asked to keep the markers level. Initially, the therapist provides verbal feedback until the patient is able to perform the movement with the pelvis level. After she is able to identify (and correct) the pelvis position, the patient practices the movement herself with **intermittent feedback** from the therapist. She also records the number of squats she performs without corrections, initially stopping and resting if she loses the position, later continuing with adjustments and recording the successful attempts.

The patient is progressed to Phase III once her weight-bearing distribution is equal, she has full range of motion, and good control of full bilateral and single-leg squats.

Progression to Jumping Reeducation and Training

Jump landing strategy reeducation is introduced, including landing using shock absorption control from all lower extremity joints with a soft landing rather than rigid co-contractions. Landing with a forward trunk encourages distribution of vertical ground-reaction forces between the hip and knee and the relative moment arm.[1–4] Instructions to land softly allow the patient to obtain immediate feedback from the sound of the landing or from the feeling of landing "hard."[1–4]

Exercise Choices

1. Double-leg vertical jumps on trampoline, progressing to single-leg jumps (trampoline helps encourage using the momentum of the downward motion to store and release the energy for the jumping action and provides immediate feedback if the patient "freezes" or stiffens during the landing).
2. Low height and depth jumps on land
3. Drop jumps (double-leg) from a small step; progress to greater height [5]
4. Split squat jumps
5. Single-leg vertical hops in place for endurance (to fatigue)
6. Run-up and jump progressing toward sports-specific drills

She has also been performing stationary double-leg jumps and stationary single-leg hops with control of her hip position. Double-leg drop jumps are introduced from a step using videotaping and verbal feedback to address landing strategies.[3] Initially, she is hesitant to absorb weight on the injured side and lands with more weight on the left leg, increasing angulation forces. After encouraging her to distribute her weight, she is asked to practice the jump landing softly and evaluating the success of the jump by the sound and elasticity of her landing.

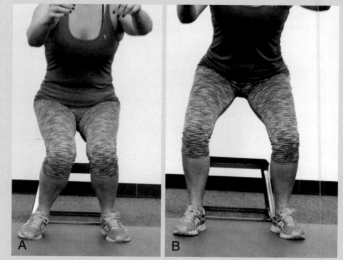

(A) Landing from drop jump with asymmetrical weight bearing and dynamic valgus. (B) Corrected landing position with improved symmetry and control of the valgus angulation.

She is also practicing single-leg hops for distance using an external focus with marks placed on the floor at 80% of her maximal single-leg hop distance.[4] The target provides immediate feedback on the achievement of the distance target, and she is also provided with verbal feedback for her landing techniques after she has performed a warm-up trial. The initial trial is videotaped, and the therapist reviews the landing form with the patient. She is then allowed to practice for 5 sets without concurrent feedback before reviewing the videotape again. At this point she is asked to review her performance before therapist provides input (fading).

References

1. Dunleavy K. Outcomes of hip resurfacing in a professional dancer: a case report. *Physio Theory Pract.* 2012;28(2):142–160.
2. Silva RS, Ferreira ALG, Nakagawa TH, Santos JEM, Serrao FV. Rehabilitation of patellar tendinopathy using hip extensor strengthening and landing-strategy modification: case report with 6-month follow-up. *J Orthop Sports Phys Ther.* 2015;45(11):899–909.
3. Munro A, Herrington L. The effect of videotape augmented feedback on landing strategy: implications for anterior cruciate and patellofemoral joint injury prevention. *The Knee.* 2014;21(5):891–895.
4. Gokeler A, Benjaminese A, Welling W, Alferink M, Eppinga P, Otten B. The effects of attentional focus on jump performance and knee joint kinematics in patients after ACL reconstruction. *Phys Ther Sport.* 2015;16(2):114–120.
5. Erickson KI, Gildengers AG, Butters MA. Physical activity and brain plasticity in late adulthood. *Dialogues Clin Neurosci.* 2013;15(1):99–108.

SEQUENCING

Learning a task can start with simple exercises and progress to more complex coordination tasks. The progression of simple-to-complex is influenced by an individual's comfort with the task, coordination, capability, and goals. The sequencing may depend on resolution of contributing impairments or improvements in mobility or muscle function (Box 7.7). For example, muscle strengthening exercises may be started in one plane of movement before performing diagonal functional strengthening (Video 7.1). If there are healing precautions for tissues in a single plane of movement or direction, exercises may be progressed within planes of movement which do not influence the structure or are within the allowed range of motion. If select local stabilizing muscles are impaired, muscle activation and anticipatory response training, followed by endurance of the local and global stabilizing muscles, should be targeted before strengthening the global movers. Usually by Phase III more complex tasks mimicking functional requirements are introduced, requiring adequate function of both the stabilizers to support joint structures and alignment and the movers to create motion and power (Videos 3.22–3.23, and 7.1). Introduction of higher level functional tasks without sufficient stability or beyond the individual's capabilities can result in muscle soreness or inflammation and slow progress. The progression of complexity is also dependent on learning capabilities, goals, and the degree of impairments and function (Clinical Example 7.9).

BOX 7.7 Sequencing, Practice, and Reinforcement

- Progressing from simple to complex is influenced by the task, coordination, capability, and goals.
- Sequencing may depend on resolving contributing impairments and improvements in mobility or muscle function.
- Exercises may be progressed within planes of movement that do not compromise the healing structure or that are within the allowed range of motion.
- Exercises to improve activation of local stabilizing muscles and training of anticipatory responses will be targeted before addressing global mover strength.
- Progressing complexity is also dependent on learning and the level of irritability.
- Biomechanical efficiency is created by adjusting lever arms, positioning weight and line of gravity relative to the base of support for increased stability or to promote motion, and the use of inertia and momentum.
- Teaching efficient movement patterns should be introduced early enough to allow the patient to develop patterns with feedback, allow time for practice, and eventually integrate the patterns into functional movement.
- Using biomechanical concepts can be particularly important if there is permanent loss of neuromuscular capability or if joint protection strategies are required.
- Learning to adjust biomechanical factors requires an understanding of concepts and the confidence to trust the new technique.
- Individuals returning to higher level sports and performance need to learn how to use forces to their advantage:
- Functional tasks are retained when practiced in context and with specificity.
- Intensive focus and instruction for teaching optimal movement is necessary early in the treatment course; then the patient progresses to practice with feedback.
- Feedback from the therapist is faded once exercise is performed well and the patient understands how to self-monitor the movement; then the patient will practice without feedback.
- Regular checks are needed to reinforce concepts and remind patients about appropriate movement strategies and dosage.
- In order to fully benefit from a home program, patients should be able to verbalize the goal of the exercise, explain what to monitor, understand if it is possible to progress parameters, and perform the exercise correctly.
- The individual's personality and tendency to do too much or to avoid the movement will influence the frequency and type of reminders.
- Reminders can include handouts, exercise drawings, videos, or written instructions.

PRACTICE AND REINFORCEMENT

Memory and Pattern Development

To establish a permanent movement pattern, movement needs to be repeated and reinforced (see Box 7.7). Learning a new pattern—particularly if there is an established maladaptive pattern—requires multiple repetitions using the correct muscle activation, position, and timing to permanently change the pattern. Retrieval also depends on context: practicing at home without distractions is different from reacting to a busy shopping environment.

Blocked Versus Random Practice

Blocked practice involves repeating movements or exercise in the same order (see Clinical Example 7.13). Movements are therefore learned in the same context and sequence. Blocked practice using the same or similar tasks may be appropriate to introduce and learn a new or adjusted pattern, often in Phases I or II. There are also times when individual characteristics will require learning the movement using a consistent order (e.g., if a patient prefers concrete sequential learning or has difficulty with complex instructions).[1]

Random practice uses a different order of tasks to challenge responses to different requirements. By changing the order of tasks and contexts, the patient learns how to respond appropriately to unexpected stimuli. Random practice provides training for the patient to reproduce the skill more consistently during activities of daily living and sport and to use the patterns in the context in which it is required. Typically, random practice is preferred for functional tasks that require transfer into circumstances where the patient needs to be able to perform movements in any situation[4] (Clinical Example 7.10).

Functional Movement Adjustment: Reinforcing Efficient Patterns

Biomechanical efficiency can be improved by adjusting lever arms, positioning body weight and line of gravity relative to the base of support (center of gravity inside the base of support for increased stability, outside the base of support to promote motion), and using inertia and momentum. Teaching efficient

---

 ## CLINICAL EXAMPLE 7.9 Sequencing

A tennis player who is recovering from a Grade I medial collateral ligament (MCL) tear might start with single-plane lunges in the sagittal plane to avoid excessive stress on the MCL in the frontal plane, followed by sideways modified lunges in the frontal plane. Only after the patient is able to perform multiple repetitions (>25) through full range is the exercise progressed to small-range lunges in diagonal planes. After increasing the speed and depth of the lunges, the movements are performed with a tennis racquet and different lunge depth to simulate movements needed to return to tennis. The exercise simulation in a controlled environment precedes returning to hitting balls against a practice wall (the athlete is able to control the excursion of the lunge) or with a coach. The return to a competitive environment requires practice and development of confidence in a progressive manner.

CLINICAL EXAMPLE 7.10 Blocked and Random Practice

Blocked Practice
The tennis player in Clinical Example 7.9 practices forwards lunges for 3 sets of 20 repetitions followed by 3 sets of sideways lunges for each exercise.

Random Practice
The complexity of the exercise is increased by the therapist instructing the patient to perform forward and sideways lunges in a random sequence. He is then asked to respond to a computerized program with random instructions to lunge in different directions. The same progression is used for return to play with forehand, backhand, and volley shots practiced in units before requiring movement to reach a ball in a random sequence.

movement patterns should be introduced early enough to allow the patient to develop patterns with feedback, allow time for practice, and then eventually integrate the patterns into functional movements with feedforward mechanisms and unconscious control.

Sometimes movement reeducation is introduced early in Phase II as improving efficiency is likely to help distribute forces and may decrease symptoms. Changing or improving movement coordination is important for all categories described in Chapter 6; however, each category will involve slightly different priorities. Patients whose primary impairments are related to hypomobility will need to learn how to adjust strategies once mobility has improved, while those with primary hypermobility will need to address neuromuscular coordination immediately to limit stress in the extreme ranges (Videos 6.14 and 6.15). Repetitive strain disorders require a complex set of priorities, including addressing causative biomechanical factors that are often a major priority in limiting future recurrence and facilitating immediate changes (Videos 4.21–4.24). Early management after surgery or traumatic injury involves teaching patients how to adhere to precautions while movement reeducation

and training is likely to be delayed with longer healing times and limitations. Applying biomechanical concepts is particularly important when a patient has permanent neuromuscular function loss or needs joint protection strategies (see Clinical Example 7.14). Learning to adjust biomechanical factors requires an understanding of the concepts and the confidence to trust the new technique (Clinical Example 7.11).

Individuals returning to higher level sports and performance activities may need to learn how to utilize forces to their advantage, particularly when inefficient movement patterns have contributed to repetitive strain injuries. The adjustments in coordination to limit excessive force on injured structures often will also help the patient learn to develop more efficient patterns for performance goals (Clinical Example 7.12).

Context and Specificity

Functional tasks are retained when practiced in the context of the functional environment or situation where the movement is needed (Videos 5.15–5.17, 7.8, and 7.9). The practice of the exact task or specificity of training is also important for retention and reinforcement of new patterns.

CLINICAL EXAMPLE 7.11 Improving Functional Movement Efficiency

The patient (Patient A from Clinical Example 3.1 and Patient B from Clinical Example 7.1) has a history of a right total hip replacement and also has right knee osteoarthritis.

Sit-to-Stand
She needs to improve her efficiency and biomechanics to move from sitting to standing. Her initial pattern is to keep her center of mass behind her feet and use her hands to help push up off the chair. To decrease the lever arm and the amount of force on the patellofemoral joint and anterior knee structures, she is asked to "Bring your feet as close as possible to the chair and move your body forward to the edge of the chair" (Video 7.6).

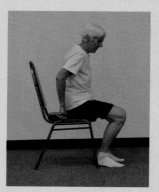

Standing from the chair using hands to assist movement.

The position of the body toward the base of support decreases the moment arm with respect to the knee joint. While leaning forward over the feet does not always feel secure, the more the patient hinges forward over the feet, the lower the forces on the knee axis and the greater efficiency of the hip extensors to assist the vertical movement.

Other strategies, such as using a higher plinth, using arm support, or leaning forward over the base with therapist assistance might be effective in preparing the patient for this task. Once the patient feels safe and realizes that she does not need to use the arms to push up, the sequence can be practiced with

feedback. The support is diminished after practicing the movement and when the patient is able to monitor the strategy independently.

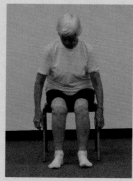

Standing from the chair leaning forward over the base of support without use of hand.

Stair Climbing/Step Training
She also needs to improve her ability to transfer her weight onto the leading leg when climbing stairs (see Clinical Example 3.1). Similar to the sit-to-stand mechanics, the displacement of the body toward the leading leg on the step (forward and slightly sideways) is established before the movement to decrease the moment arm. Instructions are adjusted to promote rapid hip extension to target the global movers, increase the power, and decrease the time in knee range flexion. The emphasis and tone of voice is used to encourage the setup, followed by rapid motion: "Move your weight forwards onto your right leg. Move upwards quickly onto the right leg" (Video 7.9).

The movement is practiced with a small step and hand support in the parallel bars, starting with the asymptomatic knee until the patient understands the concept. The amount of practice depends on pain responses. Other exercises to develop appropriate muscle activation and endurance and strength of the muscles used to stabilize the leg and limit dynamic valgus and promote hip stability are included before progressing to the movement reeducation (Exercise 7.7).

✒ CLINICAL EXAMPLE 7.12 Adjusting Running Mechanics

The patient with shin splints (see Clinical Example 7.2) is working on a progressive return to a running program. Decreasing the stride length and increasing the cadence is advocated to decrease the distance from the body weight to the anterior shin, thus limiting forces on the anterior limb while advancing the body. Setting a metronome at a faster cadence is used to provide concurrent feedback (knowledge of performance) and to decrease the stride length, rather than asking the patient to focus on shortening her stride. This type of adjustment may assist with decreasing forces contributing to repetitive strain disorders for patients with diagnoses such as shin splints.

Reinforcement and Reminders

Typically, teaching optimal movement requires intensive focus and instruction early in the treatment course. Feedback from the therapist is faded once an exercise is performed well and the patient understands how to self-monitor the movement. At this point, practice without feedback is warranted in order to reinforce the new pattern. However, regular checks to reinforce concepts and remind patients of the appropriate movement strategies and dosage are often important. In order to fully benefit from a home program, patients should be able to verbalize the goal of the exercise, perform the exercise correctly, and verbalize what to monitor (pain or swelling) and when it is appropriate to progress specific parameters (exercise dosage). The individual's personality and tendency to do too much or to avoid the movement will influence the frequency and type of reminders.

Patients may benefit from handouts or videos for more accurate recollection of the exercises to perform, proper technique, dosage, and other tips. Using a patient's smartphone to videotape home exercises is a useful and efficient tool for the therapist to record the exercise and instructions and to point out movement strategies that should be reinforced. Computer programs and apps allow video recording with superimposed angles and slow motion playback to provide feedback and monitor progress. If the patient is able to use video at home, the therapist will also be able to review the home program at the next visit. If the healthcare facility does not allow videotaping, prepared exercise video options are available on the Internet. Simple drawings and instructions can be effective, and graphics or photographs are also useful support methods for recall and reminders. An individualized handout is likely to be more helpful than a standardized exercise handout. When personalizing a written home exercise program, the therapist should keep in mind the patient's preferred learning and descriptions.

MOTIVATION

Motivation and patient "buy-in" will be influenced early in the patient encounter (Box 7.8). Explaining the goals of the exercise is important to gain the patient's **attention** and provide a target to work toward. Establishing goals that reflect the patient's interests or needs and explaining how each exercise is likely to help them attain their goals will help make the exercises more **relevant** and meaningful to the patient. **Relevance** to the patient's interests or needs can also be introduced by establishing **patient-specific**

BOX 7.8 Motivation and Confidence

- **Motivation** and patient "buy-in" will be influenced early in the patient encounter.
- Explaining the goals of the exercise is important to gain the patient's **attention**.
- **Explanations** on how the exercises will address the patient's interests or needs and reasons for choosing exercises provide **relevance.**
- Linkage to the patient's functional goals provides motivation to achieve long-term goals.
- **Confidence** is built by moving from simple to complex and providing sufficient opportunity to practice a task before advancing to a more difficult exercise.
- Positive feedback and encouragement build confidence.
- The psychological skill of coaching a patient to gain confidence in their ability to move is important.
- Fear avoidance beliefs or behaviors may require extensive time and work to address and develop confidence.
- Achieving goals assists with building confidence.
- Adherence (consistency with exercise recommendations) can be encouraged by consistent attention and supervision, as well as by promoting self-management.
- The therapist should address and minimize any personal or environmental barriers and optimize facilitating factors.

functional goals and explaining how each exercise is related to achieving their goals (Clinical Example 7.13). The patient's individual and environmental considerations can be factored into their program by using words, terminology, and images that are familiar to them. For example, a dancer is more likely to respond to demonstrations or instructions which use terms and positions related to dance (see Clinical Example 7.8). Some exercise choices are more attractive than others, and therefore giving patients a choice between exercises, or even the order of exercises, is an option to keep patients invested in their exercise program. Dyad training (pairing exercisers and having them observe each other)[15-17] and group exercise formats[18] are also methods with the benefits of observation (as discussed earlier) and the added advantage of social support.

Confidence is built through progressive scaffolding of tasks, by moving from simple to complex tasks, and by allowing sufficient opportunity to practice a task before advancing to more difficult exercise. Advancing a patient too slowly or too quickly is likely to negatively impact confidence. Making appropriate informed choices about exercises and starting points provides opportunity for encouragement, whereas selecting an exercise that is beyond a patient's capabilities will likely lead to frustration. Positive feedback and encouragement also build confidence. Therapists must develop the psychological skills to coach a patient to become independent and confident in their ability to move as part of the rehabilitation process; this will help prevent future injury. Confidence is essential for individuals to return to function without being fearful, and fear avoidance beliefs or behaviors may require extensive time and work for the patient to successfully address this component of return to function. Finally, achieving goals or knowledge of results often provides satisfaction and rewards which build confidence.

The patient–provider relationship is also likely to impact treatment outcomes and **adherence**.[19-21] Adherence refers to the

CLINICAL EXAMPLE 7.13 Motivation and Confidence

A patient who sustained right femur fractures after a motorcycle accident is evaluated 6 weeks after surgery. He has major wasting and atrophy of the quadriceps, hamstrings, and gluteal muscles, and there is still some effusion in the knee joint (Patient A in Clinical Example 7.4). There are scars on the distal lateral femur where the screws for the intramedullary rods were inserted, a scar distal to the patella where the rod was inserted through the knee joint, and a long scar in the superior lateral femur where the sliding screw was inserted for an intertrochanteric fracture. The patient is employed as a construction worker and is extremely motivated to return to work as he has no other source of income (facilitating personal factor). He does, however, tend to push himself very hard and has already attempted to ride his bicycle despite only having 20 to 90 degrees range of motion, a quadriceps lag, and major hip muscle weakness.

During the first session, his motivation to improve needs to be directed toward improving his knee and hip mobility and muscle function while adhering to precautions and preventing damage that could occur with excessive early activity and a risk of falling off his bike. The patient had access to a swimming pool and was able to begin on aquatic exercises that were more appropriate while still maintaining his motivation level (facilitating environmental factor). Stationary biking was added to address hip and knee mobility, with the explanation of the need to slowly build up the exercise without the risk of further damage.

He also responded to a challenge to fully address his quadriceps lag by the second visit (by setting specific goals). After teaching him to activate his quadriceps without compensating with his hip flexors, he was shown how to perform self-assisted knee extension using a strap, followed by isometric contractions and eccentric control. By his third visit, he was able to perform active gravity-resisted knee extension to the full passive limit.

Another technique used to maintain his motivation was constant reevaluation of his range and muscle function. During each session he was provided with a comparison to the past session and provided goals for the day. He was already very motivated to improve, so the challenge for this patient was to ensure that goals were adjusted regularly and range of motion achievements were recognized.

BOX 7.9 Motor Control and Pain

- Patients move differently when they have pain, after resolution of pain, as a precursor to pain, or if they perceive a movement may be painful.
- Addressing motor control may be critical in the management of patients who are experiencing pain:
  - Suboptimal movement that contributed to the development of pain: Address motor patterns to allow restoration of movement and progressive tissue loading.
  - Impaired movement control due to interference from pain: Reduce interference and address effects of deconditioning or movement abnormalities.
  - Modification of movement to protect an area: Decrease excessive protection and slowly reintroduce movement.
  - Modification of movement affected by pain responses: Decrease the association with pain through rational cognitive approaches or behavioral components to break the link with the pain memory.

interventions (Box 7.9). As Hodges[2] describes, patients move differently when they have pain, after resolution of pain, as a precursor to pain, or if they perceive a movement may be painful, and he proposes possible treatment approaches for each possibility (Table 7.2). Hodges[2] goes on to state that motor control may be critical in the management of patients who are experiencing pain.

Hodges[2] also emphasizes that there is no one solution to fit all patients and that patients may also require different approaches at different times. Although there is evidence of a relationship between motor control and improvement in symptoms, there is still a great deal that is not known about the ideal approaches to definitively match the right treatment approach to specific patient groups. The general approaches provided in this book can be useful to assist with clinical reasoning approaches, but it is vital for practitioners to consider new evidence as it becomes available.

patient's consistency with exercise recommendations. Strategies to improve adherence include consistent attention and supervision as well as promoting self-management.[21] Patients appreciate personalized interest, and good communication strategies are vital for a supportive relationship with the therapist.[22] Accountability and monitoring are also part of the overall treatment goal to assist patients with continuing exercise.[22] Any personal or environmental factors (see Chapter 3) that are likely barriers to adherences should be addressed and minimized while facilitating factors are optimized (see Clinical Example 7.13). The exercise program, and particularly home programs, should integrate elements to retain patient interest, build confidence, and address any barriers. Psychological contributions are especially important to consider (see Chapters 5 and 6).

MOTOR LEARNING AND CONTROL IN THE PRESENCE OF PAIN

Almost all patients experience pain as a part of their complaints, and pain behavior plays a large role in how the therapist introduces, teaches, and coaches the patient when delivering exercise

PATIENT-CENTERED APPROACHES: CONSIDERING PATIENT EXPECTATIONS AND PREFERENCES

As discussed earlier in this chapter, using the patient's preferred learning style, adapting descriptions and analogies to their background and motivating factors, and taking into account personality traits may help with buy-in. It can be very challenging to motivate patients when the patient does not want to exercise and believes that more passive treatment methods are more effective. The order, combinations, and emphasis of treatment might need to be adjusted under these circumstances (Clinical Example 7.14).

If the individual patient is presenting for treatment with a history of previous exposure to therapy or exercise, expectations may be present related to their recovery and preferences. These expectations should be considered when choosing exercises, and, fortunately, there are multiple options to provide exercise that may be preferred by a patient. Bishop and Bialosky[6] provide some guidelines for addressing patient expectations in Box 7.10.

TABLE 7.2 Motor Control Implications Related to Pain[2]

	Category	Possible Treatment Choices	Examples
1	Suboptimal movement and motor control that has contributed as a precursor to movement abnormalities, pain, and injury	Improve motor control to increase tissue loading and address movement abnormalities	Adjust movement and alignment contributors to address hamstring tendinopathy (Clinical Example 6.12) and slowly reintroduce isometric and eccentric forces to provide optimal stimulus for regeneration Provide reassurance that some pain is to be expected during exercise up to a certain point. Point out that pain is normally decreased by exercise Avoid seated exercise as this position is the most aggravating
2	Impaired movement control due to interference by actual or threatened injury or pain	Reduce interference and address effects of deconditioning or movement abnormalities	Reduce fear of movement through slow reintroduction of motion and exercise in supported positions while addressing catastrophizing after rotator cuff surgery related to a fall
3	Modification of movement to protect a painful area (or related to precautions)	Reduce excessive protection, slowly reintroduce movement and forces	Reintroduce weight bearing and reeducate alignment after precautions are lifted following a femur fracture
4	Modification of movement by a conditioned association with pain	Address conditioning response	Use graded exercise or graded exposure along with pain science education and cognitive behavioral techniques to reduce association between pain and movement

CLINICAL EXAMPLE 7.14 Addressing Patient Expectations

A patient returns after the first session of treatment for shoulder impingement and is complaining of increased pain. The initial exercises were conservative, but the patient had not exercised for some time and was also exhibiting fear-avoidance behaviors. The patient explains that she does not want to come to therapy as she has heard that it is very painful and states: "I just want the pain to go away."

The therapist may need to spend some time establishing an understanding of the extent of pain that is considered within an acceptable range and adjust to a graded exercise approach after confirming that fear avoidance is high (using the Fear Avoidance Beliefs Questionnaire [FABQ]). The understanding of exercise responses also needs to be discussed. During the discussion, the therapist asks if the patient preferred any of the initial exercises, and the upper extremity ergometer (UBE) was the most comfortable for the patient. The exercise session is started with the UBE, and the remaining exercises reassessed for dosage and potential for exacerbating the pain. The patient is closely monitored during the session and any compensation is corrected. The range of motion is decreased and weight is lowered but repetitions increased. During the session, the patient is reassured that the exercise responses are normal and that by adjusting the dosage the chance of soreness is less, but that slow progressive exercise is positive. The therapist also explains that the dosage will be continually adjusted and that the soreness is similar to starting to exercise again when there is no injury. The therapist also reassures the patient that by communicating her expectations and responses, they will be able to work together toward a positive outcome. The therapist also explains the timeframes when delayed-onset soreness is experienced and expectations of timeframes to achieve improvement.

BOX 7.10 Considering Patient Expectations While Choosing and Teaching Exercise[6]

- Portray confidence in your reasoning, choices, and belief that the exercise will assist the patient.
- Build rapport with the patient, including establishing (and honoring) patient preferences for exercise management. Give the patient options related to exercise equipment or order of exercises.
- Establish how exercise has affected the patient in the past. Any negative experience may interfere with adherence or outcomes.
- Set realistic goals and explain the potential outcomes.

BOX 7.11 Evaluation of Learning

- Evaluation of learning takes place throughout rehabilitation.
- The therapist should check whether the message was received and interpreted correctly.
- Evaluation includes constant observation of affect, reactivity, receptiveness, and appropriateness of responses.
- Asking the patient to explain what they are attempting to work on or to demonstrate the exercises at the end of the session or after performing home exercises are other options for evaluation and will help reinforce the message.
- More frequent evaluation is needed for highly skilled movement, in the presence of precautions, if there is difficulty with an exercise, or if the patient has negative attitudes toward exercise.

EVALUATION OF LEARNING FOR MODIFICATION AND ADJUSTMENT OF TEACHING METHODS

Evaluating understanding and learning occurs throughout the treatment process (Box 7.11). The patient may verbally state that he or she understands the why, how, and what elements but be unable to adequately demonstrate the exercise, even at the end of a session. The therapist needs to constantly observe affect, reactivity, receptiveness, and appropriateness of responses and recheck whether the information has been received and applied. Comparing information from the message that the therapist perceives was delivered and the receptive interpretation by the patient will help determine the extent of learning. The therapist can ask the patient to explain what he or she is attempting to work on, have the patient demonstrate the exercises again at the end of the session, and review home exercises or video performance. Verbal and nonverbal communication provides a wealth of confirming or contradictory evidence.

The goal is for the patient to be able to perform and self-monitor the exercises and responses. The reinforcement of the information and reminders can be provided in the form of written instructions, home exercise diagrams, and videos. The evaluation of understanding can be built into the delivery of this type of reminder by asking patients to provide descriptions in their own words, draw images, or record their demonstration of the home exercises on their phones or video equipment. This meets a dual purpose of reinforcing the message and assessing understanding, thus providing an opportunity to correct any misinterpretations. Those patients who are attempting to return to highly skilled movements or individuals who are having difficulty with any aspect of the exercise will require more attention from the therapist to determine if they have learned or changed their understanding of what is needed for the home exercise or to integrate the movements into functional activities. Likewise, those who need to adhere to precautions or have negative attitudes toward exercise will also need more attention. This is particularly important early on when reinforcing adjusted motor patterns or when the patient is progressing to a higher level of activity.

USING MODERATE INTENSITY EXERCISE TO PROMOTE NEUROMUSCULAR COORDINATION AND MOTOR LEARNING

While the emphasis of this chapter has been the application of teaching and learning concepts for therapeutic exercise for musculoskeletal diagnoses, there is also some recent evidence that moderate intensity cardiorespiratory exercise enhances acquisition of motor skills.[23-25] Most research has focused on longer term exercise, but even a single bout of moderate intensity activity seems to facilitate improvements in learning new skills in healthy adults.[23-25] Further research in this area is still needed, but including moderate intensity aerobic exercise as a warm-up might be useful for individuals in Phases II or III before exercise focusing on neuromuscular coordination.

▌ SUMMARY

- Learning how to perform an exercise and developing effective movement patterns involves changing and reinforcing patterns that are influenced by habit, training, pain experience, and goals.
- Initial explanations and instructions can be adjusted according to the patient's familiarity with the exercises, preferred learning style, personality, and other personal characteristics and tailored to the diagnosis, comorbidities, or impairments.
- Motor control requires a complex integration and processing of incoming sensory input, coordination, and control of movement through neurological pathways and motor output from neurological and muscle systems.
- Motor learning is the process of acquiring or adapting patterns through practice of movement or tasks resulting in permanent changes in performance ability.
- The first step in the teaching process and exercise instruction is explaining the what, why, and how of the exercise to the patient.
- A strong therapeutic alliance sets the stage for obtaining the best outcome possible.
- Goals establish the guidelines and expectations and provide further explanations of what the patient needs to achieve.
- SMART goals are Specific, Measurable, Achievable, Relevant, and have a Time set to achieve the goals.
- Internal focus is a concentration on a specific body part or a muscle action, often in isolation, and is appropriate in Phases I or II to address specific impairments. External focus is related to concentration on achieving a goal or a target external to the body and is useful during Phases II or III to address neuromuscular coordination, functional exercise, or movement training.
- Stages of learning progress from conscious cognitive control to more automatic unconscious movement patterns.
- After understanding the desired exercise structure, position, and movement, fine-tuning and correcting the performance with feedback and error detection is followed by practice.
- Error detection integrates stored memories of successful versus unsuccessful attempts at movement, allowing for adjustment of planning and processing tasks.

- Feedback mechanisms adjust future performance, whereas feedforward mechanisms occur when repeated practice allows anticipation of the required motor performance.
- Feedback and feedforward loops can be facilitated using visual, auditory, or tactile information provided by equipment, the therapist, or the patient.
- Progressing from simple to complex is influenced by the task, coordination, capability, and goals.
- Sequencing depends on resolving contributing impairments, improvements in mobility or muscle function, learning, and the level of irritability.
- Teaching efficient movement patterns should be introduced early enough to allow the patient to develop patterns with feedback, allow time for practice, and eventually integrate the patterns into functional movement.
- Learning to adjust biomechanical factors requires an understanding of concepts and the confidence to trust the new technique.
- Functional tasks are retained when practiced in context and with specificity.
- Intensive focus and instruction for teaching optimal movement is necessary early in the treatment course; then the patient progresses to practice with feedback.
- Feedback from the therapist is faded once an exercise is performed well and the patient understands how to self-monitor the movement; the patient then practices without feedback.
- Regular checks are needed to reinforce concepts and remind patients about appropriate movement strategies and dosage.
- Motivation and patient "buy-in" will be influenced early in the patient encounter and is enhanced by gaining the patient's attention, providing relevance, and facilitating confidence.
- Confidence is built by moving from simple to complex and by providing sufficient opportunity to practice a task.
- Fear avoidance beliefs or behaviors may require extensive time and work to address and develop confidence.

- Adherence can be encouraged by consistent attention and supervision, promoting self-management, minimizing personal or environmental barriers, and optimizing facilitating factors.
- Addressing motor control in the presence of chronic pain involves restoring movement with care to reduce excessive protective patterns while addressing negative pain behaviors and conditioning.

- Evaluation of learning includes constant observation of affect, reactivity, receptiveness, and appropriateness of responses, and asking the patient to explain what he or she is attempting to work on or to demonstrate the exercises at the end of the session.

REVIEW QUESTIONS

1. Define the terms *motor control* and *motor learning* and explain why these concepts are important to teach exercise and movement.
2. List the components of a SMART goal and provide an example.
3. Describe how the patient's learning style preference influences the therapist's instructions and explanations.
4. Choose an exercise and develop a script including the what, why, and how for a patient who is
   a. 75 years old and has hearing loss.
   b. 15 years old and is recovering from a thrower's shoulder injury. He wants to pursue a professional baseball career.
   c. 35 years old, a mom with three young children who has limited time to perform exercise.
5. Explain how internal and external focus are different, when the use of each is appropriate, and how you, as the therapist, would be able to provide instructions or exercise choices to encourage each form of concentration and focus.

6. Discuss the stages of motor learning and how you would adjust feedback for each stage.
7. Discuss ways you can establish a therapeutic alliance and promote motivation while teaching therapeutic exercise.
8. Describe how neuromuscular coordination sequencing is different across the phases of recovery and the factors that still need to be considered to protect an individual working under precautions.
9. Describe how functional training integrates elements of motor learning and biomechanical efficiency.
10. Describe how you would facilitate personal and environmental factors that will enhance motivation and relevance as well as minimizing the effect of inhibiting factors.
11. How would the presence of chronic pain, fear avoidance, or negative pain behaviors influence motor learning? What can you do to help facilitate learning how to move effectively and efficiently?
12. Describe how to evaluate learning components of the exercise delivery.

REFERENCES

1. Shumway-Cook A, Woollacott M. *Motor Control: Translating Research into Clinical Practice.* 5th ed. Philadelphia, PA: Lippincott Williams & Wilkins; 2017.
2. Hodges P. Motor control and pain. In: Sluka K, ed. *Mechanisms and Management of Pain for the Physical Therapist.* 2nd ed. Philadelphia, PA: IASP Wolters Kluwer; 2016:67–81.
3. Benjaminse A, Gokeler A, Dowling AV, et al. Optimization of the anterior cruciate ligament injury prevention paradigm: novel feedback techniques to enhance motor learning and reduce injury risk. *J Orthop Sports Phys Ther.* 2015;45(4):170–182.
4. McNevin NH, Wulf G, Carlson C. Effects of attentional focus, self-control and dyad training on motor learning: implications for physical rehabilitation. *Phys Ther.* 2000;80(4):373–385.
5. Bishop MD, Mintken PE, Bialosky JE, Cleland JA. Patient expectations of benefit from interventions for neck pain and resulting influence on outcomes. *J Orthop Sports Phys Ther.* 2013;43(7):457–465.
6. Bishop MD, Bialosky JE. The specific influences of nonspecific effects. In: Sluka K, ed. *Mechanisms and Management of Pain for the Physical Therapist.* Philadelphia, PA: IASP Wolters Kluwer; 2016:151–161.
7. Wulf G. *Attention and Motor Skill Learning.* Las Vegas, NV: Human Kinetics; 2007.

8. Napier C, Cochrane CK, Taunton JE, Hunt MA. Gait modifications to change lower extremity gait biomechanics in runners: a systematic review. *Br J Sports Med.* 2015;49:1382–1388.
9. McNair PJ, Prapavessis H, Callender K. Decreasing landing forces: effect of instruction. *Br J Sports Med.* 2000;34:293–296.
10. Silva RS, Ferreira ALG, Nakagawa TH, Santos JEM, Serrao FV. Rehabilitation of patellar tendinopathy using hip extensor strengthening and landing-strategy modification: case report with 6-month follow-up. *J Orthop Sports Phys Ther.* 2015;45(11):899–909.
11. Fitts PM, Posner MI. *Human Performance.* Belmont, CA: Brooks/Cole; 1967.
12. Magill RA. *Motor Learning and Control Concepts and Application.* 8th ed. New York, NY: McGraw Hill; 2007.
13. Winstein CJ, Schmidt RA. Reduced frequency of knowledge of results enhances motor skill learning. *J Exp Psychol: Learn Mem Cogn.* 1990;16:677–691.
14. Wulf G, Schmidt RA. The learning of generalized motor programs: reducing the relative frequency of knowledge of results enhances memory. *J Exp Psychol: Learn Mem Cogn.* 1989;15:748–757.
15. Shea CH, Wulf G, Whitacre CA. Enhancing training efficiency and effectiveness through the use of dyad training. *J Mot Beh.* 1999;31:119–125.
16. Shea CH, Wright DL, Wulf G, Whitacre C. Physical and observational practice afford unique learning opportunities. *J Mot Beh.* 2000;32:27–36.

17. Granados C, Wulf G. Enhancing motor learning through dyad practice, contributions of observation and dialogue. *Res Q Exer Sport.* 2007;78:197–203.

18. Dunleavy K, Kava K, Goldberg A, et al. Comparative effectiveness of Pilates and yoga group exercise interventions for chronic musculoskeletal neck pain: quasi-randomized parallel controlled study. *Physiotherapy.* 2016;102:236–242.

19. Ferreira PH, Ferreira ML, Maher CG, Refshauge Km, Latimer J, Adams RD. The therapeutic alliance between patients and therapists predicts outcome in chronic low back pain. *Phys Ther.* 2013;93(4):470–478.

20. Sluka K. Introduction: definitions, concepts and models of pain. In: Sluka K, ed. *Mechanisms and Management of Pain for the Physical Therapist.* Philadelphia, PA: IASP Wolters Kluwer; 2016:3–15.

21. Jorden JL, Holden MA, Mason EE, Foster NE. Interventions to improve adherence to exercise for chronic musculoskeletal pain in adults. *Cochrane Database Syst Rev.* 2010:CD005956.

22. Hinman RS, Delany CM, Campbell PK, Gale J, Bennell KL. Physical therapists, telephone coaches, and patients with knee osteoarthritis: qualitative study about working together to promote exercise adherence. *Phys Ther.* 2015;96(4):479–493.

23. Erickson KI, Gildengers AG, Butters MA. Physical activity and brain plasticity in late adulthood. *Dialogues Clin Neurosci.* 2013;15(1):99–108.

24. Mang CS, Snow NJ, Campbell KL, et al. A single bout of high-intensity aerobic exercise facilitates response to paired associative stimulation and promotes sequence-specific implicit motor learning. *J Appl Physiol.* 2014;117:1325–1336.

25. Statton MA, Encarnacion M, Celnik P, et al. A single bout of moderate aerobic exercise improves motor skill acquisition. *PLoS ONE.* 2015;10(10):e0141393.

BIBLIOGRAPHY

Aasa B, Berglund L, Michaelson P, Aasa U. Individualized low-load motor control exercises and education versus a high-load lifting exercise and education to improve activity, pain intensity, and physical performance in patients with low back pain: a randomized controlled trial. *J Orthop Sports Phys Ther.* 2015;45(2):77–85, B1-4.

Brumitt J, Matheson JW, Meira EP. Core stabilization exercise prescription, part 2: a systematic review of motor control and general (global) exercise rehabilitation approaches for patients with low back pain. *Sports Health.* 2013;5(6):510–513.

Bystrom MG, Rasmussen-Barr E, Grooten WJ. Motor control exercises reduces pain and disability in chronic and recurrent low back pain: a meta-analysis. *Spine.* 2013;38(6):E350–E358.

Corkery MB, O'Rourke B, Viola S, et al. An exploratory examination of the association between altered lumbar motor control, joint mobility and low back pain in athletes. *Asian J Sports Med.* 2014;5(4):e24283.

Costa LO, Maher CG, Latimer J, et al. Motor control exercise for chronic low back pain: a randomized placebo-controlled trial. *Phys Ther.* 2009;89(12):1275–1286.

Hidalgo-Perez A, Fernandez-Garcia A, Lopez-de-Uralde-Villanueva I, et al. Effectiveness of a motor control therapeutic exercise program combined with motor imagery on the sensorimotor function of the cervical spine: a randomized controlled trial. *Int J Sports Phys Ther.* 2015;10(6):877–892.

Hoeger Bement M, Sluka KA. Exercise-induced hypoalgesia: an evidence-based review. In: Sluka K, ed. *Mechanisms and Management of Pain for the Physical Therapist.* 2nd ed. Philadelphia, PA: IASP Wolters Kluwer; 2016:177–201.

Lin YL, Karduna A. Exercises focusing on rotator cuff and scapular muscles do not improve shoulder joint position sense in healthy subjects. *Hum Mov Sci.* 2016;49:248–257.

Lluch E, Schomacher J, Gizzi L, Petzke F, Seegar D, Falla D. Immediate effects of active cranio-cervical flexion exercise versus passive mobilisation of the upper cervical spine on pain and performance on the cranio-cervical flexion test. *Man Ther.* 2014;19(1):25–31.

Macedo LG, Latimer J, Maher CG, et al. Effect of motor control exercises versus graded activity in patients with chronic non-specific low back pain: a randomized controlled trial. *Phys Ther.* 2012;92(3):363–377.

Macedo LG, Maher CG, Hancock MJ, et al. Predicting response to motor control exercises and graded activity for patients with low back pain: preplanned secondary analysis of a randomized controlled trial. *Phys Ther.* 2014;94(11):1543–1554.

Macedo LG, Maher CG, Latimer J, McAuley JH. Motor control exercise for persistent, nonspecific low back pain: a systematic review. *Phys Ther.* 2009;89(1):9–25.

Magee DJ, Zachazewski JE. Principles of stabilization training. In: Magee DJ, Zachazewski JE, Quillen WS, eds. *Scientific Foundations and Principles of Practice in Musculoskeletal Rehabilitation.* St. Louis, M: Saunders Elsevier; 2007:388–414.

Meisingset I, Stensdotter AK, Woodhouse A, Vasseljen O. Neck motion, motor control, pain and disability: a longitudinal study of associations in neck pain patients in physiotherapy treatment. *Man Ther.* 2016;22:94–100.

Meisingset I, Woodhouse A, Stensdotter AK, et al. Evidence for a general stiffening motor control pattern in neck pain: a cross sectional study. *BMC Musculoskelet Disord.* 2015;16:56.

Noehren B, Scholz J, Davis I. The effect of real-time gait retraining on hip kinematics, pain and function in subjects with patellofemoral pain syndrome. *Br J Sports Med.* 2011;45:691–696.

Willy RW, Scholz JP, Davis IS. Mirror gait retraining for the treatment of patellofemoral pain in female runners. *Clin Biomech (Bristol, Avon).* 2012;27:1045–1051.

Sung W, Abraham M, Plastaras C, Silfies SP. Trunk motor control deficits in acute and subacute low back pain are not associated with pain or fear of movement. *Spine.* 2015;15(8):1772–1782.

Treleaven J, Peterson G, Ludvigsson ML, Kammerlind AS, Peolsson A. Balance, dizziness and proprioception in patients with chronic whiplash associated disorders complaining of dizziness: a prospective randomized study comparing three exercise programs. *Man ther.* 2016;22:122–130.

Tsao H, Hodges PW. Persistence of improvements in postural strategies following motor control training in people with recurrent low back pain. *J EMG Kin.* 2008;18(4):559–567.

Woodhouse A, Vasseljen O. Altered motor control patterns in whiplash and chronic neck pain. *BMC Musculoskelet Disord.* 2008;9:90.

Worsley P, Warner M, Mottram S, et al. Motor control retraining exercises for shoulder impingement: effects on function, muscle activation, and biomechanics in young adults. *J Shoulder Elbow Surg.* 2013;22(4):e11–e19.

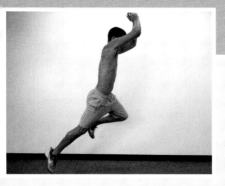

Evaluation for Adjustment of Exercise and Outcomes

Kim Dunleavy and William F. McGehee

OBJECTIVES

Upon completion of this chapter, the reader will be able to:

1. Evaluate exercise tolerance during and after exercise.
2. Describe anticipated responses to exercise, monitor tolerance, and identify responses that prompt an adjustment of the exercise choice or dosage for each of the categories discussed in Chapter 6, as well as the SINS characteristics.
3. Describe factors that may influence exercise responses and guide progression.

4. Discuss how to choose examination techniques to measure progress and develop a plan of care.
5. Describe the typical compensation patterns that a therapist should monitor when evaluating exercise tolerance.
6. Describe the critical thinking and decision-making processes used to adjust exercises.
7. Discuss how to choose and use self-reported or objective functional outcome measures to develop goals, track patient improvement, and evaluate treatment effectiveness.

EVALUATION OF RESPONSE TO EXERCISE

After the initial goals and exercise prescription have been established, the individual's responses to the exercise should be evaluated frequently (Box 8.1). The concepts discussed in the previous chapters can guide how quickly to progress exercise and the dosages within and between phases. The SINS elements (Severity, Irritability, Nature, Stage), phase of healing, tissue healing status, impairment, and functional goals, along with the categories of conditions, will help the therapist decide which tests to use and how frequently to reevaluate exercise choices.

Results from tests and measures, along with subjective responses, self-reported functional status, and functional performance measures guide clinical decision making throughout the initial evaluation, exercise testing, and prescription process. Relevant assessments are matched to the appropriate impairments and functional difficulties.

Evaluating responses to the initial exercise prescription is an ongoing process, occurring during and after the exercise session and when the patient returns for the next visit (see Box 8.1). Not all tests and measures are repeated each time, and a great deal of information can be obtained while observing and assessing the exercise performance. It is therefore important for the physical therapist to remain involved in the patient's exercise program, even if there are other personnel assisting with safety and setup. Physical therapist assistants will also be responsible for evaluating performance and communicating with the therapist if the exercises are tolerated, require adjustments, or need to be progressed. Regular communication becomes even more important when treatment time frames are limited by insurance coverage. Selected measures will be retested once enough time has passed, and the therapist will

BOX 8.1 Evaluation of Responses to Exercise: Time Frames

- Initial evaluation and exercise testing provide the baseline for comparison (see Chapter 4).
- Within a phase (individual impairments based on expected changes, functional capabilities based on impairment status or expected improvements):
  - During exercise performance
  - After exercise
  - Next visit
  - At established time frames to reevaluate short-term goals
- Between phases (impairments and functional capabilities; based on short- and long-term goals)

rely on their knowledge of expected tissue responses and current evidence to decide when to expect improvements. For example, if a patient presents with effusion, improvements in mobility would be expected during a treatment session and therefore regular reevaluation of range of motion is appropriate within the session, whereas muscle endurance and strength changes may take longer than one session to improve. Functional improvements tied to impairment expectations are likely to take more than a few sessions. Subjective responses and objective improvements should be consistently monitored during the initial exercise sessions, particularly during Phase I. As the patient progresses, the therapist will compare the patient's status to his or her baseline measurement and to evaluate whether or not the patient is ready to progress within that phase or to the next phase. This chapter will discuss how to evaluate exercise responses during, after, and across sessions, as well as using outcome measures to guide intervention and progression decisions (Clinical Example 8.1).

⚖ CLINICAL EXAMPLE 8.1   Evaluation of Responses to Exercise

A patient who sustained right femur fractures in a motorcycle accident is evaluated 6 weeks after surgery (Clinical Examples 4.10 and 7.4). His quadriceps, hamstrings, and gluteal muscles show major atrophy and wasting, and there is still some effusion in the knee joint. He presents with scars on the distal lateral femur where the screws for the intramedullary rods were inserted, a scar distal to the patella where the rod was inserted through the knee joint, and a long scar in the superior lateral femur where the sliding screw was inserted to stabilize an intertrochanteric fracture. The patient is a construction worker and is extremely motivated to return to work as he has no other source of income. He does, however, tend to push himself very hard and has already attempted to ride his bicycle, despite only having 20 to 90 degrees range, a quadriceps lag, and major hip muscle weakness.

Short-term goals:

1. Within 1 week, knee effusion will be reduced sufficiently to within 0.5 cm around the joint line in comparison to the opposite leg
2. Within 2 weeks, knee passive range of motion will increase from 10 to 110 degrees
3. Within 2 weeks, quadriceps and hamstrings activation will be sufficient to allow full support of the knee in the available passive extension range for straight leg raise without a lag for transfers
4. Within 2 weeks, the patient will be able to demonstrate quadriceps activation and endurance to allow knee extension against gravity from 45 degrees to the available passive knee extension range (>15 repetitions)
5. Within 2 weeks, the patient will be able to demonstrate hamstring activation and endurance to complete knee flexion against gravity to available passive flexion range in prone (>15 repetitions)
6. The patient will be able to demonstrate gait with crutches, demonstrating 100% adherence to partial weight-bearing precautions

Session 1: Exercise Testing and Examination

* Observe quadriceps activation
* Passive range of motion of the knee
* Active range of the motion of the knee
* Ability to perform initial exercises (repetitions, fatigue)

Quadriceps activation:

* Isometric quadriceps activation in supine (Exercise 9.39)
* Once able to properly activate his quadriceps, self-assisted knee extension using a strap is added (Exercise 9.43A), with isometric holds in full extension and eccentric control on the lowering

Evaluation of responses on the first session:

* Assess ability to perform the exercise and the patient's ability to restate the home exercise program
* Measure passive knee flexion and extension (goniometric)

Session 2: Examination at the Beginning of the Second Session

Subjective information is collected related to:

* Responses after the first visit (pain after treatment, timing of onset of pain if present, intensity and location of pain to assess delayed-onset muscle soreness and exercise tolerance)
* Ability to perform home exercise, frequency

Objective impairment measures:

* Knee passive and active range of motion: Flexion and extension
* Assess compliance with weight-bearing precautions and gait pattern

Responses After First Visit

By the second visit, he was able to perform active, gravity-resisted knee extension to the full passive limit. During the session, he was provided with the comparison to the past session and provided with goals for the day.

Reevaluation After 1 Week

Based on the short-term goals, remeasuring girth to track effusion would be completed 1 week after initial evaluation (unless improvements are noted earlier), and muscle activation and endurance would be retested at 2 weeks. However, the quality of muscle contraction and ability to move through the range of motion, as well as repetitions tolerated, would be constantly assessed during the exercise sessions to adjust dosage, parameters, or the type of exercise. The difference between active knee extension and passive range is used to reflect improvements in quadriceps activation and lag.

Monitoring Response to Exercise

Pain is one of the most common reasons for patients to seek physical therapy treatment. The patient's baseline pain levels and behavior are considered during initial evaluation, initial exercise prescription and testing, during exercise performance, and after performance. Patients are also asked to report pain intensity, frequency, and behavior at the beginning of their next visit as an indicator of how they tolerated the exercise (Box 8.2).

Pain reports can be influenced by multiple, complex factors including fear of pain, catastrophizing, depression, context of the injury, and anticipation of pain responses (see Chapters 6 and 7). While noting the patient's responses to the exercises is essential, the subjective pain reports should be interpreted within the context of these personal factors. In some cases, an increase in pain may be an indication that the exercise choice or dosage should be changed. In situations in which the psychosocial factors are an important factor, the dosage can be maintained or adjusted slightly and the emphasis switched to applying psychologically informed practice concepts such as cognitive-behavioral approaches.

The first two components of the acronym SINS—Severity and Irritability (see Chapter 1)—are useful for anticipating and determining an acceptable pain intensity during and after exercise, at follow-up visits, or at reevaluation.

Severity

Ordinal or continuous pain scales—0/10 (no pain) to 10/10 (worst pain imaginable)—or other forms of rating scales are used to determine pain severity. While there is variability in pain response based on patient perceptions, 1/10 to 3/10 is usually regarded as mild, 4/10 to 7/10 moderate, and 8/10 to 10/10 severe. If the patient's baseline pain level is severe, avoiding any increase in pain is desirable, whereas if symptoms are less severe, a small increase of 1/10 on the pain scale may be considered acceptable (Fig. 8.1, Clinical Example 8.2).

The anticipated goals for pain relief should take into account the minimally clinically important differences (MCID) to be considered relevant.[1] These values are determined from retrospective analysis of pain improvements and asking patients to complete scales reflecting the overall perception of their improvement.[1,2] On the other hand, if the patient experiences intermittent pain with specific movements, positions, or activities, the therapist may opt to monitor pain levels during any exercise with movement patterns similar to the exacerbating factors. There is recent evidence that pain with movement is a different construct to pain reports at rest. Questions to determine how the patient responds to an exercise should therefore be related to the initial pain characteristics and functional difficulties during movement.[3-6]

Depending on the severity and tendency of exacerbation, pain may be monitored during or after the exercise. These choices are based on the initial subjective examination, ongoing evaluation related to the initial testing (Chapter 4), and

progressive responses. If the mechanism of injury was repetitive strain, Magee[2] suggests using levels of severity based on the presentation of symptoms (Table 8.1), and decreasing levels of severity may be used to reflect improvement. Both the evaluation and the treatment approach will differ if the patient exhibits symptom magnification, fear avoidance, or other chronic pain-related behaviors, and the therapist may choose to monitor objective movement rather than subjective pain reports (see later section on fear avoidance).

Symptoms that are suggestive of severe consequences (red flags), such as those indicating abnormal neurological or cardiovascular responses, should be closely monitored. Under these circumstances, immediate adjustments are warranted.

BOX 8.2 Monitoring Response to Exercise

- Severity of pain during or after exercise or activity, constant pain, or pain influencing activities of daily living can be used to monitor exercise responses.
- Red flags, vital signs, neurovascular symptoms, and swelling need to be carefully monitored during and after exercise if present.
- Irritability of symptoms (timing of pain onset, pain intensity, and extent of aggravating factors) is also used to evaluate exercise, especially in the early phases or when neural irritability is present.
- Patients with active inflammatory conditions will need to be monitored carefully.
- Individuals who have a psychological component to their symptoms may require different approaches to exercises that induce symptoms.
- Delayed-onset muscle soreness is an indicator for modifying the dosage or choice of exercise.
- The specific impairment priorities for hypo- and hypermobility require different choices of outcome measures. Range of motion limitations due to effusion

can be monitored frequently along with circumferential measurements, while more established range of motion deficits are likely to show slow improvements and may not need to be measured frequently. Neuromuscular control in the presence of hypermobility may require monitoring of timing, movement symmetry, and muscle endurance and also take longer to become established. Improvements in functional activity tolerance and pain might be better choices for early outcome measures than measuring range of motion.
- Repetitive strain injuries often have multiple contributing factors, and the most relevant factors guide choice of outcome measures along with functional performance and self-report instruments.
- After surgery or trauma, healing constraints may impact the choice of functional outcome measures. There are some surgical protocols where achieving specific benchmarks allows the patient to move to the next level of exercise or functional activity.

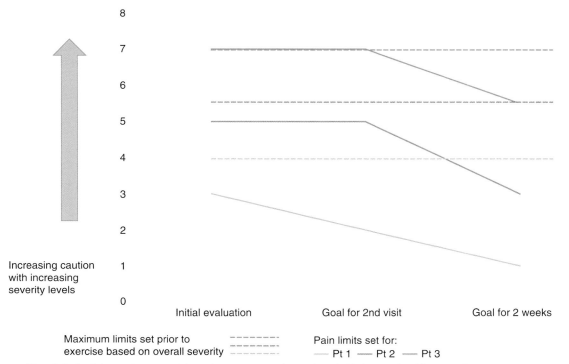

Fig. 8.1 Anticipated acceptable pain responses based on initial severity. The maximum acceptable pain responses during movement *(dotted lines)* are set apriori by the therapists based on initial severity. Note that >1.5 points on the VAS scale is a clinically important difference.

CLINICAL EXAMPLE 8.2 Severity and Irritability: Evaluation and Treatment Choices

The following patients are all seen on the second visit for neck pain.

Patient A

On initial evaluation, Patient A reported resting pain as 7/10; pain increased to 10/10 with movement in any direction and was not relieved by rest. History was significant for a whiplash incident 1 week ago, although no major damage was diagnosed in the emergency department. During the first session, isometric muscle activation of the deep neck flexors, lateral flexors, and rotators with therapist assistance was followed by gentle soft tissue mobilization of the trapezius and suboccipital muscles. Symptoms decreased slightly during the session to 6/10 with some relief of muscle spasm. On the second visit, the patient reported slight pain relief after the first session for 1 hour, with return to baseline levels with no further changes in pain the following day.

Evaluation

A report of no further increase in pain later that day or the next day would be considered a satisfactory result; continuing the exercise and soft tissue mobilization, as well as increasing repetitions to address the muscle spasm and removal of posttraumatic byproducts, would be indicated.

Patient B

On initial evaluation, Patient B's average resting pain was rated as 3/10, with increases to 5/10 after sitting for more than 3 hours. History included a gradual increase in symptoms over the past year, particularly related to desk work. During the first session, mobility exercises were selected with the goal of increasing lower cervical and upper thoracic mobility along with stretching exercises in sitting (trapezius, scalenes, levator scapulae). On the second visit, first session, the patient reported increased pain in the cervical region starting 12 hours after the first session and increasing the next day to 5/10 (constant). The pain subsided to 3/10 after 48 hours.

Evaluation

This pattern is consistent with delayed-onset muscle soreness and indicates that the intensity of the exercise was slightly too aggressive for early rehabilitation. The range and intensity of the mobility and stretching exercises were decreased.

Patient C

On initial evaluation, Patient C reported intermittent pain in the cervical region and shoulder up to 3/10 with no specific incident related to the onset of pain.

On the second visit, the patient was started on an upper extremity ergometer to promote general thoracic mobility during the initial visit. The patient reported that pain was increased in the right shoulder, accompanied by chest pain and shortness of breath.

Evaluation

The exercise was stopped immediately and vital signs assessed. His pulse was 120 and blood pressure was 150/100 mm Hg. The patient was referred for immediate medical attention related to cardiovascular symptoms.

Patient D

On initial evaluation, Patient D's symptoms included neck pain (constant 3/10) and tingling and numbness in the ulnar nerve distribution. After sitting for more than 20 minutes, symptoms increase to 6/10 with radiating pain and increased numbness in the arm. The aggravated symptoms would last for up to 2 hours and were only relieved by lying down. The patient was unable to lift light objects above shoulder level.

The patient exhibited severe forward head position, with a step-off at the C6–C7 region. Range of motion was tested in supine and sitting, with very restricted rotation and lateral flexion in sitting and with aggravation of symptoms in the arm after testing range of motion in sitting to 5/10 and some tingling in the arm. The patient was positioned in supine for the remainder of the evaluation: treatment and symptoms in the arm subsided, and pain decreased to 3/10. Initial treatment included manual therapy, soft tissue mobilization, and small-range active mid- and lower cervical flexion with the head supported to elongate the midcervical region and decrease the anterior cervicothoracic step-off. After the first session, pain and tingling in the arm decreased slightly. At the second visit, the patient reported less tingling and numbness in the arm and the ability to sit for 30 to 40 minutes without increasing symptoms.

Evaluation

Responses are indicative of high irritability for aggravation of tingling and numbness and pain in the arm related to sitting and mobility. Exercise intensity and progression is cautious to avoid aggravating arm symptoms. Because the length of time the patient is able to sit without exacerbating symptoms has increased, seated exercise could be considered for time frames less than 20 minutes or if tingling and numbness is reported.

TABLE 8.1 Pain Severity and Relationship to Activities (Repetitive Strain Injuries)

Level 1	Pain after specific activity
Level 2	Pain at start of activity resolving with warm-up
Level 3	Pain during and after specific activity that does not affect performance
Level 4	Pain during and after specific activity that does affect performance
Level 5	Pain with activities of daily living (ADLs)
Level 6	Constant dull aching pain at rest that does not disturb sleep
Level 7	Dull aching pain that does disturb sleep

From Magee DJ. *Orthopaedic Physical Assessment*. 6th ed. St. Louis, MO: Saunders Elsevier; 2014.

Shortness of breath, chest pain, or palpitations are suggestive of potentially serious cardiovascular implications, and the activity should be discontinued immediately. Vital signs should be monitored while deciding if immediate referral is necessary. Tingling, numbness, and progressive decreases in strength could indicate increased neural pressure or ischemia and require further evaluation. If numbness and tingling are reported, these symptoms may be anticipated and acceptable with chronic neurovascular mobility limitations but should be carefully monitored, along with signs of neural compression. Readers are referred to Cleland,[1] Magee,[2] Magee and Sueki,[7] and Boissonnault[8] for more details on tests necessary to rule out fractures, arterial and severe neural compression, and other conditions that should be referred for additional testing.

If symptoms are less severe, exercise progression is more rapid, and the reevaluation focus may move from primarily impairment-based measures to functional testing. The primary impairments, such as specific muscle fatigue or abnormal range of motion, determine which tests and measures are appropriate and the timing of the tests (see Clinical Example 8.2). Functional testing is appropriate when there are no precautions related to the movement (see Chapter 4). Time frames for tissue healing and for resolving impairments are also considered when deciding when to perform reassessment, selecting appropriate planes of movement, and deciding if certain directions or combinations of movement should be delayed. This is particularly important in cases of traumatic and postsurgical damage (see Chapter 2 for healing considerations and time frames, Chapter 6 for traumatic and postsurgical management).

Irritability

For a highly irritable condition, exercise choices are conservative and avoid positions, movements, or activities that aggravate symptoms. On the other hand, an individual with low irritability can be challenged with aggravating positions, movements, and activities. If the aggravating factors are introduced, the patient's responses should be closely monitored and adjustments made to the intensity, range, complexity, or biomechanics of the exercise. Tracking irritability using the questions introduced in Chapter 1 will help reduce the risk of exacerbating symptoms by anticipating the starting point and how fast to progress a patient. If the patient's symptoms are highly irritable, it is vital to also evaluate symptoms *after* exercising and at the next session. The therapist must also anticipate which movements, positions, or circumstances are likely to exacerbate symptoms and then limit the opportunity for exacerbation until the irritability decreases.

Patients with an active inflammatory condition, neural irritation, or other condition with highly irritable symptoms will follow Phase I principles for longer time frames and will progress more slowly during Phases II and III. However, someone with highly irritable symptoms usually has a poorer prognosis, and time frames for goals are likely to be longer with smaller functional improvements expected until pain and inflammatory responses are resolved. Irritability may decrease once acute inflammatory responses have subsided or once neural irritation

> ### BOX 8.3 Symptoms of Delayed Onset Muscle Soreness
>
> - Muscle or connective tissue soreness in the specific areas targeted in the exercise program
> - Pain starts 8 to 12 hours after the exercise
> - Pain increases to a maximum 24 to 48 hours after exercise
> - Pain should dissipate after 72 hours
> - The more severe the intensity and the earlier the onset, the more likely the exercise dosage and intensity need to be adjusted
> - Overall coordination can be impacted by soreness, with the potential for further damage, thus impacting activity guidelines and recommendations

or a mobility issue has been addressed. More aggressive management may then be possible.

Psychological responses can contribute to symptoms or result in responses regarded as being highly irritable. Therefore, if a patient's symptoms indicate irritability, psychological screening is very important. Under these circumstances, the therapist might focus less on the symptoms and place greater emphasis on objective improvements. A graded exposure or a graded exercise approach can be used to gradually increase exercise intensity and complexity. If the patient is able to tolerate increased resistance, repetitions, or complexity of activities, or if the patient demonstrates less fear avoidance or catastrophizing behaviors, the improvements may also allow progression using principles related to impairments or mechanism of injury (see Chapter 6). Self-reports of functional activities or objective functional tests are often used as the primary outcome measures.

Delayed-onset muscle soreness can be confused with irritability. If a patient is exhibiting increased soreness after starting exercises, the therapist must distinguish between muscle or connective tissue soreness and aggravation of symptoms related to the diagnosis. Using appropriate exercise parameters should limit soreness, but delayed-onset muscle soreness can occur after strengthening exercises or aggressive stretching, particularly when the exercise is first introduced. Patients should be instructed how to identify delayed-onset soreness symptoms (see Box 8.3) and asked to report back to the therapist, who should then reassess exercise intensity. Patients often need to be taught the difference between symptoms that are indicators of adverse responses, such as major increases in effusion, increased neural symptoms, or increased inflammation, as opposed to specific muscle soreness[9-11] (Box 8.3, Table 8.2). General guidelines for postexercise soreness have been proposed to assist with how to adjust exercise in the presence of soreness or effusion (Table 8.2). Symptoms and selected objective measures may be chosen to evaluate during and immediately after exercise and at the next session (Box 8.4).

Nature

The nature of the problem relates to the health condition component of the International Classification of Functioning (ICF) model (Chapter 3) and the general categories of disorders discussed in Chapter 6. The foundational tissue-specific healing principles introduced in Chapter 2 are used to predict the

TABLE 8.2 Soreness and Effusion Guidelines in Phase II and III[9–11]

Timing of Soreness	Dosage and Progression at Next Session
No soreness (monitored for 2 days)	Further progression of the program is possible
Some specific muscle soreness in targeted muscles present on next visit	Warm-up and monitor soreness, if soreness decreases: Maintain dosage from previous session
	Warm-up and monitor soreness, if soreness continues: Focus exercise session on other goals such as flexibility or generalized endurance without specific resistance for targeted muscles OR decrease dosage
Soreness present within 1 hour of exercise session	Rest muscle or area completely Decrease dosage to lower intensity
Trace or no effusion	Progression is possible
Increased effusion +1	Resume at same level of difficulty, continue to monitor effusion, continue home program to address effusion (ice, elevation, compression, active isometrics or isotonics in supported positions)
Increased effusion +2	Hold exercise, manage effusion with massage, ice, elevation, and compression; home program to address effusion including isometrics, isotonics in supported positions

BOX 8.4 Assessment of Exercise Responses

Therapists should consider the following factors when assessing response to exercise:

- Major subjective symptoms (pain, restricted motion, tingling, numbness, fatigue)
- Primary impairments, activity limitations, and/or participation restrictions
- Symptoms during and immediately after exercise and following exercise session including pain responses, delayed-onset muscle soreness, or effusion
- Severity and irritability to determine acceptable levels and type of symptoms during and after exercise
- Relative contributing factors
- Psychological contributions
- Understanding of the exercise and ability to reproduce the desired movements for home programs

patient's potential for tolerating various forces and types of exercise, while the therapist's understanding of pathology helps to predict the potential for improvement. Therapists are referred to Goodman's text[12] to review the implications of pathologies, such as connective tissue disorders (e.g., rheumatoid arthritis), structural conditions (e.g., scoliosis), metabolic conditions (e.g., diabetes), circulatory conditions (e.g., vascular disease), and oncological diagnoses. It is extremely common for patients to present with comorbidities that will influence the prognosis, precautions, and overall outcome expectations.

The categories presented in Chapter 6 can be used to help with hypotheses and expectations for improvement, as well as to direct exercise choices. **Hypomobility** requires further consideration of the type of restricted tissue. When connective tissue is limiting mobility, the therapist needs to evaluate the patient's tolerance to prolonged lengthening or directions of force to reach end range and access some degree of plasticity (see Chapter 2 and Chapter 6). Restricted muscle flexibility calls for an evaluation of the amount of range or "give" after full stretch of the muscle. If there are protective muscle responses to pain, the tolerance may be adjusted to address the pain responses with less aggressive stretching or repeated movement into the full range. Typically, evaluating tolerance for a patient with hypomobility involves a combination of pain response (during and after range of motion techniques) and range of motion improvements. If effusion is the primary reason that range is limited, the intervention is directed at eliminating and moving the additional fluid. Assessing circumferential measurements would be appropriate to determine if edema or effusion has decreased, along with tracking active and passive range of motion improvements. If edema or effusion increases, the exercise choices and/or the functional activities should be assessed and adjusted. New compensatory movements, especially weight-bearing avoidance, are a sign that the individual is not able tolerate the exercise intensity or choice at the time (Clinical Example 8.3).

Hypermobility can be masked by protective muscle spasm. Without the necessary passive or active restraints, pain responses are typically evoked when the area is stressed at extreme ranges. Compared to hypomobility, evaluating exercise responses can be more complex for individuals with hypermobility. Neuromuscular control (appropriate reaction times and sequencing), muscle activation, endurance, and control of static postural positions or to avoid reaching excessive ranges are all interrelated. While contributions from impairments are important, the overall movement quality and performance should be evaluated using functional performance measures. Patient self-reported functional outcome measures and pain questionnaires that cover both sustained and momentary activities are useful tools (Clinical Example 8.4).

Postural alignment or **repetitive strain injuries** can involve combinations of hypomobility and hypermobility as well as causative factors. The evaluation will therefore differ based on which components are being addressed as priorities. The choice of tests will also be influenced by patient characteristics and functional goals. The tests and measures used for repetitive strain injuries need to address contributing factors, symptoms, and functional performance. The pattern, severity, and irritability of the symptoms will be important both to direct the intensity of the exercise and for setting the limits for testing. A patient who reports symptoms with a low level of severity only after an activity may need to be monitored carefully after the activity and asked to report the pattern of symptoms at the next visit. However,

CLINICAL EXAMPLE 8.3   Evaluating Mobility Exercise for Knee Osteoarthritis

An 80-year-old woman with a diagnosis of knee osteoarthritis has decreased knee range of motion limiting functional movement. Knee osteoarthritis hypomobility is potentially related to capsular tightness, effusion, bony alignment or osteophytic formation, decreased muscle flexibility, or lack of active force closure (see also Clinical Examples 3.1 and 4.18).

The patient has effusion with a soft end feel limiting knee extension (10 degrees) and knee flexion (95 degrees). Early exercises are chosen to address the effusion and reach end range for knee extension in non–weight-bearing positions: isometrics in maximum extension with support under the ankle (Exercise 9.1B). A stationary bike is used to encourage full extension in sitting (Exercise 9.7), and active-assisted knee extension using a strap (Exercise 9.4A). Knee flexion range is encouraged by changing the seat distance on the bike, adding flexion using a slider in supine (Exercise 9.3) and flexion supported by an exercise ball (Exercise 9.4B).

Evaluation

- If her hypomobility is due to effusion, monitoring circumferential measurements as well as range of motion before and after exercise will help assess whether the exercise is effective.
- If there is no change in circumferential measurements but an improvement in the range, and the end feel is capsular, changes in the parameters and dosage are warranted. The therapist encourages the patient to reach the end range during the movement with a short hold to address capsular limitations.

Immediate progression may be possible in one session or at the next session. If, however, there is an increase in effusion and range is more restricted, the dosage will need to be adjusted to limit the range and perform motion in the midrange using a pumping action to target the effusion.

- As the patient progresses, a capsular end feel is present with minimal effusion. Exercises can be aggressive using prolonged holds and follow joint mobilization. Measuring joint range immediately after the exercise may provide information about the effectiveness; however, as connective tissue adaptations take some time, joint range should also be assessed after a home program of stretching and positioning before adjusting the dosage.
- If there is a hard end feel, goals to improve the range of motion in the specific direction are not indicated. The exercise goals would be directed toward maintaining the available range and maximizing mobility in other areas to assist the patient with function. Range of motion of the knee would only be measured intermittently, while hip or ankle range would be measured more frequently if these areas are included in the goals.
- If the effusion is easily exacerbated with weight bearing or specific ranges of motion and there is an increase in effusion after an exercise, this would indicate a change in the amount of weight-bearing load or intensity of the exercise is needed when prescribing exercises involving the aggravating factor(s).

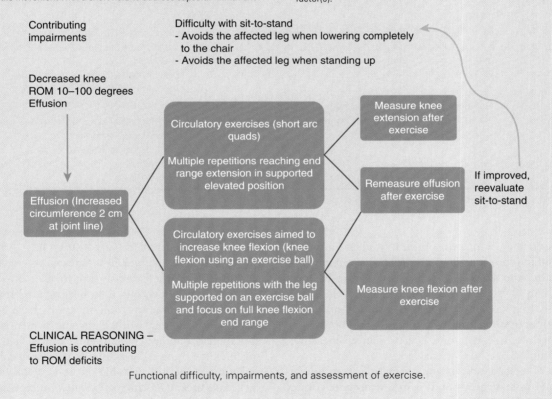

Functional difficulty, impairments, and assessment of exercise.

continued

⚡ CLINICAL EXAMPLE 8.3   Evaluating Mobility Exercise for Knee Osteoarthritis—cont'd

Contributing Impairments	Intervention	Evaluation
Capsular restriction (flexion, extension)	Bike	Measure knee flexion (goniometer) once a week until passive endfeel is hard KOOS weekly • Overall score • Sit-to-stand Relative ease of knee flexion during use of bike (during exercise) Ability to adjust seat height (during exercise) Video analysis of range during sit-to-stand (weekly)
Limited flexibility of quadriceps	Soft tissue mobilization (including patella mobilization) followed by quadriceps stretching by therapist and patient (home program)	Ely's test is remeasured 2 weeks after regular stretching is included in home program
Limited dorsiflexion contributing to difficulty with biomechanics	Stretching (belt in long sitting) (home program)	Measure weight-bearing dorsiflexion with knee flexed and extended 2 weeks after regular stretching is included in home program
Pain avoidance mechanics	Address weight-bearing distribution, adjust center of mass to decrease lever arms and stress on patellofemoral region, and decrease angulation	Observation Video analysis Pain reports
Pain responses at extreme of available flexion (100 degrees)		Weight bearing on two scales (weekly)
Decreased muscle support and force distribution during lowering	Muscle activation, endurance, and strengthening hip abductors, external rotators, hip extensors, knee extensors and flexors	Initial exercise prescription, and reevaluation at next visit for delayed-onset muscle soreness, pain responses, swelling Load for double-/single-leg press 15 RM Ability to maintain alignment (angulation, rotation), video-taping, observation during stand-to-sit and exercises
Functional difficulty	Functional training in standing to sitting, sitting to standing; home program	Number of repetitions and sets possible (every session), pain during movement 5× sit-to-stand time (every 2 weeks) Timed up-and-go KOOS weekly

KOOS, Knee Injury and Osteoarthritis Outcome Scale; *RM*, repetition maximum.

functional performance measures used to evaluate improvement will need to reproduce the activities or movements that are problematic, and functional tests may need to be more challenging than for patients with higher pain levels. Symptoms are likely to be easily reproducible for a patient having difficulty with activities of daily living and can be assessed with validated self-report and performance measures. (Clinical Example 8.5).

The primary considerations for evaluating exercise tolerance during **postsurgical and acute traumatic injury** recovery are based on the healing stage and the precautions for the damaged and repaired structures. Any increase in inflammation (pain, swelling) indicates excessive stress on the structures. Criteria for advancing to the next stage are often included in protocols based on healing time frames (Clinical Example 8.6). Some outcome measures have been used primarily with patients with a specific postsurgical diagnosis and therefore allow comparison to published evidence for specific time frames. Guidelines for postsurgical management and progression are available in the *Hospital for Special Surgery Handbook of Postsurgical Rehabilitation Guidelines for the Orthopedic Clinician*.[13]

A 13-year-old gymnast with lumbar spine hypermobility presents with localized lumbar spine discomfort. She reports pain with prolonged standing for more than 30 minutes (3/10) that decreases with movement, in the morning, or immediately after sitting down (2/10). She has pain with prolonged back bends, landing dismounts, and spinal hyperextension positions especially with simultaneous hip extension. These symptoms are consistent with low intensity and irritability. She is extremely flexible in all directions in the lumbar spine and hips, with slight pulling in the lumbar spine area with full spinal flexion in standing. She has full flexibility of the hamstrings, gluteals, hamstrings, and ankle plantarflexors, but decreased flexibility of the hip flexors The passive lumbar extension test and prone segmental instability tests were positive. Single-leg extension tests were negative and radiographs were negative for spondylolysis or spondylolysthesis.

Impairments include preferential use of the global muscles for functional movements, particularly during gymnastic activities, limited endurance of the spinal stabilizers, and habitual excessive and early lumbar lordosis while standing and during gymnastic drills and skills. Her postural alignment includes knee hyperextension and an increased lordosis. She is also unable to control her lumbopelvic position during dynamic activities including squats, landings, and single-leg balance on a beam.

Tests and Measures to Evaluate Progress

- Patient-specific functional scale
- Single-leg squat test
- Star balance and Y-balance with lumbopelvic neutral
- Visual analog score (VAS) pain (resting, upon waking, in standing, with lumbar extension)
- Time before onset of pain in standing

Evaluation

1. The patient's symptoms and objective findings are consistent with hypermobility with neuromuscular coordination impairments.
2. Phase II principles are appropriate for management with goals to improve neuromuscular coordination and proprioceptive awareness of lumbar spine position to avoid excessive, early, or prolonged lumbar extension in habitual standing and during dynamic gymnastic activities.
2. Prognosis is good for full resolution of symptoms based on limited impairments, high motivation, and no major structural conditions.
3. Expected time frames for improvement:
   - 2 to 4 weeks for improved neuromuscular coordination and timing of local stabilizer activation in supported positions and in standing in static positions
   - 4 to 6 weeks for dynamic control in gymnastic drills and performance
   - 6 weeks for improved endurance and integration of biomechanical principles

Assessment of Exercise Responses for a Gymnast With Low Back Pain and Neuromuscular Coordination Deficits

General Exercise Choices	Examples for Early Phase II Exercise Choices	Exercise Assessment Examples
Spinal stabilization, neuromuscular coordination training: awareness of neutral spine position and engaging transversus abdominus, pelvic floor, and spinal extensors with challenge from lower extremity movement	Local stabilizer activation, neutral lumbar lordosis (Exercise 11.20) Challenge neutral spine on foam roller with arm movements (Exercise 11.22) Bicycle (with head support; Exercise 11.23) Prone (forearm support): leg lifts (Exercise 11.27) Four-point kneeling over ball: weight shifting, alternating leg lifts (Exercise 11.28) Prone plank from BOSU (Exercise 11.28) Abdominal curls (Exercise 11.33) Diagonal curl-ups (Exercise 11.34)	Ability to achieve and maintain lumbopelvic neutral using pressure biofeedback Timing of spinal stabilizers and anticipatory control; visual observation for lower extremity challenges and four-point kneeling leg lifts Timed prone plank Number of abdominal curls/diagonal curl-ups before fatigue and loss of transversus control
Postural reeducation to minimize excessive forces at end range (control lordosis and knee hyperextension) Active force closure and muscular activation while maintaining spinal alignment and force closure	Correction of standing posture Partial double-leg squats to lift object (Exercise 11.43) Stride lunges to lift object (Exercise 11.44) Neuromuscular reeducation: Reversal of flexed position (Exercise 11.38) Seated upright posture challenges with pulleys on an exercise ball (Exercise 11. 39) Latissimus dorsi pull-downs (Exercise 10.32)	Ability to actively control degree of lordosis and knee hyperextension using video analysis Angular measurements recorded using video without feedback Ability to distribute motion without early hinging in lumbar spine Pain in standing
Spinal extensor and abdominal endurance with external challenges focusing on anticipatory activation and maintenance of positions in double- and single-leg activities Proprioceptive control and ability to maintain position with unstable surfaces and upper extremity challenges using progressive motor learning principles	Hinged positions: upper extremity challenge (Exercise 11.37) Double- and single-leg squats; lunges on stable and unstable surfaces (Exercise 9.30) Balance activities on the balance beam, maintaining lumbopelvic position, progressing into modified gymnastic activities	Time that the patient is able to maintain hinge position Time and repetitions for double- and single-leg squats with neutral lumbopelvic position Ability to recognize and correct loss of lumbopelvic position during and/or after movement on videotape Timed plank position Timed side plank Timed balance on unstable surface (one leg with gymnastic routine arm or leg positions) Patient-specific functional scale items related to standing endurance or balance Y-balance, star balance test; symmetry and maintenance of lumbopelvic position with multiple repetitions
Decreased flexibility hip flexors	Hip flexor stretching (Exercise 9.8)	Ely's test

BOSU, Both Sides Up Balance Trainer.

CLINICAL EXAMPLE 8.5   **Repetitive Strain Injury**

Patient A

Patient A is 78 years old, with hip and knee osteoarthritis. She reports fatigue and pain after walking two blocks. The Timed Up and Go Test, a Six-Minute Walk Test, perceived exertion scale after the Six-Minute Walk Test, and a visual analogue pain scale could be used to record functional improvement. The Lower Extremity Functional Scale or the Western Ontario and McMaster Osteoarthritis Scale (WOMAC) are used to track self-reported functional status. Hip and knee range of motion, muscle endurance, and strength are also measured to reflect changes in impairments but are completed less frequently; the emphasis is on the functional measures.

Patient B

Patient B is a 25-year-old marathon runner with patellofemoral dysfunction who can run for 3 km before the onset of symptoms. Functional self-reported outcome measures include the Lower Extremity Functional Scale, as well as the distance before onset of pain. If the major contributing factors include overstriding, dynamic valgus, and excessive internal rotation during stance and limited hip external rotator endurance, the measures used to reflect improvements should reflect any

improvements in these impairments as well as running. Stride length and cadence might be monitored using video recording on the treadmill after the patient has run 3 km. The lower extremity dynamic valgus angle may be chosen to reflect hip stabilizer endurance or a more defined impairment-based measure, such as a handheld dynamometer, can be used to reflect maximal muscle strength.

Comparison of Patients A and B

The major outcome measures for Patient A will be self-reported measures and objective functional outcome measures with less emphasis on range of motion and strength impairments. Her age and the potential for fixed range of motion deficits decrease the expectation for major changes, although even a few degrees of range of motion or any endurance improvements are likely to impact her function. Patient B is already at a high functional level, and there may be a ceiling effect when using the Lower Extremity Functional Scale. Identifying the possible contributing impairments can be used to help with changing the patterns used while running and may be useful for his goal-setting. The distance before pain onset is likely to be an outcome measure that will help with motivation.

 CLINICAL EXAMPLE 8.6   **Evaluation of Progress for Return to Sport/Military Requirements**

A 23-year-old female cadet in the Reserve Officer Training Corps (ROTC) program sustained an anterior cruciate ligament (ACL) tear 4 months previously and underwent surgical reconstruction with a hamstring graft 2 weeks later. She has been progressing rapidly through her rehabilitation without complications. At 18 weeks postoperatively, she was required to submit documentation of her status to the ROTC medical supervisor to be eligible for continuation of her scholarship. The letter includes the following information:

Ms. Gordon is progressing extremely well after surgical reconstruction using a hamstring graft. At 18 weeks post surgery, she is currently able to meet the required ROTC running time and required number of sit-ups and push-ups. She has started with more advanced balance and response time training and is working toward being able to respond to all forms of external balance challenge on unsteady or uneven surfaces. Her prognosis is extremely good: she has achieved symmetry for the functional tests performed up to this point and is extremely motivated, works very hard, and has a high level of coordination.

On reevaluation 18 weeks after surgery, she has achieved the following:

- Normal and equivalent range of motion for all hip, knee, and ankle range with the exception of a zero-degree extension on the surgical side while she has 5 degrees of hyperextension on the nonsurgical knee
- Equal stationary timed single-leg hop test (133 repetitions in 1 minute)
- Equal timed single-leg squat test (56 in 1 minute)
- Equal timed step-up test (39 L compared to 41 R in 1 minute)
- Surgical leg reach on the Y-balance test slightly greater than on the R in all directions
- No swelling, some clicking (painless) with squats

In the past 4 weeks, she reports running 1.5 miles in 11 minutes, thus meeting the ROTC running requirements. She is increasing the intensity and time for running every second day and has had no adverse responses. Her self-selected speed on the treadmill is 6.6 mph, with equal symmetry. On the International

Knee Documentation Committee self-reported functional outcome measure she reports slight pain when kneeling directly on the left knee, but no other functional problems. Her Lower Extremity Functional Scale is reported as 77/80 with a little difficulty with hobbies, hopping, and sharp turns when running fast.

Her present exercise program consists of weight-bearing functional strengthening (squats, single-leg hops in place, modified Burpees, mountain climbers, step-ups, single-leg balance on unstable surfaces), a graduated running program, strengthening exercises in the gym, and response time and proprioceptive training. She was recently able to add single-leg stationary hopping to her program and both hopping, dynamic balance and running will be progressed to add progressive motion in frontal and diagonal directions. Changes in direction for running and hopping will be progressed after she has achieved symmetry for all planes of movement.

Recommendations and Revised Goals

Her present physical therapy impairment and functional goals will be adjusted to meet the following in 6 weeks:

1. Achieve at least 80% quadriceps strength of her nonsurgical leg
2. Adapt to all outside unexpected challenges while standing on unstable surfaces 100% of the time without loss of postural stability or compensations
3. Increase her knee hyperextension range to match her nonsurgical leg
4. Increase her running speed and endurance to presurgical status
5. Achieve equivalent progressive hop distance and time (triple-hop, single-leg hop for distance in all directions, crossover hop)
6. Achieve equivalent time for star shuttle runs with outside directional challenge
7. Return to running with weight (20 lb) for 5 miles

We anticipate that she will need to continue with supervised progression for another 2–3 months but with intermittent monitoring.

Stage

Evaluation of the impairments, stage of healing, and functional capability helps decide where to start and when to progress the exercise prescription while adhering to healing precautions. The general criteria to enter phases and typical interventions for each phase are illustrated in Figs. 8.2A and B. Inflammation should be resolved before progressing from Phase I to Phase II (Fig. 8.2A). Progressing from Phase II to Phase III is gradual, with the focus moving from impairment-based management to functional recovery (Fig. 8.2A). Precautions and contraindications will influence Phase I and Phase II, and most precautions are lifted before entering Phase III. Stages are sometimes defined using time frames for resolving impairments or approximate healing time frames. Following surgery, the progression to the next phase can be time-based and broken down into smaller phases, with common considerations for healing during treatment (Clinical Example 8.7). If higher-level functional goals are a requirement to return to sport or physically demanding work, additional conditioning requires full resolution of impairments before starting high-intensity training programs (Fig. 8.2B).

EVALUATING COMPENSATIONS AND MOVEMENT PATTERNS

Compensations can occur in multiple regions simultaneously, and those in the spine influence the extremities and vice versa (Box 8.5). Compensations can be caused by insufficient range of motion, muscle weakness or fatigue, poor habits, pain, or fear of pain. Evaluation findings such as muscle activation patterns, joint and soft tissue restrictions, or postural misalignment are used to determine if the exercise choice or parameters need modification or if movement coordination should be addressed (Videos 4.12–4.14). The biomechanical considerations for different areas of the body can be found in the corresponding section of the workbook chapters. Each exercise and functional activity should be observed for signs of fatigue during repeated movements. Typically, compensations related to muscle strength or endurance can be detected by a trained observer before the patient reports fatigue.

Fear avoidance patterns will also include regional compensations, but they are often identified by incongruent movement patterns (Box 8.5), reports of fear of movement, and nonverbal communication of discomfort before movement. In these cases,

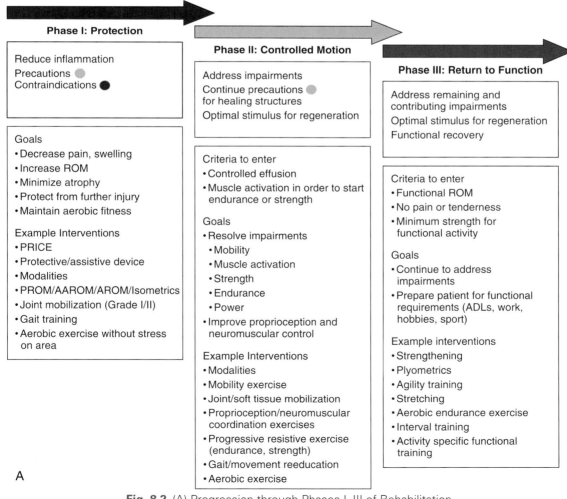

Fig. 8.2 (A) Progression through Phases I–III of Rehabilitation.

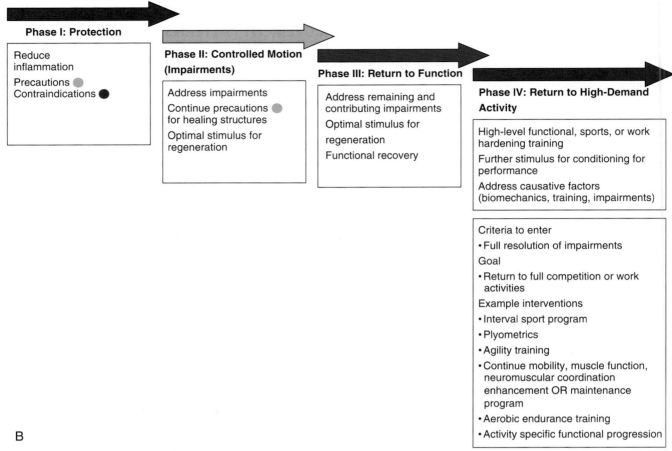

Phase I: Protection

Reduce inflammation
Precautions ●
Contraindications ●

Phase II: Controlled Motion (Impairments)

Address impairments
Continue precautions ● for healing structures
Optimal stimulus for regeneration

Phase III: Return to Function

Address remaining and contributing impairments
Optimal stimulus for regeneration
Functional recovery

Phase IV: Return to High-Demand Activity

High-level functional, sports, or work hardening training
Further stimulus for conditioning for performance
Address causative factors (biomechanics, training, impairments)

Criteria to enter
• Full resolution of impairments
Goal
• Return to full competition or work activities
Example interventions
• Interval sport program
• Plyometrics
• Agility training
• Continue mobility, muscle function, neuromuscular coordination enhancement OR maintenance program
• Aerobic endurance training
• Activity specific functional progression

B

Fig. 8.2, cont'd (B) Progression through Phases I–IV (high demand). (Modified with permission from Dr. Theresa Chmielewski.)

⚖ CLINICAL EXAMPLE 8.7   Gait Speed as an Outcome Measure

The patient is a 75-year-old woman who is being seen after a hip fracture (open reduction and hemi-arthroplasty) 10 weeks ago.

Long-term goal: In 4 weeks, the patient will be able to ambulate safely in the community, including crossing a street at a light, walking at a speed of 1.3 m/sec.

Initial Evaluation
• The patient is weight bearing as tolerated but still using a walker.
• She is able to stand with good balance reactions and without loss of balance.
• She can walk in the parallel bars (10 m) at a speed of 2 m/sec using the 10-meter walk test with stand-by assistance but is cautious and holds onto the bars repeatedly

At 2 Weeks Post Initial Evaluation
After treatment 3 times a week (aquatic therapy, strengthening exercises, balance activities, gait reeducation):
• She is able to walk short distances at home without a walker.
• Single-leg balance is possible for 5 seconds.

Evaluation
Single-leg balance time associated with good dynamic balance and normal gait patterns in adults between 70 and 79 years old is, on average, 14 seconds.[1] Further

improvements are still needed. New short-term goal for 2 weeks is to be able to stand on one leg for 14 seconds. (Change will exceed the MDC of 7 seconds.)[2,3] She can walk in the parallel bars (10 m) at a speed of 1.8 m/sec using the 10-meter walk test without assistance and only holds onto the bars when turning.

Average community gait speed requirement is 1.3 m/sec; further improvements are needed. New short-term goal for 2 weeks is to be able to walk independently outside the bars at a speed of 1.4 m/sec to exceed an MDC of 0.25 seconds[4] compared to the gait speed measured in the initial evaluation (2.0 m/sec). The 6-week goal is set at 1.2 m/sec to reach community ambulation requirements.

References
1. Bohannon R, Larkin P, Cook A, Singer J. Decrease in time balance test scores with aging. *Phys Ther.* 1984;64:1067–1070.
2. Naylor JM, Hayen A, Davidson E, Hackett D, Harris IA, Kamalsina G, Mittal R. Minimal detectable change for mobility and patient-reported tools in people with osteoarthritis awaiting arthroplasty. *BMC Musculoskelet Disord.* 2014;15:235.
3. Carcia CR, Perera S, Mody S, Woodman RC, Studenski SA. Meaningful change and responsiveness in common physical performance measures in older adults. *J Am Geriatr Soc.* 2006;54:743–749.
4. Hollman JH, Beckman BA, Brandt RA, et al. Minimum detectable change in gait velocity during acute rehabilitation following hip fracture. *J Geriatr Phys Ther.* 2008;31:53–56.

BOX 8.5 Evaluating Compensations

- Compensations occur in multiple regions simultaneously.
- Compensations can be due to range of motion or flexibility restrictions, habit, muscle activation, endurance, strength or power impairments, coordination patterns due to pain or fear, reinforcement due to habit or training, or from neurological impairments.
- Observation is used to identify and correct patterns, with some objective tests that are used for symmetry, sequencing, or fine-motor coordination.
- Compensations may be different between patients and within an exercise course.
- Fear avoidance may be observed by hesitancy or refusal to move, stopping movement without symptoms of fatigue, difficulty performing a movement, asymmetrical weight bearing, or inconsistencies between functional movement capabilities and available range and strength noted during impairment testing.

BOX 8.6 Evaluation of Home Programs

- Home programs can be started at different time frames, with more conservative and delayed home exercise if the patient's condition is irritable or there are more precautions.
- A patient who has symptoms that are less severe, of lower irritability, and chronic will be able to start a home program earlier.
- Regular assessment and updating of home exercises are needed.
- Home exercise programs should be chosen based on the individual's motivation, access to equipment, functional needs, and learning characteristics.

early identification of the compensations is key so that the therapist can address the fear of movement and initiate instruction in proper exercise technique without avoidance compensations.

As patients improve and new exercises are selected or progressed, compensations can also be indicators of excessive load or complexity beyond the patient's capabilities rather than fear. Patients should be educated about their altered movement patterns and how to correct and monitor themselves, particularly during any exercise where endurance is required.

EVALUATION FOR CHOICE OF HOME PROGRAM EXERCISE PRESCRIPTION

Deciding which exercises should be included in a home exercise program and when to start exercises is always individualized to the patient (Box 8.6). The SINS categories are used to determine how easily the problem is exacerbated: if a patient has high severity, high irritability, or a condition with more precautions, home exercises should be more conservative, and the therapist should provide the patient with clear instructions about what circumstances call for discontinuing the exercise. Low severity and irritability and a chronic condition may not require as much caution. Assessing the patient's personality and likelihood of doing too much is as important in determining the number and difficulty level of exercises. A patient who is very motivated to return to sport or recover from surgery who is still in Phase I will need exercises that are very unlikely to cause increased stress on the injured structure. However, as the patient progresses through Phases II and III, including exercises similar to those required for return to sport is important, as long as any precautions are maintained. The amount of time a patient has to devote to a home exercise program is also an important consideration, so home exercises should be modified, replaced, and prioritized as the patient improves. Conversely, patients who have time limitations may need to be guided to select exercises that optimize the patient's time. One of the most important aspects of a home program may be assessing patients' understanding of goals and how to avoid compensation. Home exercise program performance should be assessed soon after exercises are introduced to ensure that exercises are being performed correctly.

When choosing home exercises, the therapist should consider the patient's environment, available equipment, and preferences for type of exercise. For example, if the patient has a gym membership or has a treadmill at home, the therapist could provide a home program utilizing the available equipment (Videos 2.3, 3.21, and 6.27) versus prescribing simple home exercises with bodyweight or elastic resistance (Videos 2.15 and 2.26). Home program instruction should also include instructions for modifying exercises if pain is elicited or how to adjust activities of daily living so that there is less stress on the tissues. This type of education is an important component of Phase I management. If the patient has financial or insurance restrictions for rehabilitation, home exercise programs should be introduced as soon as possible, and options to space out the individual therapy sessions with detailed home programs might be considered.

Home programs can help promote optimal tissue regeneration and improve muscular or cardiovascular endurance as well as reinforce patient and treatment goals. Home exercises that reinforce goals are more relevant to the patient, but the patient must be able to perform multiple repetitions without compensations using correct form in order to effectively reinforce the desired movement (see Chapter 7). Typically, home programs are needed to maintain range of motion that was gained during individualized treatment sessions and should be started as soon as possible. Parameters such as the desired end range, position, and amount of pressure should be included in the instructions, along with preferred frequency and hold time for each exercise.

OUTCOME MEASURES

Outcome measures (see Tables 8.3–8.5) are used to track a patient's improvement and treatment effectiveness but, in some cases, can also be used to guide treatment focus or predict prognosis. Relevant outcome measures are selected during the initial examination and evaluation process based on the patient's health condition and region of impairments as well as the type of impairments and functional difficulties (Fig. 8.3). Using validated outcome measures allows the therapist to compare results to normative data and provide a mechanism for determining the extent of impairments, activity limitations, or participation restrictions. The interpretation of measures also allows the therapist to use the results to set goals and informs the choice of other examination techniques. Some outcome measures are also useful predictors of prognosis or for identifying of risk of injury such as falls.

Other tools provide additional information about psychological status, which can help guide the type of motivational or

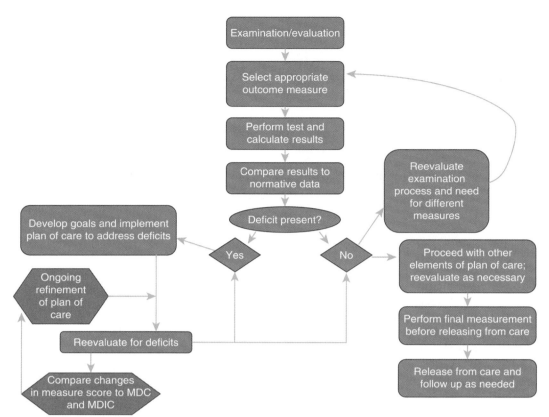

Fig. 8.3 Outcome measure decision-making algorithm. *MDC*, Minimum detectable change; *MCID*, minimum clinically important difference.

psychologically informed approaches to exercise prescription. The number of available of functional outcome measures (self-reported and objective measures) has dramatically increased, and there are multiple outcome measures for specific diagnoses, patient populations, and regions.[1,2]

Both self-reported outcome measures and objective functional outcome measures should be reliable (repeatable across administration), valid (reflect results accurately for the patient population or compared to a gold standard), and sensitive (shows appropriate changes in the instrument with patient improvement). It is also important that the instruments have been tested in similar patient populations and do not have ceiling or floor effects for the patient characteristics. The psychometric properties and advantages/disadvantages of the selected outcome measures are described in Magee and Sueki and in Cleland.[1,2,7] An important psychometric property of any outcome measure is the **minimum detectable change (MDC)** or the amount of error which needs to be exceeded in order to show true change. The MDC is reported in the same units of measurement, and therefore the clinician can gauge whether any change can be considered to be above the expected error, which is inherent with variability in measurement techniques, tester error, and patient variability. The smaller the MDC or the **relative percentage MDC (MDC%)**, the more attractive the instrument. As important is the **minimum clinically important difference (MCID),** which is the amount of change perceived as important by patients.[1] The amount of change within the 95% confidence interval is described at the MDC_{95} or at the 90% confidence interval as the MDC_{90}. All of these properties should be considered when selecting the appropriate outcome measure.

As described in Chapter 3, specific functional deficits can be linked with impairments and tracked across treatment sessions, and this helps with the clinical reasoning associated with treatment choice. Individual rating scores can be used to provide treatment goals and assist with communicating the relevance of treatment to the patient. Using functional outcome measures over the course of rehabilitation is a valid and reliable method of measuring progress over time. Functional measures are being mandated by both public and private payors at increasing rates. Using appropriate outcomes measures consistently, and applying the requisite clinical judgment to interpret them, is essential to successfully comply with insurance reporting requirements. Although insurance requirements are an important element of providing care, the primary justification for functional measures is to inform decision making and progression of management for optimal care.

Self-Reported Outcome Measures

Self-reported measures reflect the patient's perspective of his or her status and improvement (Table 8.3). The advantage of these instruments is efficiency (patients may complete the questionnaires while waiting for treatment), and most measures have been tested for reliability and validity. Self-reported measures can include symptoms, perception of a patient's functional status, and attitudes. While self-reported functional measures are useful reflections of the patient's perception of his or her physical function, a patient's ability to perform a movement is not always measured with self-reported measures. Other disadvantages of self-reported measures are literacy limitations and

TABLE 8.3 Self-Reported Functional Outcome Questionnaires

Functional Outcome Questionnaires	Description	MDC/MCID
Disabilities of the Arm, Shoulder and Hand Questionnaire (DASH)[1,14] Short form DASH[1,15]	Full questionnaire consists of 30 Likert-style questions, including 21 physical function of the upper extremity items, 5 pain items, and 4 items related to participation Short 11-item questionnaire addresses physical function and symptoms.	MCID 10 points (full questionnaire) [1,14] 8 points (short form) out of 100[1,15]
Lower Extremity Function Scale (LEFS)[1,16]	Likert-style questions of difficulty with 20 tasks requiring lower extremity function with a total score of 80	MDC and MCID 9 points out of 80[1,16]
Oswestry Disability Index (ODI)[1,17] Modified ODI[1,18]	Ratings of difficulty with 10 functional tasks used for patients with lumbar or thoracic spine diagnosis. Modified Oswestry replaces the question related to sexual activity with an item related to homemaking or employment	MCID Oswestry 11 points[1,17] Modified Oswestry Index 6 points[1,18]
Neck Disability Index (NDI)	Similar to the ODI with 10 functional tasks influenced by cervical pain	MDC $_{90}$ 5 points out of 100 (chronic neck pain) 7; MCID 7.5 in patients after spinal fusion[19]
Patient-Specific Functional Scale (PSFS)	Can be used to address functional difficulties for multiple regions; patients select the major functional activities that are problematic	MDC 2 points for neck pain[20]
Western Ontario and McMaster Universities Osteoarthritis Index (WOMAC)	24 items related to pain, stiffness, and physical function used for individuals with osteoarthritis	16% reduction [21] with OA, 15 points out of 100 for TKR [22]
Short Form SF36	Patient-reported outcome measure covering 8 domains (physical functioning, role limitation [physical and emotional], bodily pain, general health, vitality, social functioning, mental health) used to measure health-related quality of life	MDC $_{95}$ 19–45 depending on domain in patients with parkinsonism[23]; MDIC 4.9 points for the physical component summary domain of the SF-36 in patients with low back pain[24]

MDC, Minimum detectable change; *MCID*, minimum clinically important difference; *OA*, osteoarthritis; *TKR*, total knee replacement.

TABLE 8.4 Questionnaires Assessing Presence and Magnitude of Psychological Elements

Questionnaire	Description	Indications
STarT Back Tool	Tool designed to screen patients with low back pain in primary care. Eight questions involve characterizing back pain and response to it. One question assesses distress. Scores range from 0 to 9. Recently validated for use in other anatomic regions.[25]	Use with patients experiencing low back pain to assess risk for poor outcome and to classify for appropriate treatment. Categorized as low, medium, or high risk. Higher scores indicate higher risk.[26–28]
Fear Avoidance Beliefs Questionnaire (FABQ)	Items related to agreement with statements about influence of back pain on physical activity (4 items) and work (7 items).	High scores indicate high fear avoidance beliefs and the need to address psychological components during exercise prescription, motivation, and goal setting.[29–31] MDC 6.1 for FABQ-PA scale in patients with pelvic girdle pain[32]; MDC 13 for FABQ-W and MDC 8 for FABQ-PA in workers with upper extremity injury.[33] MCID: 13 points in patients with lower back pain.[31]
Tampa Kinesiophobia Questionnaire	Seventeen-item scale originally designed to measure fear of movement/reinjury in patients with chronic low back pain. Has been expanded to other patient populations.	Higher scores indicated higher degree of kinesiophobia. Scores range from 17 to 68. Greater than 37 considered high. MDC 4.8.[28,29]

MDC, Minimum detectable change; *MCID*, minimum clinically important difference.

language barriers that can influence patient understanding of the questions. The individual's psychological status and attitude toward movement can influence the results and may necessitate using screening tools such as the STarTBack or Orbero Musculoskeletal Pain Screening Questionnaire, or specific psychological measures such as the Fear Avoidance Beliefs Questionnaire or the Tampa Kinesiophobia Scale (Table 8.4).

Objective Functional Performance Outcome Measures

Objective functional performance measures are used to quantify distance, speed, repetition, time sustained, or level of difficulty with movements required for everyday activity (Table 8.5).

Most objective measures are easily reproducible and can be performed without sophisticated equipment (see Clinical Example 8.7). When choosing an outcome measure, therapists should consider the precautions, healing phase, and the patient's ability to safely complete the testing. In some postsurgical protocols, the clearance to move to the next phase of treatment is based on achieving specific criteria (Tables 8.6 and 8.7). The progression of exercise choices is also built on achievement of criteria along with the patient's history, extent of tissue damage and healing, and surgical procedure (Clinical Examples 8.6 and 8.8). The test results can also be used to establish short- and long-term goals and evaluation for discharge decisions (Clinical Examples 8.1, 8.6, and 8.9).

TABLE 8.5 Functional Performance Measures

Functional Test	Description	MDC/MCID	Purpose and Interpretation
Single-leg or one-legged stance test (Video 8.1)	Patient is asked to stand on one leg with the opposite leg flexed without touching the supporting leg. Can be completed with eyes open or closed.	MDC_{90} 7 seconds (affected limb), 11 seconds (unaffected limb) in patients with hip osteoarthritis.[34]	Patients unable to perform the one-leg stand for at least 5 seconds are at increased risk for injurious falls. Age-related norms are available.[35]
Timed up-and-go (Video 8.2)	Patient starts in a seated position, stands, and then walks 3 m or 10 ft, turns around, walks back to chair, then sits. Time to complete task from command to go until patient sits back into the chair is recorded.	MDC_{95} is 1.1 seconds in patient with knee OA[36]	Tests ability and power to move from sit-to-stand, walking speed, coordination to turn around, and return.
5× sit to stand	Patients stand from a seated position and returns 5 times, moving as fast as they can. They are instructed to keep their hands folded across their chest. Time to complete this task is recorded.	MDC: 2.5 seconds in older females[37] MCID: 1.7 seconds in patients with COPD[38]; 2.3 seconds in patients with vestibular disorders[39]	Tests lower extremity strength, dynamic functional movements, and balance. Also used to determine fall risk.
Six-minute walk test	Patient walks at a self-selected pace for 6 minutes. Distance is measured.	MDC: 79 m in patients awaiting knee arthroplasty; 81.5 m in patient awaiting hip arthroplasty[40] MDC = 58.21 m older adults[41] MCID: 50 m in older adults[41]	Reflection of distance within set time, tests both endurance and speed.
10-meter walk test	Patient walks 10 m on level surface. Patient is timed over middle 6 m.	MDC: 0.18 to 0.82 m/sec post hip fracture[42,43] MCID: 0.05 to 0.25 m/sec depending on population[41,44]	Tests gait speed.
Star excursion test (Video 8.3)	Patient stands on one leg in center of star-shaped grid made from intersecting strips of tape that are 6 to 8 feet in length. While standing on one limb, patient is asked to reach as far as possible with the free limb in eight different directions.[45] Stance foot alignment and hand position (on the hips or reaching forward) influences the results and should be standardized.[46] Results can be normalized as a percentage of the reach distance to the leg length.[46]	MDC is not available. Normal asymmetry ranges from 3% to 8% in collegiate athletes.[45]	A dynamic balance and postural stability test that requires strength, flexibility, and proprioception. A dynamic balance measure that provides significant challenge to athletes and those who are physically active.[45] Can be used to assess postural control, symmetry, and risk for lower extremity injury (4 cm left/right anterior reach difference increases risk of injury ×3).[47] Used to identify chronic ankle instability (2–4% difference)[46,48–51] or altered neuromuscular control at knee and hip.[51,52] Can be used for neuromuscular control and symmetry training; score improves with other forms of training.[51,52]
Y balance test (Video 8.4)	Abbreviated form of the star balance test; can be performed using a sliding device. Patient stands on the center point while reaching behind in either direction or in front[53,54]	MDC is not available.	Can be used to assess postural control, symmetry, and risk for lower extremity injury. Anterior asymmetry of more than 4 cm for anterior reach increases the odds of non-contact injury in Division 1 athletes by 2.33 (95% CI, 1.15–4.76)[54] and distinguishes between individuals with or without previous history of injury.[45] The test can also be used to identify lower extremity flexibility and flexibility asymmetry.[53]
Standing heel rise test	Number of heel rises possible standing on one leg; represents plantarflexor strength.	SEM 2.1 to 3.4[55–58] 2.07 repetitions[55]	Represents plantarflexor strength (28 repetitions is considered normal for the dominant limb) and is related to functional balance, gait ability, and walking speed.[55–58]
Step-up tests (Video 3.20)	Count how often the subject can step up onto a 15-cm block and down again leading with the same leg in 15 seconds. Number of whole repetitions is recorded for each leg. A Six-Minute Step Test has also been validated compared to the 6-minute walk test and is a moderate predictor of lower extremity strength.[59]	15-second test: MDC 3 (affected limb), 4 (unaffected limb) in patients with hip osteoarthritis.[34]	Designed to assess advanced changes in base of support (dynamic balance), lower extremity strength, and endurance (Six-Minute Step Test) Single-leg step up and down and lateral step-down can be used to evaluate movement quality and kinematics.[60,61]

TABLE 8.5 Functional Performance Measures—cont'd

Functional Test	Description	MDC/MCID	Purpose and Interpretation
Hop tests	Timed test. Patient is timed while hopping 6 m on uninjured followed by injured leg.[62] Single-leg hop test for distance; distance is measured and compared to the opposite side when hopping as far as possible on one leg. The athlete starts in a semi-crouched position, swings the arms, and then hops as far as possible to land safely (Video 3.24). Triple hop: Distance measured for three consecutive hops on the same leg when attempting to hop as far as possible in a straight line; total distance is recorded (Video 8.5). Crossover hop: The same procedures are used as with the triple-hop, with the additional challenge of crossing a line on each hop. Total distance is recorded (Video 8.6).	SEM for 6-meter timed test 0.06 second for healthy young men.[63]	Total time taken is compared between legs. Indicator of functional reaction time, ability to repeatedly produce sufficient power, and dynamic balance. Single-leg hop for distance and triple-hop tests reflect explosive power and dynamic balance when landing. The triple-hop also reflects the ability to regenerate power and is a progression.[64] The crossover hop also reflects proprioceptive ability and includes a frontal plane challenge. Single-leg hop, triple-hop, and crossover hop are able to detect asymmetries and potential functional deficits in individuals after anterior cruciate ligament (ACL) reconstruction.[65] Dynamic tests also allow evaluation of movement strategies.[66,67] Athletes should demonstrate 90% of the performance on the uninjured leg before return to sport after ACL reconstruction.[66]
Vertical jump or drop jump	Patient is asked to jump as high as possible; distance to the tips of the fingers is recorded. Drop jumps are conducted from a step.	MDC% 11% to 33% in middle-aged healthy individuals.[69]	Reflects strength and power to produce vertical motion for jumping athletes[68]

COPD, Chronic obstructive pulmonary disease; *MDC,* minimum detectable change; *MCID,* minimum clinically important difference; *OA,* osteoarthritis; *SEM,* standard error mean.

TABLE 8.6 Phases Post–Knee Microfracture Surgery[13]

Phase	Precautions	Outcome Criteria for Advancement
Phase I: Weeks 0–6	No weight bearing, knee maintained at zero degrees in brace to allow microfractures to heal and bleeding to fill cartilage deficits	Clearance for weight bearing from physician (based on extent of injury, location of defect relative to weight-bearing surfaces, presence of swelling) Range of motion 0–120 degrees Hip strength equivalent to unaffected leg Straight leg against gravity without a quadriceps lag
Phase II: Weeks 6–12	Avoid excessive passive stress on healing structures (vertical compression), especially with descending stairs, squats in extreme ranges Monitor for extreme swelling and pain responses and adjust exercise load and difficulty accordingly	Range of motion within normal limits (equivalent to opposite side and for functional activities) Normal symmetrical gait pattern Ability to ascend 8-inch step Normal patellar mobility
Phase III: Weeks 12–18	Monitor for swelling and pain responses and adjust exercise load and difficulty accordingly Only progress to running and impact activities once adequate strength and partial weight-bearing endurance are present using equipment which does not load the joint maximally (bike, leg press, elliptical)	Ability to descend 8-inch steps with good control and no pain (10–15 repetitions) 85% limb symmetry on isokinetic testing and forward step-down test
Return to sport: Week 18+[a]	Monitor for swelling and pain responses and adjust exercise load and difficulty accordingly Avoid any sports activity until adequate strength develops and physician clearance is given	Hop test with at least 85% symmetry Lack of apprehension with sport-specific movement (Fear-avoidance beliefs questionnaire or Tampa Kinesiophobia questionnaire) Flexibility required for sports Able to perform home program and adjust exercises safely

[a]Some protocols include more than three phases, especially if there is a need to return to sport or high-level work activities (see Fig. 8.2A,B).

TABLE 8.7   Phases of Post–Rotator Cuff Repair[13]

Phase	Precautions	Treatment	Criteria for Progression to Next Phase
Phase I: Maximum protection (weeks 0–3)	Immobilize in a sling to minimize gravitational forces No active movement Maintain range of motion precautions established by the surgeon according to extent and location of tear	Patient education for activities of daily living and sleeping to protect shoulder Pendular exercises in sling (if allowed by surgeon) Passive range of motion within precautions AAROM if allowed by surgeon Distal joint active range of motion	Time, following surgeon's requirements for progression based on early healing
Phase II: Moderate protection (weeks 3–7)	No active elevation against gravity No maximal rotator cuff activation Range of motion limitations as determined by surgeon	Progress passive range of motion, active-assisted range of motion Scapula muscle initiation and stabilization Isometric shoulder exercises (in supported positions, submaximal force)	Ability to activate rotator cuff and deltoid without pain 80% of range of motion (flexion, external rotation)
Phase II: Early strengthening (weeks 7–13)	Limit activities or exercises that stress the repaired muscles Limit forces or time spent in impingement positions Restore scapulohumeral rhythm and scapulothoracic connection before increasing load at higher ranges Gradual return to light activities of daily living below 90 degrees	Continue focusing on improving range of motion including functional ROM exercises (hand behind back, dressing, bathing) Scapula muscle strengthening (isotonic, isometric progressive resistance) Rotator cuff strengthening low-load, high-repetition active range of motion in the scapular plane, supported positions, progress to gravity resisted Rhythmic stabilization Progress to closed-chain exercises (isometric) Upper body ergometer as strength improves	Minimal pain Full passive range of motion Proper muscle activation and ability to perform exercises midrange progressive loads Normal scapulohumeral rhythm below 90
Phase II: Late strengthening (weeks 14–19)	Only progress to overhead activities when proximal stability and mechanics are observed Limit excessive forces at end ranges Limit forces when impingement is possible	Continue to progress strengthening to higher loads with lower repetitions (scapula and rotator cuff muscles) Add resistance exercises using weight machines if part of home exercise program plan (lat pull-downs chest press, rows) with appropriate mechanics Progress closed-chain exercises to include plyometrics if appropriate	Normal scapulohumeral rhythm through full range of motion Full strength equivalent to other side (dynamometer)
Phase III: Return to sport (weeks 20–24)	Avoid pain with exercise, activity, or sport Surgeon's clearance	Progressive sports-specific strengthening and flexibility Plyometrics or reaction training Interval and periodization training	Independence with home program Return to sport

AAROM, Active-assisted range of motion; *ROM,* range of motion.

🏃 CLINICAL EXAMPLE 8.8   Post SLAP Repair Outcome Evaluation for Progression

A 22-year-old lacrosse player was diagnosed with a SLAP tear after repeated shoulder trauma including falls on an outstretched arm and external force from another player while her arm was elevated. The type II tear extended from approximately 11 to 2 o'clock, with separation of the labrum from the glenoid but no biceps tendon tear.

Precautions

Phase I precautions for between 3 and 4 weeks include using an immobilizer at all times except when bathing or performing exercise, no active biceps contraction or tension through the biceps tendon, and caution with external rotation to avoid stress on the labrum (limited to neutral).

Phase I Goals[1,2]

1. Reduce pain and inflammatory by-products
2. Improve passive range to 90 degrees of flexion, external rotation to neutral
3. Adherence to precautions for all functional activities
4. Promote muscle activation in protected ranges without stress on sutured tissue

Exercise Choice[1–3]

- Distal range of motion and muscle activation and endurance in supported positions: wrist active movement with the arm supported in the immobilizer or on a table, wrist and finger resistance with toning balls (Exercise 10.34), and grip strength (Exercise 10.35)
- Submaximal deltoid and rotator cuff isometrics (self-resisted arm supported on a table to limit tension; Exercise 10.19)
- Passive (Exercise 10.52) and active-assisted external rotation to neutral (supported on a table, with modification; Exercise 10.33), active-assisted flexion in scaption using a T-bar (Exercise 10.4) and with pulleys (Exercise 10.5)

Evaluation

The criteria to advance the range of motion are achievement of neutral external rotation and 75 degrees of shoulder flexion in scaption without pain or resistance to passive movement with minimal pain (<2/10).[1–3] The normal timeline is between 3 and 4 weeks before advancing range.[1,2] The patient achieves the criteria by 3 weeks and is able to progress range of motion while still adhering to healing requirements.

CLINICAL EXAMPLE 8.8 Post SLAP Repair Outcome Evaluation for Progression—cont'd

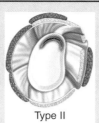

Type II

A type II labral tear. (From Rynders S, Hart J. *Orthopaedics for Physician Assistants*. Philadelphia: Saunders; 2013.)

Precautions

For Phase II, from weeks 3 to 6, no biceps strengthening or tension until week 8. Slow progression with load and tension on rotator cuff. Based on the history of the injury, compressive forces and full external rotation should be introduced slowly.

Exercise Choices

Early Phase II Progression (Weeks 3–6)[1-3]

- Continue forward flexion in scaption to 90 degrees and increase passive external rotation up to 30 degrees in the scapula plane at 45 degrees of abduction (supported)
- Progress active assisted movement using pulleys and hydrotherapy to slightly less than passive limits
- Wean sling immobilization with slow discontinuation of support when standing or working

- Introduce scapula muscle activation and endurance exercises without excessive stress on rotator cuff (Exercise 10.14 and with the arm supported in side lying; Exercise 10.51, aquatic therapy)
- Rotator cuff isometric endurance and alternating rhythmic stabilization in supported positions midrange (Exercises 10.16 and 10.18)

Evaluation

Criteria for Progression in Weeks 5–8[1-3]

- Progress flexion to up to 145 degrees if pain-free passive and active movement is available above 90 degrees in scaption
- Progress external rotation in mid-abduction to 60 degrees if pain-free passive and active movement is available to 30 degrees
- Minimal pain
- Isometric activation and endurance is progressing without pain exacerbation; initiate small-range isotonics in open-chain positions

References

1. Levinson M. Superior labrum anterior to posterior (SLAP) repair. In: Cioppa Mosca J, et al., ed. *Handbook of Postsurgical Rehabilitation Guidelines for the Orthopaedia Clinician. Hospital for Special Surgery.* St. Louis, MO: Mosby Elsevier; 2008.
2. Dodson C, Altchek D. SLAP lesions: an update on recognition and treatment. *J Orthop Sports Phys Ther.* 2009;39(2):71–80.
3. Wilk KE, Reinold MM, Dugas JR, Arrigo CA, Moser MW, Andrews JR. Current concepts in the recognition and treatment of superior labral (SLAP) lesions. *J Orthop Sports Phys Ther.* 2005;35(5):273–291.

CLINICAL EXAMPLE 8.9 Choosing Outcome Measures to Match Functional Goals

A 53-year-old woman is seen on postoperative day 4 after a total hip arthroplasty. The therapist uses the Timed Up and Go (TUG) and 10-meter walk test as part of the initial evaluation. At the 2.5 week reevaluation, these basic functional activities have improved and the patient has met her initial goals for transfers and gait speed. A new functional outcome measure, the Lower Extremity Functional Scale (LEFS), was chosen to reflect her status for higher-level skills needed to meet her long-term goals of being independent and returning to work. The LEFS assesses 20 multidimensional functional activities reflecting a broader range of functional activities compared to only using the TUG and 10-meter walk test and assesses more advanced function. The LEFS uses a scale of 0 (extreme difficulty or unable to perform activity) to 4 (no difficulty) on each item. The MDC for the LEFS is 10 points and the MDIC is 9 points.[1]

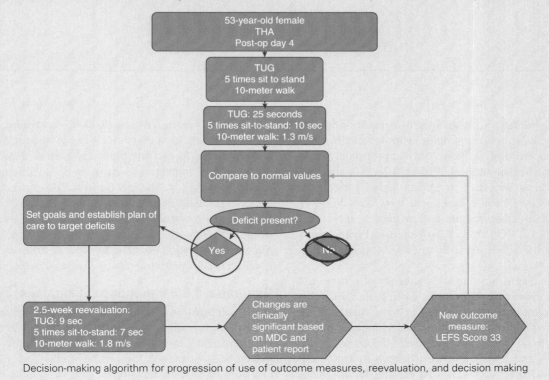

Decision-making algorithm for progression of use of outcome measures, reevaluation, and decision making

CLINICAL EXAMPLE 8.9 Choosing Outcome Measures to Match Functional Goals—cont'd

The focus of interventions for this patient, based on the items on the LEFS of importance to her, was to improve her rating of the following activities: usual work (as a healthcare provider), hobbies and recreational activities, squatting, lifting an object from the floor, and walking a mile. She reported moderate difficulty with work, hobbies, squatting, and lifting an object from the floor (2/4 on a scale of 0–4/4 with 0/4 = extreme difficulty or unable to perform and 4/4 = no difficulty) on the relevant items of the LEFS. She also reported extreme difficulty with walking for a mile (1/4).

Goals were aligned with the items on the LEFS so that she would be able to perform work and recreational activities, squatting, and lifting objects from the floor with minimal difficulty (3/4) within 4 weeks. The goal to walk a mile with minimal difficulty was set for 8 weeks.

Reference

Binkley JM, Stratford PW, Lott SA, Riddle DL. The lower extremity functional scale (LEFS): scale development, measurement properties, and clinical application. North American Orthopaedic Rehabilitation Research Network. *Phys Ther.* 1999;79:371–383.

LEFS Score 33

Weaning from assistive device
High-resistance exercises
Obstacle course training
Outdoor gait training
Mini-squats with resistance
Work task simulation training
Treadmill training

Reevaluate

Patient has met all goals; LEFS score 70

Release from care and follow up as needed

Decision-making algorithm for reevaluation and discharge decision making.

Some functional tests are vigorous and require adequate range of motion and functional strength without eliciting pain or swelling, thus making the tests only appropriate during late Phase II or III rehabilitation (Videos 3.24, 8.5, and 8.6). Screening criteria are available to guide whether patients are ready to participate in some functional tests (see Box 4.7). There are tests intended for specific patient groups, such as the Timed Up and Go (TUG [Video 8.2]), functional reach, or 5× Sit-to-Stand Tests that are primarily intended for older adults (Table 8.3).

The therapist must determine the frequency of testing, and some functional performance measures are repeated only after an adequate amount of time has passed to allow change. If the outcome measure is similar to actual exercise technique, improvements are easier to document. For example, if the single-leg hop (Videos 3.24, 8.5, and 8.6), Y balance (Video 8.4), or the star excursion test (Video 8.3) is used as an exercise for an athlete whose goal is to return to basketball, it is relatively easy to evaluate the performance at every visit. The Six-Minute Walk Test may not be suitable to measure individual session improvement but are suitable for an interim reevaluation due to the amount of time required for the test. The MDC and MCID as measures are also useful to guide the decision on frequency of testing. For example, a measure with a smaller MDC and MCID and greater sensitivity would be preferred to guide proper progression of an exercise, and more frequent testing would be appropriate if the measure is likely to reflect small amounts of change (Tables 8.3–8.5).

Generalized Combinations of Functional Tests

Some combinations (often called a *battery*) of tests used to screen fitness level or functional performance may be useful for comparison to normative values or for injury prevention strategies. For example, the Senior Fitness Test includes combinations of tests for functional range of motion, balance, and strength and provides age-related normative comparisons.[69] The Dynamic Gait Index includes a series of tests that reflect mobility, balance, and reaction time. The Functional Movement Screen also includes tests for functional range of motion, flexibility, and strength, but it is designed for screening for injury potential in athletes.[70,71]

Other combinations of tests can be created using specific drills, although the results are individual and not always reliable. Shuttle runs, carioca drills, and obstacle courses can be used during Phase III management for challenging three-dimensional movement, speed, and functional coordination. While these drills are useful for individual goals, there are no valid comparisons for prior function. Occasionally, higher-level athletic or performance requirements are very specific, and there are no reliable and valid tests available for the given population. For example, a rhythmic gymnast needs extreme mobility and rapid reaction times to safely return to practice. A series of drills mimicking the required movements or reaction speeds in the required extreme ranges of motion would be a more useful outcome than one of the functional tests tested with athletes without these requirements. Often contralateral limb measurements or normative values for the average age ranges will have to be used for comparison purposes.

Rehabmeasures.org (http://www.rehabmeasures.org) is a comprehensive online database.[72] This repository is consistently updated to reflect current research and should serve as a valuable resource for students, faculty, and practicing clinicians. There are also extensive resources for multiple self-reported and objective measures, interpretation, and psychometric properties in Magee's *Orthopaedic Physical Assessment* (6th ed., 2014).[1] The American Physical Therapy Association's PTNow website provides an online resource for tests and measures, and it is updated regularly (http://www. ptnow.org/tests-measures).[73]

SUMMARY

- Evaluation of responses to exercise is an essential ongoing process that must occur frequently.
- Factors used to assess responses to exercise and guide progression of an exercise program include:
  - Primary subjective symptoms and history including assessment of severity, irritability, nature of the problem, and stage
  - Primary impairments, activity limitations, and/or participation restrictions
  - Symptoms during and immediately after exercise or following an exercise session, including pain responses, delayed-onset muscle soreness, or effusion
  - Psychological contributions
  - Patient's understanding of the exercise
  - Ability to reproduce the desired movements for home programs
- The results of the ongoing evaluation guide clinical decision making, including exercise selection, outcome measure choice, and plan of care development.

- Compensations and abnormal movement patterns can be indicative of inappropriate dosing of exercise or ineffective patient education on the correct exercise form.
- Home exercise prescription is an essential component of a comprehensive therapeutic exercise intervention to promote tissue regeneration, improve muscular or cardiovascular endurance, and reinforce patient and treatment goals. Factors such as the phases of healing, patient compliance, cognitive status, likelihood of over- or underdosing the exercise, and the patient's environment need to be considered when prescribing a home exercise program.
- Outcome measures, either self-reported, objective functional performance, or a combination of both, are used to establish the extent of impairments, activity limitations, and participation restrictions. Choosing the correct measure or measures will assist the therapist in evaluating a patient's improvement and treatment effectiveness. Selected outcome and impairment measures guide treatment focus or predict prognosis.

REVIEW QUESTIONS

1. Describe how the SINS characteristics influence exercise progression, including the prescription of a home exercise program.
2. Describe how pain and symptom response is used to guide the choice of exercises and the decision on when and how to progress an exercise regimen.
3. Explain the importance of compensation and abnormal movement patterns during the performance of exercise and how to use information on these patterns to adjust exercise dosage.
4. Describe how factors such as the phases of healing, patient compliance, cognitive status, likelihood of over- or underdosing the exercise, and the patient's environment influence home exercise program prescription.
5. What are the important factors to consider when choosing an outcome measure?
6. How would you use MCID and MDC for a given outcome measure when assessing the effectiveness of your exercise prescription or patient progress?
7. Describe the similarities and differences between a self-reported outcome measure and an objective functional performance measure.

REFERENCES

1. Cleland JA, Koppenhaver S. *Netter's Orthopaedic Clinical Examination - An Evidence-based Approach*. 2nd ed. St Louis, MO: Saunders Elsevier; 2011.

2. Magee DJ. *Orthopaedic Physical Assessment*. 6th ed. St. Louis, MO: Saunders Elsevier; 2014.

3. Mankovsky-Arnold T, et al. Measures of spontaneous and movement-evoked pain are associated with disability in patients with whiplash injuries. *J Pain*. 2014;15(9):967–975.

4. Srikandarajah S, Gilron I. Systematic review of movement-evoked pain versus pain at rest in postsurgical clinical trials and meta-analyses: a fundamental distinction requiring standardized measurement. *Pain*. 2011;152(8):1734–1739.

5. Sayers A, et al. Rest pain and movement-evoked pain as unique constructs in hip and knee replacements. *Arthritis Care Res*. 2016;68(2):237–245.

6. Parker P. Systematic review of movement-evoked pain versus pain at rest in postsurgical clinical trials and meta-analyses: a fundamental distinction requiring standardized measurement. *Pain*. 2012;153(1):250.

7. Magee DJ, Sueki D. *Orthopedic Physical Assessment Atlas and Video: Selected Special Tests and Movements*. 6th ed. St. Louis, MO: Elsevier Saunders; 2011.

8. Boissonnault WG. *Primary Care for the Physical Therapist: Examination and Triage*. 2nd ed. St. Louis, MO: Elsevier Saunders; 2016.

9. Arundale A, Silvers H, Logerstedt D, Rojas J, Snyder-Mackler L. An interval kicking progression for return to soccer following lower extremity injury. *Int J Sports Phys Ther*. 2015;10(1):114–127.

10. Axe M, Wickam R, Snyder-Mackler L. Data-based interval throwing programs for little league, high school, college, and professional baseball pitchers. *Sports Med Arthrosc*. 2001;9:24–34.

11. White K, Di Stasi S, Smith A, Snyder-Mackler L. Anterior cruciate ligament-specialized post-operative return-to-sports (ACL-SPORTS) training: a randomized control trial. *BMC Musc Dis*. 2013;14(1):108.

12. Goodman CC, Fuller KS. *Pathology: Implications for the Physical Therapist*. 4th ed. St. Louis, MO: Saunders; 2015.

13. Cioppa-Mosca J, Cahill JB, Tucker CY, eds. *Handbook Of Postsurgical Rehabilitation Guidelines For The Orthopaedic Clinician*. St. Louis, MO: Elsevier Saunders; 2008.

14. Roy JS, MacDermid JC, Woodhouse LJ. Measuring shoulder function: a systematic review of four questionnaires. *Arthritis Rheumatol*. 2009;61:623–632.

15. Mintken PE, Glynn P, Cleland JA. Psychometric properties of the shortened disabilities of the arm, shoulder, and hand questionnaire (QuickDASH) and numeric pain rating in patients with shoulder pain. *J Shoulder Elbow Surg*. 2009;18(6):920–926.

16. Binkley JM, Stratford PW, Lott SA, Riddle DI. The Lower Extremity Functional Scale (LEFS): scale development, measurement properties, and clinical application. *Phys Ther*. 1999;79:371–383.

17. Lauridsen HH, Hartvigsen J, Manniche C, et al. Responsiveness and minimal clinically important difference for pain and disability instruments in low back pain patients. *BMC Musculoskeletal Disord*. 2006;7:82.

18. Fritz JM, Irrgang JJ. A comparison of a modified oswestry disability questionnaire and the quebec back pain disability scale. *Phys Ther*. 2001;81:776–788.

19. Carreon LY, Glassman SD, Campbell MJ, Anderson PA. Neck Disability Index, short form-36 physical component summary, and pain scales for neck and arm pain: the minimum clinically important difference and substantial clinical benefit after cervical spine fusion. *Spine J*. 2010;6:469–474.

20. Westaway MD, Stratford PW, et al. The patient-specific functional scale: validation of its use in persons with neck dysfunction. *J Orthop Sports Phys Ther*. 1998;27:331–338.

21. Hmamouchi I, Allali F, et al. Clinically important improvement in the WOMAC and predictor factors for response to non-specific non-steroidal anti-inflammatory drugs in osteoarthritic patients: a prospective study. *BMC Res Notes*. 2012;5:58.

22. Escobar A, Quintana JM, et al. Responsiveness and clinically important differences for the WOMAC and SF-36 after total knee replacement. *Osteoarthritis Cartilage*. 2007;15(3):273–280.

23. Steffen T, Seney M. Test-retest reliability and minimal detectable change on balance and ambulation tests, the 36-item short-form health survey, and the unified Parkinson disease rating scale in people with parkinsonism. *Phys Ther*. 2008;88(6):733–746.

24. Copay AG, Glassman SD, Subach BR, Berven S, Schuler TC, Carreon LY. Minimum clinical important differences in lumbar spine surgery patients: a choice of methods using the Oswestry Disability Index, Medical Outcomes Survey Questionnaire Short-Form 36, and Pain Scales. *Spine J*. 2008;8(6):968–974.

25. Butera K, Lentz TA, Beneciuk JM, George SZ. Preliminary evaluation of a modified STarT Back screening tool across different musculoskeletal pain conditions. *Phys Ther*. 206;96:1251–1261.

26. Beneciuk JM, Fritz JM, et al. The STarT Back Screening Tool for prediction of 6-month clinical outcomes: relevance of change patterns in outpatient physical therapy settings. *J Orthop Sports Phys Ther*. 2014;44(9):656–664.

27. Beneciuk JM, Bishop MD, et al. The STarT back screening tool and individual psychological measures: evaluation of prognostic capabilities for low back pain clinical outcomes in outpatient physical therapy settings. *Phys Ther*. 2013;93(3):321–333.

28. Fritz JM, Beneciuk JM, et al. Relationship between categorization with the STarT Back Screening Tool and prognosis for people receiving physical therapy for low back pain. *Phys Ther*. 2011;91(5):722–732.

29. Cleland JA, Fritz JA, et al. Psychometric properties of the Fear-Avoidance Beliefs Questionnaire and Tampa Scale of Kinesiophobia in patients with neck pain. *Am J Phys Med Rehabil*. 2008;87(2):109–117.

30. Swinkels-Meewisse EJ, Swinkels RA, et al. Psychometric properties of the Tampa Scale for kinesiophobia and the fear-avoidance beliefs questionnaire in acute low back pain. *Man Ther*. 2003;8(1):29–36.

31. George SZ, Fritz JM, et al. Fear-avoidance beliefs as measured by the fear-avoidance beliefs questionnaire: change in fear-avoidance beliefs questionnaire is predictive of change in self-report of disability and pain intensity for patients with acute low back pain. *Clin J Pain*. 2006;22(2):197–203.

32. Grotle M, Garratt AM, Jenssen HK, Stuge B. Reliability and construct validity of self-report questionnaires for patients with pelvic girdle pain. *Phys Ther*. 2012;92(1):111–123.

33. Inrig T, Amey B, Borthwick C, Beaton D. Validity and reliability of the Fear-Avoidance Beliefs Questionnaire (FABQ) in workers with upper extremity injuries. *J Occup Rehab*. 2012;22(1):59–70.

34. Choi YM, et al. Interrater and intrarater reliability of common clinical standing balance tests for people with hip osteoarthritis. *Phys Ther*. 1994;(5):696–704.

35. Springer BA, Marin R, et al. Normative values for the unipedal stance test with eyes open and closed. *J Geriatr Phys Ther.* 2007;30(1):8–15.

36. Alghadir A, Anwer S, Brismee JM. The reliability and minimal detectable change of Timed Up and Go Test in individuals with grade 1-3 knee osteoarthritis. *BMC Musculoskelet Disord.* 2015;16:174.

37. Goldberg A, Chavis M, Watkins J, Wilson T. The five times sit to stand test: validity, reliability, and detectable change in older females. *Aging Clin Exp Res.* 2012;24(4):339–344.

38. Jones SE, Kon SS, Cananvan JL, et al. The five-repetition sit to stand test as an functional outcome measure in COPD. *Thorax.* 2013;68(11):1051–1020.

39. Meretta BM, Whitney SL, Marchetti GF, Sparto PJ, Muirhead RJ. The five times sit to stand test: responsiveness to change and concurrent validity in adults undergoing vestibular rehabilitation. *J Vestib Res.* 2006;16(4-5):233–243.

40. Naylor JM, Hayen A, Davidson E, et al. Minimal detectable change for mobility and patient-reported tools in people with osteoarthritis awaiting arthroplasty. *BMC Musculoskeletal Disord.* 2014;15:235.

41. Carcia CR, Perera S, Mody S, Woodman RC, Studenski SA. Meaningful change and responsiveness in common physical performance measures in older adults. *J Am Geriatr Soc.* 2006;54:743–749.

42. Hollman JH, Beckman BA, Brandt RA, et al. Minimum detectable change in gait velocity during acute rehabilitation following hip fracture. *J Geriatr Phys Ther.* 2008;31:53–56.

43. Latham N, Mehta V, Nyugen AM, et al. Performance-based or self-report measures of physical function: which should be used in clinical trials of hip fracture patients? *Arch Phys Med Rehabil.* 2008;89:2146–2155.

44. Loo Van, Moseley AM, et al. Test-retest reliability of walking speed, step length and step width measurement after traumatic brain injury: a pilot study. *Brain Inj.* 2004;18(10):1041–1048.

45. Stiffler MR, Sanfilippo JL, et al. Star excursion balance test performance varies by sport in healthy division I collegiate athletes. *J Orthop Sports Phys Ther.* 2015;45(10):772–780.

46. Cug M. Stance foot alignment and hand positioning alter star excursion balance test scores in those with chronic ankle instability: what are we really assessing? *Physiother Theory Pract.* 2017;33(4):316–322.

47. Plisky PJ, Rauh MJ, et al. Star excursion balance test as a predictor of lower extremity injury in high school basketball players. *J Orthop Sports Phys Ther.* 2006;36(12):911–919.

48. Hertel J, Braham RA, Hale SA, Olmsted LC. Simplifying the Star Excursion Balance Test: analyses of subjects with and without ankle instability. *J Orthop Sports Phys Ther.* 2006;36: 131–137.

49. Olmsted LC, Carcia CR, Hertel J, Shultz S. Efficacy of the star excursion balance tests in detecting reach deficits in subjects with chronic ankle instability. *J Athl Train.* 2002;379(4):501–506.

50. Gribble PA, Hertel J, Denegar CR, Buckley WE. The effects of fatigue and chronic ankle instability on dynamic postural control. *J Athl Train.* 2004;39(4):321–329.

51. Hale SA, Hertel J, Olmsted-Kramer LC. The effect of a 4 week comprehensive rehabilitation program on postural control and lower extremity function in individuals with chronic ankle instability. *J Orthop Sports Phys Ther.* 2007;37(6):303–311.

52. English T, Howe K. The effect of Pilates exercise on trunk and postural stability and throwing velocity in college baseball pitchers: single subject design. *NAJSPT.* 2007;2(1):8–19.

53. Overmoyer GV, Reiser 2nd RF. Relationships between lower-extremity flexibility, asymmetries, and the Y balance test. *J Strength Cond Res.* 2015;29(5):1240–1247.

54. Smith CA, Chimera NJ, et al. Association of y balance test reach asymmetry and injury in division I athletes. *Med Sci Sports Exerc.* 2015;47(1):136–141.

55. Carcia CR, Martin RL, Houck J, Wukich DK. Achilles pain, stiffness, and muscle power deficits: achilles tendinitis clinical practice guidelines linked to the international classification of functioning, disability, and health from the orthopaedic section of the American physical therapy association. *J Orthop Sports Phys Ther.* 2010;40(9):A1.

56. Lunsford BR, Perry J. The standing heel-rise test for ankle plantar flexion: criterion for normal. *Phys Ther.* 1995;75:694–698.

57. Silbernagel KG, Gustavsson A, Thomee R, Karlsson J. Evaluation of lower leg function in patients with Achilles tendinopathy. *Knee Surg Sports Traumatol Arthrosc.* 2006;14:1207–1217.

58. Ross MD, Fontenot EG. Test-retest reliability of the standing heel-rise test. *J Sport Rehabil.* 2000;9:117–123.

59. Arcuri JF, Borghi-Silva A, et al. Validity and reliability of the 6-minute step test in healthy individuals: a cross-sectional study. *Clin J Sport Med.* 2016;26(1):69–75.

60. Rabin A, Portnoy S, et al. The association of ankle dorsiflexion range of motion with hip and knee kinematics during the lateral step-down test. *J Orthop Sports Phys Ther.* 2016;46(11): 1002–1009.

61. Rabin A, Portnoy S, et al. The Association between visual assessment of quality of movement and three-dimensional analysis of pelvis, hip, and knee kinematics during a lateral step down test. *J Strength Cond Res.* 2016;30(11):3204–3211.

62. Booher LD, Hench KM, Worrell TW, et al. Reliability of three single leg hop tests. *J Sports Rehab.* 1993;2:165–170.

63. Ross MD, Langford B, et al. Test-retest reliability of 4 single-leg horizontal hop tests. *J Strength Cond Res.* 2002;16(4): 617–622.

64. Cliborne AV, Wainner RS, et al. Clinical hip tests and a functional squat test in patients with knee osteoarthritis: reliability, prevalence of positive test findings, and short-term response to hip mobilization. *J Orthop Sports Phys Ther.* 2004;34(11):676–685.

65. Myer GD, Schmitt LC, Brent JL, et al. Utilization of modified NFL combine testing to identify functional deficits in athletes following ACL reconstruction. *J Orthop Sports Phys Ther.* 2011;41(6):377–387.

66. Roos PE, Button K, et al. Altered biomechanical strategies and medio-lateral control of the knee represent incomplete recovery of individuals with injury during single leg hop. *J Biomech.* 2014;47(3):675–680.

67. Bley AS, Correa JC, et al. Propulsion phase of the single leg triple hop test in women with patellofemoral pain syndrome: a biomechanical study. *PLoS One.* 2014;9(5):e97606.

68. Ditroilo M, Forte R, et al. Intra- and inter-session reliability of vertical jump performance in healthy middle-aged and older men and women. *J Sports Sci.* 2011;29(15):1675–1682.

69. Adamo DE, Talley SA, et al. Age and task differences in functional fitness in older women: comparisons with senior fitness test normative and criterion-referenced data. *J Aging Phys Act.* 2015;23(1):47–54.

70. Teyhen DS, Shaffer SW, et al. The Functional Movement Screen: a reliability study. *J Orthop Sports Phys Ther.* 2012;42(6): 530–540.

71. Perry FT, Koehle MS. Normative data for the functional movement screen in middle-aged adults. *J Strength Cond Res.* 2013;27(2):458–462.
72. Rehabmeasures.org http://www.rehabmeasures.org. Accessed April 24, 2017
73. American Physical Therapy Association. PTNow online resource for tests and measures. http://www.ptnow.org/tests-measures.

BIBLIOGRAPHY

Angst F, Aeschlimann A, et al. Smallest detectable and minimal clinically important differences of rehabilitation intervention with their implications for required sample sizes using WOMAC and SF-36 quality of life measurement instruments in patients with osteoarthritis of the lower extremities. *Arthritis Rheum.* 2001;45(4):384–391.

Bohannon R, ELeary K. Standing balance and function over the course of acute rehabilitation. *Arch Phys Med Rehab.* 1995;76:994–996.

Cavanaugh JT, Williams HA. Microfracture procedures of the knee. In: Cioppa-Mosca J, Cahill J, Young Tucker C, eds. *Handbook of Postsurgical Rehabilitation Guidelines for the Orthopaedic Clinician.* St Louis, MO: Mosby Elsevier; 2008:297–302.

Chatman AB, Hyams SP, et al. The patient-specific functional scale: measurement properties in patients with knee dysfunction. *Phys Ther.* 1997;77:820–829.

Cibulka M, White D, Woehrle J, et al. Hip pain and mobility deficits: hip osteoarthritis: clinical practice guidelines linked to the international classification of functioning, disability, and health from the orthopaedic section of the APTA. *J Orthop Sports Phys Ther.* 2009;39(4):790–797.

Clark NC. Functional performance testing following knee ligament injury. *Phys Ther Sport.* 2001;(2):101.

Cleland JA, Whitman JM, et al. Psychometric properties of selected tests in patients with lumbar spinal stenosis. *Spine J.* 2012;12:921–931.

Gill SD, de Morton NA, et al. An investigation of the validity of six measures of physical function in people awaiting joint replacement surgery of the hip or knee. *Clinical Rehabil.* 2012;26:945–951.

Haber M, Golan E, Azoulay L, Kahn S, Shrier I. Reliability of a device measuring triceps surae muscle fatigability. *Br J Sports Med.* 2004;38:163–167.

Hall MP, et al. Neuromuscular evaluation with single-leg squat test at 6 months after anterior cruciate ligament reconstruction. *Orthop J Sports Med.* 2015;3(3).

Hamilton RT, Shultz SJ, Schmitz RJ, Perrin DH. Triple-hop distance as a valid predictor of lower limb strength and power. *Athletic Training.* 2008;43(2):144–151.

Hammer A, Nilsagard Y, et al. Evaluation of therapeutic riding (Sweden)/hippotherapy (United States). A single-subject experimental design study replicated in eleven patients with multiple sclerosis. *Physiother Theory Pract.* 2005;21:51–77.

Harrison E, Duenkel N, Dunlop R, Russell G. Evaluation of single-leg standing following anterior cruciate ligament surgery and rehabilitation. *Phys Ther.* 1994;74(3):245–252.

Hefford C, Abbott JH, et al. The patient-specific functional scale: validity, reliability, and responsiveness in patients with upper extremity musculoskeletal problems. *J Orthop Sports Phys Ther.* 2012;42:56–65.

Impellizzeri FM, et al. A vertical jump force test for assessing bilateral strength asymmetry in athletes. *Med Sci Sports Exerc.* 2007;39(11):2044–2050.

Kennedy DM, Stratford PW, Robarts S, Gollish JD. Using outcome measure results to facilitate clinical decisions the first year after total hip arthroplasty. *J Orthop Sports Phys Ther.* 2011;41(4):232–241.

Krause DA, et al. Reliability and accuracy of a goniometer mobile device application for video measurement of the functional movement screen deep squat test. *Int J Sports Phys Ther.* 2015;10(1):37–44.

Lim LI, Van Wegen EE, et al. Measuring gait and gait-related activities in Parkinson's patients own home environment: a reliability, responsiveness and feasibility study. *Parkinsonism Relat Disord.* 2005;11(1):19–24.

Loudon J, Weisner D, Goist-foley H, Asjest C, Loudon K. Intrarater reliability of functional performance test for subjects with patellofemoral pain syndrome. *Sports Rehabil Phys Ther.* 2002;37(3):256–261.

MacDermid JC, Walton DM, Avery S, et al. *J Orthop Sports Phys Ther.* 2009;39(5):400–417.

Marchetti GF, Lin CC, et al. Responsiveness and minimal detectable change of the dynamic gait index and functional gait index in persons with balance and vestibular disorders. *J Neurol Phys Ther.* 2014;38(2):119–124.

Maschi RA, Fives G. Rotator cuff repair: arthroscopic and open. In: Cioppa-Mosca J, Cahill J, Young Tucker C, eds. *Handbook of Postsurgical Rehabilitation Guidelines for the Orthopaedic Clinician.* 2008:383–392.

Maughan EF, Lewis JS. Outcome measures in chronic low back pain. *Eur Spine J.* 2010;9:1484–1494.

Outermans JC, Van Peppen RP, et al. Effects of a high-intensity task-oriented training on gait performance early after stroke: a pilot study. *Clin Rehabil.* 2010;24(11):979–987.

Peer MA, Lane J. The Knee Injury and Osteoarthritis Outcome Score (KOOS): a review of its psychometric properties in people undergoing total knee arthroplasty. *J Orthop Sports Phys Ther.* 2013;43(1):20–28.

Reid A, Birmingham TB, Stratford PW, Alcock GK, Giffin JR. Hop testing provides a reliable and valid outcome measure during rehabilitation after anterior cruciate ligament reconstruction. *Phys Ther.* 2007;87(3):337–349.

Resnik L, Borgia M. Reliability of outcome measures for people with lower-limb amputations: distinguishing true change from statistical error. *Phys Ther.* 2011;91:555–565.

Romero S, Bishop MD, et al. Minimum detectable change of the Berg Balance Scale and Dynamic Gait Index in older persons at risk for falling. *J Geriatr Phys Ther.* 2011;34(3):131–137.

Roos EM, Toksvig-Larsen S. Knee injury and osteoarthritis outcome score (KOOS): validation and comparison to the WOMAC in total knee replacement. *Health Qual Life Outcomes.* 2003;1:17.

Sassi RH, et al. Relative and absolute reliability of a modified agility T-test and its relationship with vertical jump and straight sprint. *J Strength Cond Res.* 2009;23(6):1644–1651.

Schenkman M, Cutson TM, et al. Reliability of impairment and physical performance measures for persons with Parkinson's disease. *Phys Ther.* 1997;77(1):19–27.

Silbernagel KG, Thomee R, Eriksson BI, Karlsson J. Full symptomatic recovery does not ensure full recovery of muscle-tendon function in patients with Achilles tendinopathy. *Br J Sports Med.* 2007;41:276–280.

Silbernagel KG, Thomee R, Thomee P, Karlsson J. Eccentric overload training for patients with chronic Achilles tendon pain–a randomized controlled study with reliability testing of the evaluation methods. *Scand J Med Sci Sports.* 2001;11:197–206.

Smithson F, Morris ME, et al. Performance on clinical tests of balance in Parkinson's disease. *Phys Ther*. 1998;78(6):577–592.

Steffen T, Hacker T, Mollinger L. Age and gender related test performance in community-dwelling elderly people: six-minute walk test, berg balance scale, timed up and go test and gait speeds. *Phys Ther*. 2002;(82):128–137.

Stratford P. Assessing disability and change on individual patients: a report of a patient specific measure. *Physiother Can*. 1995;47:258–263.

Suni J, Pekka O, Laukkanen R, Miilunpalo S, Pasanen M, Vuori I. Health-related fitness test battery for adults: aspects of reliability. *Arch Phys Med Rehab*. 1996;77:399–405.

Vellas B, Wayne S, Baumgartner R, Rubenstein L, Garry P. One-Leg Balance is an important predictor of injurious falls in older persons. *J Amer Ger Soc*. 1997;45(6):735–738.

PART II

Therapeutic Exercise Prescription Workbook

The workbook chapters are organized by regions—the lower extremity, the upper extremity, and the spine—and are divided into four of the categories introduced in Chapter 6: hypomobility, hypermobility, repetitive strain injuries, and postsurgical conditions. The workbook chapters begin with general biomechanical concepts and functional requirements applicable for the given region of the body. Exercises used frequently for rehabilitation purposes are organized by mobility and trauma categories and overall goals. There are countless exercise options. The options, alternatives, and modifications in these chapters are not meant to be all inclusive but rather to provide ideas and examples so the reader can build a repertoire and framework to work with and expand on. Each section includes the general exercise approaches for the category, precautions and contraindications, general parameters, tests and measures, and compensations. The purpose, position, exercise description and actions, teaching tips, advantages, alternatives, and progressions are listed for each exercise. Some exercises are also suitable for other categories or other regions; in such cases, references to progressions or alternatives are provided. Figures and selected videos illustrate the exercise, alternatives, progressions, compensations, or modifications.

Expanded case studies are presented at the end of each section, with explanations of exercise choices and application of the concepts and principles. Along with illustrating choices for the category, the cases have been designed to apply concepts presented in the foundational chapters, presenting different elements such as progression, choices appropriate for phase of healing, and concepts for the final category (chronic pain behaviors and psychological elements).

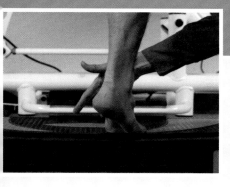

9

Lower Extremity Workbook

Jason Roberts, Kim Dunleavy, and Amy Kubo Slowik

STRUCTURAL AND BIOMECHANICAL

BACKGROUND TO BE CONSIDERED FOR LOWER EXTREMITY EXERCISE

The lower extremity functional requirements to support the body in upright positions and to transport the body for gait and other functional activities require a great deal of muscular strength and power. The linkage of the lower extremity to the trunk consists of muscle attachments from the lumbar spine and pelvis to the femur and the hip joint. Alignment of the lower extremity is influenced by the angles of the femur and tibia, as well as by the rearfoot and forefoot relationships. Exercise implications of these factors are outlined in Table 9.1.

TABLE 9.1 Biomechanical Concepts for Lower Extremity Exercises

Biomechanical Concepts	Exercise Implications
Core Position	
Lumbopelvic position influences the **location of center of gravity** with respect to the lower extremities in standing.	Monitor lumbopelvic orientation as well as position of pelvis relative to the base of support in weight-bearing positions (standing, kneeling, lunging) and dynamic movement.
Lumbopelvic relationship influences **hip muscle alignment** and efficiency.	The lumbopelvic position is maintained by active muscle support and influences the ability of lower extremity muscles originating from the pelvis or lumbar spine to create torque.
Decreased hip mobility or muscle flexibility often results in compensations in the lumbar spine and pelvis position.[1,2]	Decreased hip mobility or muscle flexibility of muscles attaching to the pelvis often results in pelvic tilting (anterior or posterior) and lumbar motion. Observation for compensations and cueing to monitor and correct the position are necessary for most exercises. Restricted hip extension or hip flexor flexibility: Anterior pelvic tilt Restricted hip flexion or hip extensor flexibility: Posterior pelvic tilt The relationship between the pelvis and the femur is maintained by hip muscle activity in weight-bearing positions.
Core muscle activation provides support for the trunk and decreases the amount of vertical load placed on lower extremities in weight-bearing positions or movement (standing, squatting, kneeling).	Early trunk muscle activation (and upper extremity muscle activation if appropriate) can be used to assist with support when vertical loading is problematic.
Lower Extremity Neuromuscular Stabilization	
Pelvic position is reliant on hip abductor and adductor **frontal plane stabilization** for single-leg stance or when transferring weight from one leg to another, with the hip rotators contributing to rotational stability in the transverse plane.[2]	Observe for loss of pelvic position in the frontal and transverse planes in weight-bearing activities. Cueing to maintain alignment as well as specific exercises to promote activation and endurance of the stabilizers are often part of exercise programs to promote biomechanical alignment and force distribution.
Knee hyperextension can be reduced by active control of the posterior muscles around the knee including the hamstrings, the gastrocnemius, and the popliteus (to unlock the joint).	With excessive knee hyperextension, active unlocking of the knee using the hamstrings and popliteus muscles can be used to promote force distribution and vertical alignment in standing.
The intrinsics, peroneals, tibialis posterior and anterior, and toe flexors help support and control the **arches of the foot**, although most of the arch support is provided by the fascia and ligamentous structures.[2]	Excessive or early pronation can indicate inadequate activation or endurance of the stabilizing foot muscles.

Continued

TABLE 9.1 **Biomechanical Concepts for Lower Extremity Exercises—cont'd**

Bony and Dynamic Alignment

Genu valgus is defined as >9–10 cm between the ankles when patellae are facing forward [3] or a lateral angle of <170 degrees between the femur and tibia in the frontal plane[2] (Table Fig. 9.1; see Fig. 2.34A).

Genu varus is defined as >4 cm between the knees when the ankles are together[3] or a lateral angle that is greater than 180 degrees[2] (see Table Fig. 9.1).

Genu recurvatum is defined as greater than 10 degrees of hyperextension (Table Fig. 9.2).[2]

Leg length discrepancies and **scoliosis** impact the alignment of the femoral-pelvic region and the muscle attachments from the lumbar spine and pelvis (Fig. 4.11).

Normal hip anteversion angle is 8–15 degrees[1,2,4] (Table Fig. 9.3–9.5; see Fig. 4.12). The femoral torsion is measured with Craig's test [4] (Table Fig. 9.4). Increased anteversion leads to toeing-in with increased medial rotation and less lateral rotation.

The patella alignment is influenced by the hip and femoral alignment with extremes of anteversion or retroversion impacting muscle position and angulation.

Mid position of the natural bony alignment (evaluated in non–weight-bearing positions) places the muscles in optimum position for force distribution.

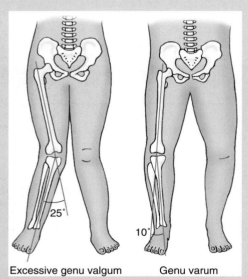

Excessive genu valgum   Genu varum

Table Fig. 9.1 (From Muscolino JE. *Kinesiology.* 2nd ed. St. Louis, MO: Mosby; 2011.)

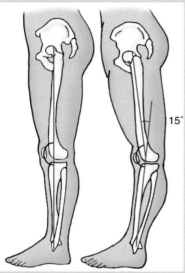

Table Fig. 9.2 (From Muscolino JE. *Kinesiology.* 2nd ed. St. Louis, MO: Mosby; 2011.)

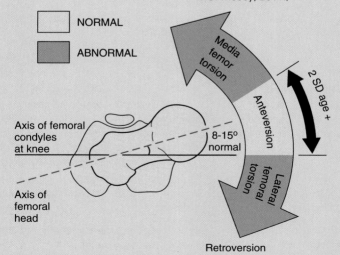

Table Fig. 9.3 Normal and abnormal femoral torsion. (From Magee DJ. *Orthopedic Physical Assessment.* 5th ed. St. Louis, MO: Elsevier Saunders; 2007.)

TABLE 9.1   Biomechanical Concepts for Lower Extremity Exercises—cont'd

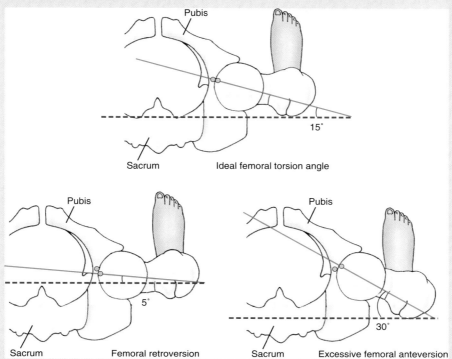

Table Fig. 9.4 (From Muscolino JE. *Kinesiology.* 2nd ed. St. Louis, MO: Mosby; 2011.)

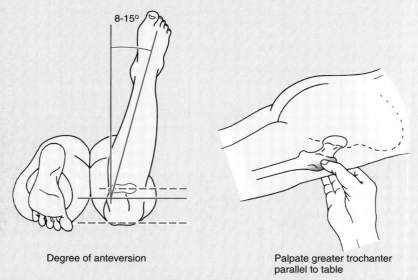

Table Fig. 9.5 Clinical measurement of anteversion using Craig's Test. (From Magee DJ. *Orthopedic Physical Assessment.* 5th ed. St. Louis, MO: Elsevier Saunders; 2007.)

Continued

TABLE 9.1 Biomechanical Concepts for Lower Extremity Exercises—cont'd

Tibial external rotation (torsion)

- The tibia is externally rotated with respect to the femur ranging between 12 and 18 degrees in adults.[4] The angle is usually less acute in children (>5 degrees).[1] In a midline, non–weight-bearing position, less tibial rotation will result in the feet facing toward each other or straight forward. Extreme tibial or femoral rotation (torsion) in either direction contributes to angulation of the patella tendon or patellofemoral complex[1,5,6] (Table Figs. 9.6 and 9.7).
- Weight-bearing alignment will be influenced by multiple factors: femoral and tibial bony alignment, foot position influencing the tibial position, soft tissue flexibility throughout the lower extremity chain, muscle balance/imbalances, and pain or fear avoidance.

Natural tibial external rotation places the foot in a slightly externally rotated position ("toed-out"). The natural bony position should be assessed in non–weight-bearing positions and the position adjusted in standing so that the patella faces forward.

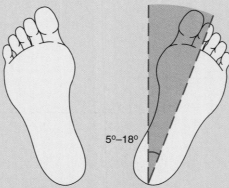

5°–18°

Table Fig. 9.6 (From Magee DJ. *Orthopedic Physical Assessment*. 5th ed. St. Louis, MO: Elsevier Saunders; 2007.)

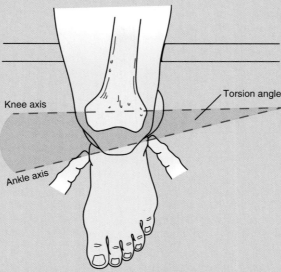

Knee axis

Torsion angle

Ankle axis

Table Fig. 9.7 (From Magee DJ. *Orthopedic Physical Assessment*. 5th ed. St. Louis, MO: Elsevier Saunders; 2007.)

TABLE 9.1   Biomechanical Concepts for Lower Extremity Exercises—cont'd

Rearfoot and forefoot varus and valgus

- The static foot pronation or supination position in standing influences tibial position and overall lower extremity rotation. Early, excessive, or prolonged pronation during gait or running increases lower extremity rotational forces with more force absorbed by soft tissue (see Fig. 4.15A). Excessive supination or lack of pronation through the foot decreases shock absorption with more forces absorbed higher in the lower extremity chain (see Fig. 4.15).
- The longitudinal arch normally drops approximately 7 mm (healthy males) in standing.[7] The connective tissue of the fascia and the midfoot joints support some of the vertical forces and stores energy in a "spring" action, helping with shock absorption and elasticity to adapt the foot to the ground[2] (Table Fig. 9.8).
- The foot posture index, has been recommended as a method to assess foot position in standing.[1,10–12]
- The loads on the foot during weight-bearing positions increase from 1.2 times the body weight in walking to 2 times the body weight in running and 5 times the body weight jumping down from a height of 60 cm.[1]

Orthotics or taping can be used to support excessive static or dynamic pronation or inadequate shock absorption during weight-bearing exercise for short-term pain relief.[8–10]

Normal arch

Dropped arch

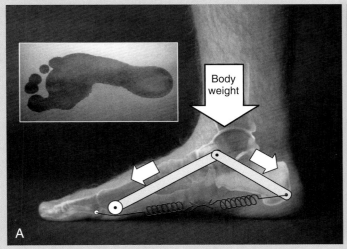
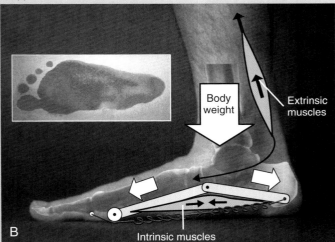

Table Fig. 9.8 Longitudinal foot arch. (From Neumann DA. Kinesiology of the *Musculoskeletal System*. 3rd ed. St. Louis, MO: Elsevier; 2017.)

Closed pack positions[1]

- Hip: Full extension, medial rotation, abduction
- Knee: Full extension, lateral rotation of the tibia
- Ankle: Full dorsiflexion
- Foot: Full supination

Closed pack positions can be used to provide a relatively stable position provided by joint congruency and capsule tension.

Resting position[1]

- Hip: 30 degrees flexion, 30 degrees abduction, slight lateral rotation
- Knee: 25 degrees flexion
- Ankle: 10 degrees plantar flexion, mid eversion and inversion
- Foot: Neutral

If there is intraarticular effusion, the resting position is often assumed as there is less tension on the capsule and ligaments. Early Phase I mobility exercises and isometrics may be started in the resting position with progression of range as the effusion decreases. Joint mobilization for pain relief and oscillations for pain relief can also be started in the resting position.

Continued

TABLE 9.1   Biomechanical Concepts for Lower Extremity Exercises—cont'd

Patellofemoral joint alignment and mechanics

- The patella contacts the femoral condyles at 30 degrees of flexion with progressive articular congruency in the femoral condyles (Table Fig. 9.9A) and with compression forces reaching maximum compressive load between 60 and 90 degrees flexion.[2] Maximum stress (force/area) is greatest in this range but is higher on the lateral aspect of the patella with malalignment or increased lateral forces transmitted through the iliotibial band and lateral retinaculum[2] (Table Fig. 9.9B).
- Patella tendon tension increases with greater degrees of flexion and maximal tension in full flexion (Table Fig. 9.9C).
- If the inferior pole of the patella compresses the infrapatellar fat pad, the fat pad may become enlarged, irritated, and painful with symptoms reproduced in terminal extension.

Patients with patellofemoral complex syndromes may need to avoid full flexion in loaded or weight-bearing positions initially.[13]

Pain with terminal extension related to enlarged fat pads; avoid terminal extension initially.[13]

Minimizing angulation and rotation of the patellofemoral complex may require adjustment of the pelvis, femoral rotation, or foot position.[1,2]

Active force closure is required to maintain and control the lower extremity rotation and angulation, with the hip and foot positions playing a vital role for rotation and frontal plane stability.[2]

Forces related to the range of motion of the patellofemoral complex will need to be considered when selecting exercises, particularly with single-leg weight-bearing exercises such as squats, lunges and step-ups/step-downs.[13,15]

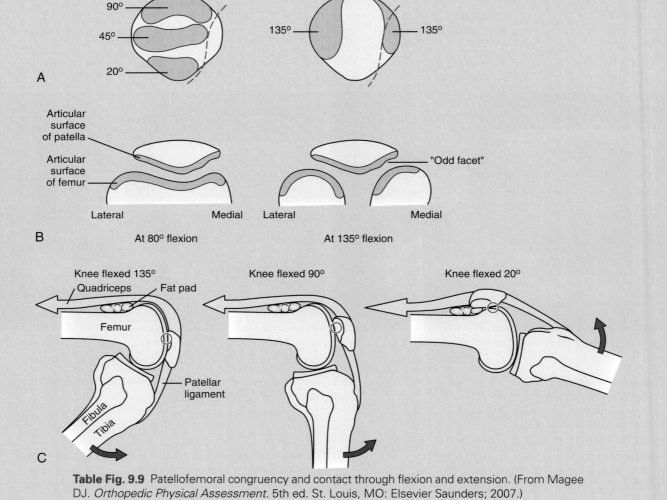

Table Fig. 9.9 Patellofemoral congruency and contact through flexion and extension. (From Magee DJ. *Orthopedic Physical Assessment.* 5th ed. St. Louis, MO: Elsevier Saunders; 2007.)

TABLE 9.1   Biomechanical Concepts for Lower Extremity Exercises—cont'd

- Alignment of the patellofemoral complex depends on the femoral-tibial angle with increased angulation with genu valgus. Femoral anteversion/retroversion, tibial and femoral torsion, and foot position also impact the angulation and rotation from the proximal or distal relationship. Both the patella tendon angulation and patellofemoral compressive force change with progressive knee flexion and with generalized lower extremity rotation[2,14] (Table Fig. 9.9C and D).
- Q angle: The line between the ASIS to midpoint of the patella and tibial tuberosity to midpoint of the patella is a reflection of the overall quadriceps alignment and influenced by proximal and distal static bony alignment. Average Q angle is 13–18 degrees (SD 4.5 degrees) and is larger in females due to the wider pelvis than males.[1,2,15]
- Compressive forces on the patellofemoral joint increase 2.5–3.5× body weight with stair climbing and up to 7× body weight with deep squats.[1,2,6]

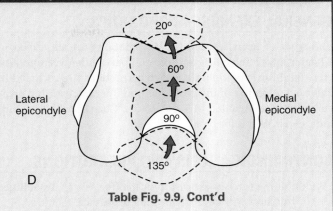

D

Table Fig. 9.9, Cont'd

Functional Requirements of the Lower Extremity

Most functional requirements for lower extremity motion involve closed chain strength, power, and balance.

Functional strength and mobility at extreme ranges are required for some sports/hobbies (gymnastics, dance).

Range of motion or strength goals to achieve functional range appropriate for age, occupation, hobbies. As range of motion increases, exercises will need to be adjusted to maintain range and develop strength in the new ranges.

Lower extremity closed-chain function is more important in upright positions required for functional movement.

If endurance is required at higher ranges or for specific movements, exercises should integrate these positions.

SECTION 9.1: HYPOMOBILITY

GENERAL EXERCISE APPROACHES

The types of exercise used for hypomobility are described in Chapter 6 (see Table 6.3) and the comparison between parameters used for hypomobility and hypermobility are included in Table 6.4. A review of the goals, methods, parameters, and measurements are included in Table 9.2 See Chapter 6, Table 6.2 for indications for specific type of exercises.

CONTRAINDICATIONS AND PRECAUTIONS

1. Mobility exercises are not indicated for severe instabilities or fractures without early healing or surgical fixation.
2. Determine if adequate healing is present after trauma (fractures, meniscus, labrum, tendon, or ligament tears).
3. Acute inflammation requires caution (e.g., with acute inflammation and osteoarthritis of the knee).
4. Address swelling and edema first.
5. Use care with amount of force and load in the presence of muscle spasm and guarding.
6. Avoid excessive strain with inflammatory conditions (e.g., rheumatoid arthritis).
7. Limit weight-bearing forces if there is evidence of effusion or history or suspected arthritis
8. Use care with extreme range of motion with suspected labral or meniscus tears.
9. See Section 9.4 for postsurgical precautions.
10. Monitor responses to extreme range or load and adjust if pain or spasm increases during treatment.
11. Decrease extent of load and strain on the following visit if soreness increases within 8 hours after mobility exercise.

GENERAL PARAMETERS

Reach end range with:
- Oscillations *OR*
- Low load, high repetitions *OR*
- Prolonged hold

TESTS AND MEASURES

See Magee,[1] Magee and Sueki,[4] and Cleland[16] for more detailed description of available tests and measures, interpretation, and psychometric properties; see Reese and Bandy[17] for range of motion testing and values.

1. Goniometric range of motion (active or passive)
2. Pain reports at end range of motion
3. End feel with passive movement relative to amount of range of motion
4. Muscle flexibility special tests
5. Functional movement outcome measures for functional mobility (e.g., standing lunge, dynamic squat)
6. Ability to perform activities without compensations or to perform home programs independently
7. Functional mobility measures (hand behind back or hand behind head compared to opposite side, ability to dress, or reach)
8. Lower extremity functional scale (LEFS)
9. Region-specific (e.g., Knee Outcome Scale), general health (e.g., SF36), or diagnosis-specific outcome measures (WOMAC). See Chapter 8 for selected outcome measures and Magee Orthopedic Assessment.[1]

OBSERVATION FOR COMPENSATIONS AND RESPONSES

- Observe for and adjust to limit compensations in areas of relative mobility in surrounding regions.
- Stabilize proximal and distal segments.
- Use supported positions if there is any chance of loss of balance or excessive compensations.
- Ask patients to report any discomfort.
- Monitor for delayed-onset muscle soreness, increased effusion, or edema after treatment

TABLE 9.2 Goals, Methods, Parameters, and Measurement when Hypomobility Is the Primary Impairment			
Goals	**Methods**	**Parameters**	**Measurement**
Decrease swelling (edema or effusion), muscle spasm, and related pain symptoms	Circulatory "pumping" exercises (open chain) Moving joint actively in mid to end range (does not have to reach end range) without compensation and excessive pain Isometric contractions with adequate relaxation to create "pumping" effect	Multiple repetitions (>30) Low loads Supported positions Adequate rest periods between sets Repeat frequently throughout the day Pain should decrease with continued repetitions	Circumferential measurements in areas Goniometric measurement of range of motion Pain reports (at rest, with activity, and related to movement toward end range) Functional range of motion measurement (video or functional tests)
Increase body temperature before mobility exercise to maximize improvements	General aerobic exercise	Equipment set to allow repeated motion within available range Low to moderate resistance Intensity set to achieve perceived exertion of 11–13 but no increase in pain during exercise Initially time set for warm-up rather than aerobic endurance, progress to aerobic endurance	Perceived exertion Pain intensity during and after exercise

TABLE 9.2 Goals, Methods, Parameters, and Measurement when Hypomobility Is the Primary Impairment—cont'd

Goals	Methods	Parameters	Measurement
Increase capsule and/or connective tissue mobility	Non–weight-bearing, open chain exercise to end range (therapist-assisted, self-assisted, equipment-assisted) using: Oscillatory motion reaching end range Active, active-assisted motion, or resisted movement through range to limits without compensation Passive positioning Prolonged stretch (to address connective tissue and muscle length)	High repetitions (>25) Low load Controlled speed Reach end range	Goniometric measurement of range of motion Functional range of motion measurement (video or functional tests) End feel and relative amount of motion before end feel (passive motion, joint play) Selective tissue tension evaluation; relationship between amount of active and passive range of motion
Improve muscle flexibility (including two-joint muscles)	Passive positioning Prolonged stretching (performed by therapist or self-stretch by patient) at end range of joint motion reaching full length of muscle–tendon complex at one or both ends in direction of fibers Contract-relax Hold-relax	Sustained hold (15–30 seconds) OR multiple repetitions to end range Low loads Contract-relax or hold-relax uses maximal resistance for target muscle groups followed by immediate relaxation and motion into the maximal length of target muscle Range should increase with time held or repetitions	Goniometric measurement of range of motion Functional range of motion measurement (video or functional tests) End feel with passive movement relative to amount of range of motion Muscle flexibility special tests
Increase neural mobility with specific neural stretching techniques	Neural gliding and/or stretching techniques	Motion targeted to increase mobility of specific neural tissue with range and hold dependent on severity and irritability Multiple repetitions with motion to end range or within range short of symptom reproduction OR starting to reproduces symptoms Prolonged hold if low severity and irritability	Goniometric measurement of range of motion Neural tension tests Functional range of motion measurement (video or functional tests) Symptom reproduction with combined functional positions
Improve lower quarter mobility	Generalized or specific joint mobility	Capsule or connective tissue (see connective tissue section above) Muscle flexibility (see muscle flexibility section)	Functional range of motion measurement (video or functional tests) Range of motion (inclinometer or goniometer) End feel with passive movement relative to amount of range of motion Muscle flexibility special tests
Improve lower quarter proximal support, postural awareness, and endurance	Generalized lower quarter and spinal postural positioning and endurance during all exercises	High repetitions (>15 repetitions) OR Prolonged hold in position (timed) before loss of position, fatigue, or compensation in order to provide optimal alignment	Ability to maintain optimal alignment during exercise or function Time able to maintain optimal alignment before fatigue or compensations Perceived exertion/degree of specific fatigue during prolonged position or exercise
Increase muscle activation and endurance in newly available range gained from other techniques joint mobilization, joint mobility exercise, or muscle flexibility	Muscle activation in new ranges; may be gravity-assisted, -eliminated, or -resisted positions Progressive resistive exercise for endurance and tissue stimulus in new range	High repetitions (>30) Low load Newly obtained range End range if possible Facilitate muscle activation in specific range after mobility exercises	Movement observation Ability to activate through available passive range Number of repetitions reaching end of possible range
Improve and maintain dynamic mobility and extensibility of tissue Teach active methods to maintain and improve functional mobility	Functional training Self-stretching or mobility exercise	Motor control concepts; practice with specificity to use available range, training concepts for practice with precision and monitoring	Ability to perform functional movement through range without compensations or feedback Functional mobility measures Functional movement self-reports (e.g., Lower Extremity Functional Scale)

EXERCISES

PASSIVE, ACTIVE-ASSISTED, OR ACTIVE MOBILITY

GENERALIZED AEROBIC MOBILITY

SELF-STRETCHING FLEXIBILITY

PROGRESSIVE RESISTIVE EXERCISE IN NEW RANGE

EXERCISE DESCRIPTIONS

PASSIVE, ACTIVE-ASSISTED, OR ACTIVE MOBILITY

9.1 Passive and active low-load knee extension

9.1A Passive stretch in supine with ankle weight above the knee

See Fig. 9.1A.

Purpose
* To restore passive knee extension, with low loads, in a fully supported position

Position
* Long-sitting or supine, with towel roll or a half foam roll under the Achilles tendon
* Cuff weight (weight to tolerance) placed on the distal thigh, superior to patella

Action
* Passive knee extension with prolonged hold

Advantages
* Allows prolonged stretching under a low-load, to increase ROM
* Can be used as part of a home exercise program using weight bags or cuff weights

Teaching tips
* A hot pack can be added to assist with pain relief and muscle relaxation while stretching.

* Monitor and test to determine a load (weight) that can be tolerated for 30 seconds without increasing muscle spasm.

Specific parameters
* Prolonged hold can be started at 30 seconds and build up to 3 minutes if tolerated.
* Short holds followed by releasing the position should be repeated to reach a total of 3–5 minutes.

Alternatives
* Supine active knee extension (Exercise 9.1B)
* Prone passive knee extension off the table with the weight below the knee (Exercise 9.1C: Prone knee hangs)
* The patient can provide a self-stretch using manual pressure on the anterior thigh.

Progression
* Increase duration of stretch and decrease number of repetitions to prolong effect of stretch.
* If the patient is only able to tolerate short holds, increase the number of sets.
* Increase load above knee without increasing pain or inducing guarding of hamstrings to prevent knee extension.
* Increase height of support under ankle.
* Progress to active terminal knee extension (or supplement with active extension) without substitution of psoas and/or gluteus maximus.

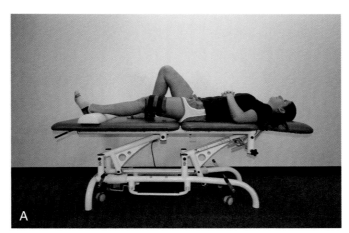

Fig. 9.1A

9.1B Active isometric terminal knee extension

Purpose
- Increase extension range of motion

Position
- Supine or long sitting, leg extended in front of the patient
- Place a small towel roll or soft support under the back of the knee to provide support in the available extension range and prevent knee hyperextension.

Action
1. Engage the quadriceps, cueing the patient to press the back of the knee down into the towel and lift the heel, without lifting the thigh off the table.
2. Adding ankle dorsiflexion increases the stretch for the gastrocnemius, providing additional stretch for the knee capsule.

Advantages
- This exercise can be done combined with manual mobilization (mobilization with movement).
- The last few degrees of extension are vital for normal stance and gait patterns. This exercise provides isometric challenge in this specific terminal range.
- The action promotes elongation and stretching of the posterior knee structures.
- Promotes muscle activation in a position where active control can be difficult due to the length–tension relationship.

Teaching tips
- Instruction example:
  - "Tighten up your quadriceps by pulling your knee cap toward your hip and press the back of your knee down into the towel."

- The therapist can provide additional proprioceptive input by looping an elastic resistance band under the knee, placing his or her hand under the knee, or tapping on the quadriceps. Ask the patient to press into the elastic band or hand or to focus on using the quadriceps while tapping the muscle.

Specific parameters
- Time is established based on the amount of time the contraction can be held and increased progressively.
- Short holds followed by releasing the position are repeated to reach a total of 3–5 minutes.

Alternatives
- The therapist can passively stretch the knee into extension followed by active terminal extension.
- The towel can be placed under the ankle to assist with regaining hyperextension (Fig. 9.1B).
- Prone hang or passive extension (Exercise 9.1C) with a weight followed by isometric terminal knee extension
- Standing with elastic resistance band looped above the knee joint and anchored in front at knee height. The patient actively extends the knee against the resistance of the band (Exercise 9.16).

Progression
- Increase range
- Increase duration
- Hold/relax prone for knee extension
- Short arc quadriceps activation and endurance through new range
- Eccentric control for terminal extension

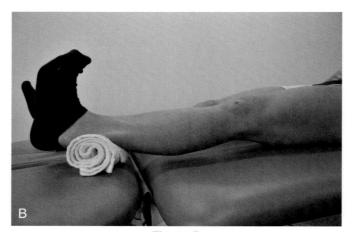

Fig. 9.1B

9.1C Passive knee extension in prone (prone knee hang)

See Fig. 9.1C

Purpose
- Increase knee extension range of motion

Position
- Prone, thigh relaxed on table
- Lower leg suspended off edge of table
- Ensure that the patella is off the edge of the table or place a folded towel under distal thigh to avoid compressing the patella.
- Placing a pillow under the abdomen while a patient is in a prone position will help the patient maintain lumbar spine in a neutral position.

Action
- Passive knee extension using the weight of leg and gravity to provide the stretch

Advantages
- Allows low-load, long-duration stretch to improve mobility

Teaching tips
- Instruct the patient to crawl forward onto the table rather than bending the knee when finishing the stretch. Immediately reversing the stretch does not allow the tissues to accommodate and will be very uncomfortable.
- The patient can place weighted objects in a purse or tote bag and hang it on his or her ankle over the edge of the bed to replicate the exercise at home. Bags of dried goods such as rice or beans are packaged by weight, often in 1-pound increments and can be added to the bag for increased challenge.

Specific parameters
- Prolonged hold can be started at 30 seconds and built up to 3 minutes, as tolerated.
- Short holds followed by releasing the position should be repeated to reach a total of 3–5 minutes.

Alternatives
- Supine passive extension stretch (Exercise 9.1A)
- Hold/relax in prone (Exercise 9.2)

Progression
- Add cuff weight to ankle to increase stretch.
- Increase duration.
- Progress to active extension exercises.

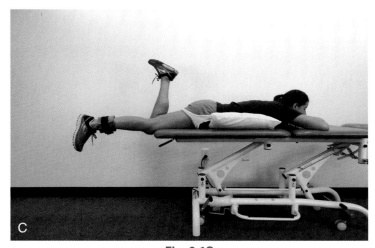

Fig. 9.1C

9.2   Hold/relax prone for knee extension

See Fig. 9.2.

Purpose

- Increase knee extension ROM

Position

- Prone, pillow under abdomen
- Thigh relaxed on table
- Towel roll under the distal quadriceps above the patella

Action

1. The therapist stabilizes the patient's thigh above the knee with one hand (Fig. 9.2A).
2. The patient is instructed to engage his or her hamstrings to flex the knee against submaximal resistance provided by the therapist on the distal tibia and hold for 8–10 seconds.
3. The patient relaxes while the therapist presses the knee into maximal extension and then holds the stretch for 20–30 seconds (Fig. 9.2B).

Teaching tip

- Instruction example:
  - "Try to bend your knee against my resistance and hold it. Completely relax, then let me try to straighten your knee again."

Advantages

- Manual contact allows the therapist to detect muscle guarding and to modify the amount of force delivered for resisting the hamstrings or providing the stretch.

Specific parameters

- The emphasis is reaching the available range and increasing the stretch toward the maximum elastic end feel.
- As the range increases, and if no swelling is present, the amount of time held at full extension is slowly increased.
- Resistance can be adjusted to allow knee flexion (contract/relax) if the full extension range is painful.

Alternatives

- Active isometric knee extension in sitting (Exercise 9.1B)
- Prone knee hangs (Exercise 9.1C)
- Hamstring stretching (Exercise 9.9)

Progression

- Increase duration of stretch.
- Increase range.
- Increase amount of resistance or length of time of contraction.
- Active or active assistive knee extension in supine or sitting to access the newly available range and train neuromuscular activation patterns.

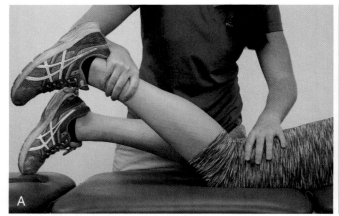 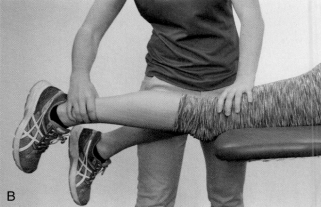

Fig. 9.2

9.3   Active supine heel slides with slider (extension and flexion mobility)

See Fig. 9.3.

Purpose

- Increase or maintain hip or knee range of motion with minimal stress on knee joint
- Decrease knee joint effusion by low-load repetitive range of motion creating a muscle pumping action
- Decrease pain
- Initiate proprioceptive input and stability/control of knee and hip. Isolation of the movement to sagittal plane will help the patient maintain proper lower extremity alignment during functional exercises.

Position

- Supine with head supported or long sitting, depending on patient comfort
- Hip and knee flexed (on both sides if possible)
- Pelvis level and neutral spine
- Ankle and foot are placed on a surface with limited friction (such as tile or hardwood floor) using a sock or material to assist sliding (Fig. 9.3A). A furniture slider (Fig. 9.3B) or a roller board (Fig. 9.3C) will decrease friction between the foot and supporting surface, or the exercise can be performed on a sliding board.

Action

1. Slide the heel toward the body to flex the hip and knee, keeping the heel in contact with the supporting surface.
2. After reaching end range of knee flexion, reverse the motion by sliding the heel away until the hip and knee are fully extended.

Teaching tips

- Common errors to correct:
  - Allowing the leg to move in and out of the sagittal plane (no abduction/adduction)
- Methods to address or prevent compensations:
  - Teach the patient to maintain the plane of movement in the sagittal plane using the hip internal and external rotators to prevent the knee drifting inward or outward. If the patient is having difficulty, using a strap or band is useful in the early stages of rehabilitation (Exercise 9.4A).

Advantages

- Low load and stress on joints and tissues
- Requires minimal muscle activation
- Decreasing friction reduces the amount of muscle activation needed while allowing the primary goal of mobility to be addressed.

Alternatives

- Use a strap around the ball of the foot to assist knee flexion or under the distal thigh to assist with hip flexion.
- Sit with the foot on the floor (tile or wooden floor) using a sock or sheet to assist the motion.

Progression

- Increase the range of motion as swelling and pain decrease.
- Hold the end range 8–10 seconds for increased stretch.
- Perform motion with heels on an exercise ball, which increases feedback to stabilize the leg in the sagittal plane and is more challenging to control (Exercise 9.4.B).
- Progress from an exercise ball to a smaller ball (e.g., basketball or inflatable ball), which offers less support.
- Perform active knee flexion in standing or prone.

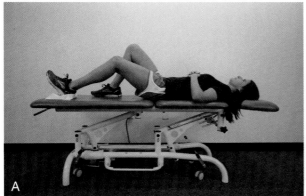
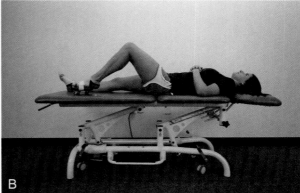
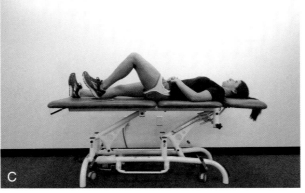

Fig. 9.3

9.4 Active-assisted knee extension or hip and knee flexion

9.4A Active-assisted knee extension using a strap

See Fig. 9.4.

Purpose
- Increase or maintain knee extension, knee flexion, or hip flexion range of motion
- Increase quadriceps activation through terminal extension
- Pumping action to assist with edema resolution

Position
- Supine or long-sitting on a treatment plinth, with towel roll, pillow, or bolster under knee (Fig. 9.4A)
- The patient's foot is placed in the strap while holding on to the other end (Fig. 9.4A).
- A dog leash, belt, sheet, or towel can be used as a substitute for a strap to continue this exercise at home.

Action
1. The patient activates the quadriceps to straighten the knee and lift the heel off table.
2. The patient uses the strap to assist lifting the foot until the knee is fully extended.
3. Slowly lower the foot while controlling the movement with an eccentric contraction of the quadriceps.

Advantages
- Assistance for knee extension prevents compensation of psoas major, iliacus, or gluteus maximus

Teaching tips
- Instruction example:
  - "Concentrate on the muscle contraction and watch as your quadriceps extend your knee." (Seeing the muscle contract provides instant feedback and increases the visual input to strengthen the neuromuscular connection.)

Alternatives
- The therapist can assist the movement until the patient understands the purpose of the exercise.
- Electrical stimulation or biofeedback can be used at the same time to facilitate activation (see Exercise 9.39).
- Pulley-assisted knee extension in sitting: A strap is attached behind the patient's lower leg with the pulley assisting the extension movement. The patient first initiates flexion, then relaxes into extension (contract-relax) (Fig. 9.4B).

Progression
- Decrease rest periods between contractions.
- Increase repetitions.
- Reduce assistance.
- Increase the range by positioning the knee over a bolster, foam roller, or foam cushion.
- Progress to active small-range extension assisted through the movement and then slowly lower the leg, reducing the amount of support.
- Increase range of extension against gravity by having patient sit on edge of table or in a standard chair with the leg starting from the ground.

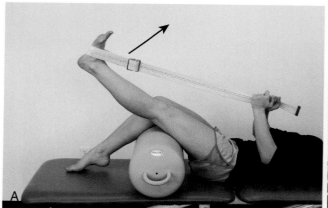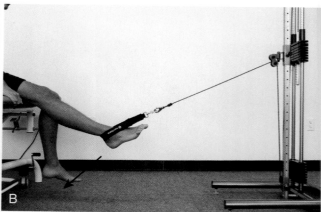

Fig. 9.4

9.4B Active hip and knee flexion on an exercise ball or knee flexion using a strap

See Fig. 9.4C–E.

Purpose
- Increase knee and hip flexion
- Challenge proprioceptive ability while performing sagittal plane motion

Position
A. Active hip and knee flexion with the leg supported on an exercise ball
   - Supine, with lower half of lower leg resting on an exercise ball (55 or 65 cm depending on the patient's leg length) (Fig. 9.4C, D)
   - Neutral spine, level pelvis
   - Ankle in neutral position
B. Using a strap for self-assisted hip flexion or knee flexion
   - Strap placed behind the back of the thigh to increase hip flexion (supine; Fig. 9.4E)
   - Strap placed around the ankle to increase knee flexion (in prone or standing) (Fig. 9.4F and G)

Action
A. Active hip and knee flexion with the leg supported on an exercise ball
   1. Activate the hamstrings to roll the ball toward the hips (Fig. 9.4D; Video 1.8).
   2. Maintain a neutral position of ankle by co-contracting the ankle dorsiflexors and plantarflexors (isometric contraction).
   3. Control the position of the ball (in the sagittal plane) throughout the movement.
   4. Reverse the movement to extend the hip and the knee.
B. Using a strap for self-assisted hip flexion or knee flexion
   1. Use upper extremities to pull the leg toward the body using the strap to assist with motion as needed (Fig. 9.4E–G).

Advantages
- Low load/stress on the knee and hip
- Visual and tactile input for flexion range
- The exercise ball decreases friction and supports the weight of the leg.
- The strap can be used to assist mobility for a full passive stretch.

Teaching tips
- Instruction example:
   - "Keep the ball moving in a straight line without crossing an imaginary line between your legs."
- Common errors to correct:
   - Losing the sagittal alignment or creating excess rotation or valgus stress once the end range is reached
- Methods to address or prevent compensations:
   - Ask the patient to maintain the ball moving in line with the hip (sagittal plane) to challenge proprioception and maintain lower extremity alignment.
   - Placing the heel on the ball and pushing down gently encourages active knee flexion using the hamstrings and the gastrocnemius.

Alternatives
- Heel slides with the feet on wall, or rolling a ball on the wall, encourages flexion with gravity assistance.
- The size of the ball can be selected to encourage hip flexion (larger ball with the lower leg supported) or to encourage controlled knee extension (smaller ball).
- A fully inflated ball will provide more support for the weight of the leg.
- Small motion toward full flexion range can be used to increase knee flexion.
- Prone or standing with the strap placed around the ankle to increase knee flexion (Fig. 9.4G)

Progression
- Increase range by adjusting the starting position of the ball with respect to the body: move the ball closer to the body to increase hip and knee flexion or further away to increase extension.

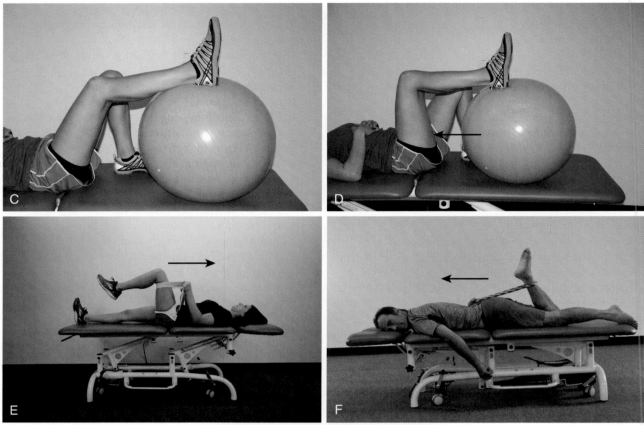

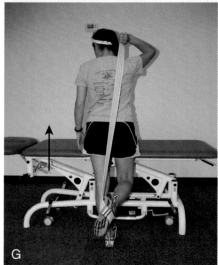

Fig. 9.4, Cont'd

9.5 Active hip internal and external rotation on a swivel stool

See Fig. 9.5.

Purpose

- Restore or maintain hip rotation range of motion

Position

- Standing, with the knee of the involved leg flexed to 90 degrees and positioned in the center of a swivel stool (Fig. 9.5A)
- The hip is in a neutral flexion/extension.
- Involved leg (femur) is lined up with the central axis of the stool.
- If the patient has knee pain, the patella can be positioned over the edge of the stool.

Action

1. Activate the trunk stabilizers to keep the pelvis level and avoid placing excessive vertical forces through the leg on the stool. (Do not let the patient rest too much body weight through the stool.)
2. Activate the hip rotators to spin the stool clockwise or counterclockwise while keeping the trunk still (Fig. 9.5B, C).

Advantages

- Low weight-bearing load on the hip while performing isolated rotation
- Rotation mobility is restored in neutral, functional position of hip.

Teaching tips

- Instruction example:
  - "Keep your pelvis facing forward while turning your leg inward and outward."
- Common errors to correct:
  - Watch for generalized trunk motion rather than hip rotation or pelvic rotation rather than hip rotation
  - Watch for Trendelenburg position
- Methods to address or prevent compensations:
  - The height of the stool should be adjusted to keep the pelvis level, with limited body weight supported on the knee.
  - The supporting leg can be flexed to keep the pelvis level.

Alternatives

- Supine, legs extended, active internal and external rotation of the hip
- Gravity-assisted rotation in prone with the knee flexed to 90 degrees

Progression

- Increase range.
- Increase repetitions.
- Increase hold at the end range.
- Clam shells to increase activation, endurance, or strength through external rotation range against gravity (Exercise 9.26A)

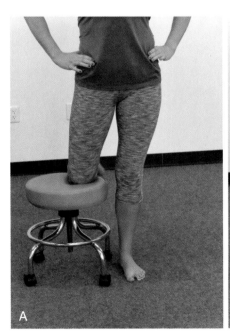
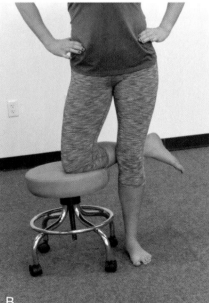
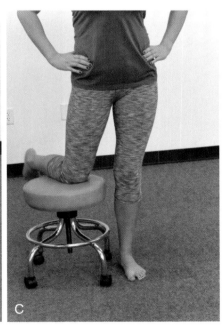

Fig. 9.5

9.6   Active hip abduction in supine on a sliding board

See Fig. 9.6.

Purpose

- Restore or maintain hip abduction in a gravity-eliminated position

Position

- Supine, lower leg and/or foot on sliding board or heel on friction-minimizing fabric/surface or foot resting on a sheet to reduce friction
- Knee extended

Action

- Activate hip abductors to slide the leg into abduction on the board without moving the trunk.

Advantages

- Low load on hip and gravity eliminated
- Abduction mobility in a neutral position of the hip (required for stance) without balance requirements or high levels of muscle activation

Teaching tips

- Common errors to correct:
  - Watch for generalized trunk motion rather than hip abduction.

- Methods to address or prevent compensations:
  - The patient can flex the uninvolved leg and place some pressure through the foot to help stabilize the pelvis.
  - The patient can place his or her hands on the pelvis to help monitor for motion.

Alternatives

- Placing the foot on a roller skate provides the same assistance.
- Buoyancy-assisted movement (with a float on the lower leg or without if standing) if there are no contraindications for aquatic therapy.

Progression

- Increase range.
- Increase repetitions.
- Increase hold at the end range.
- Reduce assistance by removing sliding board or friction-minimizing surface.
- Gravity-resisted abduction in standing holding onto the plinth or a table requires good standing balance, and the patient should be closely monitored for trunk compensations.
- Progress to standing or side-lying abduction to improve muscle activation, endurance, and strength (Exercise 9.26B).

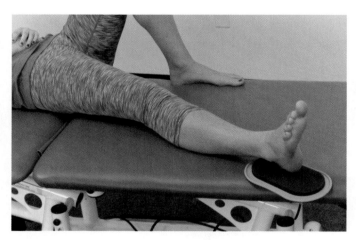

Fig. 9.6

GENERALIZED AEROBIC MOBILITY

9.7   Stationary bike: mobility focus

See Fig. 9.7A–C.

Purpose
- Increase range of motion
- Warm-up before mobility exercise or manual techniques
- General endurance

Precautions
- Use care with range of motion if there are hip flexion precautions after hip surgery (total hip replacement) or with hip labral tears.

Position
- Seated on bike
- Adjust seat height so the knee is slightly flexed (~10 degrees) when the foot is at the lowest point of the pedal cycle and ensure patient can move pedal throughout the entire cycle range.
- Toe straps may be used to promote ankle motion.

Action
1. Controlled forward and backward pedal motion to end-range/restriction through a half or quarter revolution
2. Emphasis can be changed to hip, knee, or ankle motion by changing the seat height or by cueing.

Advantages
- The bike can be used for long-duration, repetitive movement.
- The de-loaded position is useful for individuals with osteoarthritis, or meniscus or other cartilage damage.
- The consistent movement is useful for reducing effusion and for warm-up.
- The exercise can be adjusted for various range of motion deficits.
- The exercise can also be used for muscle endurance or generalized endurance if needed.
- Weight-bearing movement compensations are not as prevalent.

Teaching tips
- Common errors to correct:
    - Avoid hiking the hip as the knee flexes at the top of the pedal cycle or laterally flexing away from the hypomobile side.
    - Avoid letting the hips rotate instead of the knee and hip flexion; keep the legs in the sagittal plane.

Alternatives
- Recumbent bike
- Seated pedal
- Elliptical (Exercise 11.41)
- Airdyne bike (Exercise 10.29)

Progression
- Full revolutions
- Increase seat height to target hip and knee extension.
- Decrease seat height to target hip and knee flexion.
- Change foot position on the pedal to target plantar flexion (toes on pedal) or dorsiflexion (heel on pedal).
- Increase duration.
- Increase resistance.

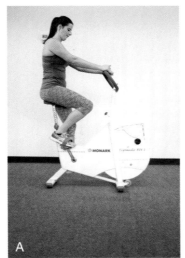

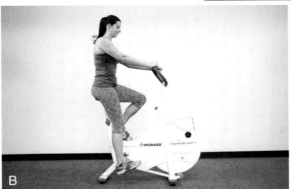

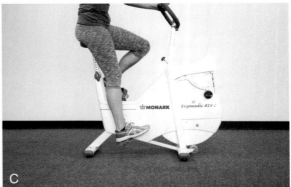

Fig. 9.7

SELF-STRETCHING FLEXIBILITY

9.8 Hip flexor stretch

Purpose
- Increase flexibility of hip flexors to increase hip extension

Position
- Sitting with the hips supported at the edge of the table, legs over the edge of the table See (Fig. 9.8A)

Action (Video 6.8)
1. The patient flexes one leg and holds below the knee or behind the thigh with both hands.
2. While still holding the leg, the patient rolls back to a supine position.
3. The position is held with the involved leg hanging off the table, using gravity to provide an assisted stretch.
4. The hip should remain neutral in the sagittal plane.

Advantages
- Supine position allows the patient to control the position of the pelvis while gravity provides the stretch.
- Flexing the opposite hip limits the amount of lumbar motion.

Teaching tips
- Common compensations to correct:
  - Hip abduction during the stretch, especially if the tensor fascia latae or iliotibial band is tight.
  - Lumbar extension or pelvic rotation are common compensations.

- Methods to prevent or address compensations:
  - If the hip abducts or externally rotates during the stretch, the therapist can provide manual assistance to correct the position.
  - Correct the pelvis position manually until the patient is aware of how to self-correct.
  - Instruct the patient to stabilize the lumbopelvic region using abdominal muscle activation throughout the stretch.

Alternatives
- Manual stretch from the therapist (Video 6.7)
- Half-kneeling position while stabilizing the pelvis in the sagittal plane using gluteal and abdominal muscle contraction (Fig. 9.8C, D, F). (Pressing hands onto top knee can help facilitate the abdominal muscles).
- Weight is shifted forward to the front leg while keeping the spine and pelvis from rotating. Avoid tilting the pelvis anteriorly by opposing the movement using the abdominals (Fig. 9.8F).
- The stretch can be performed standing but there is a higher risk of compensations (Fig. 9.8B).
- Figure-4 stretch (Exercise 9.12)

Progression
- Increase duration of the stretch.
- Increase hip extension range by actively contracting the hip extensors.
- Use additional force (therapist-assisted).

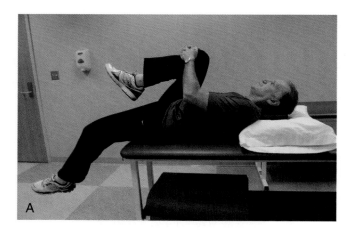

Fig. 9.8

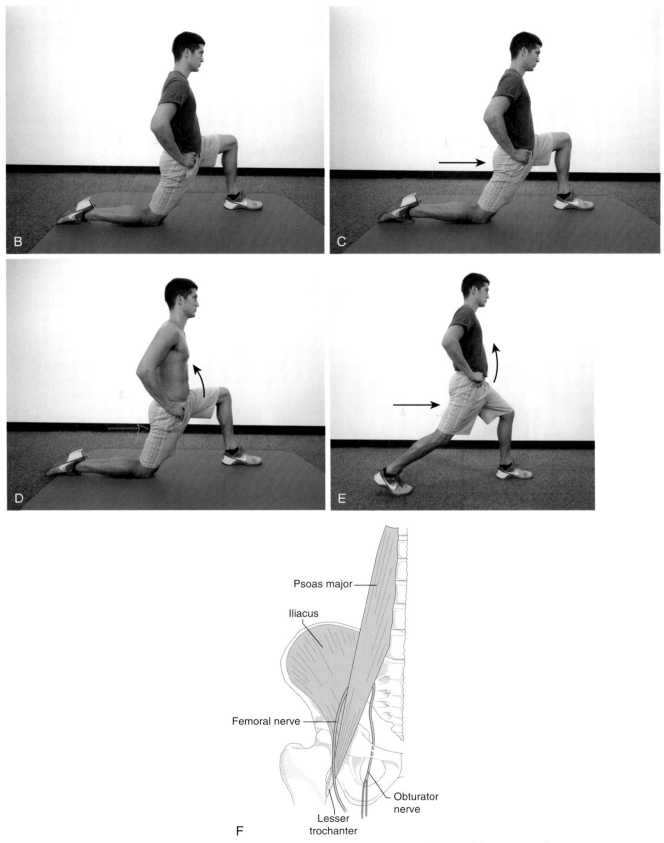

Fig. 9.8, Cont'd (F from Palastanga N, Soames R. *Anatomy and Human Movement—Structure and Function.* 6th ed. Edinburgh: Churchill Livingstone Elsevier; 2012.)

9.9 Hamstring stretch

Purpose

- Increase hamstring flexibility

Precautions

- The stretch should be felt in the hamstrings, behind the knee or thigh. If the patient reports shooting pain, numbness, or tingling, neural tension may be present and neural tension testing, as well as the lumbar spine testing, should be done.

Position

- Supine, neutral pelvis position (Fig. 9.9A)
- One leg starts with 90 degrees hip flexion, hands supporting the leg behind the thigh.

Action (Video 9.9A)

1. Keep the hip flexed to 90 degrees and the upper thigh stationary (Fig. 9.9A).
2. Straighten the knee until a stretch is felt behind the back of the knee and/or thigh.

Advantages

- Can be performed as a home exercise.
- Performed correctly, the exercise will isolate the posterior leg stretch and not allow lumbar spine movement.

Teaching tips

- Instruction example:
  - "Keep your pelvis heavy and hip still while straightening your knee until you feel a stretch behind the thigh."
- Common error to correct:
  - Observe for posterior tilt or rotation of the pelvis while extending the knee (Video 9.9B).
- Method to address or prevent compensations:
  - Point out the possibility of movement of the pelvis (rotation or tilting) for the patient to monitor and avoid.

Alternatives

- Use a rope or strap to support the thigh at 90 degrees of hip flexion while straightening the knee to the maximum stretch (Video 6.11).
- Use the rope or strap around the foot to lift the leg, flexing the hip to 90 degrees with the knee extended. This is more challenging to stabilize the lumbar spine than the previous alternative version.
- Standing with one foot in front of the body on a step, hinge at the hips leaning forward. This stretch may be necessary for situations where lying supine is not possible (Fig. 9.9B).

Progression

- Increase duration.
- Increase range.

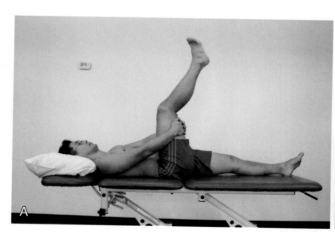
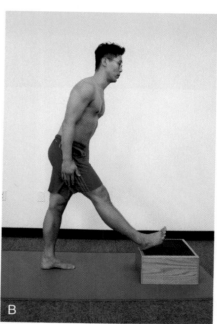

Fig. 9.9

9.10   Gluteal stretch

See Fig. 9.10.

Purpose

- Increase flexibility of the gluteus maximus muscle and posterior hip capsule

Precaution

- If a patient has a torn labrum or femoro-acetabular impingement, extreme flexion may compress the labrum or bony extensions and the stretch may cause pain in the groin. If the patient experiences pain inside the hip joint or in the anterior groin region with full flexion, further evaluation may be needed to rule out impingement. If the patient does have an impingement, placing a small towel roll in the fold of the hip during the stretch may reduce the pain.

Position

- Supine
- Involved leg is flexed toward the body, opposite leg extended.
- Neutral spine position

Action (Video 9.10)

1. Grasp the leg behind the thigh on one side
2. Use the arms to bring the leg toward the body to obtain full hip flexion with some adduction.
3. Adjust the angle of the stretch to fully stretch the gluteal muscles fibers in multiple diagonal directions.
4. Maintain a neutral lumbar spine position.

Advantages

- Can be done independently as home program.
- The patient monitors the degree of stretch.

- The pelvis is somewhat stabilized by the position of the opposite leg, although pelvic position still needs to be monitored.

Teaching tips

- Instruction example:
  - "Keeping your pelvis still and a little space under your lower back, bring your knee up toward your chest until you feel a stretch under your hip."
- Common errors to correct:
  - Watch for lumbar side bending, posterior pelvic tilt.
- Methods to address or prevent compensations:
  - Monitor motion of the lumbar spine and pelvis and point out compensations to the patient.

Alternatives

- The patient can grasp under the thigh rather than around the shin if it is difficult to fully flex the knee or knee flexion is painful.
- Sitting with the involved leg crossed over the uninvolved leg, the patient grasps the crossed leg around the knee to bring the leg further across midline.
- Quadruped can be used to increase range past 90 degrees hip flexion by shifting the pelvis toward the feet while maintaining a neutral spine position.
- Piriformis stretching with hip external rotation and using the opposite leg to assist the flexion (Exercise 9.11).

Progression

- Increase duration.
- Increase range.
- Change angle of the stretch to address the direction with the greatest limitation.

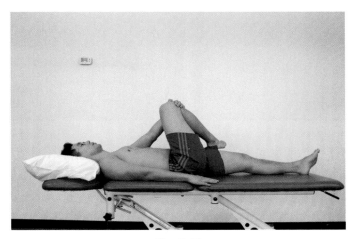

Fig. 9.10

9.11 Piriformis stretch

Purpose

- Improve posterior hip flexibility to increase external rotation and flexion
- Decrease muscle spasm

Position

- Supine with both hips and knees flexed
- Ankle of involved leg is crossed over the opposite knee, with the hip externally rotated.

Action

1. The patient grasps behind the uninvolved leg with both hands and pulls the femur toward the body.
2. Involved hip is flexed passively by the motion of the opposite leg.
3. External rotation is maintained during the stretch by the patient, providing a downward force on the thigh of the leg being stretched.

Advantages

- Can be done as a home program.

Teaching tips

- Common error to correct:
  - Observe for lumbar spine lateral flexion compensations.
  - Avoid extreme lumbar flexion; the hip should only be flexed to the point of stretch in the gluteal region.

Alternatives

- Perform the exercise while sitting with the ankle of involved leg crossed over the opposite knee. Keeping the lumbar spine neutral and the hip externally rotated, lean forward from the hip with the spine stabilized.
- Use the arms only (Video 9.11) or keep the uninvolved leg on the table (Fig. 9.11 A and B).

Progression

- Increase duration.
- Increase range.

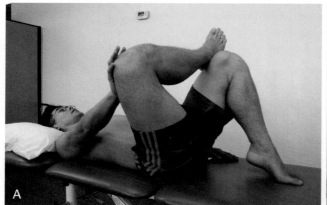
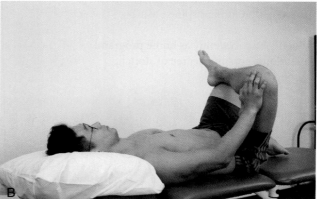

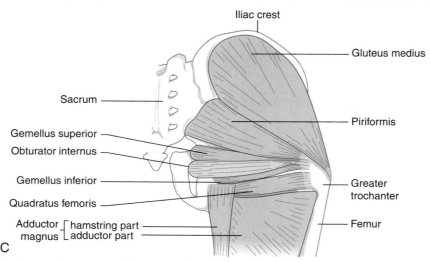

Fig. 9.11 (C from Palastanga N, Soames R. *Anatomy and Human Movement—Structure and Function.* 6th ed. Edinburgh: Churchill Livingstone Elsevier; 2012.)

9.12 Figure-4 anterior hip stretch

See Fig. 9.12.

Purpose
- Increase flexibility of anterior hip to increase external rotation and extension range of motion

Precautions
- Use care with amount of stretch and position the knee off table. If there is pain on the medial aspect of the knee, patellofemoral pain or instability or medial knee joint instability may be indicated.

Position
- Prone, with the involved hip externally rotated, knee hanging off the side of the table
- Tuck the ankle of the involved leg under the opposite knee.

Action
- Contract the gluteal muscles to move the pelvis toward the mat and stretch the anterior hip.

Advantages
- Uses body weight and gravity to provide an anterior hip stretch.
- The prone position can be used to maintain the pelvis position and limit stress placed on the spine by concentrating on the contact with the table.

Teaching tips
- Instruction examples:
  - "Stabilize your low back by engaging your abdominal muscles, then move the front of your pelvis toward the mat. Try not to arch your back."
  - "Engage your gluteal muscles and try to lift your bent knee toward the ceiling. Keep the front of your body on the table."

Alternatives
- Hip flexor stretch (Exercise 9.8) without external rotation (if hip extension is the major limitation)
- Supine, allowing gravity to assist external rotation if rotation is extremely limited
- Piriformis stretch (Exercise 9.11) if the external rotation limitation is greater in flexion and related to gluteal muscle flexibility

Progression
- Increase duration.
- Increase range.
- Increase hip external rotation range and neuromuscular control by lifting the bent knee.

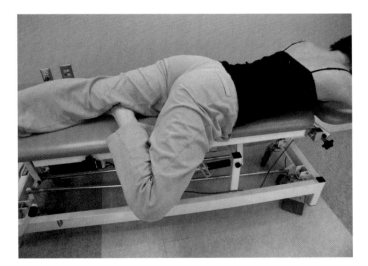

Fig. 9.12

9.13   Gastrocnemius/soleus stretch

See Fig. 9.13A
Purpose
- Increase flexibility of gastrocnemius, soleus, and Achilles tendon complex
Position (Fig. 9.13A)
- Standing, split stance with the involved lower extremity (back leg) straight, front knee flexed in a semi-lunge position
- Weight is on the back foot.
- Subtalar joint neutral; a small pad can be placed under the arch, if needed, to prevent excessive pronation and angulation of the muscle complex.
- Hands supported on counter, table, or wall
Action
1. Maintaining the alignment and weight on the back foot, the patient leans forward keeping the back heel on floor and the knee extended to stretch the gastrocnemius.
2. Maintaining the weight on the back foot, flex the knee while still leaning forward, to stretch the soleus.
Advantages
- Can be done anywhere, including at home or work.
Teaching tips
- "Facing the wall, start with lunge position. Keeping the back knee straight and front knee slightly bent, put most of your weight on the back leg. Using the wall for support, lean slightly forward at the hips until a stretch is felt behind your lower leg to stretch gastrocnemius."
- "In the same position, bend the back knee slightly to stretch soleus."
- Common errors to correct:
  - Lifting the back heel off the ground or shifting the weight to the front foot (Fig. 9.13B)

- Rotating or dropping the pelvis
- Flexing the knee when trying to stretch the gastrocnemius
- Dynamic valgus
- Pronating the foot excessively
- Not performing the stretch in the natural tibial or femoral rotation alignment
- Methods to address or prevent compensations:
  - Initial position should maintain the patient's natural bony alignment of the lower leg. For example, if the patient has 15 degrees of tibial external rotation, maintain the external rotation rather than facing the foot straight forward in the sagittal plane to keep the origins/insertions of the gastrocnemius–soleus complex in alignment.
  - If the patient normally wears orthotics, he or she should wear them while stretching.
Alternatives
- If there are weight-bearing precautions, this exercise can be performed sitting or supine by pulling back on a strap placed under the ball of the foot.
- If the muscle complex is extremely tight, a small pad can be placed under the heel until there is more flexibility.
- If the patient is having difficulty with the stretch, a sloped wedge placed under the forefoot may be useful to increase the dorsiflexion without requiring as much forward lean.
Progression
- Increase range.
- Increase duration.
- Progress to a standing lunge stretch without holding onto support.

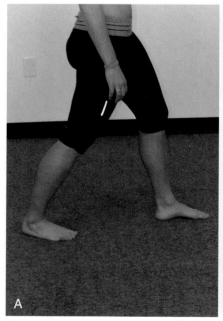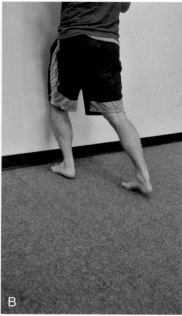

Fig. 9.13 Gastrocnemius/soleus stretch. (A) The patient keeps her weight on the back leg with the knee extended while flexing the front knee. (B) Note that while the patient is moving toward the wall without keeping the weight on the back foot, the knee is flexed and the heel is lifted.

9.14 Iliotibial (IT) band stretch

See Fig. 9.14.

Purpose
- Increase flexibility of tensor fascia latae (TFL) and IT band

Position
- Side-lying on uninvolved side
- Knees and hips flexed to 90 degrees

Action
1. Grasp the involved (top) ankle.
2. Extend the hip.
3. Adduct thigh toward floor.

Teaching tips
- Instruction example:
  - "Keep your pelvis still while you move your leg backward, stopping just before you feel a stretch on the front of the leg. Drop the knee toward the table. You should feel a stretch on the side of your hip or leg."
- Common errors to correct:
  - Lumbar spine hyperextension or side-bending
  - Allowing the pelvis to tilt anteriorly
  - Allowing the femur to rotate (internal or external) or the hip to flex
  - Pelvis rolling backward toward the involved leg
- Methods to address or prevent compensations:
  - A pillow or towel roll placed under the waist may help control side-bending.
  - If the patient is unable to hold the ankle, a belt can be used to reach the leg backward.

Advantages
- This version of the exercise is not as difficult as standing stretches, but compensations in the pelvis are still common.

Alternatives
- Standing, with weight shifted onto the involved leg, the uninvolved leg is crossed in front. Side-bend trunk away from the involved leg.
- In side-lying, use a strap placed above the ankle if the patient has limited knee flexion or difficulty grasping the lower leg.
- Figure-4 (anterior hip) stretches (Exercise 9.12), general hip flexor stretching (Exercise 9.8), or gluteal muscle stretches (Exercise 9.10). Increasing the flexibility of muscles attaching to the iliotibial band improves overall mobility of the connective tissue and helps with alignment of forces.

Progression
- Increase range.
- Increase duration.

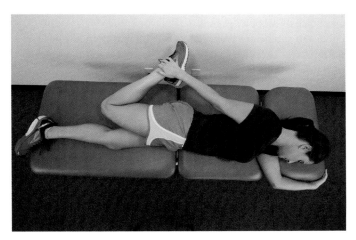

Fig. 9.14

9.15   Neural mobility (slump position)

See Fig. 9.15.

Purpose

- Increase gliding of neural structures between surrounding tissues
- Positive neural mobility slump, or straight leg raise tests indicate the need for improved neural gliding and/or mobility

Position

- Sitting, knees flexed with legs off the edge of the treatment table

Precaution

- This exercise requires caution if there is any neural irritability, and range is adjusted (or holds) to avoid exacerbating symptoms excessively.

Action

1. Flex the spine forward, and then extend the knee on the involved side to the point of, or slightly before, reproduction of symptoms (referred pain, tingling, hot/cold sensations) (Fig. 9.15A).
2. Dorsiflex and plantarflex the ankle (Fig. 9.15B).
3. Release the cervical spine flexion or slump position if the symptoms are too severe (Fig. 9.15C). The sequence of the movements can be changed by using proximal (cervical/trunk) movement and prepositioning the lower extremity just short of the symptomatic range or alternatively prepositioning the trunk and moving the lower extremity.
4. Monitor the type and region of symptoms and use the information from the selective tissue tension and neural mobility tests to select the appropriate position and choice of mobility exercise. Hamstring stretching and neural glides in supine are preferred if there are excessive neural symptoms (Exercise 9.9).

Teaching tips

- Instruction examples:
  - "Keep your knee straight and look down while you bring your foot and toes up and then point the foot and toes down. You should feel a gentle stretch, but not pain, on the back of your leg. If it hurts, then make the movements smaller."

Advantages

- The seated versions of the slump neural mobilization can be performed easily throughout the day.

Specific parameters for neural mobility

- Range and sequence can be adjusted to target symptom avoidance or reproduction:
  - "Flossing," moving through range without reaching the end range to promote movement
  - Move to end range, or the point of symptom reproduction, and then reverse the movement without holding.
  - Holding the end range
- The parameters are selected based on SINS, *especially* irritability. Peripheral nerve sensitization can result in increased symptoms during or after the movement; therefore, it is very important to monitor the degree of irritability and responses.

Alternatives

- Supine or side-lying
- Start without cervical motion or slump
- See Chapter 11 Section 4 (Exercise 11.51) for further alternatives for neural mobility.

Progression

- Increase range by increasing motion at the ankle, knee, hip, or spine.
- Increase repetitions.
- Increase frequency.
- Add cervical flexion or generalized slump.

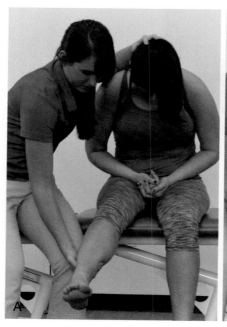
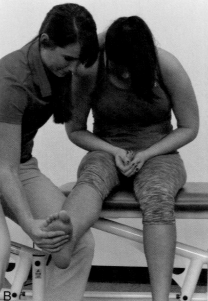
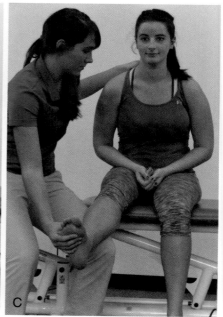

Fig. 9.15

PROGRESSIVE RESISTIVE EXERCISE IN NEW RANGE

9.16   Closed chain terminal knee extension in standing

See Fig. 9.16.

Purpose
- Increase strength of the quadriceps and hamstrings in end-range extension

Position
- Standing, facing the anchor point of an elastic resistance band or a cable column pulley
- Resistance band or cable cuff above the knee
- Knee is slightly flexed with tension on the resistance band or pulley system (Fig. 9.16A).

Action
- Activate the quadriceps and hamstrings to fully extend the knee (Fig. 9.16B).

Teaching tips
- Instruction examples:
  - "Press your heel into the ground and straighten your body by pushing your knee into the band/cuff."

- Common error to correct:
  - Observe for excessive movement of the pelvis and trunk forward or backward; compensations can place stress on the lumbar region

Advantages
- Closed chain movements produce less shear loads on the knee joint than open chain movements.
- Exercising in standing is functional and the movement is useful to prepare for standing from a chair or for going up steps when terminal extension is needed on one leg.
- The cuff or band placement above the knee emphasizes hip extension, which is helpful for patients having difficulty activating their hip extensors.

Alternatives
- Seated short arc quad (Exercise 9.43A)

Progression
- Step-up or squats while fully extending the knee using the band or pulleys to provide feedback
- Weight shift toward one side with the opposite heel lifted as a precursor to single-leg stance terminal knee extension (Fig. 9.16C)

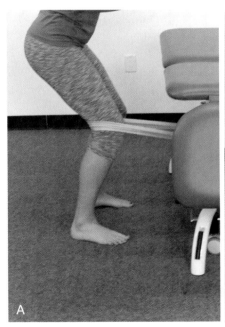 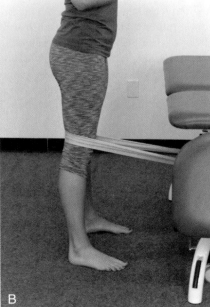 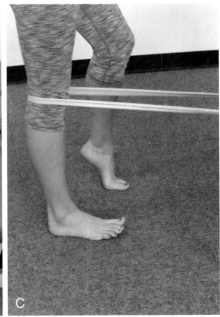

Fig. 9.16

9.17 Terminal hip extension

See Fig. 9.17.

Purpose

- Activate the hip extensors in terminal range and challenge the muscle using activation, endurance, or strengthening parameters to increase, or maintain, hip extension ROM.
- Used after hip mobilization or hip flexor stretching

Precautions

- Avoid lumbar extension.

Position

- Patient is prone with a pillow under the stomach to help avoid lumbar hyperextension.

Action

- Stabilize the lumbopelvic region, then activate the gluteus maximus to lift the leg while keeping the knee straight (Fig. 9.17A, B).

Teaching tips

- Instruction example:
  - "Engage your abdominals, then lift your entire leg, as one unit, off the table. Only lift as high as you can keep your pelvis still."
- Common error to correct:
  - Anteriorly tilting the pelvis or hyperextending the lumbar spine (Video 9.17A)
  - Pelvic/abdominal rotation toward the extended leg (Video 9.17B)
- Methods to address or prevent compensations:
  - If the patient is lifting higher than he can stabilize his lumbopelvic region, instruct him to: "Think about lengthening your leg and reaching out with your foot, rather than how high you can lift your leg. Keep the front of your pelvis (the bony parts) in contact with the mat."

Advantages

- Low load on hip joint and lumbar spine
- Core stability and supported leg stability are also part of the exercise in addition extending the hip.

Alternatives

- This exercise can be done with the hip externally rotated (Video 9.45A) or neutral (Video 9.45B). Gluteus maximus and biceps femoris are emphasized when externally rotated. The semimembranosus and semitendinosus are emphasized when neutral. Externally rotating the hip reduces the tension of the rectus femoris when extending the hip, so it is less challenging to stabilize the pelvis from anteriorly tilting when lifting the leg. If this variation is used, rotation of the lumbar spine or pelvis is common: the patient needs to be aware of the position with respect to the treatment plinth.
- If the patient is having difficulty maintaining a stable neutral lumbar spine position, prone over a Both Sides Up (BOSU) balance trainer (Video 9.17C) or exercise ball allows greater hip extension range and lumbar motion is less likely.
- Positioning the patient over the edge of the table with the pelvis supported is useful if there is very limited hip extension or the patient has lumbar spine pain. The position is sometimes easier to assume than starting over a BOSU or prone on the table and can also be used for home exercise with the body supported on a bed (Fig. 9.17C).
- Closed chain bilateral hip extension can be performed in prone over a BOSU (Fig. 9.17C, D), exercise ball (Video 6.18), or bolster. Both feet are kept on the floor while extending both hips and knees or only one side. By keeping the ankle and toes on the floor, hip and knee extension will take place using both the gluteal muscles and hamstrings for terminal hip and knee extension.

Progression

- Add resistance using elastic resistance band or cuff weight.
- Increase range.
- Progress to closed chain squats in supported positions on equipment or in standing.

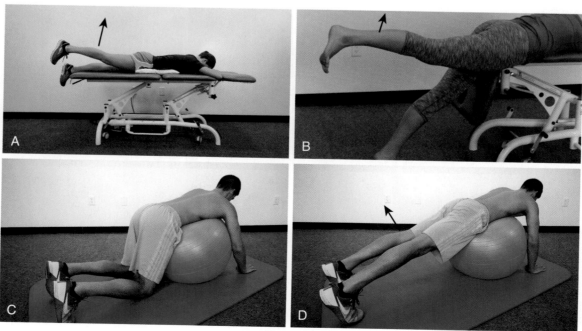

Fig. 9.17

◎ CASE STUDY 9.1: KNEE OSTEOARTHRITIS

This case study illustrates the concepts related to hypomobility as well as selective tissue tension test implications for exercise.

A 56-year-old man is diagnosed with right knee osteoarthritis and is referred to physical therapy to manage his knee pain. The patient leads an active lifestyle but is moderately overweight. His main goal is to be able to tolerate standing to complete his job duties as an assembly line worker at an auto plant. He would also like to return to recreational activities including deer hunting, golf, yardwork, and walking his dog.

Functional status and goals

- *Functional outcome scales*: Lower extremity functional scale 47/80, Western Ontario and McMaster Arthritis Index (WOMAC) 30/96 = 31%

Patient's goals

1. Stand at work for 8–10 hours/day
2. Negotiate one flight of stairs at home
3. Climb up one flight of steps to the deer stand and stand for up to 6 hours within the confines of a small space. The patient is concerned that his balance is not sufficient for his favorite hobby. Hunting season starts in 2 months.
4. Walk the dog around one block.

Subjective complaints

See Box 9.1 for interpretation of subjective complaints and implications for intensity and type of objective examination and exercise choices.

He reports that his knee pain started 8 years ago and has gradually progressed from intermittent to constant pain. Initially, his pain presented following more aggressive activities, but lately

---

BOX 9.1 Interpretation of Subjective Information

- His symptoms are MODERATELY severe, with LOW irritability for weight-bearing activities, but high irritability for twisting. The anticipated pain levels that are acceptable during objective examination are no more than 5/10. Weight-bearing activities will be included in the examination, but pain and effusion will be monitored during and after the treatment. No weight-bearing combined with twisting activities will be introduced during functional assessment due to HIGH irritability for combined rotation and weight-bearing.
- His symptoms are consistent with osteoarthritis.[16] Selective tissue tension assessment will be important to confirm contributions of different structures to impairments during the objective examination. The end feel, comparison of active versus passive range of motion, effusion, and weight-bearing patterns will be helpful to determine relevant impairments and contributions from pain and effusion. Reports of effusion indicate the need for girth measurements.
- Functional activities that need to be evaluated and linked to possible impairments include standing (alignment, pain, tolerance, weight-bearing), stairs, gait, and transitional movements (sit-to-stand, single-leg standing balance).
- The therapist should also address weight loss as part of the treatment plan.[17–20]

---

pain is present every day. His chief complaints are medial joint line pain, cramping and tightness (in the hamstrings, quadriceps and calf), stiffness upon waking, and knee effusion at the end of the day.

- *Severity*: Fluctuating pain 3/10 to 7/10 at the medial knee joint line. The highest pain levels occur at the end of the day after standing all day (5/10) or with twisting while standing on the affected leg.
- *Irritability*: Standing and walking for 4 hours (by midday) increases pain to 5/10, but pain decreases after sitting for 5 minutes. Increased pain due to twisting decreases to baseline level within 10 minutes after a twisting incident.
- *Nature*: Pain and joint effusion increase after standing or walking, especially if prolonged. Stiffness is worse in the morning or with increased effusion. Symptoms are consistent with arthritis or joint pathology.
- *Stage*: Chronic, Phase II

Objective findings

- *Posture/alignment:*
  - Mild pronation on left, moderate on right
  - 40/60% weight-bearing on the right versus left
  - Genu valgum right more than left
- *Girth measurement:*
  - Swelling right knee: 2 cm increased diameter at the knee joint line, 1 cm greater above the joint line
- *Range of motion*: See Table 9.3 and Box 9.2 for selective tissue tension interpretation.
- *Muscle length:*
  - Decreased flexibility of the quadriceps Ely's test: R 30 flexion: some pulling pain, L 45 degrees)
  - Hamstrings 90/90 test: R knee 45 degrees, L 30 degrees flexion (90 degrees hip flexion)
  - Gastrocnemius-soleus complex: 2 degrees plantarflexion with full knee extension
- *Muscle function:*
  - Right lower extremity strength is decreased for quadriceps, hamstrings, hip extensors, abductors, and external rotators.
  - Specific strength testing with dynamometer:
    - Right 30% less than left for knee extension at 45 degrees of extension in sitting
    - 20% less than left for knee flexion at 45 degrees of flexion.
  - Hip abduction, extension and external rotation at 10 degrees of flexion in prone is 20% less than the left.
  - Quadriceps extension is painful at end range.
- *Palpation and joint play:*
  - Tenderness to palpation along medial joint line. Medial hamstrings are tender and tightness on palpation.
  - Knee joint effusion is present.
  - Patellofemoral joint compression; slight pain and soft effusion end feel.
  - Lateral retinaculum soft tissue mobility is limited.
  - Lateral tilt of the patella is present and medial glide is decreased.

TABLE 9.3   Range of Motion for Case Study 9.1

		RIGHT		LEFT	
		Active	Passive	Active	Passive
Primary Area of Complaints/Dysfunction					
Knee	Extension	−10*	−10 (soft)*	0	0 (hard)
	Flexion	125	125 (elastic springy tissue stretch some pulling pain over the anterior knee)	135	135 (elastic tissue stretch)
Surrounding Areas Impacting Lower Kinetic Chain					
Hip	Extension	0	2 extension (capsular hard endfeel)	5 extension	5 (elastic tissue stretch)
	Flexion	125	125 (soft tissue approximation)	125	125 (soft tissue approximation)
	Abduction	Within normal limits			
	External rotation	Within normal limits			
	Internal rotation	Within normal limits			
Ankle	Dorsiflexion (with knee extension in sitting)	−2	0 (elastic muscular)	10	10 (elastic muscular)
	Plantarflexion	40	40	40	40

*Lacks 10 degrees of extension

BOX 9.2   Selective Tissue Tension Interpretation and Linkage to Functional Mobility Requirements

- Primary mobility deficit knee extension. Active and passive knee extension are equivalent for the right knee, with a soft end feel and effusion present with girth measurement. Effusion contributes to decreased extension, and end feel and range will need to be reevaluated after effusion has been addressed. Goals will be set to match the left leg at zero degrees of knee extension to assist with gait and standing alignment.[21–23]
- Knee flexion is limited but within functional limits for all required activities with the exception of deep squats.
- Hip extension is limited bilaterally with contributions from impaired flexibility of hip flexors and quadriceps. Goals will be established to increase bilateral hip extension range of motion to 10 degrees of hyperextension to assist with gait, distribution of forces in standing, and right-to-left symmetry.[22]
- Ankle dorsiflexion is limited on the right with limited gastrocnemius flexibility. Limitations are likely to impact stance phase, stairs, and squats. Goals will be set to increase dorsiflexion range of motion to 10 degrees to allow normal gait and limit stress during stairs and squats to match the left leg.

- Gait and movement analysis:
  - Unequal step length with a shorter right stance time and smaller left step length
  - Antalgic gait pattern
  - Decreased knee extension in mid-to-terminal stance
  - Gait speed 1.5 m/sec
  - Right Trendelenburg in stance phase
  - Unable to stand on right leg for >10 seconds due to pain
  - Stand-to-sit: avoids right leg when sitting down
  - Functional testing: 5× sit-to-stand completed in 15 seconds, majority of weight on left leg with increased pain (5/10) after 2 repetitions
  - Pain increases with step-ups from 3/10 to 5/10, and he avoids weight-bearing on the right leg on step-downs. Repeated testing is delayed.

- *Radiographic findings:* Medial compartment and patellofemoral joint space narrowing, sclerosis, osteophytes.

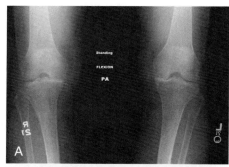

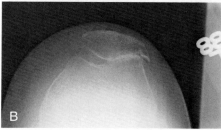

From Rynders SD, Hart JA. *Orthopaedics for Physician Assistants.* Philadelphia: Elsevier; 2013.

Evaluation

See Box 9.3 and Box 9.4 for implications for exercise choices.

- *Physical therapy diagnosis:* Right knee hypomobility, difficulty walking (antalgia, decreased step length, decreased hip and knee extension in stance), difficulty with stairs.
- *Contributing impairments:* Decreased load-bearing tolerance, limited flexibility (hip flexors, quadriceps, gastrocnemius), decreased range of motion (hip and knee extension, ankle dorsiflexion), and muscle endurance/strength (20–30% less on than the left side), pain and effusion. Bony alignment contributions from genu valgum.

BOX 9.3 Implications for Exercise Choices

Implications of medical diagnosis (body structure) for exercise choices:
- Use open chain and de-loaded or partial loaded positions to avoid increasing joint stress.[28]
- Promote equal weight-bearing and proximal support to distribute forces.[29]
- Genu valgum will limit long-term prognosis but needs to be considered during exercise set up and during functional activities.[30]

- Promote joint gliding and circulatory exercises to assist with effusion removal.[31]
- Teach the patient to avoid angulation or rotation while weight-bearing.[32]
- Promote proximal force distribution with hip and trunk strengthening exercises and muscle strengthening and endurance for knee muscles to provide force closure.[33]

BOX 9.4 Implications of Hypomobility Impairments (Effusion, Knee Joint Capsule, Gastrocnemius, Hip Flexor, Quadriceps, Hamstring Mobility Limitations) for Exercise Choices

- Effusion is contributing to decreased range of motion and should be monitored after exercise in the clinical setting and at home with particular attention to when effusion increases related to activity and exercise.
- One of the primary goals is to decrease effusion. Teaching the patient to manage and monitor effusion after exercise or functional activity will be important.
- Mobility exercises to address early morning stiffness will be included in the program.
- After increasing joint range of motion, focus on improving muscle activation, endurance, and strength to support the knee and to distribute forces.

- Mobility exercises should follow mobilization and manual stretching during treatment sessions.
- Exercise parameters to promote mobility are indicated for knee extension, hip extension, and ankle dorsiflexion.
- Muscle stretching is indicated to increase hip extension (hip flexors), ankle dorsiflexion (gastrocnemius). Quadriceps and hamstring contributions to range limitations will need to be reevaluated once effusion decreases and the patient's knee range of motion allows full stretch of the two-joint muscles.
- Progressive neuromuscular endurance and strengthening should be performed in positions with lower loads and less compressive forces on the knee.[34]

Precautions

- Poor load-bearing tolerance with increased swelling/pain: limit weight-bearing loads during initial exercise, use open chain exercise to promote optimal muscle function.
- Monitor effusion after exercise and adjust exercise choices, parameters, and dosage if the patient has increased effusion for any reason.

Prognosis

Good prognosis for partial reduction of symptoms and improved function. Genu valgum and radiographic findings of decreased joint space and subchondral medial joint line and patellofemoral sclerosis limit long-term prognosis for complete resolution.[24–27]

The patient is motivated and willing to start exercising regularly. The patient may benefit from losing weight to improve the prognosis for resolving pain.[17]

Treatment and exercise choices for initial treatment session

Initial treatment choices

1. Manual traction to tibiofemoral joint, patella glides
2. Soft tissue mobilization: quadriceps and hamstrings
3. Exercise choices (Table 9.4)
4. During the first session, exercise tolerance is assessed to establish baseline dosage.

TABLE 9.4   Initial Exercise Choice Examples

Exercise	Goal	Parameters	Rationale and Modifications
Generalized Mobility Exercise			
Bike (Exercise 9.7)	Promote intraarticular motion to assist with effusion, fluid removal Decrease pain Improve circulation and removal of waste products	Low resistance, seat height set to limit extension to 10 degrees knee extension for 5 minutes, lower height of the seat to target knee flexion for 5 minutes	Progress range within session as the patient becomes more comfortable. Monitor pain and ease of movement. Primary goal is to obtain relatively pain-free range of motion and promoting intraarticular movement to decrease effusion without pushing past available extension. Also decreases load, weight-bearing.
Small-Range Repeated Active Movement to Improve Circulation and Decrease Effusion			
Active-assisted ball exercises in supported positions (Exercise 9.4B)	Decrease pain, promote removal of inflammatory exudate, decrease muscle spasm	Multiple repetitions, relaxation in between sets	Primary goal to decrease pain, activate muscles to decrease spasm, and increase circulatory responses. The unstable support from the ball requires muscle activation throughout the movement while the "pumping" action is important to provide gliding motion without weight-bearing.
Active Range of Motion/Active-Assisted, Range of Motion			
Active isometric extension with ankle supported (Exercise 9.1B) Active-assisted knee extension with a strap (Exercise 9.4A)	Maintain any range improvements obtained with mobilization and bike and continue to increase mobility limited by effusion while promoting active quadriceps activation Decrease muscle spasm and protective reactions to allow further ROM	End of available range of motion, maintaining position with active quadriceps contraction	Start with short hold at end of range, monitoring pain levels (no higher than 5/10). These active and active-assisted exercises are suitable for an early home program to maintain (and improve) terminal extension and should be repeated frequently (at least daily) to maximize connective tissue plasticity.
Gravity-Assisted			
Prone knee hang (Exercise 9.1C)	Maintain and increase range of motion	End of range, hold until tolerated (starting point 20–30 seconds). No increase in knee pain above a 5/10 (to prevent increasing protective muscle spasm)	Prone knee hang is after the active exercises targeting capsular restrictions. This exercise is also used as a home program with progressive increase in time held and weight as the patient is able to tolerate the position and load.
Muscle Flexibility Exercises			
Gastrocnemius-soleus stretching (supine with strap) (Exercise 9.13) Hip flexor stretching (Thomas stretch) (Exercise 9.8) Quadriceps stretching (Thomas stretch with knee flexion) (Exercise 9.8)	Increase muscle flexibility	Open chain, non–weight-bearing End range: start by reaching end range without a hold, progress to 15–20 second hold Monitor for pain. Stretching sensation of the target muscle is acceptable	Avoid compensations or increasing knee pain.
Muscle Activation and Early Endurance in Terminal Ranges			
Terminal knee extension (Exercise 9.17) Terminal knee extension with straight leg raise (Exercise 9.42)	Promote activation to maintain new range	Reach and hold at end range to fatigue. During initial testing, the patient is only able to hold for 5 seconds and the patient is taught to combine the action with self-assisted knee extension with the strap (Exercise 9.4A) using active movement as much as possible to hold for 20+ seconds. Progressive hold at maximum range	Open chain or modified closed chain exercise is chosen to avoid loading and compression at the knee.

SECTION 9.2: HYPERMOBILITY

GENERAL EXERCISE APPROACHES

The overall goal is to promote force closure (neuromuscular control, muscle function) to distribute forces and initiate muscle activation. See Table 6.3 for descriptions of the types of exercises used to address hypermobility and Table 6.4 for the comparison between parameters used for hypomobility and hypermobility. In the lower extremity, typical diagnoses in this category are:

- Specific hip, knee, or ankle instability related to congenital structural alignment or previous trauma (posterior hip subluxation, patellar dislocation, generalized knee instability related to connective tissue laxity, chronic ankle instability)
- Generalized instability (e.g., Ehlers-Danlos syndrome, genetic hypermobility)

When hypermobility is identified in a patient following surgical intervention, apply these guidelines once the initial precautions have been lifted with time for adequate tissue healing and recovery (Phase II and III) (see Section 4). A review of the goals, methods, parameters, and measurements are included in Table 9.5.

TABLE 9.5 Goals, Methods, Parameters, and Measurement When Hypermobility Is the Primary Impairment

Goals	Methods	Parameters	Assessment/Measurement
Initiate muscle activation of local stabilizers and improve neuromuscular timing	Promote neuromuscular control using motor control principles Closed chain and multiple forms of sensory input (visual, tactile including taping) Use of balance responses or oscillations to promote muscle activation, alternating contractions	Supported positions progressing to unsupported Inner to midrange for specific instability, midrange for generalized instability or hypermobility Timing of local stabilizers before use of global movers (anticipatory sequencing) Multiple repetitions with adequate rest *OR* alternating movement High repetition or prolonged hold with specificity of contractions Parameters progressed based on motor learning to maintain position or control of range without exacerbation of symptoms	Ability to maintain axis of motion (observation of neuromuscular coordination, or time held in position) Analysis of biomechanics for distribution of forces (visual analysis of timing, axis of motion) Ability to hold isometric contractions (timed) or number of repetitions Pain responses Amount of feedback and correction needed
Improve ability to maintain midrange joint position; muscle endurance, progress to muscle strengthening	Isometrics, progress to isotonics Small range isotonics Promote neuromuscular control using motor control principles Closed chain and multiple forms of sensory input (visual, tactile including taping)	Progression from isometrics to multiple angle isometrics to controlled small range isotonics Prolonged contraction for isometrics Low load/high repetition to fatigue (endurance), progressing to higher load/low repetition (strength) High repetition for small-range isotonics, progress to controlled motion without compensations and increasing load, low repetitions. Monitor for fatigue and compensations Use of local or global stabilizers	Ability to maintain axis of motion (observation of neuromuscular coordination, or time held in position) Analysis of biomechanics for distribution of forces (visual analysis of timing, axis of motion) Ability to hold isometric contractions (timed) or number of repetitions Achieving a targeted position for a length of time Amount of feedback and correction needed Pain responses Functional tasks requiring maintaining a position Lower extremity functional scale
Improve ability to withstand external forces and avoid reaching extreme end range or combinations of directions	Promote neuromuscular control using motor control principles Multiple forms of sensory input (visual, tactile including taping) Progress to eccentric control Progress to dynamic motion and balance	Slow progression into controlled end range Eccentric control to limit end range Progress to higher loads, low repetitions (isometric or isotonic)	Achievement of targets (% of successful trials) Amount of feedback and correction needed Lower extremity functional scale
Improve neuromuscular coordination and response time for functional requirements	Promote neuromuscular control using motor control principles	Reaction time and controlled movement	Achievement of targets Amount of feedback and correction needed Speed and reaction time Lower extremity functional scale

CONTRAINDICATIONS AND PRECAUTIONS

1. Intensity, difficulty, and level of exercise depends on severity, irritability, and if the symptoms are acute.
2. Protect passive structures from excessive stress or strain, limit end ranges, and amount of stress.
3. Avoid excessive range (may be direction-specific).
4. No stretching.
5. Specific precautions are listed with individual exercises.
6. Pain responses and muscle spasm can mask underlying hypermobility, and, once the pain decreases, caution with active range of motion control may be necessary.
7. Sensory input is often impaired with hypermobility and patients may not be able to monitor position or range limits without additional feedback (tactile, verbal, or visual).

GENERAL PARAMETERS

- Midrange (joint or muscle)
- Use supported positions and progress to unsupported
- Closed chain to promote centralized axis of motion
- Dosage starts with low load/high repetitions (>25) or low loads/prolonged holds for isometric contractions before fatigue, with an emphasis on appropriate timing, sequencing, and targets for muscle activation and endurance.
- Dosage progresses to higher load/lower repetitions (<15) in midrange with the ability to maintain the position as a requirement before increasing the load.
- Focus on neuromuscular coordination throughout the treatment progression with high specificity and targets.
- Correction of movement patterns is essential to protect the area and distribute forces.
- Oscillations may be used to activate neuromuscular responses to provide force closure and support the hypermobile joint.
- Progressing the range is the last priority. Full range of motion is *not* necessarily the goal, but rather the ability to *control* the functional range is important.

- Progress to challenging control through range (eccentric control or proprioceptive challenges).
- In Phases II and III, improving reaction time and strength to control end range and limit excessive movement may be appropriate for athletes or work-related functional requirements.

TESTS AND MEASURES

See Magee[1] and Magee and Sueki[4] for more detailed descriptions of available tests and measures, interpretation, and psychometric properties.

1. Pain reports
2. Functional movement outcome measures for endurance or strength
3. Ability to perform activities without compensations or home programs independently
4. Lower Extremity Functional Scale (LEFS)

OBSERVATION FOR COMPENSATIONS AND RESPONSES

- Emphasize maintaining the joint position in the area of concern as the first priority, but also observe overall alignment at proximal and distal areas that will influence the forces on the joint.
- Observe for loss of static or dynamic alignment.
- Observe for delayed muscle activation, muscle imbalances, or inefficient timing of neuromuscular responses.
- Observe for signs of muscle fatigue with progressive deterioration of form and coordination.
- Observe for common dynamic compensations (see Chapter 4).
- Ask patients to report any discomfort *during* or *after* the exercise.
- Monitor for delayed-onset muscle soreness, increased effusion or edema after treatment.

EXERCISES

INITIATE MUSCLE ACTIVATION, INCREASE ABILITY TO MAINTAIN MIDRANGE USING ISOMETRICS OR ISOTONIC SMALL-RANGE

MID-RANGE MUSCLE CONTROL, ABILITY TO WITHSTAND EXTERNAL FORCES: PROGRESSIVE ENDURANCE AND STRENGTHENING

IMPROVE NEUROMUSCULAR COORDINATION AND RESPONSE TIME, PROPRIOCEPTIVE CHALLENGE (PERTURBATIONS AND POSITIONAL CHALLENGE)

EXERCISE DESCRIPTIONS

INITIATE MUSCLE ACTIVATION, INCREASE ABILITY TO MAINTAIN MIDRANGE USING ISOMETRICS OR ISOTONIC SMALL-RANGE

9.18   Multidirectional ankle isometrics against elastic resistance

Purpose
- Multidirectional isometric activation
- Increase muscle endurance
- Increase strength
- Improve circulation to resolve effusion and edema during early Phase I

Precautions
- Specific direction(s) may be contraindicated in the presence of unstable fractures.

Position
- Long sitting with the talocrural joint in the neutral position (or resting position if effusion is present); the ankle can be off the table or supported (Fig. 9.18A).
- Elastic resistance band is wrapped around patient's midfoot.

Action
1. Therapist provides resistance in a variety of directions.

2. The patient resists tension from elastic resistance band without ankle motion.

Advantages
- Very low stress on talocrural joint
- Minimal stress on ligamentous structures in mid-position
- Proprioceptive training and neuromuscular reeducation

Teaching tips
- Instruction example:
  - "I am going to use this band to pull your ankle in different directions but I want you to keep your ankle perfectly still."

Alternatives
- Manual resistance; one direction at a time
- Patient provides self-resistance with the band with the injured leg flexed and crossed over the opposite leg in sitting (Fig. 9.18A, B).

Progression
- Increase speed of changes in direction of resistance (activation, neuromuscular coordination).
- Change and add multiple directions of resistance (neuromuscular coordination).
- Increase duration of hold (endurance).
- Increase amount of self-resistance (strength).
- Increase sets (endurance or strength).
- Increase range (isotonics) in plantarflexion, dorsiflexion, or eversion in sitting (Fig. 9.18 C).

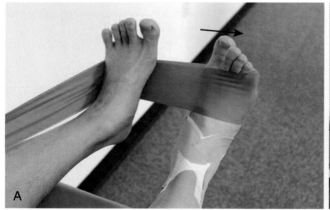
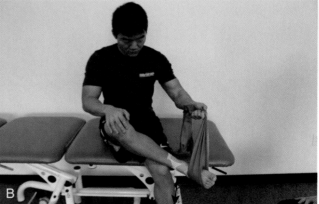
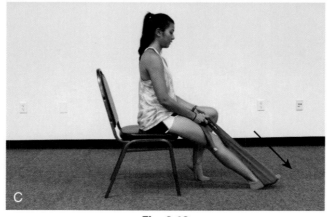

Fig. 9.18

9.19 Reclined squats on resistance equipment (leg press, Total Gym, Rebounder, Pilates Reformer machine)

See Fig. 9.19.

Purpose
- Increase lower extremity muscle endurance.
- Increase strength.
- Improve proprioceptive of the lower extremity using closed chain exercise in a supported position.

Position
- Patient is reclined on the machine with legs hip-distance apart and aligned in the patient's natural bony alignment.
- Weight is set at load appropriate for endurance or strength parameters.

Action (Video 9.19)
1. Patient pushes feet into foot platform without moving the platform (isometric co-contraction) (Fig. 9.19A).
2. Patient pushes feet into foot platform to move the sled away from platform (isotonic motion) (Fig. 9.19B).
3. The exercise can be performed with the foot in dorsiflexion or starting with the ankle plantarflexed to challenge the ankle and foot muscles (Fig. 9.19C).
4. The patient should maintain the lower extremity alignment in the sagittal plane avoiding dynamic valgus or generalized internal rotation.

Teaching tips
- Instruction examples:
  - For isometric exercise: "Press into your heels, but don't move the sled."
  - For isotonic exercise: "Press into your heels, then straighten your hips and knees. Think of your legs traveling in the same line without your knees moving inward or outward."
- Common error to correct:
  - Patients may tend to internally rotate and adduct their legs while moving the sled in or externally rotate and abduct their legs while pushing the sled away from the foot board.

Advantages
- Closed chain activity minimizes shear forces and facilitates co-contraction, and provides proprioceptive input.
- Supine position supports the trunk and upper body, allowing patient to focus on developing neuromuscular control of the lower extremity.

Alternatives
- Lie supine with hips and knees flexed; the therapist holds an exercise ball on the wall and asks the patient to hold it in place with his or her feet (Fig. 9.19D).
- Use a resistance band tied (or crossed and held by the patient) around the outside of the thighs to emphasize alignment of the lower extremities and activate the hip abductors and external rotators by maintaining tension on the band during the movement (Fig. 9.19E).
- Use a resistance band placed behind one leg at a diagonal held with the opposite hand to emphasize the hip extensors and external rotators or on the same side of the body to emphasize the hip extensors. Placing the band around one leg is useful to encourage weight-bearing and proprioceptive awareness of the leg with the additional sensory input.

Progression
- Progress to one leg isometrics.
- Progress to movement through range (isotonics).
- Emphasize eccentric control on the return.
- Increase repetitions.
- Increase load.
- Progress to weight shift, followed by alternating weight shift then extending the hip and knee.
- Progress to active ankle plantarflexion and dorsiflexion.

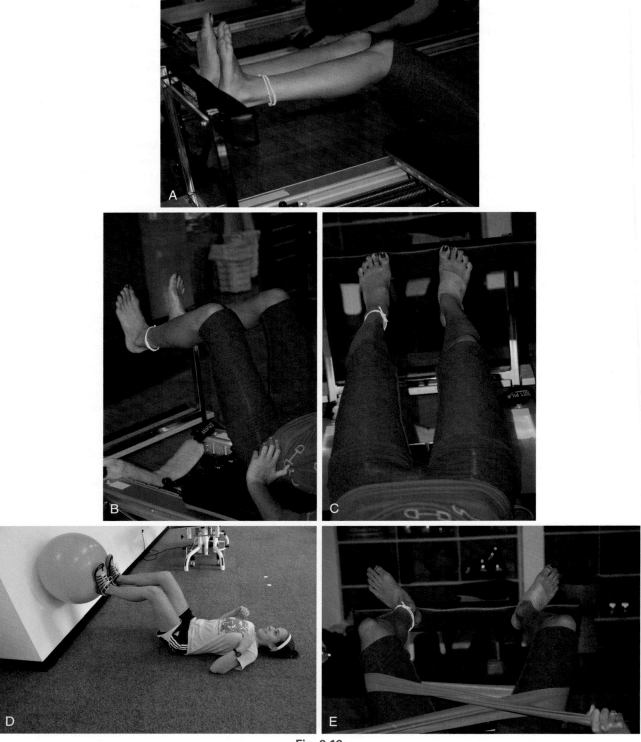

Fig. 9.19

MID-RANGE MUSCLE CONTROL, ABILITY TO WITHSTAND EXTERNAL FORCES: PROGRESSIVE ENDURANCE AND STRENGTHENING

9.20   Multi-hip machine using affected/unaffected leg

See Fig. 9.20.

Purpose

- Improve hip, knee, and ankle proprioception
- Increase endurance or strength of hip muscles
- Improve single-leg stability (support leg)

Position

- Standing on one leg with the other leg in contact with the resistance arm of the machine
- The chest and trunk are positioned over the supporting leg.
- Neutral lumbopelvic position
- Ankle and subtalar joint are neutral.

Action

1. Maintaining balance on the supporting leg, the opposite leg moves against the resistance arm of the machine. The direction of the movement is adjusted for hip flexion, extension, abduction, or adduction to allow clearance of the moving leg and resistance arm of the equipment.
2. The patient should stabilize the core and keep the pelvis level while moving his or her leg.
3. The patient can target different muscle groups by adjusting placement of the resistance arm and by facing different directions on the machine.

Teaching tips

- Common error to correct:
  - Excessive movement of the pelvis and lumbar spine
- Method to address or prevent compensations:
  - Dosage should be adjusted if signs of fatigue or compensations are detected.
  - Moving through a small range of motion is often sufficient to challenge balance on the standing leg.

Advantages

- Exercise can be used to improve hip muscle strength or endurance either leg.
- Can be used during non–weight-bearing precautions for open chain strengthening.
- Challenges balance on the supporting leg with arm support and proximal resistance.
- Allows resistance training in a functional position.
- Closed chain activity (on the supporting leg) minimizes shear forces and facilitates co-contraction, and provides proprioceptive input.

Progression

- Increase resistance.
- Increase range of moving leg.
- Increase repetitions.
- Remove arm support.

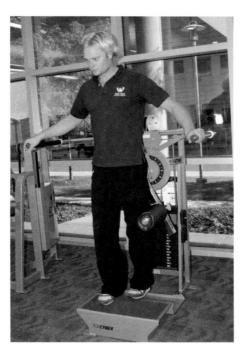

Fig. 9.20

9.21 Bridging

See Fig. 9.21.

Purpose

- Improve hip extensor and core stability, endurance, or strength
- Isolating hip extension movement without spinal motion
- Increase strength of hip extensors
- Improve frontal plane muscle stabilization at the ankle (invertors/evertors), hip (abductors, adductors, rotators)

Position

- Supine, hook-lying position with arms at side
- Lower extremity natural bony alignment
- Lumbar spine and pelvis are neutral

Action (Video 9.21A)

1. Patient presses the heels into table or floor to activate gluteus maximus, then lifts the pelvis and spine off the supporting surface (Fig. 9.21A, B).
2. The shoulders, hips, and knees should form one diagonal line (Fig. 9.21C, D).

Teaching tips

- Instruction example:
  - "Stabilize your spine, then lift your hips until you form one long line between your shoulders, hips, and knees."
- Common errors to correct and methods to correct them:
  - Watch for ankle inversion: posteriorly tilting the pelvis and/or flexing the spine as the patient bridges off the supporting surface.
- Methods to address or prevent compensations:

- Instruct patients to keep pressure on the big toe as they lift their pelvis, or put a ball between the knees and instruct patients to keep pressure on the ball as they lift their pelvis.
- Wrap elastic resistance around the upper leg to encourage hip external rotator and abductor stabilization (Fig. 9.21A–D).

Advantages

- Closed chain activity minimizes shear forces on hip and knee joints, facilitates co-contraction, and provides proprioceptive input.
- Stable position for lower extremity strengthening with limited balance challenge.
- Early weight-bearing activity in supported position.

Alternatives

- Supine with legs supported on a ball or on a chair
- Add an elastic resistance band located above the knees to provide tactile input for hip external rotator and abductor stabilization (Fig. 9.21A–D).
- Position can be adjusted to accommodate limited ankle dorsiflexion range.

Progression

- Add resistive loads to increase strength challenge.
- Change hip and knee range.
- Add an unstable surface to challenge stability (Video 9.21B; Fig. 9.21F, G).
- Shift weight from foot to foot once the hips are elevated.
- Plantarflex the ankle after the weight shift.
- Increase repetitions.
- Increase resistance of the band.
- Progress to single-leg bridging (Fig. 9.21C–G; Video 5.8).

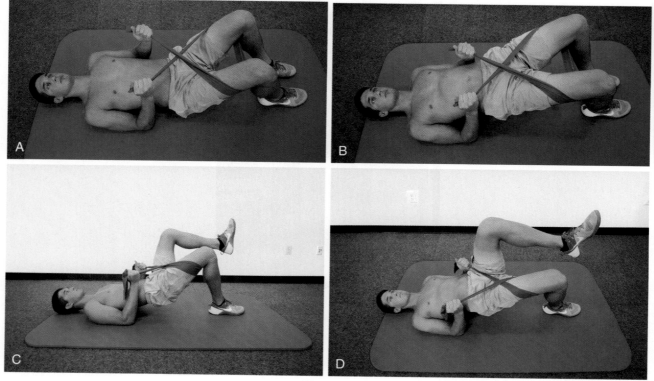

Fig. 9.21

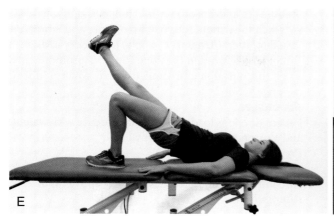

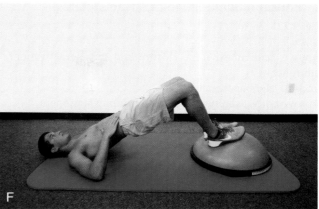

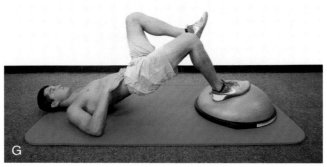

Fig. 9.21, Cont'd

9.22   Partial loading lunge or stride stance

See Fig. 9.22.

Purpose

- Improve generalized force closure and muscle activation/ endurance
- Graded weight acceptance
- Improve body awareness of lower extremity alignment
- Improve neuromuscular control

Position

- Stride stance position (lunge or natural step length distance)
- Involved leg forward.

Action

1. Patient shifts weight onto front (involved) leg to point of tolerance (symptom-free load).
2. As the weight is shifted onto the front leg, the back heel is allowed to lift off the floor (Fig. 9.22A–C).
3. Patient holds position 3–5 seconds, then shifts weight back to starting position.

Teaching tips

- Instruction examples:
  - "Keep your weight across all five toes as you shift your weight forward. Then hold the position for 5 seconds."
  - "Aim your knee over your second toe as you shift your weight forward. Feel the muscles on all sides of your knee as you hold the position"
- Common error to correct:
  - Losing the alignment of the leg

- Methods to address or prevent compensations:
  - Teach the patient to avoid hip or knee adduction or internal rotation (dynamic Q-angle) by placing an elastic resistance band around the upper thigh to promote activation of the hip abductors and external rotators during the lunge action.

Advantages

- Patient develops load tolerance, confidence with weight shift, and awareness of need to shift weight.
- Pre-gait training activity
- Closed chain activity minimizes shear forces and facilitates co-contraction, and provides proprioceptive input.

Alternatives

- Perform exercise inside parallel bars or walker for stability or to decrease load.
- Sitting on the edge of a raised plinth with involved leg forward. Transfer from sitting to standing, shifting weight from back leg to front leg.

Progression

- Progress to adding arm movement using the opposite arm forward to simulate normal gait pattern.
- Follow with arm reach in front to the body to further increase weight shift.
- Add load in the arm.
- Add an unstable surface for one or both legs (e.g., foam or a BOSU; Fig. 9.22D–F).
- Teach weight shift to progress to single-leg stance stability.

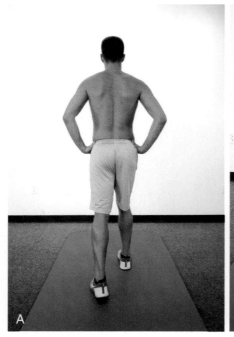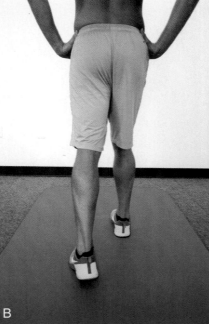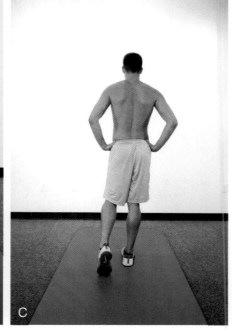

Fig. 9.22

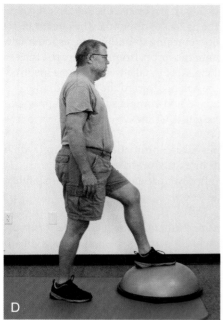
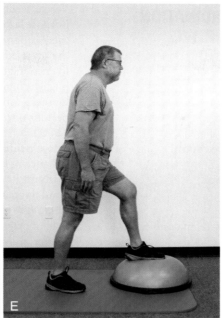
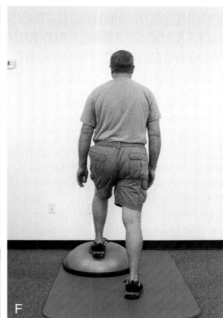

Fig. 9.22, Cont'd

IMPROVE NEUROMUSCULAR COORDINATION AND RESPONSE TIME, PROPRIOCEPTIVE CHALLENGES (PERTURBATIONS AND POSITIONAL CHALLENGE)

9.23   Perturbation training

See Fig. 9.23.

Purpose

- Develop neuromuscular and proprioceptive control
- Improve lower extremity stability
- Improve reaction time to changes in direction
- Improve standing balance

Position

- Standing on a rocker board or unstable surface, in double-leg stance hip distance apart with weight distributed equally on both legs (Fig. 9.23A)
- Knees and hips slightly flexed
- Chest aligned over the forefoot

Action (Video 9.23)

1. Therapist provides push and pull forces to the rocker board to challenge the patient's balance reactions (Fig. 9.23B).
2. Patient maintains static standing position while responding to perturbation.

Teaching tips

- Instruction example:
  - "I am going to move the rocker board: you will need to respond and keep your balance. I will not push you too hard or let you fall."
- Methods to address or prevent compensations:

- Verbal feedback is not necessary during the exercise; the purpose is for the patient to respond to the outside forces. If there is difficulty returning to midline or responding with the involved limb, the forces from the therapist may need to encourage the patient to take weight on the involved leg by disturbing the balance toward the involved side.
- Observe for fatigue and compensations and provide rest periods once fatigue is visible.

Advantages

- Develops neuromuscular coordination and control with limited chance of falls or excessive stress
- Opportunity to improve patient confidence in ability to respond to outside forces

Alternatives

- Instead of external perturbation, the patient performs upper extremity movement in various planes outside the base requiring balance responses.
- A mirror can be used for feedback.
- If there is a need to promote hip muscle activation in the frontal plane to prevent dynamic valgus, elastic resistance can be used around the upper thighs to provide additional tactile input. Another option to facilitate responses from the involved leg is to place the uninvolved leg on a stable surface with the injured foot on the rocker board (see Clinical Example 7.6).
- Initially, the patient is aware of the timing and possible directions. The therapist can move out of the visual field requiring the patient to respond without anticipating challenges.

Progression

- Perform activity with eyes closed.
- Change hip and knee range of motion.
- Progress to split stance and then single-leg stance.

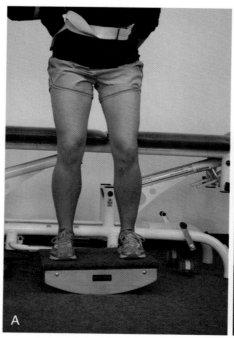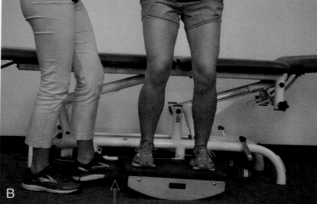

Fig. 9.23

9.24 Single-leg standing balance

See Fig. 9.24.

Purpose

- Improve generalized force closure and muscle activation (particularly frontal plane hip and ankle stabilizers) using balance challenges
- Improve single-leg stability and neuromuscular coordination after weight bearing precautions or injury (Fig. 9.24A, B)
- Challenge ankle and foot stability on unstable surfaces (foam)
- Improve standing balance
- Improve response time

Precautions

- Use upper extremity support if difficulty standing on one leg without loss of balance (Fig. 9.24B).
- Test single-leg balance with guarding before starting the exercise or progressing to more unstable options (Video 9.24A).

Position

- Standing on the involved leg with the knee slightly flexed
- Chest over forefoot
- Subtalar joint neutral, natural bony alignment
- Center of mass is over the midfoot

Action (*Fig. 9.24C; Video 2.15*)

- Patient shifts weight to the involved leg and lifts the uninvolved leg from floor, maintaining initial alignment on stance leg with or without arm support.

Teaching tips

- Instruction example:
  - "Stabilize your core and pelvis before lifting your leg. Keep your pelvis level."
- Common errors to correct (Fig. 9.24D–F):
  - Hiking the pelvis on the side of the free leg is a common compensation for lack of hip abductor and adductor stabilization on the standing leg (Fig. 9.24E; Video 4.27)

- Pelvic rotation
- Hip drop (Fig. 9.24D)
- Methods to address or prevent compensations:
  - Instruct the patient to focus on a specific object across the room with help with accessing righting reactions.
  - Pressing the free leg against the supporting leg is less challenging than holding the leg close to, but not touching the other leg.

Advantages

- Proprioceptive training
- Isometric muscle activation
- Balance responses
- Endurance

Alternatives

- Double-leg standing balance with shift to the involved leg to achieve 75%/25% by lifting the heel of the involved leg, or a split lunge stance can be used if the patient is unable to manage single-leg balance for long (Video 4.24).
- Electronic systems, such as the Balance Master or Nintendo Wii, can provide concurrent feedback on the overall stability and targets to maintain the center of mass inside the limits of stability.

Progression

- Start on stable surfaces and progress to unstable surfaces (Fig. 9.24G; Video 9.24B; Clinical Example 7.7).
- Add upper extremity motion or weights.
- Add sports-specific activities or ranges of motion.
- Add external challenges to challenge neuromuscular control and reaction time (Exercise 9.27).
- Increase load during activity.
- Increase speed.
- Increase distance outside of the base for reaching or catching.
- Change directions of challenges randomly.

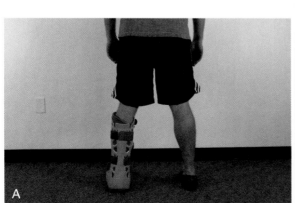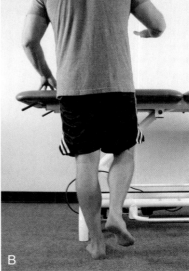

Fig. 9.24 (A and B) Single leg standing balance after weight-bearing precautions are lifted prior to gait training.

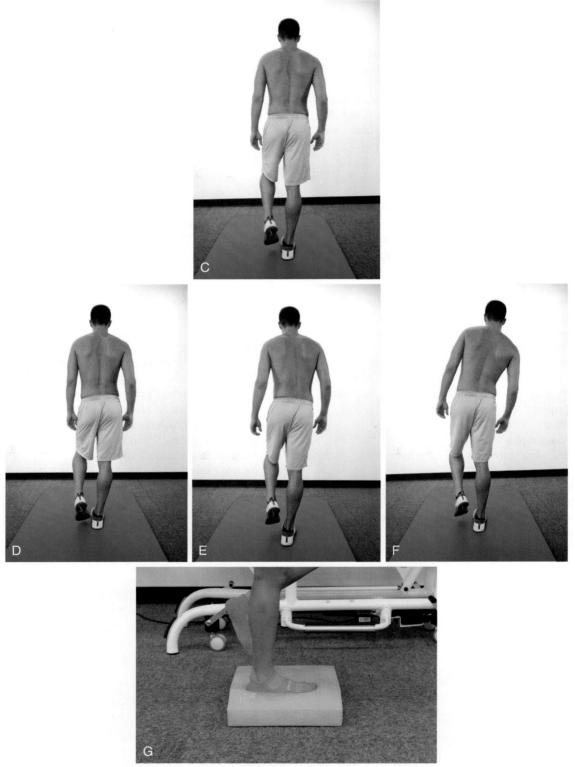

Fig. 9.24, Cont'd (C) Ideal single-leg standing balance position with level pelvis. (D–F) Compensations in single-leg stance. (D) Trendellenberg or dropped pelvis on L. (E) Reverse Trendellenberg or lateral side bending on the left leg to compensate for lack of hip stabilization in the frontal plane or pain. (F) Lateral trunk lean to compensate for lack of hip stabilization or pain. (G) Unstable surfaces challenge single-leg balance.

9.25 Rocker board motion

See Fig. 9.25.

Purpose

- Improve reaction time
- Improve proprioception
- Improve neuromuscular coordination
- Improve standing balance

Precautions

- Balance precautions: provide appropriate guarding and options for the patient to use his or her arms if needed (Fig. 9.25A).

Position

- Standing on rocker or Balance and Proprioception System (BAPS) board with the surface level (Fig. 9.25A)
- Hips and knees slightly flexed

Action (Video 9.25)

- The patient is asked to move the board through different directions (Fig. 9.25B).

Teaching tips

- Common errors to correct:
  - Allowing the rocker board to move using momentum rather than actively controlling the movement
  - Unequal weight-bearing or limited weight shift
  - Lack of hip or trunk stabilization
- Methods to address or prevent compensations:
  - Instruct the patient to control the movement through the desired range of motion without allowing the board to drop suddenly.

- Show the patient how to use the balance board in sitting before asking him or her to stand on it.
- Use a mirror and ask the patient to concentrate on keeping the hips level.
- Instruct the patient to not allow the board to touch the ground or allow it to drop quickly.
- Use arm assistance, such as the parallel bars or a plinth, until the patient is able to control the movement. Gradually remove arm support.

Advantages

- Challenges dynamic or static balance reactions to outside forces

Alternatives

- BAPS board with weights
- Change the direction of the rocker board to provide more or less stability (Fig. 9.25C)
- Foam

Progression

- Progress to single-leg stance.
- Perform with eyes closed.
- Increase the speed of alternating movement.
- Start in planes that do not stress the injured structures and progress to planes of movement in which more active control is needed. For example, for a patient with a lateral ankle sprain, start with placing the rocker board so that plantarflexion and dorsiflexion is allowed but medial and lateral motion is not possible (Fig. 9.25A, B) and then progress by adjusting the rocker board so that the unstable direction is in the frontal plane (Fig. 9.25C).

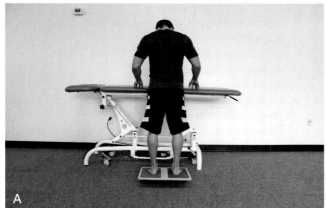
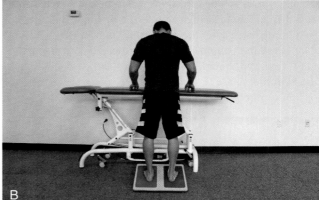
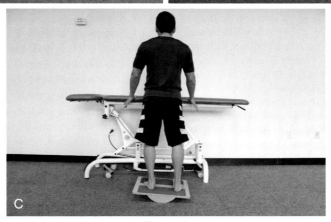

Fig. 9.25

◎ CASE STUDY 9.2: LOWER EXTREMITY HYPERMOBILITY

This case illustrates exercise choices for hypermobility and related impairments as well as parameters chosen to adhere to healing precautions after ligament injury.

A 27-year-old female nurse sustained a Grade II tear of the right anterior cruciate ligament (confirmed with magnetic resonance imaging [MRI]) while transferring a patient 4 months ago. She would like to avoid surgery. Her knee is swelling intermittently, and she has had one incident of the knee buckling since the original incident.

Functional status and goals

She is having difficulty supporting patients during transfers and is wearing a brace for work. Her goals are to work safely without being apprehensive about her knee "giving way," to return to running, and to avoid surgery.

- *Functional outcome scale:* LEFS 45/80

Subjective complaints

- *Severity*: She reports pain in the right anterior and medial knee (3–6/10) with intermittent swelling when standing or walking for long periods, negotiating stairs, or with change in directions. She also reports a sensation of instability and with quick movements or twisting.
- *Irritability*: Pain improves with decreased loading (at times her pain is a 1/10 on her days off from work) and increases to 4/10 when there is increased swelling. Occasionally, her pain exacerbates to 6/10 with increased activity and functional activities especially with changing directions when she is distracted and does not think about being careful. The pain levels go down almost immediately after the aggravating movement.
- *Nature*: Previous trauma with anterior cruciate ligament grade II tear, hypermobility
- *Stage*: Chronic, Phase II

See Box 9.5 for interpretation of subjective complaints.

BOX 9.5 Interpretation of Subjective information

The patient's history of effusion and feeling as if the knee is going to give way (without actual buckling) indicates the need to evaluate for instability and to screen for the potential to respond to conservative management.[35,36] LOW to MODERATE pain levels and LOW irritability allows functional testing, but testing should be discontinued or adjusted if pain increases to more than 3/10 during exercise or she reports symptoms of buckling or giving way. Effusion should be measured and monitored during and after testing and treatment. If effusion increases, the intensity of exercise should be adjusted. The patient's ability to maintain the centralized axis of motion should be carefully monitored. Ligamentous tests and neuromuscular coordination assessment tests are indicated. As her job requires lifting patients, some bending and twisting motions are unavoidable. Therefore, the exercise program should build to include higher level squat and lunge functional strengthening as well as teaching safe methods to lift without placing excessive stress on the knee during the healing time frames.

Objective

- *Posture and alignment*: Slight tibial torsion and genu varum, she stands with most (75%) of her weight on her left leg, pelvis is rotated.
- *Girth measurement*: No major effusion is noted, and circumferential measurement around the knee joint is equal. There is moderate atrophy of the quadriceps with a 1 cm difference compared to the non-injured limb when measured 5 cm above the knee joint.
- *Range of motion and muscle length*: The patient has full range of motion (5 degrees of hyperextension, 130 degrees of knee flexion) and full muscle length.
- *Muscle function*: Patient is able to activate right quadriceps in terminal range but is unable to sustain extension for more than five seconds against gravity. Dynamometer assessment: 40% less quadriceps strength tested at 30 degrees of extension, 35% less strength tested at 45 degrees of extension, and 15% less at 60 degrees of extension. Hamstring strength is relatively equivalent (5% less on the right); right hip abduction is slightly less than the right (5%). All other hip muscle isometric tests are equivalent to the left side.
- *Special tests*:
  - Positive Lachman's and anterior drawer tests with increased anterior motion, positive Slocum test for anterior-lateral instability[1,4]
  - Negative varus and valgus laxity tests, 90/90 posterior sag tests
  - Negative McMurray's, Appley's tests for meniscus damage
- *Palpation and joint play*:
  - Patella mobility is within normal limits and equal to the left side.
  - No pain on palpation of the joint line, patella retinaculum, or peri-patellar region.
- *Gait and movement analysis, functional tests*:
  - Gait is slightly asymmetrical with decreased stance time on the right.
  - Difficulty maintaining single-leg balance on the right for more than 10 seconds.
  - Step-ups and -downs were painful on the right leg with some subjective instability, dynamic valgus and pelvic rotation compensations. Only able to perform four repetitions before pain increasing to 5/10.
  - Single-leg weight acceptance was slower than on the left; single-leg balance 10 seconds compared to >30 seconds on the left (eyes closed).
  - Double-leg squat: Early weight shift, dynamic valgus. Able to perform 26 repetitions from 45–60 degrees without increasing pain.
  - Single-leg isometric squat at 45 degrees: Only able to perform six seconds on the right leg secondary to fatigue and loss of control, 35 seconds on the left.

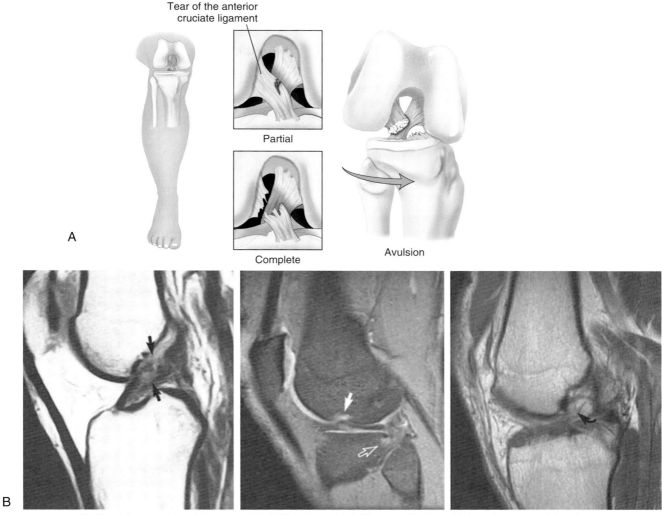

Tear of the anterior cruciate ligament

Partial

Complete

Avulsion

A

B

(A) Partial, complete ACL tear. (B) MRI of partial ACL tear. (A from Rebar C, Ignatavicius D, Heimgartner N, et al. *Medical-Surgical Nursing*. 10th ed. St. Louis, MO: Elsevier. B from From Taylor JA, Hughes TH, Resnick D. *Skeletal Imaging*. 2nd ed. Philadelphia: Saunders Elsevier; 2010, Fig. 9.47.)

Evaluation

See Box 9.6 and Box 9.7 for implications for exercise choices.

- *Medical diagnosis*: The patient's history, subjective complaints, and objective findings are consistent with a Grade II anterior cruciate ligament sprain and knee instability.[35]
- *Physical therapy diagnosis*: Anterior-lateral instability and movement coordination impairments: (hypermobility)[35]
- *Contributing impairments*: Significant loss of muscle strength (quadriceps, hamstrings) and slight deficits in right hip abduction strength. Pain, neuromuscular coordination, and proprioceptive deficits (especially with rotational movements), difficulty with functional balance in single-leg stance and stairs, gait compensations, and compensatory patterns. Difficulty controlling the knee

BOX 9.6 Implications for Exercise Choices

Implications of anterior cruciate ligament partial tear (body structure and medical diagnosis) and hypermobility

- Use closed chain exercise to promote proprioceptive input and a centralized axis of motion with early strengthening in double-leg positions for squats and closed chain weight equipment (leg press, squats).[37,38] Higher loads are possible from 90–45 degrees where there is less strain on the anterior cruciate ligament,[37,38] with a slow increase in stress to promote tissue adaptation.[42]
- Use sensory feedback (tactile, visual, balance) to accommodate for decreased afferent input from capsule and ligamentous structures.[43]

position in weight-bearing activities and decreased confidence with functional requirements including lifting and turning.

BOX 9.7 Implications of Impairments for Exercise Choices

- Initial dosage and parameters are chosen to facilitate muscle activation for force closure, and tolerance is monitored carefully. If there is any exacerbation exercise to decrease effusion would be included (unloaded, repetitive, motion through range) and more aggressive exercise delayed for one to two sessions.
- Neuromuscular coordination principles are indicated to develop force closure using alternating perturbations, unstable surfaces, and balance challenges.[36,40,41]
- Emphasize and progress neuromuscular activation, endurance, strength, and power to enhance force closure to enable knee joint stability in response to outside forces and limit shearing/rotation.[35,37]
- Use motor control principles to assist with neuromotor retraining and coordination.[43]

- Weight acceptance and response time training will be started early with progression from double- to single-leg stance and then from one leg to the other as tolerated.[39]
- Improving confidence with weight acceptance and lower extremity support will be important, and the psychological support will be built into a slow progression of endurance and strengthening exercises from more supportive positions to positions simulating functional activities.[44]
- Muscle strength dosage will be slowly progressed in ranges where there is less strain on the ACL using parameters that enhance proprioceptive input.
- Treatment Plan: Exercise choices for first 2 weeks are listed in Table 9.6.

TABLE 9.6 Hypermobility Exercises, Positions, Parameters, Modifications, and Rationale

Exercise	Parameters	Rationale and Modifications, Common Compensations
General Lower Extremity Warm-Up, Effusion Resolution, and Lower Extremity Muscle Endurance		
Bike (Exercise 9.7)	Seat height is set to allow full cycle from 45–80 degrees knee flexion. Resistance on the bike is moderately high to challenge lower extremity strength with fatigue within 2 minutes. Alternating cycles of 2 minutes with moderately high resistance to low resistance for 10 minutes.	Strengthening dosage in higher degrees of flexion for early exercise program. Bike places relatively low tensile strain on the ACL.[45]
Improve Muscle Function: Activation, Endurance, Strength		
Closed Chain Lower Extremity Strengthening		
Leg press (Exercise 9.19)	Double-leg supported isotonic squats from 90–45 degrees of knee flexion on the leg press against 50 kg; sufficient load to fatigue within 14 repetitions on initial test. Three sets of 12, 10, and 8 repetitions are used for the first session.	Elastic resistance is used around the upper thigh to promote alignment with instructions to keep weight on both feet and monitor fatigue on the injured side or movement toward the unaffected leg. Dosage is progressed on the next visit if there is no swelling or major delayed onset soreness by increasing the number of repetitions to 12 for all 3 sets. Closed chain exercise on a leg press with 40% of body weight produces less ACL strain than open chain knee extension [37] The position also provides a stable surface for early strengthening that can provide feedback and encourage symmetry.
	Single-leg isometrics at 45 degrees of knee flexion on affected leg against 20 kg for as long as possible.	Single-leg exercise is only performed on the affected side. Range is limited to 45 degrees to limit stress on the ACL.[37,38]
Open Chain Hip Muscle Strengthening		
Straight leg raise (Exercises 9.42, 9.45, or 11.28)	Open chain hip strengthening using strap-on weights (2 kg) with sufficient load to fatigue between 8 and 12 repetitions. Starting position for anterior straight leg raise is in supine, hip abduction in side-lying on the unaffected leg, hip adduction on the affected side, and standing with the torso supported on the plinth (modified prone) with unaffected leg support for hip extension.	Strap-on weights are placed around the ankle with a longer lever arm challenging hip muscle contractions. If the patient is unable to maintain the full knee extension throughout the anterior straight leg raise, the weight may be decreased to set the dosage for knee extensor fatigue. Once the patient is performing the exercise without compensations and the dosage is established, this exercise can be performed as part of her home program (2–3 times per week when not attending physical therapy).
Multi-hip machine standing on affected leg with the knee unlocked; slight knee flexion (Exercise 9.20)	Closed chain strengthening, single-leg support endurance, neuromuscular control, and proprioceptive challenge. Dosage and range is set to challenge the positional control and specific fatigue of the supporting leg for endurance of the supporting leg (time to maximum fatigue; at least 10 seconds). The patient is asked to support her weight by holding onto the arm supports and to monitor the weight-bearing alignment.	The initial loads are low to challenge single-leg endurance. Dosage can be increased relatively quickly once she is able to self-monitor her weight-bearing alignment. Excessive speed or range is likely to cause rotation or angulation of the weight-bearing leg, and compensations from lumbopelvic motion are also common.

TABLE 9.6 Hypermobility Exercises, Positions, Parameters, Modifications, and Rationale—cont'd

De-loaded squats using a latissimus dorsi bar and pulley resistance (Exercise 9.29)	The patient is asked to keep the latissimus dorsi bar just below 90 degrees of shoulder flexion. The load on the pulley system is sufficient to assist the movement slightly on ascent. The squat is performed from 30 to 60 degrees of knee flexion[38] with the emphasis on equal alignment.	The bar provides feedback for symmetry,[43] along with trunk muscle activation to decrease the vertical loads on the lower extremity. She is asked to point her legs forward toward lines set on the floor to provide external focus.[43] Symmetry and minimal compensations with multiple repetitions are used initially along with feedback to promote neuromuscular coordination.
Improve Lower Extremity Muscle Strength, Neuromuscular Coordination, and Weight Acceptance		
Double-Leg Neuromuscular Coordination Training		
Double-leg squats on unstable surfaces (rocker board and foam) (Exercise 9.30 alternatives)	Isotonic squats from 45 to 60 degrees, using visual and verbal feedback to ensure symmetry[37,38] Isotonic small-range. Initial dosage set based on point where weight distribution on both legs is lost (3 sets 15 + reps).	Sensory stimulus and balance challenges are used to promote quadriceps and hamstring coactivation in midrange and develop neuromuscular coordination responses to limit the need for ligament control at the end of range[36,40,41] Emphasis is on weight-bearing symmetry and alignment. Midrange of the hamstring and quadriceps muscles is used as a starting point.
Increase Weight-Bearing Tolerance and Control		
Partial loaded positions in partial forward lunge-isometric (stride stance) (Exercise 9.22)	The front foot placed on a BOSU with 30–45 degrees of knee flexion to limit load on the anterior cruciate ligament.[46,47] The body weight is moved forward onto the injured leg. The isometric contraction is held for 10–15 seconds or as long as possible before losing alignment or fatigue. The BOSU requires micro-adjustments of the lower extremity position and also limits knee extension. Time on injured leg and different degrees of knee flexion range are added as neuromuscular control and endurance improves before increasing speed and isotonic lunges.	Maintain neutral knee alignment, controlling valgus movement and tibial and femoral internal rotation by asking the patient to point the knee forward toward an object placed in front of the body.[43] The patient is instructed on the forward lunge position with a trunk lean to decrease loading on the anterior cruciate ligament.[46–48]
Single-Leg Balance Training		
Single-leg balance (Exercise 9.24)	Hold position for as long as possible; initial time is used as the outcome comparison. Goals are set to be able to maintain up to 60 seconds (eyes open), 30 seconds (eyes closed) on a stable surface.	Challenge stability and control of lower extremity during activity. Elastic resistance bands can be used to challenge or promote proprioceptive control of the lower extremity alignment (dynamic valgus, rotational control).
Weight Transfer to Affected Leg		
Partial loading lunge or stride stance (Exercise 9.22)	Motor control concepts; feedback is provided for trials with complete weight acceptance followed by practice without feedback.	Neuromuscular coordination and sensory feedback to promote weight acceptance.[39]

Precautions

- Avoid loaded tibiofemoral rotation during functional movements and exercise.
- Limit anterior shear forces of the tibia on the femur especially at extreme strain.[37,38]
- Monitor responses to weight-bearing (pain and effusion).
- Progress movements requiring response time and ability to accept weight slowly.[39]

Prognosis

The patient has moderate potential for conservative management of her partial ACL tear due to lack of concomitant meniscus and articular cartilage or other ligament damage, younger age, and high motivation level. She has had only one episode of giving way, but reports subjective instability and is unable to stand on one leg or complete other functional movements tests 4 months post injury, decreasing the overall prognosis for higher level physically demanding activity.[35,36,40,41] As she does not want to return to competitive running or high-level contact sport, conservative management may be appropriate for her functional needs.

Progression at 2 weeks

The patient is tolerating the exercise program well with no effusion. Some exercises are progressed and open chain strengthening is added to the program (Table 9.7).

TABLE 9.7 Additional Exercises and Progression at 2 Weeks

Exercise	Parameters	Rationale
Improve Muscle Function: Activation, Endurance, Strength		
Closed Chain Lower Extremity Strengthening		
Leg press (Exercise 9.19)	Resistance increased to 60 kg (bilateral) with fatigue by 10 repetitions for each set.	
	Single-leg closed chain exercise from 90–45 degrees against 25 kg is tolerated well.	Single-leg exercise is only performed on the affected side. Range is limited to 45 degrees to limit stress on the ACL.[37,38]
Open chain hip muscle strengthening Straight leg raise (Exercises 9.42, 9.45, or 11.28)	Weight is increased to 3 kg.	Exercise is used for her home program (2–3 times per week when not attending physical therapy).
Multi-hip machine standing on affected leg with the knee unlocked; slight knee flexion (Exercise 9.20)	Time is increased to allow standing on the injured leg for up to 20 seconds. Resistance for the moving leg is increased by 5 kg.	Hip muscle endurance on the standing leg is addressed to assist with force distribution.
De-loaded squats using a latissimus dorsi bar and pulley resistance (Exercise 9.29)	The amount of assistance is decreased by lowering the load. The squat is performed from 30 to 60 degrees of knee flexion[38] with the emphasis on equal alignment.	
Open chain weight machine resistance strengthening knee extension (Exercise 9.43), knee flexion (Exercise 9.44)	Dosage is set to challenge muscle strength with sufficient resistance to fatigue the target muscles from 90 to 45 degrees for knee flexion with the machine application pad closer to the knee to decrease the leverage and from 45 to 90 degrees for knee flexion (point of application at the ankle).[38] After initial testing, load that can be lifted smoothly for 8–12 repetitions is chosen with 2 sets performed for 6–10 repetitions for each set. If there is no delayed-onset muscle soreness, the repetitions are increased with exercise to fatigue, followed by increasing the load once the patient can perform 15 repetitions.	Muscle strengthening to assist with knee control and hip muscle force distribution. Anterior cruciate ligament strain is lower in more flexed positions. Strengthening dosage can be higher when there is lower tensile strain.[38] Although the injury was 4 months ago, ligament healing can take up to 1 year for complete connective tissue replenishment. The use of combinations of open and closed chain strengthening is recommended strongly in the APTA Clinical Practice Guidelines for knee ligament sprain.[35]
Improve Lower Extremity Muscle Strength, Neuromuscular Coordination and Weight Acceptance		
Double-Leg Neuromuscular Coordination Training		
Double-leg squats on unstable surfaces (rocker board and foam) (Exercise 9.30 alternatives) *Progression:* Perturbations on the rocker board (Exercise 9.25)	Perturbations are added once the patient is able to achieve equal weight-bearing distribution with isometric holds at different ranges.	Sensory stimulus and balance challenges are used to promote quadriceps and hamstring co-activation in midrange and develop neuromuscular coordination responses to limit the need for ligament control at the end of range.[36,40,43] Emphasis is on weight-bearing symmetry and alignment with return to the midline position.
Single-Leg Balance Training		
Isometrics single-leg balance (Exercises 9.24 and 9.27)	Maintain balance progressing from stable position to unstable surface (foam, rocker board). Hold position for as long as possible; initial time on the unstable surface is used as the outcome comparison.	Challenge stability and control of lower extremity during activity with balance challenges.
Weight Transfer to Affected Leg		
Partial loading lunge or stride stance with increased speed (Exercise 9.22)	Weight transfer is progressed from eyes open using visual feedback progressing to eyes closed.	Neuromuscular coordination and sensory feedback to promote weight acceptance.[39]

SECTION 9.3: REPETITIVE STRAIN

GENERAL EXERCISE APPROACHES

The types of exercise used to address repetitive strain injuries are described in Chapter 6, and a review of the goals, methods, parameters, and measurements are included in Table 9.8. When treating repetitive strain injuries, the priority is to reduce the strain by adjusting the movement biomechanics to allow tissue recovery. The overall goals are to distribute forces to avoid excessive force on inflamed, irritated, or degenerated tissue and to promote alignment and optimization of biomechanical efficiency, as well as to promote symmetrical and efficient muscle function. In order to address other contributing factors, improving flexibility and length of restricted soft tissue or joint motion and promoting

overall endurance are also included in the intervention strategies. If hypermobility is present, the goals for hypermobility take precedence over those for hypomobility, and additional care is warranted to avoid stresses on the area of concern.

Typical diagnoses in this category include:
- Tendinopathy (patellar tendon, Achilles, gluteal, iliotibial band (ITB), flexor hallucis longus, plantar fasciitis, patella tendinopathy)
- Degenerative conditions (hip, knee, ankle, toe osteoarthritis, labral tears, patellofemoral osteoarthritis, patellofemoral syndrome)
- Stress fractures

If surgical intervention is necessary, it is appropriate to apply these guidelines in conjunction with the postsurgical precautions and recovery (Phases II and III).

TABLE 9.8 Goals, Methods, Parameters, and Measurement When Repetitive Strain Is the Primary Mechanism of Injury

Goals	Methods		Parameters	Assessment/ Measurement
Distribute forces to avoid placing excessive force on inflamed, irritated, or degenerated structures.	Muscle activation and endurance exercise for areas surrounding the affected region		Open chain or isometric activity around affected area if closed chain Apply resistance in an area that will not place stress on affected region. Utilize other planes of motion or other joints rather than affected region. Specificity of activation and timing before motion Low load, high repetitions without pain responses from affected area Range depends on the requirements for functional activity and the ranges where stress is likely to be placed on other structures Isometric or isotonic	Pain responses after exercise (delayed-onset muscle soreness) Specific muscle function capabilities (amount of load and repetitions before fatigue) Movement patterns during exercise and functional tests Functional tests
Address causative factors increasing forces on structures and impairments resulting from compensations.	Decreased joint mobility or muscle flexibility	Muscle flexibility (stretching) Joint mobility focus	End range (joint or muscle) Low loads with sustained holds Maximal length of affected tissue Progress time of hold or load Allow some time to accommodate to new lengths before progressing load. Goals to achieve functional range	Pain responses during and after exercise (delayed-onset muscle soreness) Range of motion (goniometric or functional tests) End feel (especially for muscle guarding)
	Address muscle imbalances (decreased muscle activation, endurance or strength)	See section on distributing forces to avoid excessive forces on inflamed, irritated, or degenerated structures; applied to surrounding regions and to affected area.		
	Training factors	Adjust training intensity, frequency, or type to decrease local stress while maintaining conditioning. Alternate exercise selected (cross-training) Cardiovascular or muscle endurance exercise	De-loaded positions RPE 11–13 if possible without increasing symptoms. Multiple repetitions, low load, if possible without increasing symptoms	Pain responses during, and after exercise (delayed-onset muscle soreness) Time before onset of symptoms Functional measures LEFS or other functional outcome measures Time or intensity for endurance exercise

Continued

TABLE 9.8 Goals, Methods, Parameters, and Measurement When Repetitive Strain Is the Primary Mechanism of Injury—cont'd

Goals	Methods	Parameters	Assessment/ Measurement
Adjust dynamic biomechanical alignment.	Promote neuromuscular control using motor control principles Multiple forms of sensory input (visual, tactile, including taping) Progress to eccentric control Progress to dynamic motion and balance	Slowly progress into ranges where increased biomechanical stress is likely. Loads less than normal functional requirements with high repetitions (supported or unsupported) Progress to higher loads, low repetitions (isometric or isotonic) in pain-free ranges.	Achievement of targets (% of successful trials) Amount of feedback and correction needed Pain responses or movement quality through range or with repetitions Dynamic movement assessment
Promote tissue healing and optimal regeneration.	Tendon; slowly progress isotonic exercise and eccentric loading	Progress from low-load/high repetition to higher load/low repetitions. Midrange and progress to end range Maintain alignment of tendon (plane and direction of movement).	Monitor symptoms (pain, edema) Functional tests Resistive or special tests LEFS or other functional outcome measures
	Bone; slowly progress loading forces	Progress from low-load/high repetition to higher load/low repetitions Use intermittent loading, then slowly increase time of sustained loading (without additional angulation or rotational forces).	Monitor symptoms (pain, edema) Functional tests Special tests LEFS or other functional outcome measures
	Cartilage; slowly progress gliding and intermittent compression and decompression with decreased weight-bearing	Low-load/high repetition; allow adequate rest periods.	Monitor symptoms (pain, edema, effusion) Functional tests Resistive or special tests LEFS or other functional outcome measures
Improve neuromuscular coordination and response time for functional requirements.	Promote neuromuscular control using motor control principles. Closed chain or open chain, depend on functional requirements and stage of recovery. Feedback for adjustment of movement strategies (auditory, visual, tactile, including taping)	Supported positions progressing to unsupported, movements depending on functional requirements. Multiple repetitions after desired movement strategy has been achieved Parameters progressed based on motor learning to maintain position or control of range without exacerbation of symptoms.	Analysis of biomechanics (visual analysis of timing, axis of motion) Ability to perform movement correctly (timed) or % of repetitions performed before fatigue or compensation Amount of feedback and correction required % of targets achieved

LEFS, Lower extremity functional scale; *RPE,* rating of perceived exertion.

CONTRAINDICATIONS AND PRECAUTIONS

- Avoid combined forces resulting in microfailure (specific directions, or type of forces, ranges, specific movements, or adjusting biomechanical factors).
- Avoid angulation or rotation in extreme ranges combined with high loads (see stress–strain curve in Chapter 2).
- Introduce forces to the damaged tissue slowly.
- Specific precautions for:
  - Bone (stress fractures): Avoid rotation and high impact forces
  - Tendinosis: Avoid high loads with extreme ranges
  - Cartilage damage (osteoarthritis): Avoid high weight-bearing forces

GENERAL PARAMETERS

- Correcting biomechanical alignment and force distribution is a priority and dosage is determined by the ability to achieve optimal position, fatigue, or symptoms.
- Supported positions progressing to unsupported
- Closed chain is used to promote a centralized axis of motion.
- Open chain is used to increase range of motion or flexibility.
- Dosage starts with from low load/high repetitions (>25) or low loads/prolonged holds for isometric contractions before fatigue, with an emphasis on appropriate timing, sequencing, and targets for muscle activation and endurance.

- The patient must demonstrate the ability to maintain the given position before increasing the load, and then dosage progresses to higher load/lower repetitions (<15).
- Emphasize neuromuscular coordination throughout the treatment progression by choosing exercises and parameters to address specific muscle activation, sequencing, intensity, and timing. Along with specificity, achievable targets and correcting movement patterns are important for return to function and to meet the patient's goals, but also to prevent further injury.
- Progressing the range is based on functional requirements or alleviating contributing factors without increasing symptoms.

TESTS AND MEASURES

See Magee[1] and Magee and Sueki[4] for more detailed description of available tests and measures, interpretation, and psychometric properties.
1. Pain reports
2. Functional movement outcome measures for endurance or strength
3. Movement observation (qualitative)
4. Functional outcome measures for symmetry, repetition, or functional requirements
5. Ability to perform activities without compensations or home programs independently
6. LEFS, Patient Specific Functional Scale

OBSERVATION FOR COMPENSATIONS AND RESPONSES

- Keep the area of concern supported with active neuromuscular control as the first priority, but observe for overall alignment at proximal and distal areas influencing the forces on the joint.
- Monitor proximal areas and adjust position and muscle activation to address moment arms as well as excessive angulation or rotation.
- Observe for loss of position or muscle activation with fatigue and monitor symptom reproduction.
- Use supported positions when needed.
- Ask patients to report any discomfort during or after the exercise.
- Monitor for delayed-onset muscle soreness, increased effusion, or edema after treatment.

EXERCISES

DISTRIBUTE FORCES TO REDUCE LOCALIZATION OF FORCE ON INFLAMED, IRRITATED, OR DEGENERATED STRUCTURES

ADDRESS CONTRIBUTING FACTORS (IMPAIRMENTS, BIOMECHANICS, COMPENSATIONS)

- Mobility and flexibility exercise (see section on Lower Extremity Hypomobility exercise)
- Muscle activation, endurance, strength (see Section 2: Lower Extremity Hypermobility and Section 4: Post Surgical Management)

ADJUST DYNAMIC BIOMECHANICAL ALIGNMENT

- See also lower extremity hypermobility exercises and post-surgical exercises

PROMOTE TISSUE HEALING AND OPTIMAL REGENERATION: ECCENTRIC STIMULUS FOR TENDON

IMPROVE NEUROMUSCULAR COORDINATION AND RESPONSE TIME FOR FUNCTIONAL REEDUCATION

- Lifting techniques (see Lifting reeducation, Exercises 11.43–11.45)

EXERCISE DESCRIPTIONS

DISTRIBUTE FORCES TO REDUCE LOCALIZATION OF FORCE ON INFLAMED, IRRITATED, OR DEGENERATED STRUCTURES

9.26A Clam shells

See Fig. 9.26A and B.

Purpose

- Facilitate specific activation or increase endurance/strength of the hip external rotators and posterior fibers of gluteus medius

Position

- Side-lying, with hips, knees, and shoulders stacked on top of each other
- Hips are flexed 45 degrees, and knees are flexed 60–90 degrees.
- Lumbar spine is in a neutral alignment.
- Head supported with underside arm or pillow, resting in alignment with thoracic spine.

Action (Videos 4.32 and 4.34)

1. Engage the spinal stabilizers and lift the waist using the oblique muscles to align the lumbopelvic region (Exercise 11.29).
2. Keeping the feet together, activate hip external rotators of top leg to lift the top knee as high as possible without rotating the pelvis or lumbar spine (Fig. 9.26A).

Teaching tips

- Instruction example:
  - "Keeping your feet together, open your top knee."
- Common errors to correct:
  - The pelvis should not rotate backward as the top leg lifts.
  - Ensure that the starting position of the pelvis is in the correct plane to provide a stable base for the external rotators and that the lumbar spine does not move during the exercise.
- Methods to address or prevent compensations:
  - Instructions to: "Keep your top hip pressing forward as you lift your top knee to avoid rocking the pelvis."

Advantages

- Open chain hip muscle activation, endurance, or strengthening exercise allows positioning to facilitate external rotator activation against gravity but with minimal load on the hip and knee joints.
- Isolation of the hip external rotators is possible without requiring balance and control of lower extremity alignment in standing.
- The supporting surface provides the patient with tactile feedback if the torso and pelvis are not stabilized and starts to rotate when rotating the hip.

Alternatives

- Supine, bilateral hip external rotation against elastic resistance from a band tied around the thighs above the knees (Fig. 9.26B; Video 9.26)

Progression

- Elastic resistance band above the knees

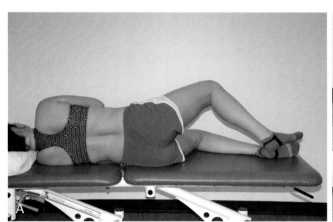

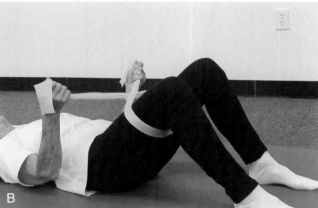

Fig. 9.26

9.26B   Side-lying hip abduction

See Fig. 9.26C and D.

Purpose

- Facilitate specific activation or increase endurance/strength of the hip abductors

Position

- Side-lying, with hips, knees, and shoulders lined up
- Hips and knees are in neutral
- Lumbar spine is in a neutral alignment
- Head supported with underside arm or pillow, resting in alignment with thoracic spine.

Action (Video 2.16)

1. Engage the spinal stabilizers and lift the waist using the oblique muscles to align the lumbopelvic region (Exercise 11.29).
2. Activate the hip abductors of top leg to lift the leg, keeping the patella facing forward and the leg in line with the body without rotating the pelvis or lumbar spine.

Teaching tips

- Instruction example:
  - "Keeping your knee straight, lift your top leg without letting your pelvis rock."
- Common errors to correct:
  - The pelvis should not rotate backward as the top leg lifts.
  - Ensure that the starting position of the pelvis is in the correct plane to provide a stable base for the external rotators and that the lumbar spine does not move during the exercise.
  - Watch for using the tensor fascia latae or quadriceps instead of the gluteus medius, if the anterior muscles are used to lift the leg the hip will rotate or flex during the movement.

- Methods to address or prevent compensations:
  - Demonstrate the area where the patient should be feeling fatigue or have the patient palpate the area during the exercise (Fig. 9.26D).
  - Ask the patient where he or she is feeling the muscle action. The patient should report fatigue of the gluteus medius not the anterior hip flexors or quadriceps.

Advantages

- Open chain hip muscle activation, endurance, or strengthening exercise allows positioning to facilitate hip abductor activation against gravity but with minimal load on the hip and knee joints.
- Isolation of the hip abductors is possible without requiring balance and control of lower extremity alignment in standing.
- The supporting surface provides the patient with tactile feedback if the torso and pelvis are not stabilized and starts to rotate.

Alternatives

- Hip abduction can be performed in supine with the leg on a roller board or sliding board if there is severe hip muscle weakness.

Progression

- Elastic resistance band above the knees
- Standing closed chain single-leg balance without losing the pelvis position (Exercise 9.24, 9.27)
- Side stepping with or without elastic resistance tied around the legs (Exercise 9.28)
- Standing, single-leg open chain abduction against pulley or elastic resistance

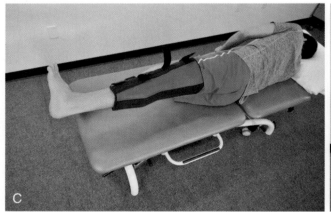 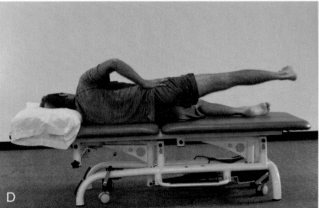

Fig. 9.26

9.27 Single-leg balance with external challenges

See Fig. 9.27.

Purpose

- Develop lower extremity static stability
- Promote neuromuscular control and local stabilizer activation (hip and foot stabilizers)
- Promote static balance reactions
- Promote early activation and/or endurance of hip, ankle, and foot stabilizing muscles
- Increase functional ankle and hip control

Position

- Standing on the involved leg, with the knee slightly flexed to unlock the knee, subtalar joint neutral
- The opposite leg is off the ground with the knee and hip slightly flexed to clear the leg without touching the supporting leg.
- Weight is equally distributed across the stance foot.
- The patient can use the upper extremities for support if needed.

Action

1. The focus is to maintain lower extremity *and* pelvic alignment while performing:
   - Upper extremity activities: Catching a ball, pushing, pulling light loads
   - Moving the opposite leg in various directions, off the ground with or without resistance from elastic resistance or pulleys (Fig. 9.27A, B; Video 2.5)
2. The direction of the challenge is adjusted and changed to promote control against external load in different planes of movement (Fig. 9.27C–G).

Advantages

- Static balance reactions require local stabilizer activity around the hip and foot.
- Proprioceptive training and body awareness use balance reactions.
- Closed chain activity minimizes shear forces and facilitates co-contraction, thereby increasing stability through force closure.

Teaching tips

- Instruction examples:
  - "Watch your pelvis and keep it level and facing in the same direction."
  - "Keep your balance on one leg with your pelvis level."
- Common errors to correct:
  - Losing the pelvic alignment by dropping the pelvis (Trendelenburg position)
  - Hiking the pelvis on the side of the free leg
  - Allowing pelvic rotation
- Methods to address or prevent compensations:
  - While the challenge is to maintain balance, the muscle activation patterns used to maintain stability are the major goal of the exercise. Observe the patient's ability to maintain the proximal hip and trunk position during the activities and stop the exercise if compensations are noted.

Alternatives

- Stand in unloading harness to take compressive loads off hip, knee, and ankle.
- Use the parallel bars to provide upper extremity support for one hand.
- Shift 75% of weight to the supporting leg with similar upper extremity reaction challenges.
- Split stance (lunge position)
- Start in double-leg stance, shift weight to unilateral stance as the upper body challenge is initiated. (e.g., shifting to one leg when catching a ball). This challenges weight shift, balance, and reaction speed.
- Use perturbations for the upper extremity movement (Bodyblade or shaking a ball) to elicit and challenge balance reactions (Exercise 10.22).

Progression

- Increase speed of movement.
- Increase range of motion of the upper extremity and trunk movement.
- Change the single-leg balance in full knee extension to slightly flexing the hip and knee joints (maintaining a mini-squat).
- Increase speed of changes in direction of external forces (unstable surfaces; (Fig. 9.27H and I; Video 3.13).
- Move from anticipated challenges to unanticipated challenges (Fig. 9.27C–G, J–P).
- Elastic resistance direction can be varied to challenge balance.
- Additional elastic resistance can be attached to the same leg to promote stabilization activity of the hip abductors or external rotators.
- Increase load by changing the lever arm of the resistance.
- Add unstable surfaces (Fig. 9.27H–P; Video 3.13).
- Challenge neuromuscular coordination by closing eyes to remove visual input.

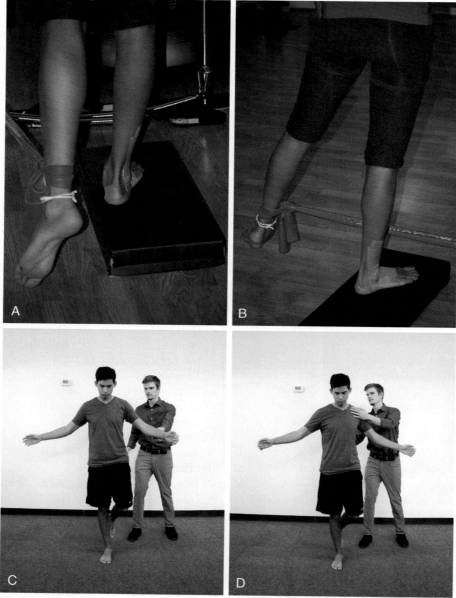

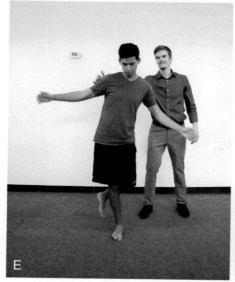

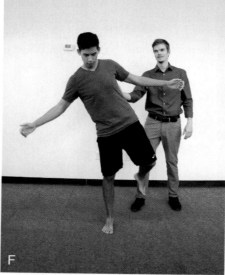

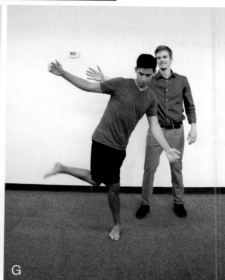

Fig. 9.27

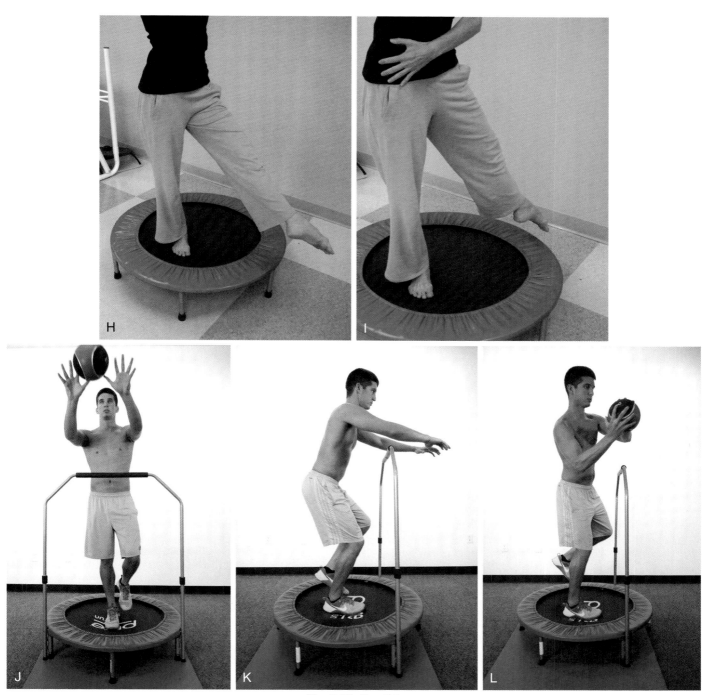

Fig. 9.27, Cont'd.

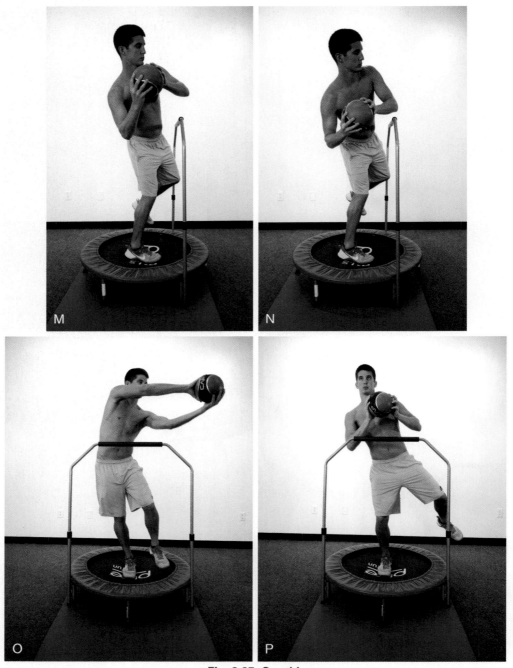

Fig. 9.27, Cont'd.

9.28 Side-stepping against elastic resistance

See Fig. 9.28.

Purpose
- Increase hip abductor strength
- Teach patient to initiate lateral movement with hip abductors
- Neuromuscular reeducation to improve frontal or rotational dynamic control for gait or for preparation for sports activities requiring sideways movement

Position
- Standing, mini-squat position with hips and knees slightly flexed, feet hip-distance apart.
- Elastic resistance band is tied around legs, just above the knees or ankles
- The band should be stretched in the starting position, but allow the legs to abduct slightly with movement

Action (Video 9.28A)
1. The patient initiates the movement by shifting the weight from the standing leg and abducting the free leg (Fig. 9.28A)
2. The trunk moves with the leading leg and is placed over the foot when it is set on the ground. (Fig. 9.28B)
3. After transferring the body weight to the leading leg, the patient takes a small step in the same direction with the other leg, placing the initial supporting leg under the body
4. Continue in the same direction for 10–15 steps, and then change direction.

Advantages
- Standing posture is functional
- This exercise can easily be assigned as a home exercise
- Simultaneous open and closed chain activity
- The side stepping action is important for athletes
- The elastic resistance challenges hip stability and can be used to train hip stabilization during weight transference.

Teaching tips
- Tying the elastic resistance band in a bow rather than a knot, allows for quicker adjustments to the band and easier donning and doffing
- Instruction examples:

  - "Keeping your pelvis level, take a step to the side followed by a smaller step with the other leg. Keep 12 to 18 inches between your feet at all times."
  - "Bring your body with your moving leg."
- Common errors to correct:
  - Avoid side-bending the trunk or hip hiking during this exercise
  - Watch for general trunk, pelvis, or hip rotation; dynamic lower extremity rotation (Video 9.28B); or valgus
  - If the trunk does not move over the supporting leg or the step is too big, dynamic valgus or rotation of the leading leg is likely
  - It is important to shift weight from one leg rather than lifting the hips to create the movement
  - Watch for signs of fatigue (the patient will start taking smaller steps and switch directions)
- Methods to prevent or address errors:
  - Teach the patient to observe for dynamic valgus, pelvis position, and rotation in a stationary squat first (Exercise 9.30), then use small steps sideways before progressive sideways steps
  - Ask the patient to be aware of the position of the pelvis and kneecaps facing forward during the movement
  - Place markers on the floor to help with the size of the step
  - Use a mirror or laser system around the pelvis to help with external focus
  - Check the amount of resistance on the band or change the position of the band to above the knees instead of the ankles

Alternatives
- Remove the band (Fig. 9.28C)
- Standing (Exercise 9.27) or side-lying hip abduction (Exercise 9.26) with resistance around ankle

Progression
- Increase resistance.
- Increase speed.
- Change directions more frequently.
- Hold a dumbbell or kettlebell in one hand with arm at 90 degrees of shoulder and elbow flexion.

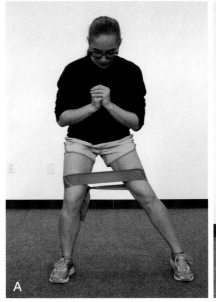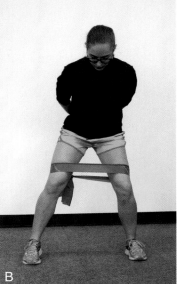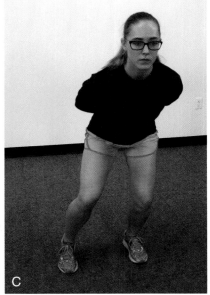

Fig. 9.28

ADJUST DYNAMIC BIOMECHANICAL ALIGNMENT

9.29   De-loaded squats

See Fig. 9.29.

Purpose

- Early vertical loading for individuals requiring slow progression of compression forces (osteoarthritis or after long periods of inactivity)
- Closed chain activity to strengthen multi-joint muscles of the lower extremities for patients who are unable to tolerate squats without increasing pain
- Functional training with decreased compressive loads
- Can be used to improve weight-bearing distribution
- Useful for individuals with evidence of fear avoidance

Position

- Standing, supported by a harness applied around the trunk and attached to a cable column (or mechanical device) to provide vertical support
  OR hold a latissimus pull-down bar pulled toward the chest or in front of the body with some resistance
- The amount of vertical load absorbed by the apparatus is determined by the patient's body weight and the amount of weight that provides symptom relief.

Action

1. Lower the body by flexing the hips and knees.
2. Maintain optimal lower extremity alignment of foot, ankle, knee, and hip in the sagittal plane (avoiding internal rotation and valgus throughout the movement) while maintaining equal weight-bearing on both legs.
3. On the upward motion, the patient presses through the feet, extends the hips and knees to return to standing, focusing on equal push through right and left foot.

Advantages

- Lower compressive forces at knee, hip, and ankle
- Functional training for transfers and squatting to the ground
- De-loaded exercise for patients with joint and cartilage damage or during recovery after fractures
- Closed chain activity minimizes shear forces and facilitates co-contraction, thereby increasing stability and providing proprioceptive input to the hip, knee, and ankle

Teaching tips

- See mini-squats (Exercise 9.30) and eccentric squats (Exercise 9.32) for instructions and common errors.
- The harness is positioned in line with the line of gravity to avoid leaning or tilting toward the line of pull of the harness.

Alternatives

- Perform on leg press machine or Pilates Reformer machine under very light load (less than body weight) or on Total Gym with low percentage body weight (closer to horizontal position).

Progression

- Decrease amount of support.
- Progress to full body weight double-leg mini-squat.
- Progress to single-leg squat with body weight support.
- Progress to single-leg squat without body weight support.

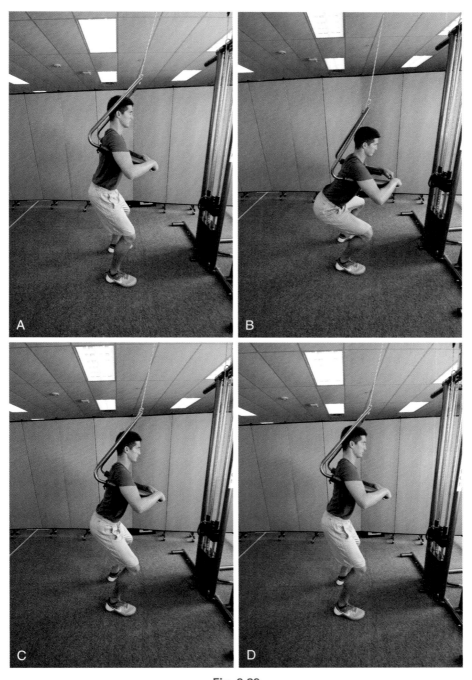

Fig. 9.29

9.30 Mini-squats with elastic resistance

See Fig. 9.30.

Purpose

- Train neuromuscular coordination for squat mechanics and alignment to avoid dynamic valgus or generalized internal rotation
- Challenge hip external rotator, abductor, and foot stabilizer activation and neuromuscular control
- Increase muscular endurance or strength of hip and knee extensor muscles
- Retrain neuromuscular coordination for sit-to-stand, squatting, or equal weight distribution

Position

- Standing, with hips, knees, and feet aligned with weight equally distributed between legs
- Elastic resistance band tied around the legs, above the knees
- Ensure that the bony alignment is in the patient's natural bony alignment (hip mid-position). Each person's mid-position will vary. Placing the foot "straight" or directly in the sagittal plane will not be the optimal position for most individuals because the tibia has some natural external rotation (10–15 degrees) resulting in a slightly toed-out position (see Table 9.1).
- If necessary, evaluate bony alignment in supine before standing.

Action (Video 3.12)

1. Lower the body as if sitting down in a chair. The hips and knees should flex simultaneously, with the trunk hinging forward (hip flexion) while maintaining the weight over the center of the feet (Fig. 9.30A).
2. Maintain pressure into the elastic band with the distal thighs to help prevent genu valgus during squat.
3. Activate the gluteus maximus and hamstrings to return to standing.

Advantages

- Functional training of the squat pattern controlling angulation and rotational forces
- Elastic resistance band provides feedback to increase proprioceptive feedback and facilitate hip abductor and external rotator muscle activation to maintain alignment.
- Closed chain activity minimizes shear forces and facilitates co-contraction, thereby increasing stability. Closed chain actions provide enhanced proprioceptive input to the hip, knee, and ankle than open chain movement.

Teaching tips

- Instruction examples:
  - "Press into the band and maintain the tension in the band as you squat and on the return."
  - "Maintain weight across all five toes as you squat."
- Common errors to correct:
  - Increased dynamic Q angle during squatting motion (increased pronation, genu valgus, tibial, and femoral internal rotation, hip adduction; Video 4.18).
  - Hip flexion and knee flexion should occur simultaneously.

- The pelvis should be level, with weight equally distributed, and symmetrical hip rotation. If there is less tension on the band from one leg, pelvic rotation or asymmetrical weight-bearing can be observed from the front (Fig. 9.30B).
- Observe for the position of the trunk behind the feet; if the center of mass is behind the base the relative external moment arm increases force on the patella (Video 3.25; see Chapter 2).
- One of the common misperceptions of ideal squat mechanics is the belief that the knees should not go "past the toes." Athletic movements and lifting an object from the floor will both require the patient to move their knees beyond their toes while squatting. The depth of the squat will determine the amount of knee flexion and hip flexion: the deeper the squat, the more the knees should be moving slightly past the toes. If the trunk is inclined forward, the overall forces at the hip and knee are distributed and the forces on the patellofemoral joint are lower than if the trunk is positioned behind the base of support (see Fig. 9.30C and D). The one circumstance when the knees should not go "past the toes" is after an ACL injury or repair in the healing time frames when anterior translation stress should be limited in the early stages of healing (especially in ranges between 0 and 45 degrees).
- The knee alignment is based on the individual's natural bony structure. Each person's mid-position may be slightly different. Typically, if the patella is facing forward in the sagittal plane, the patellofemoral complex is aligned within relative to the individual's bony structure. There is some natural tibial external rotation (10–15 degrees), and therefore placing the foot position "straight" or in the sagittal plane is not the optimal position for most individuals.
- Methods to prevent or address compensations:
  - Use lines in front of the body to guide the patient's visual target for the knee alignment.
  - Use a laser strapped to the thigh to visualize alignment sagittal alignment.
  - Use a mirror to demonstrate the desired movement or for the patient to monitor the alignment.
  - Ask the patient to hold the arms in front of the body to move the center of mass further forward over the base of support.
  - Use a small ball between the legs to maintain the distance between the legs instead of the resistance from the band (instruct the patient to "Squat while maintaining the ball between the knees" rather than squeezing the ball between the knees).
  - Stand with body against a gym ball on the wall and allow the ball to guide combined hip and knee flexion with a more forward trunk incline during the movement (Fig. 9.29E–G see Clinical Example 7.1).

Alternatives

- If the patient is unable to squat past 30 degrees with equal weight-bearing on a leg press, then a Total Gym, or Pilates Reformer machine with elastic resistance band around knees is an alternative to decrease load on the patellofemoral joint (Exercise 9.19) or de-loaded squats (Exercise 9.29).

- Mini-squats standing on a rocker board or foam can be used to challenge neuromuscular responses. The exercise can be performed with small-range squat action or isometrics at different ranges (see Clinical Example 7.6).

  Progression
- Increase range.
- Hold weights or a weighted bar in front of the body or next to the side.

- Add upper extremity arm movement with the squat (biceps curls, lateral raises).
- Hold the position at different ranges.
- Eliminate the elastic resistance band (less proprioceptive feedback).

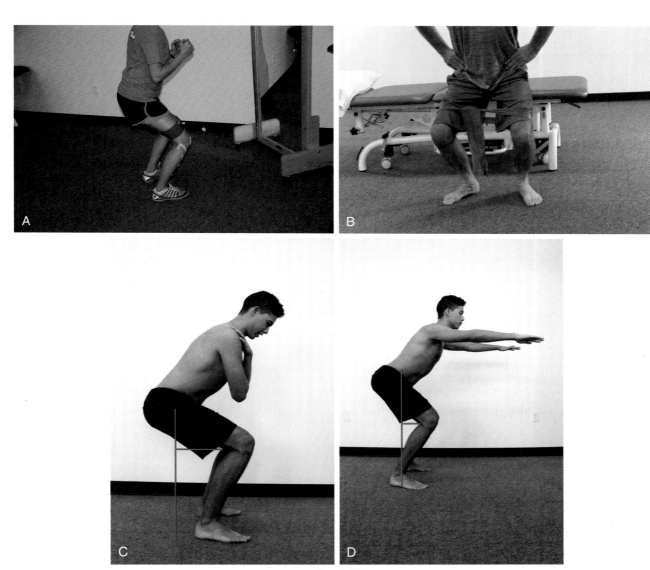

Fig. 9.30

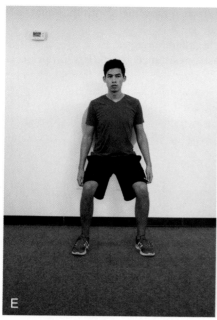
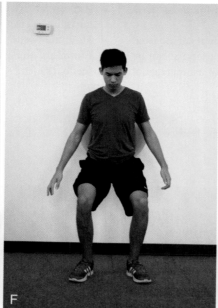
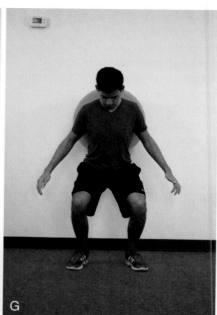

Fig. 9.30, Cont'd.

9.31 Step-ups and step-downs

See Fig. 9.31.

Purpose

- Increase strength of quadriceps, hamstrings, and gluteal muscles
- Functional training

Specific Precautions

- If the patient's dorsiflexion range of motion is limited, it will impact the knee and hip biomechanics during step-ups and -downs, but particularly during step-downs (Video 3.7). The ankle range of motion should be addressed as a priority before using this exercise, especially for primary patellofemoral diagnoses.

Position

- Standing behind the step
- Height of step is variable based on the patient's height and available range of motion, start with 2- to 4-inch step

Action

1. Place the foot of the involved leg on top of the step.
2. Maintain a neutral pelvis and supported trunk, but shift the trunk forward and slightly diagonally over the foot on the step.
3. Use both the hip and the knee to extend the supporting leg, pressing into the foot to lift the body vertically and diagonally forward up onto the step and over the front foot (Fig. 9.31A; Video 9.31A).
4. Step-down: The unsupported leg is moved toward the ground as the supporting leg controls the body weight by flexing the hip and knee. The center of mass should stay over the foot on the step until the patient is about to place weight on the leading leg (Video 9.31B).

Advantages

- Closed chain, functional movement to prepare for stair climbing
- Closed chain activity minimizes shear forces and facilitates co-contraction, thereby increasing stability and providing proprioceptive input.

Teaching tips

- Practice closed chain dorsiflexion on the ground before attempting the step-down exercise. Step-downs (and going down stairs) require full ankle dorsiflexion range of motion (10–15 degrees of dorsiflexion) to be able to control the body weight over the supporting leg.
- A typical household step is ~8 inches high.
- The average number of steps in a flight of stairs is 12.

- Pressing the heel into the step can help facilitate the gluteus maximus and hamstring muscles. This is particularly important for patients with a quad-dominant muscle activation pattern.
- The patient can be taught to push off with the bottom leg to assist the top leg when ascending stairs.
- Instruction examples:
  - "Lean forward as you go up the stairs. Press through your heel and you should feel your gluts, hamstrings and quadriceps working to lift you up the step, not just your quadriceps."
  - "Keep your weight over the foot on the step as you go down. Only move onto the foot on the ground at the end of the movement."
- Common errors to correct:
  - Watch for increased dynamic valgus angle (Video 4.16), early pelvis drop, or rotation during step-down due to decreased hip control or as a compensation for inadequate dorsiflexion (Fig. 9.31B).
  - Patients often hold their body weight back behind the leading leg in an attempt to avoid the pain. In this situation, the patient may need to practice the forward weight shift on a small step or on the ground before the step-up.

Alternatives

- Perform toe taps without moving through full range (Video 9.31C and D).
- Perform with an unweighting harness or buoyancy of water in a pool.
- Allow the patient to hold onto a counter or wall for support.
- Use a cane or practice in a stairwell with a handrail.
- Side step-up or step-down requires less dorsiflexion.
- Use an elastic resistance band for proprioceptive feedback for the leading leg (step-up) or the supporting leg (step-down) to cue hip muscle activation and neuromuscular control for alignment (see Clinical Example 7.1 and Fig. 9.31B, C; Video 7.8 and 9.31E).

Progression

- Increase repetitions (Videos 3.20 and 7.9).
- Increase speed or time the number of steps in a minute.
- Progress to step-up followed by step-down (step-up and over the step).
- Go up steps backward.
- Side step-ups.
- Increase height of step.

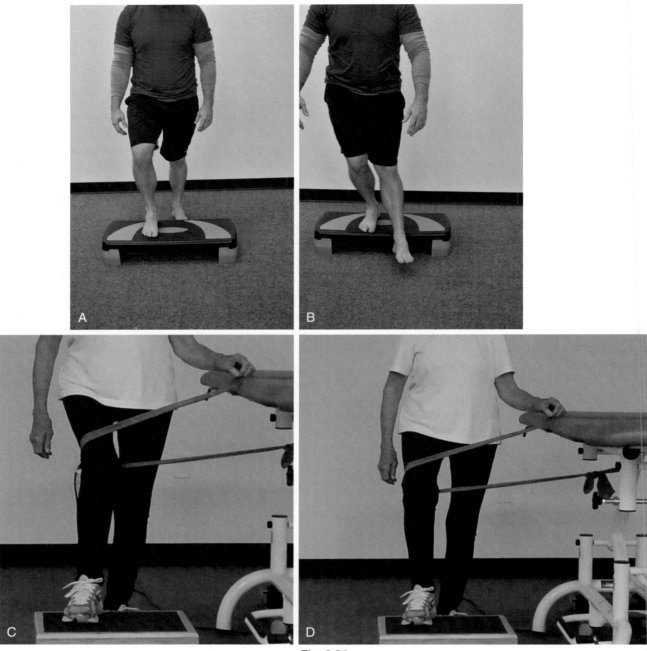

Fig. 9.31

PROMOTE TISSUE HEALING AND OPTIMAL REGENERATION: ECCENTRIC STIMULUS FOR TENDON

9.32 Eccentric control squats

See Fig. 9.32.

Purpose

- Provide tensile stimulus for patellar tendon regeneration
- Train eccentric control of the quadriceps and hip extensor muscles
- Functional alignment training for slower motion and descending actions
- Preparation for jump training (Fig. 9.32A–D; Videos 5.12–5.14)

Precautions

- The patient should demonstrate good control in the frontal and transverse planes throughout the desired squat range before introducing eccentric control squats.
- Control through a smaller range, short of excessive pain reproduction, can be used as a starting point.
- Evaluate pain during, immediately following, and in the subsequent days after introducing this exercise.
- If there is pain related to fat pad enlargement, avoid the terminal extension range, which may increase compression and reproduce pain.

Position

- Standing, with neutral lower extremity alignment (see mini-squats)
- Subtalar joint neutral (activate the intrinsic foot muscles to support the arch if there is excessive pronation)
- Weight is centered over the middle of the feet with symmetrical distribution between legs.

Action (Videos 4.21 and 4.22)

1. Slowly lower the body with control, flexing the hips and knees (eccentric phase).
2. Maintain equal weight-bearing and optimal lower extremity alignment of foot, ankle, knee, and hip in the sagittal plane (avoiding internal rotation and valgus throughout the movement).
3. Return to upright, pressing through the feet, extending the hips and knees to return to an upright posture, focusing on

equal push through each foot (concentric phase; this phase can be faster).

Advantages

- Specific stimulus for patella tendinopathy
- Functional activity
- Closed chain activity minimizes shear forces and facilitates co-contraction, thereby increasing stability and providing proprioceptive input to the hip, knee, and ankle.

Teaching tips

- See teaching tips for mini-squats
- Using an elastic resistance band to promote hip stabilization will provide proprioceptive feedback to maintain alignment (see mini-squats) (Fig. 9.32E and F; see Fig. 9.30A and B)
- Instruction example:
  - "Slowly control the squat on the way down, the slower the movement, the more the challenge."
- Common error to correct:
  - Watch for dynamic valgus and internal rotation particularly with fatigue (Fig. 9.32G).
- Methods to address compensation:
  - Add elastic resistance band above knees (placed under the feet and holding the ends of the band [Fig. 9.32A–D], tied around the ankles (Fig. 9.32E), or under the feet to add foot intrinsic control (Fig. 9.32F) and instruct patient to press into the band to avoid dynamic valgus (Video 3.12).
  - Use a mirror and ask the patient to concentrate on keeping the knees the same distance apart throughout the movement (Video 3.12).
  - Use a laser strapped above the knee and ask the patient to keep the laser pointing in the same direction throughout the movement.

Alternatives

- Provide assistance with an unweighting harness or hold onto a latissimus dorsi pull-down bar if unable to tolerate body weight load (Fig. 9.32C, D–G).

Progression

- Increase repetitions.
- Increase range or depth of the squat.
- Add external load.

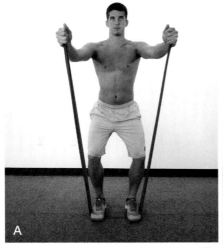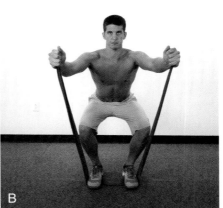

Fig. 9.32

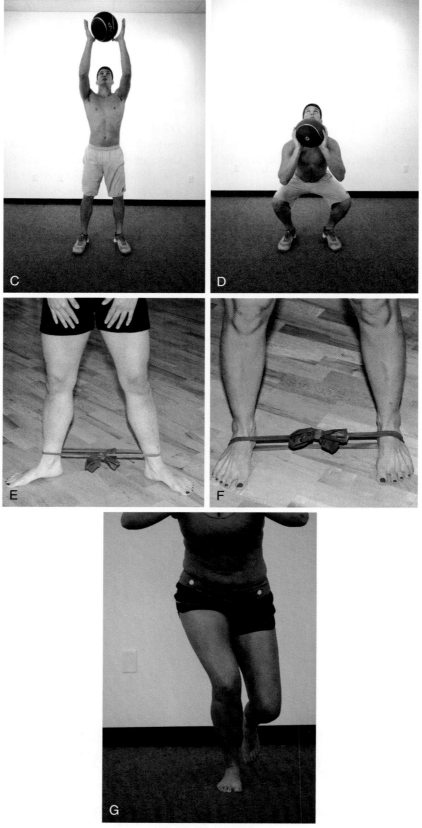

Fig. 9.32, Cont'd.

9.33 Eccentric control heel raises

See Fig. 9.33.

Purpose

- Concentric and eccentric strengthening of gastrocnemius/soleus complex, with specific loading to the Achilles tendon complex
- Challenge ankle and foot stability through the movement

Position

- Standing with the legs hip-width apart in the patient's natural bony mid-position and the knees unlocked at 0–5 degrees of flexion.
- The exercise can be conducted on the ground (Fig. 9.33A) or with the heels off a step (Fig. 9.33B–F).

Action (Video 2.4C and 9.33)

1. Shift weight forward onto balls of feet and activate gastrocnemius soleus complex to lift the heels (concentric control).
2. Slowly lower the heels toward the ground (eccentric control).

Advantages

- Functional strengthening
- Closed chain activity minimizes shear forces and facilitates co-contraction, thereby increasing stability and providing proprioceptive input to the hip, knee, and ankle.
- Does not require any equipment and can be easily replicated as a home exercise.

Alternatives

- Open chain plantarflexion against an elastic resistance band (Exercise 9.18)
- Reclined position on resistance equipment: leg press, Total gym or Pilates Reformer machine (Video 2.3)

Teaching tips

- A small wedge can be placed under the heel if the gastrocnemius complex flexibility is limited or if there is pain related to insertional tendinopathy at the end of range.
- If the patient has poor balance, start the exercise in the parallel bars or with hand support on a raised treatment table/counter.
- Instruction example:
  - "Keeping equal weight on all five toes, shift your weight forward and lift your heels off the ground."
  - "Slowly lower the heels using your calf muscles to control the movement"
- Common error to correct:
  - Loss of ankle stability. Rolling to the outside of the foot results in ankle inversion and rolling to the inside of the foot results in ankle eversion.
  - Allowing the heels to drop rapidly without eccentric control
  - Locking the knees or hyperextending the knees
- Methods to prevent or address compensations:
  - Manual correction of the foot position (Fig. 9.33B)
- Ask the patient to count through the lowering eccentric movement using twice the time compared to the concentric heel raise.

Progression

- Single-leg heel raise in standing (Fig. 9.33B)
- Add handheld weights.
- Decrease the speed of eccentric descent.
- Increase range for the lowering off the edge of a step (Fig. 9.33F).

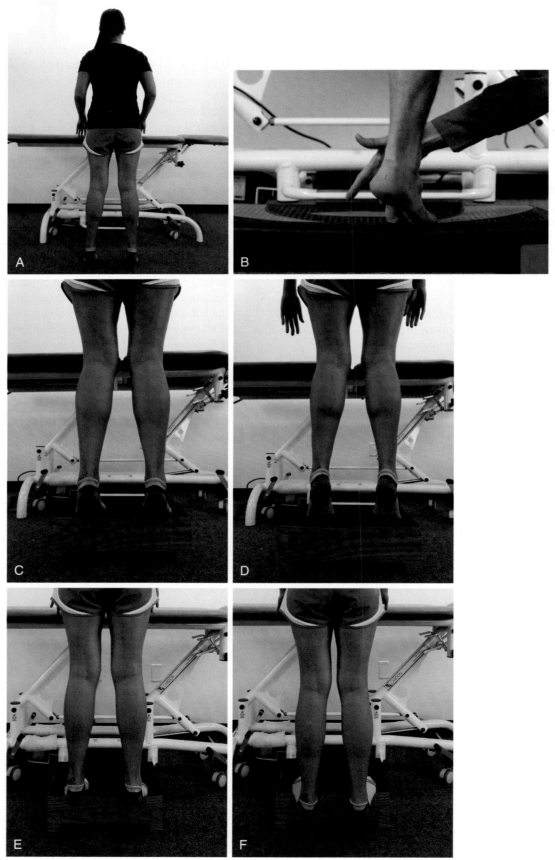

Fig. 9.33

9.34 Hip hinges

See Fig. 9.34.

Purpose
- Increase strength of gluteus maximus and hamstrings (eccentric and concentric gluteus maximus and hamstring activity occurs as the pelvis moves forward and backward on the head of the femur).
- Train dissociation of hip from lumbopelvic motion. Stabilizing the spine as the pelvis moves forward teaches the patient how to bend forward at the hips rather than through the spine.
- Provide stimulus for hamstring tendon insertion regeneration through eccentric tensile loading

Position
- Standing, feet hip distance apart
- Hold a 36-inch dowel against contact points of spine— sacrum, thoracic, and back of head— with one hand behind head stabilizing dowel high and one hand behind back stabilizing dowel against sacrum.

Action
1. Flex the hips (by leaning forward from the hips) without changing contact of the spine against the dowel (Fig. 9.34A).
2. Continue the movement until the hips are flexed to 60 degrees (Fig. 9.34B).
3. Using the hip extensors, return the trunk to a vertical position without changing the contact points on the dowel (Fig. 9.34C).

Advantages
- Closed chain activity minimizes shear forces and facilitates co-contraction thereby increasing stability and providing proprioceptive input to the hip, knee, and ankle.
- Functional movement to teach forward bending with correct body mechanics.

Teaching tips
- Instruction examples:
  - "This exercise will teach you to move from your hips as opposed to your spine when you are bending forward. Control the movement slowly on the way down using the muscles at the back of the leg."
  - "Keep the dowel in contact with your spine as you bend forward from your hips."
- Common errors to correct:
  - Hyperextending the knees
  - Excessive weight shifting posteriorly onto the heels while hinging forward at the hips
  - Losing or changing contact points on the dowel is indicative of spinal flexion.
- Methods to prevent or address compensations:
  - Start with knees slightly flexed to avoid hyperextending knees.

Alternatives
- Teach hip hinge in sitting before doing the exercise in standing. The patient can learn how to differentiate hip motion from lumbopelvic motion before adding the challenge of stabilizing the lower extremities in standing

Progression
- Decrease speed during hip flexion to challenge eccentric control using the hamstrings.
- Once able to stabilize spine correctly, perform the exercise without the dowel.
- Reach one or both hands in line with the body during the hinging motion to increase overall leverage and challenge spinal stability.
- Hold a weight to further increase the load.
- Single-leg hip hinges are used to target hamstring and gluteal strengthening or optimal stimulus for the hamstring tendon with eccentric control past 45 degrees of hip flexion. The opposite leg can be extended behind the body to increase leverage and load (single-leg deadlift [Video 2.11, 2.14]) (Fig. 9.34E).
- Reach in multiple directions to add directional stimulus.
- Hold an elastic resistance band in each hand and add a rowing action as the patient returns to vertical to challenge trunk extension. The band can be anchored at waist-height and then lowered to knee- or ankle-height.

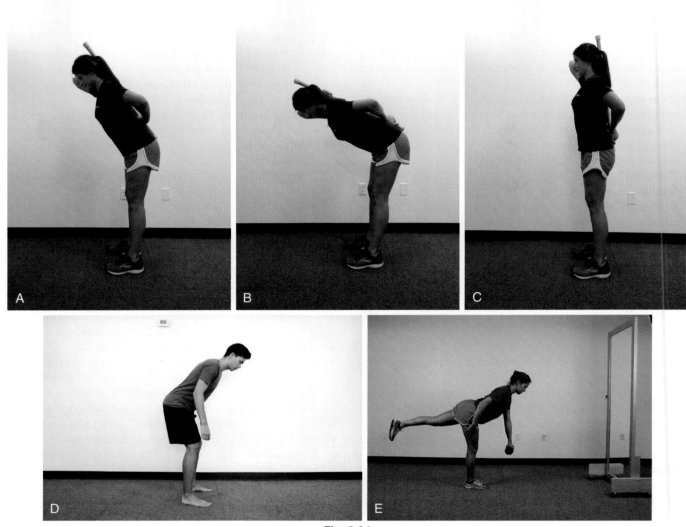

Fig. 9.34

IMPROVE NEUROMUSCULAR COORDINATION AND RESPONSE TIME FOR FUNCTIONAL REQUIREMENTS

9.35   Star balance

See Fig. 9.35.

Purpose
- Improve balance
- Increase lower extremity proprioception and stability
- Increase strength
- Increase endurance
- Challenge pelvic and lower extremity dynamic alignment

Position
- Standing on involved leg, hip and knee slightly flexed, chest over foot, pelvis neutral
- Subtalar joint neutral (activate the intrinsic foot muscles to support the arch if there is excessive pronation)
- Adjust the standing foot alignment with respect to the tape if there is tibial torsion.
- The exercise can be performed on the floor with tape placed in a variety of planes to provide targets.

Action (Fig. 9.35A–D)
1. Maintaining stance posture on injured limb, flex the supporting knee and hip and reach the unsupported leg forward, sideways, and backward or at a diagonal as far as possible.
2. The task for this exercise is to maintain balance on the standing leg while reaching with the free leg.

Advantages
- Closed chain activity minimizes shear forces and facilitates co-contraction thereby increasing stability and providing proprioceptive input to the hip, knee, and ankle.
- Closed chain activity has lower shear forces and co-contraction and challenges proprioception.
- The reaching activity provides an external target while challenging single-leg control.
- Challenges lower extremity and pelvic stability, neuromuscular coordination, and proprioception

Teaching tips
- Instruction examples:
  - "Maintain your balance on your supporting leg and reach your opposite heel toward each line."
  - "Touch the heel (or toe) lightly on the tape but return to a balanced position each time."
- Common errors to correct:
  - Patients will often try to reach as far as they can and allow the standing leg to compensate to achieve a greater distance for the reach.
- Methods to address or prevent compensations:
  - Therapists should encourage accuracy and ask patients to maintain the alignment; only reward larger distance if the alignment is maintained.

Alternatives
- Add an elastic resistance band around the support leg to provide feedback.
- Knee extended instead of flexed (supporting leg); the reach will be smaller
- Different trunk and lower extremity relationships (e.g., leaning forward in skating position)
- Balancing on one leg, reach hand toward target on the star line instead of the foot
- Y balance position instead of the star using tape on the floor or the measurement device (Fig. 9.35E–G)

Progression
- Increase speed.
- Change the order of directions.
- Add an elastic resistance band.
- Respond to instructions for different directions.
- Alternate support limb followed by reaching.
- Add a dynamic weight shift onto the foot followed by a single-leg reach.
- Add lunges in different directions (Video 9.49).
- Add jumps to land in different directions (Video 9.51).

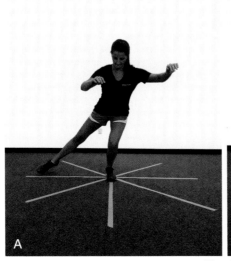
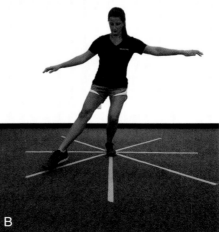

Fig. 9.35

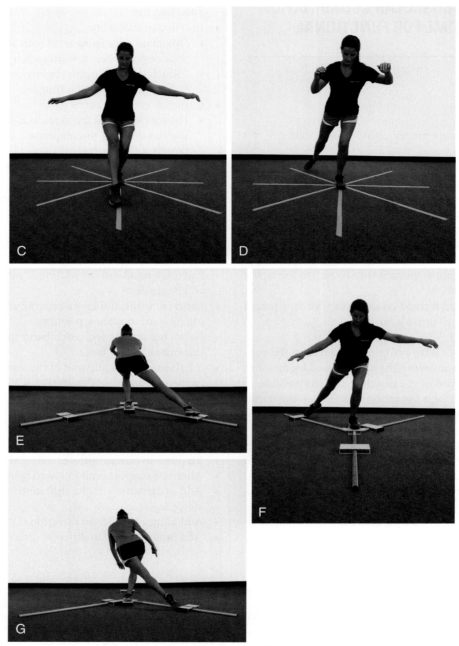

Fig. 9.35, Cont'd.

9.36   Functional movement reeducation: running

See Fig. 9.36.

Purpose

- Improve running mechanics using neuromuscular and visual input
- Minimize energy loss
- Increase tissue tolerance to ground reaction forces
- Graded return to forward running.

Position

- Stand, preferably in front of a mirror
- Place a line of tape down center of mirror for patient to assess alignment and movement.
- Treadmill

Action

1. Videotape walking (without instructions) and running on the treadmill in front of a mirror.
2. Assess foot strike position, lateral weight shift of hips, vertical displacement of trunk, position of trunk relative to foot strike, and trunk lean. Hip, knee, and ankle angles can be measured, along with qualitative analysis of the movement pattern by the therapist.
3. The patient is asked to observe and comment on symmetry.
4. Gradually increase walking speed while continuing assessment of preceding movements. Average normal values for males = 1.37 m/sec (3 mph), females = 1.5 m/sec [22]; fast speed is considered as between 3 and 4 mph.
5. As speed increases, foot strike pattern should narrow toward midline. Observe for excessive vertical displacement and lateral movement and provide corrections.
6. After identifying gait and fast speed gait deviations, provide 1–2 external cues for corrections if needed. Practice for 5–10 minutes with the patient observing the pattern in the mirror.
7. Remove mirror and see if the pattern is retained. Videotape for 30 seconds and compare, pointing out the desired patterns and deviations to the patient.
8. Continue until able to perform the patterns, then start to introduce running. Running is characterized by periods when both feet are off the ground.
9. Run in place for 1 minute and then return to walking speed for 1 minute. Continue to alternate running and walking for 10 minutes.

Advantages

- Encourages independence and transitioning to discharge from physical therapy by teaching patient to detect and modify gait deviations.
- Easy to modify durations.

Teaching tips

- Instruction examples:
  - "Lean forward slightly at the hips; allow your body to help your forward movement."
  - "Keep your feet under your body as much as possible."
- Common errors to correct:
  - Hip drop or Trendelenburg
  - Asymmetrical stance time
  - Limited pelvis/trunk rotation
  - Reaching with the lead leg in front of the body
  - Leaning backward or a vertical trunk rather than a slight forward lean from the hips
  - Slow cadence
  - Prolonged stance time or heavy landing
- Methods to address or prevent compensations:
  - Gait deviations while walking on level terrain should be resolved before introducing running.
  - Use a metronome to set higher cadence goals for the patient.
  - Use a mirror or videotape the patient and display on a smartphone or television screen to provide concurrent feedback.

Alternatives

- Decrease load if unable to control compensations by running in a pool, or use an unweighting device with a harness.

Progression

- Practice walking on level terrain, increasing the cadence or velocity first.
- Increase time.
- Decrease time walking, increase time running.
- Increase speed (gait or running).
- Add change of directions or sports specificity if needed.
- Increase slope last.

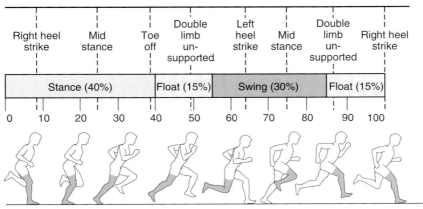

RUNNING

Fig. 9.36 (From Magee DJ. *Orthopedic Physical Assessment*. 5th ed. St. Louis, MO: Elsevier Saunders; 2007.)

◎ CASE STUDY 9.3: LOWER EXTREMITY REPETITIVE STRAIN PATELLOFEMORAL SYNDROME

This case study illustrates (1) a progression of exercises from Phase I through Phase III for a repetitive strain injury, (2) use of subjective information to guide objective testing choices, and (3) functional movement assessment and training.

A 36-year-old accountant is referred to physical therapy with a diagnosis of patellofemoral syndrome and patella tendinopathy (Unn Fig. 9.3). He reports an onset of intermittent bilateral knee pain approximately 1 year ago with progressively increasing frequency of symptoms.

Patient Goals

He wants to be able to sit for at least an hour, to negotiate stairs without pain, and return to basketball.

Subjective Complaints

- *Severity*: In the past 2 weeks, the pain in the right knee has progressed from intermittent to constant (3/10) and is significantly limiting his function. He reports pain going down stairs, running, or landing from jumps (6/10). Sitting for longer than 30 minutes requires moving (4/10).

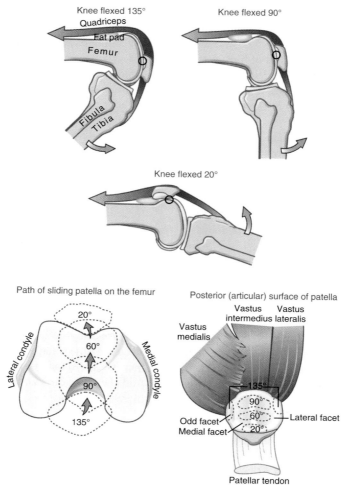

From Neumann DA. *Kinesiology of the Musculoskeletal System.* 3rd ed. St. Louis, MO: Elsevier; 2017.

Functional Status

In the past 2 weeks, he has not been able to negotiate stairs, run, or play basketball. He is also having difficulty sitting for more than 30 minutes and reports puffiness and swelling in the kneecap region. The lower extremity functional scale (LEFS) self-reported measure is 46/80.

- *Irritability*: Pain returns to pre-exercise levels 30 minutes after playing basketball. Pain with sitting for more than 30 minutes decreases when he stands up and walks around for 5 minutes.
- *Nature*: Symptoms are consistent with patellofemoral syndrome (repetitive strain).
- *Stage*: Phase I, chronic

See Box 9.8 for interpretation of subjective information.

BOX 9.8 Interpretation of Subjective Information

The patient's symptoms are consistent with patellofemoral syndrome.[49,50] His MODERATE severity (pain levels, increasing difficulty with stairs, running) and MODERATE irritability for higher level forces (running and jumping) indicate the need to limit testing for movements that increase pain above 4/10, and running or jumping are not planned for the initial evaluation. A history of repetitive strain injury calls for full consideration of contributing impairments at the hip, knee, and ankle. Static and dynamic bony alignment should be assessed first, followed by range of motion, flexibility, and muscle function in supine, sitting, or prone. Functional testing in upright loaded positions (sit-to stand, squats, steps, single-leg balance, and gait) will be limited to assessing dynamic movement patterns without increasing pain levels above 4/10. Functional endurance and strength tests will be delayed until the severity and irritability decreases.

BOX 9.9 Treatment Focus for Early Treatment

- Flexibility exercises to improve ankle dorsiflexion and hip extension are indicated to help distribute forces, while soft tissue mobilization and manual patella mobilization is used to assist local mobility.[51]
- Introduce quadriceps and patellar tendon loading in inner range to limit strain on tendon while promoting tissue recovery but avoid full knee extension due to fat pad enlargement.[13] Early hip muscle strengthening is introduced without high loads on the knee, especially with the moderate severity and irritability.[56–60]
- Limit angulation and rotation and address biomechanics to limit force on the patellofemoral region.[52,54,55]

Objective Findings

- *Posture/alignment*: Bilateral pronation, tibial varus and torsion (lateral external rotation 20 degrees), knee hyperextension. Equal leg length and femoral rotation within normal ranges.
- *Girth*: There is moderate effusion around the suprapatellar region (1 cm difference above the patella and at the joint line) and both fat pads are enlarged.
- *Range of motion and muscle length*:
  - *Ankle*: Decreased gastrocnemius flexibility bilaterally (lacks 10 degrees of dorsiflexion)
  - *Knee*: Within normal limits, but very painful with active extension (5/10) from 10 degrees of flexion to 0 degrees. The asymptomatic knee range is 135 degrees to 10 degrees of hyperextension.
  - *Hip*: Within normal limits except for positive Ober's test (iliotibial band mobility) and restricted gluteal flexibility at 110 degrees of hip flexion combined with adduction, tight tensor fascia latae.
  - *Palpation*: The patellofemoral joint, infrapatellar fat pad, and retinaculum are tender to palpation, with the right knee being more painful than the left. The lateral retinaculum mobility is restricted, as is iliotibial band and quadriceps mobility. The fat pads are enlarged bilaterally, and there is pain with patella medial, lateral, and superior glide.
- *Muscle function*:
  - *Manual muscle testing*: all resisted tests 5/5, but resisted knee extension reproduces pain in the patella tendon region of the right knee.
- *Local and global stabilizer activation and muscle endurance testing for right hip muscles*:
  1. Hip abductors: Completes eight repetitions of side-lying hip abduction with correct form before showing signs of fatigue
  2. Hip external rotators: Completes 14 repetitions of hip external rotation in side-lying before showing signs of specific fatigue
  3. Hip extension: Completes >25 repetitions in standing with support for the upper body on the plinth without fatigue, able to perform 15 repetitions using a 2 kg cuff weight without increasing knee pain and 8 repetitions with a 4 kg cuff weight
- *Functional tests (dynamic alignment, movement patterns, pain)*:
  - Bilateral squat reproduces pain the patella tendon region (5/10) at 45 degrees of flexion, progressively increasing

with increased flexion to 6/10 at 60 degrees. Dynamic valgus and overall internal rotation occurs early in the squat at 45 degrees with excessive posterior shift of his center of mass (behind his feet.) The squat is discontinued and repetitions are not tested; single-leg squats are not tested due to the severity and irritability of his symptoms.
  - Single-leg balance is unsteady and increases his pain to 4/10.
  - He sits with his right knee flexed 30 degrees and primarily uses his left leg to stand up from sitting.
  - Antalgic gait with short stride length on the left, short stance and no push-off on the right

Evaluation

- *Physical therapy diagnosis*: Patellofemoral joint syndrome with fat pad enlargement and possible patella tendinopathy.[13,49,50]

Contributing Impairments

- Bony alignment (tibial varus and torsion, pronation)[14]
- Limited dorsiflexion (gastrocnemius/soleus flexibility)[51]
- Decreased gluteal and tensor fascia latae muscle flexibility
- Decreased soft tissue mobility around the lateral aspect of the knee, iliotibial band, and lateral retinaculum
- Enlarged fat pad and effusion contributing to pain in terminal extension as well as pain with resisted knee extension, consistent with patella tendinopathy and fat pad irritation[13]
- Decreased hip muscle endurance/strength of the hip abductors, extensors, and external rotators[52,53]
- Neuromuscular coordination and compensatory patterns for squats, sit-to-stand, gait: antalgia, dynamic valgus, internal rotation, body weight is positioned behind his base.[52–54]

Precautions

- Limit knee angulation and rotation, limit exercise in terminal extension and loads in weight-bearing positions with flexion more than 60 degrees.

Prognosis

- Good for resolution of symptoms with less aggressive activities secondary to motivation and potential for improvement in ankle dorsiflexion and hip muscle flexibility. Patient was able to correct dynamic alignment with correction in first visit.
- Enlarged fat pad may prolong time for pain-free full extension (see Box 9.9).[13]

TABLE 9.9 Local and Global Stabilizer Endurance and Strength to Distribute Forces[53,56-60]

Exercise	Parameters	Rationale and Modifications
Side-lying hip abduction to increase muscle activation and endurance of the left gluteus medius (Exercise 9.26B)	Six repetitions of side-lying hip abduction with correct form 3 sets at zero degrees extension in bony alignment, open chain to limit forces on patellofemoral region in full extension based on natural bony alignment	Global stabilizer strength aimed to distribute forces from the knee and to support the femoral-pelvic relationship
Clamshell to increase left hip external rotation activation, muscle endurance (Exercise 9.26A)	Twelve repetitions of hip external rotation in side lying before specific fatigue 3 sets	Local stabilizer endurance aimed to distribute forces from the knee and to limit angulation and dynamic valgus
Hip extension supported by plinth (Exercise 9.45 alternative: Hip extension with torso supported by plinth)	Six to eight repetitions with 4-kg strap-on weight 60–0 degrees	Global mover strengthening in preparation for neuromuscular training in closed chain activities to decrease force on the patellofemoral joint
Single-leg stance balance activities in subtalar joint neutral stance for neuromuscular retraining to improve rotational control in left lower extremity (Exercise 9.27)	Single-leg balance on foam; 3 sets for as long as possible: able to manage 20–30 seconds	Medial-lateral stability, foot position control, and facilitation of local stabilizer activation
Reclined double-leg squats on a leg press (Exercise 9.19)	Double-leg squats in the patient's natural alignment with elastic resistance around the upper thighs to provide sensory input to encourage hip external rotator and abductor engagement. Resistance equivalent to 50% of the patient's body weight provides sufficient challenge for quadriceps fatigue after 16 repetitions from 60 to 10 degrees.	The supported position limits the need for balance responses and reduces the resistance from the patient's body weight. The proprioceptive support and position also allows the patient to observe his legs to decrease angulation while the elastic resistance helps with feedback.

Initial Exercise and Treatment Choices

For flexibility and soft tissue mobility treatment choices (Table 9.9)
- Dorsiflexion standing lunge stretch with alignment matching the natural bony position and maintaining weight over the side being stretched. Alignment is modified to accommodate tibial torsion and a pad is used under the midfoot to limit pronation (Exercise 9.13).
- Gluteus maximus stretching (Exercise 9.10)
- ITB stretching without knee flexion (Exercise 9.14)
- Soft tissue mobilization (lateral retinaculum and quadriceps insertions into iliotibial band)
- Taping for de-loading and pain relief of the fat pad and patella tendon during early sessions

Muscle activation, endurance, and strengthening choices: (see Table 9.9)

After 2 Weeks (Box 9.10)

Subjective Complaints

His knee pain is more intermittent; he is able to tolerate sitting for 45 minutes with less pain (3/10) and has less pain when negotiating stairs (pain 4/10).

Objective Findings

- *Flexibility and soft tissue mobility*: While his dorsiflexion is still limited (2 degrees), and the Ober's test is still positive, he has less difficulty and tension with the gastrocnemius, gluteal, and ITB stretching. There is less difficulty and pain with patella glides and soft tissue mobility techniques.

BOX 9.10 Interpretation of Status at 2 Weeks

- Pain at rest and with movement has decreased.
- Flexibility is improving but still needs further improvements.
- Knee extension has improved but still needs 5 degrees of hyperextension.
- Squat mechanics and pain responses have improved, but single-leg squat tolerance is difficult and, if added to the exercise program, may need additional arm support.[55,56,60]
- Step-ups on a 2-inch step are possible with adjustments of his movement to a forward trunk position.[61-63] Step-down exercise is slowly introduced once the step-up exercise is mastered.[55]

- *Range of motion*: Active knee extension is less painful up to zero degrees of extension. Five degrees of hyperextension is possible but painful.
- *Functional movement testing*:
  - *Bilateral squat*: Movement is still painful, but pain has decreased to 4/10 starting at 60 degrees of flexion, and he is able to squat to 80 degrees without further increase in symptoms. He is able to complete 12 repetitions without additional increase in pain.
  - *Single-leg quarter-squat*: Pain 4/10 on right compared to 3/10 on left, but he is able to squat further (45 degrees) on the left. He maintains the line of gravity behind the knee throughout the movement and presents with a dynamic valgus in both legs, but greater on the right than the left. He is able to perform five single-leg quarter-squats on either leg with increased pain to 6/10 on the right compared to 5/10 on the left.

- *Step-up/down*: On a 4-inch step, step-up is somewhat painful (4/10), and step-down is very painful (6/10). His normal movement pattern is to maintain his center of mass behind the knee throughout movement. He is able to manage a 2-inch step with 3/10 pain for step-ups, and his pain decreases to a 1/10 if his trunk is inclined forward over his leading leg.

Exercise and Treatment Progression From 2 to 6 Weeks (Phase II)

1. Continue *flexibility exercises* as a home program, increasing the range and time held in the fully stretched position.
2. Continue *soft tissue mobilization* and teach self-mobilization with a foam roller and massage balls for the lateral retinaculum.
3. Assign *open chain strengthening exercises* as a home program, increasing load as the patient is able to perform more than 10 repetitions before specific muscle fatigue.
4. Increase *specific load for patella tendon* stimulus by increasing resistance using *closed chain exercise*. Reclined *double-leg partial squats* are performed up to 60 degrees of flexion (isotonic) and isometrics are performed with slightly higher resistance at 30 and 45 degrees of flexion on a Pilates Reformer (Exercise 9.19). The range and position produces less compressive force on the patellofemoral joint[64] and less tension on the tendon,[13] and the equipment provides loads less than body weight. Initial isometric loads are established to fatigue the quadriceps between 20 and 30 seconds for the isometric holds and to fatigue the quadriceps between 15 and 20 repetitions as long as there is no pain increase during or after the exercise. Loads are gradually increased to target strength and additional tissue adaptations if there are no adverse responses to the exercise. Once there is no pain with isometrics at various angles and minimal pain (<3/10), isotonic exercises are included in small ranges, progressing the range as tolerated.[13] Range is limited to less than 60 degrees of flexion and up to 0 degrees. Load is set for endurance (15–20 repetitions), progressing to loads with fatigue between 6–10 repetitions.
5. *Single-leg open chain isometric knee extension* at 30 degrees is performed using a leg extension machine (maintaining alignment to minimize tendon angulation). Resistance that induces fatigue within 20–30 seconds is used for initial dosage (Exercise 9.43). Load is increased first, to the level where fatigue occurs within 10–15 seconds. Isotonic exercise is added next, initially with small-range concentric extension then with eccentric control on the return.
6. *Single-leg standing balance exercise* is progressed by maintaining isometric knee flexion (30 degrees) while challenging the stability using pulley resistance (or a multi-hip machine) for hip flexion/extension, abduction/adduction for the opposite leg (Exercise 9.20).
7. *Functional movement adjustments* are introduced for sit-to-stand mechanics (Exercise 9.47) and step-ups (Exercise 9.31), moving the center of mass over the foot early by leaning the trunk forward.[61,62] Similar to the step-up mechanics, the forward lean decreases the lever arm, placing the body weight further forward over the foot. Movement sequence and force distribution is also adjusted by encouraging the patient to use the hip extensors for the vertical movement. The hip abductors and rotators are also important to limit angulation and rotation, and visual feedback can be provided using mirrors or visual targets to maintain the lower extremity alignment; tactile input using elastic resistance is helpful in the early practice phases.[43] The range and repetitions are increased as the movement becomes less painful, and the patient is able to perform the movement using the appropriate mechanics. Single-leg lunges are added to the program (isometrics and isotonics) with a forward trunk lean.[63]
8. *Promote sagittal plane alignment to match bony position while preventing dynamic valgus and early pronation* using elastic resistance to promote external rotator and abductor activation during sit-to-stand, step-ups, and isometric squat positions. Motor learning concepts are applied to teach the desired pattern with concurrent feedback, progressing to self-monitoring using a mirror.[63]

Exercise Progression and Return to Function at 6 Weeks (Phase III)

As the patient progresses, remaining impairments are addressed to prepare the patient to return to playing basketball. The load is increased and functional training is progressed to multiple planes with higher-level challenges and increased speed.

1. During Phase III, the patient continues the mobility and flexibility exercises as a home program.
2. The muscle function exercise load is increased throughout range while still teaching neuromuscular control to promote force distribution and minimize angulation focused at the patellofemoral complex. Double-leg squats are progressed to single-leg squats on the equipment and then progressed to standing. Step-ups are progressed by increasing the height, the speed of the movement, and ensuring accuracy of the alignment, followed by step-downs and emphasizing control during the eccentric phase of the squats and the step-downs.
3. This phase emphasizes restoring functional capabilities, and more time is allocated during treatment sessions for progressively challenging speed, complexity, and directional changes. Malliaras[13] describes the next stage of progression toward full functional movement and sport for patella tendinopathy as "addressing energy-storage." In order to prepare for this stage, Malliaris[13] suggests that patients wanting to return to jumping should be able to perform single-leg leg-press or similar exercises against approximately 150% of body weight for 8–10 repetitions without increasing pain during or after the exercise (within 24 hours), as well as performing single-leg squats without difficulty. The patellar tendon must absorb a considerable amount of force when landing from a vertical jump; around 5 times body weight is absorbed within a very short time frame.[65] Important parameter considerations for this stage are speed, height of jumping or lowering, rest periods, and complexity of directions and movement.[13,65–67]

Squat Progression. *Double- and single-leg squats*: Speed of the upward motion is increased, but the movement is slowed down during the return phase to target eccentric lengthening contractions with progressive load targeting the connective tissue regeneration. Squat mechanics should be corrected to ensure adequate hip flexion and a forward trunk lean without dynamic valgus.[68]

Return to Running. The patient is encouraged to maintain a forward trunk position during running to decrease stress on the patellofemoral region and encourage the forward momentum.[69] He is encouraged to adjust his heel strike landing pattern to more midfoot contact by decreasing his anterior reach in front of his body.[70] His running cadence is increased using a metronome while running on the treadmill with real-time feedback from a live-streamed video projected in front of him to a television screen. A paced running program is introduced with walk/jog intervals every other day, followed by increasing time and then increasing the length of the jogging intervals.

Jump Progression on Equipment (Box 9.11).

1. Double-leg jumps are started on a Pilates Reformer (with a trampoline). Range is limited to 60 degrees. Dosage is established using light springs, low repetitions, and adequate recovery time between sets. Therapy sessions are scheduled once a week to allow adequate time for the tendon to recover and regenerate.[13]
2. The number of jumps is based on quadriceps fatigue and alignment rather than stopping movement for low levels of pain (3/10 or less). The therapist observes the patient carefully and suggests corrections if the patient does not maintain proper alignment or weight-bearing symmetry. The

number of sets is progressed slowly with at least 2 minutes recovery time between sets.

Jump Progression.

- Double-leg vertical jumps on trampoline, progressing to single-leg jumps (trampoline helps encourage using the momentum of the downward motion to store and release the energy for the jumping action and provides immediate feedback if the patient "freezes" or stiffens during the landing).
- Low height and depth jumps on land
- Drop jumps (double-leg) from a small step, progress to greater height.
- Split squat jumps
- Single-leg vertical hops in place for endurance (to fatigue)
- Run-up and jump progressing toward sports-specific drills

BOX 9.11 Jumping Reeducation and Training

- Teaching a patient to land jumps properly includes strategies for controlling shock absorption, utilizing *all* lower extremity joints (not just the knees) and a soft, eccentric landing rather than rigid co-contractions.[66,67]
- Landing with the trunk pitched slightly forward helps distribute vertical ground-reaction forces between the hip and knee and reduces the relative moment arm for the patellofemoral joint and patella tendon tension.[65-67]
- The sound, or feeling of landing "hard" or "soft" will provide immediate feedback about whether or not the patient has achieved a soft landing.

SECTION 9.4: POSTSURGICAL MANAGEMENT

GENERAL EXERCISE APPROACHES

The major priorities after surgery or trauma are to protect the injured or surgically repaired structures from excessive force and tension, with slow progressive introduction of forces suitable to stimulate new tissue regeneration over the course of treatment. Treatment follows principles for phases of management with different timelines based on the type of tissue, surgical incisions, and type of surgery. While the damaged tissue recovers, early exercise will focus on preventing loss of range of motion and minimizing atrophy during weight-bearing or movement restrictions. Postsurgical management will progress from protective management and resolving range of motion in the healing phase, to restoring motion, strength, and function as the healing constraints and postsurgical protocol allows. Principles outlined in the preceding sections may be appropriate to regain sufficient range of motion or flexibility (Section 9.1); promote muscle activation, endurance, and strength related to limited structural stability (Section 9.2); and address contributing factors such as biomechanical alignment and neuromuscular coordination or impairments related to prolonged immobilization or weight-bearing restrictions (Section 9.2).

Typical postsurgical diagnoses in this category for the lower extremity include:
- Joint arthroplasty (hip, knee, and ankle replacement)
- Arthroscopic joint debridement, microfracture (hip, knee, ankle)
- Meniscus repair or meniscectomy
- Hip labral repair
- Ligament repair or reconstruction (anterior cruciate, posterior cruciate, medial or lateral collateral ligaments knee, medial or lateral collateral ligaments ankle)
- Tendon repair (Achilles tendon, patella tendon)
- Fracture internal or external fixation
- Osteotomy (femoral, tibial, bunionectomy)
  Trauma diagnoses:
- Ligament tears (knee, ankle)
- Tendon tears (patella, tibialis posterior, Achilles tendon)
- Muscle tears (hamstring, adductors, quadriceps, gastrocnemius)

CONTRAINDICATIONS AND PRECAUTIONS

During the early healing time frames, weight-bearing or specific range of motion may be avoided completely or limited (see Chapter 2). Forces are introduced slowly after early healing is present.

Precautions are specific for the tissue properties including the type of force, direction, and length of tissue:
- Bone: Avoid rotation, angulation, or shear specific to type of fracture and internal fixation and high-impact forces.
- Tendon: Avoid high loads with extreme ranges (stress and strain), especially combined with angulation or rotation, rapid contraction in closed chain positions.
- Cartilage repair or debridement, microfracture for joint surface regeneration: Avoid excessive compressive (weight-bearing) forces or compressive and shear forces.
- Ligament: Avoid extreme strain (angulation, rotation).

GOALS

- Promote force closure around surgical site to distribute forces and allow healing.
- Address any possible causative factors (impairments and movement patterns) that were related to presurgical dysfunction.
- Restore functional range of motion.
- Restore muscle activation, endurance, strength, and power after muscle and neuromuscular adaptations related to weight-bearing or movement precautions.
- Promote functional return and neuromuscular coordination while following healing precautions.
- Address psychological components (fear avoidance beliefs and pain behavior).

TESTS AND MEASURES

See Magee,[1] and Magee and Sueki [4] for more detailed description of available tests and measures, interpretation and psychometric properties.
1. Pain reports (with movement, functional activity or positions)
2. Functional movement outcome measures for endurance, strength, neuromuscular coordination (symmetry, repetition, timed tests): Single-leg standing balance, sit-to-stand, ambulation or running distance, symmetry, speed, step-up tests, single-leg hop tests, Y balance, star excursion test, squat tests
3. Movement observation (qualitative)
4. Functional outcome measures for symmetry, repetition, or functional requirements
5. Ability to perform activities without compensations or home programs independently
6. LEFS, Patient Specific Functional Scale, region specific measures

OBSERVATION FOR COMPENSATIONS AND RESPONSES

- Monitor the plane, specific ranges, and directions involving the injured or surgically repaired structure.
- Limit motion resulting in accumulation of force or high stress/strain on the injured structures while allowing motion in other planes.
- Keep the area of concern supported with active neuromuscular control as the first priority, but observe for overall alignment at proximal and distal areas influencing the forces on the joint.
- Monitor proximal areas and adjust position and muscle activation to address moment arms as well as excessive angulation or rotation.
- Observe for loss of position or muscle activation with fatigue and monitor symptom reproduction.
- Use supported positions when needed.
- Ask patients to report any discomfort during or after the exercise.
- Monitor for delayed-onset muscle soreness, increased effusion or edema after treatment.

DOSAGE (SPECIFIC DOSAGE FOR IMPAIRMENTS AS WELL AS BY PHASE)

- Phase I: Circulation and edema, restoration of functional mobility and muscle function prevention of deconditioning
- Phase II: Dosage for impairments with slower progression for surgically incised tissues
- Phase III: Continued progression of loads for injured tissue to provide optimal stimulus
- Progress toward functional activities while adhering to healing time frames and surgical protocols.
- Timelines to enter Phase III will differ based on healing status of surgically incised or healing tissue.

EXERCISES

PHASE I

PHASE II

PHASE II/III

EXERCISE DESCRIPTIONS

PHASE I

9.37   Ankle pumps

See Fig. 9.37.

Purpose
- Stimulate blood flow, which in turn mobilizes swelling and increases venous return
- Decrease risk of deep vein thrombosis
- Improve lower extremity circulation and venous return

Precautions
- Recent increase in edema, redness, and pain in the lower leg may require further evaluation for the presence of deep vein thrombosis.

Position
- Supine with leg elevated above level of heart using pillows, bolsters, foam wedge, or small exercise ball

Action (Video 9.37)
- Activate lower leg muscles to dorsiflex and plantarflex the ankles

Advantages
- Muscle contraction with elevation enhances swelling reduction

Teaching tips
- Common error to correct:
  - Avoid inverting or everting ankle if there is a need to protect ankle ligaments.

Alternatives
- Decrease range if very swollen or start with toe movement and progress to ankle movement.
- Can be performed after applying ice or ice baths to assist with circulation and pain reduction.
- Can be performed with compression (bandage or tubing).
- Use rocker board (Exercise 9.38).

Progression
- Add elastic resistance band around the ball of the foot.
- Place a small ball under the lower leg to provide an unstable surface.
- Ankle pumps at end-range extension of short arc quadriceps contraction: maintain the knee in full extension while performing ankle pumps.
- Ankle pumps while holding leg in straight leg raise position (6 inches off table) (see straight leg raise), or hip abduction in side-lying, hip extension in quadruped.
- BAPS board in sitting: plantarflexion and dorsiflexion in sagittal plane only

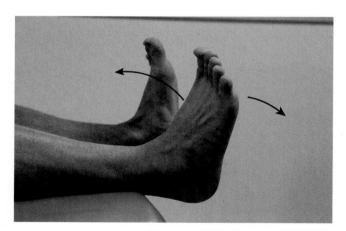

Fig. 9.37

9.38 Rocker or Balance Board active ankle motion

See Fig. 9.38.

Purpose
- Decrease effusion and edema
- Increase ankle range of motion
- Decrease risk of deep vein thrombosis
- Improve lower extremity circulation and venous return

Position
- Sitting with body weight supported on the plinth, one or both feet resting on the rocker board or BAPS (Balance and Proprioception System) board.
- No body weight supported through the foot/feet on the rockerboard

Action
1. Plantarflex and dorsiflex the ankle(s).
2. Move the rockerboard at a steady speed using multiple repetitions.

Teaching tips
- Common error to correct:
  - Avoid placing excess weight on the rockerboard, the board should move easily with a steady rhythm.

Advantages
- Minimal stress or loading on joint or ligaments

Alternatives
- Active range of motion in sitting without weight
- Active plantar and dorsiflexion against light elastic band resistance

Progression
- Increase range.
- Increase repetitions.
- Single-leg activity (injured foot)
- BAPS board, plantar and dorsiflexion, inversion and eversion, or combinations if there are no precautions for specific directions
- The exercise can be progressed to standing or with partial body weight and arm support on the plinth or parallel bars to introduce weight-bearing forces and muscle activation (Fig. 9.38 C, D).

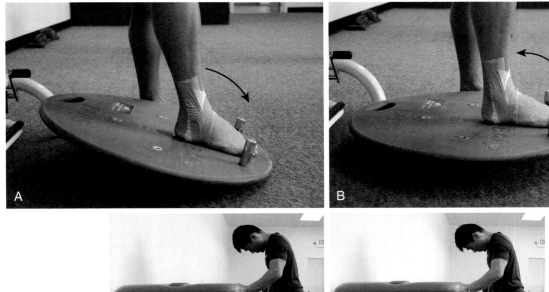

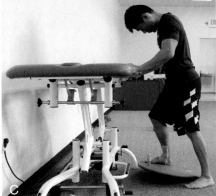
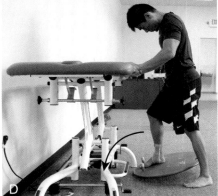

Fig. 9.38

9.39   Quadriceps isometrics

See Fig. 9.39.

Purpose
- Activate quadriceps
- Improve neuromuscular coordination in terminal extension
- Avoid disuse atrophy of quadriceps muscle
- Increase isometric strength of the quadriceps muscle

Position
- Long sitting with leg extended, small towel roll under knee to avoid hyperextension.

Action (Video 1.6)
- Activate quadriceps muscle.

Teaching tips
- Example instructions:
  - "Tighten up the muscle on the front of your thigh, think of pulling your kneecap up toward your hip."
  - "Push the back of your knee toward the table while you lift the ankle off the mat. Pull your toes toward your body."
- Common errors to correct:
  - If there is swelling in the knee joint, activation in terminal extension is more difficult. Often patients will attempt to contract the quadriceps but only use the hip flexors or substitute with hamstring activity.
- Methods to address or prevent compensations:
  - The therapist can place a hand behind the knee to encourage terminal knee extension (Video 3.10).

- A small ball or towel under the knee also provides additional proprioceptive feedback.
- If the patient is having difficulty activating the quadriceps, using electrical stimulation or watching the muscle may assist with muscle contraction (Video 3.11).

Advantages
- Low load exercise on knee joint and patellofemoral joint
- Minimal shear or compressive loading
- Can be easily assigned as a home exercise

Alternatives
- Supine or standing position
- Use functional electrical stimulation at the same time as the exercise to assist muscle recruitment.
- Use a small ball or towel under the knee to assist proprioceptive feedback for terminal knee extension.

Progression
- Place the knee in varying degrees of knee flexion/extension to facilitate muscle activation throughout the range (multiangle isometric contractions).
- Short arc quadriceps isotonic contraction or contraction through range (Exercise 9.43A)
- Closed chain, standing with elastic resistance band wrapped behind slightly flexed knee and anchored in front of patient at knee level. The patient presses into the band, extending the knee (Exercise 9.16).
- Use resistance against pulleys or machine resistance at different angles of knee flexion/extension.

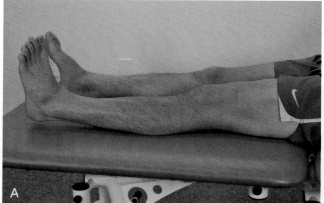
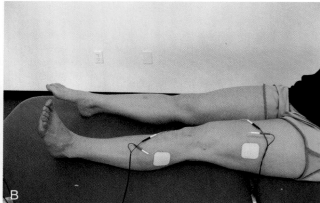

Fig. 9.39

9.40   Hamstring isometrics

See Fig. 9.40.

Purpose
- Activate the hamstrings after surgery or trauma
- Avoid disuse atrophy of the hamstring muscles
- Promote circulatory responses for the knee and lower extremity

Position
- Supine hook-lying with knee and hip flexed
- Heel on the table

Action
1. Activate the hamstring muscles by pushing the heel into table and attempting to flex the knee without moving.
2. Maintain a neutral foot and lower leg position.

Advantages
- Very low load on knee joint structures.

Teaching tips
- Instruction example:
  - "Push your heel down into the table as if you are bending your knee. You should feel the muscles on the back of your thigh tighten up. Hold for 5 seconds."

- Common errors to correct:
  - Lifting the hip using the gluteals without isometric hamstring contraction.

Alternatives
- Sitting in a chair, push the heel into the floor. This option allows isometrics at different ranges of knee flexion.
- Prone with knee flexed and therapist providing manual resistance
- Supine, with legs resting on a stability ball (Exercise 9.4B small-range or isometric)
- Small range active or self-assisted hip and knee flexion (Exercise 9.3 or 9.4)

Progression
- Multi-angle isometrics
- Active assistive range of motion hip and knee flexion (Exercise 9.4) or on a slider (Exercise 9.3) with an emphasis on muscle activation and circulatory parameters

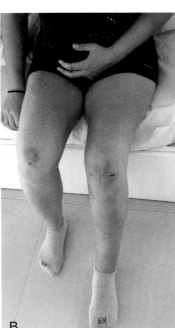
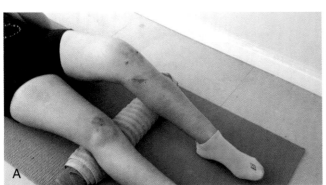

Fig. 9.40

9.41   Gluteal isometrics

Purpose

- Initiate gluteus maximus activation
- Facilitate body awareness of hip extensors
- Avoid disuse atrophy of the gluteus maximus muscle
- Promote circulation through muscle contraction

Position

- Supine with legs extended

Action

- Activate the gluteal muscles bilaterally, tightening the buttocks and trying to create external rotation of thighs without necessarily moving the legs.

Advantages

- Muscle activation without hip or lumbar joint stresses.

Teaching tips

- Instruction example:
  - "Squeeze your gluts together, hold for 3–5 seconds and then relax."
- Common error to correct:
  - Avoid flexing the lumbar spine or tucking the pelvis to create movement.

Alternatives

- Standing or prone position.

Progression

- Multi-angle isometric contractions
- Active assistive hip extension
- Active hip extension

9.42 Straight leg raise

See Fig. 9.42.

Purpose

- Increase strength of quadriceps, hip flexors, and dorsiflexors

Position

- Supine with involved leg straight, uninvolved leg flexed up, foot flat, arms at sides

Action (Video 3.10)

1. Activate the quadriceps muscle to straighten the knee.
2. Lift the leg to the height of the uninvolved thigh.
3. Keeping the ankle dorsiflexed helps with maintaining the knee extension.
4. Slowly lower the leg toward the table to a count of 5.

Advantages

- Very low load, maintains muscle strength throughout limb

Teaching tips

- Instruction example:
  - "Pull your toes up and tighten up the muscle on the front of your thigh to straighten the knee. Then press your arms and opposite leg down into the table as you lift your straight leg off the table."

- Common errors to correct:
  - Allowing the pelvis to move; hiking or posterior rotation during the leg lift or on the lowering.
- Methods to address or prevent compensations:
  - Stabilizing the core and the opposite leg will provide a proximal base for muscles to lift the leg.

Alternatives

- Ankle pumps combined with straight leg raise
- Hip extension straight leg raise in four point (Exercise 9.45)
- Hip abduction in side-lying (Exercise 9.26B)

Progression

- Slow eccentric lowering
- Increase repetitions.
- Add cuff weight above the ankle.
- Single-leg straight leg raise with bridging (Fig. 9.42B)

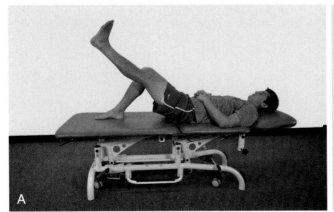
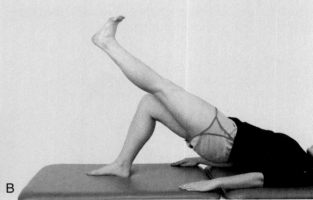

Fig. 9.42

9.43   Open chain knee extension

See Fig. 9.43.

Purpose

- Increase strength of quadriceps without loading through lower extremity joints

Position

- Supine, long sitting, or upright sitting
- Knee is flexed between 0 and 90 degrees

Action

A. *Short arc quads:*
  1. Exercise is started between 45 and 30 degrees.
  2. Instruct the patient to push the knee down against the bolster or towel, initiate quadriceps contraction and extend the knee.
  3. Focus on full extension at the end of the range.
  4. If the patient is unable to achieve full active extension, the therapist moves the knee passively to full extension, then asks the patient to contract and hold the position followed by slowly releasing the support while asking the patient to maintain the position. Eccentric activity is likely to promote muscle activation in the terminal range.

B. *Full knee extension:*
  1. Activate the quadriceps muscle to fully extend knee through the available range.
  2. Hold the maximal extension for 2–5 seconds, then lower foot back down to starting position.

Advantages

- Isolated quadriceps strengthening
- Appropriate exercise when non–weight-bearing
- Important exercise after surgery, particularly when there is a lack of quadriceps activation due to effusion or pain or if there is a quadriceps lag

Teaching tips

- Instruction example:
  - "Straighten your knee using the muscle on the front of your thigh, drawing your kneecap up with the muscles on either side of your kneecap."

Alternatives

- Use functional electrical stimulation to facilitate quadriceps contraction.
- Active-assisted knee extension using a strap

Progression

- Knee extension against elastic resistance, pulleys, or machine resistance
- Add weight.
- Eccentric control through small ranges with a weight strapped to the lower leg or with isometric holds against higher loads.
- Progress to straight leg raise (Exercise 9.42).
- Progress to weight-bearing strengthening once range of motion is controlled through active muscle contraction.

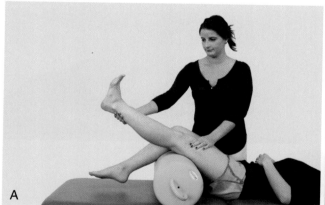 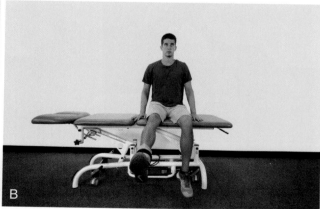

Fig. 9.43

9.44   Open chain knee flexion

See Fig. 9.44.

Purpose
- Increase hamstring activation and eccentric control

Position
- Standing on uninvolved leg or prone

Action
1. Activate hamstring muscle group to bend knee, bringing heel(s) toward buttocks.
2. Hold for 3 seconds, then slowly lower the foot toward the ground or the treatment plinth, controlling the movement with the hamstrings (eccentric control).

Advantages
- Isolated hamstring strengthening with minimal load or stress

Teaching tips
- Common error to correct:
  - Not stabilizing lumbopelvic region in standing
  - Allowing the leg to move too quickly with gravity assistance

Alternatives
- Use a strap-on cuff weight (around the ankle) to provide resistance.
- Isometric hamstring contractions (Exercise 9.40)
- Bridging (Exercise 9.21)
- Concentric contractions against pulley resistance, resistance bands, or strap-on weights in prone

Progression
- Increase weight using machine, pulley, or elastic resistance (leg curls) in sitting or prone.
- Increase repetitions.

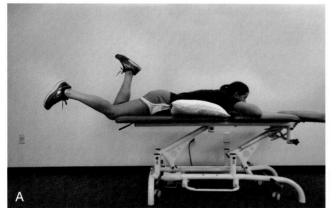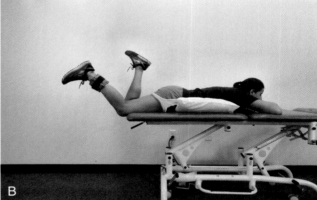

Fig. 9.44

PHASE II

9.45   Four-point kneeling hip extension

See Fig. 9.45.

Purpose

- Increase strength of gluteus maximus and hamstrings while stabilizing the trunk

Position

- Four-point kneeling, with knees hip distance apart
- Hands are under shoulders with elbows slightly flexed.
- Spine is in neutral.

Action (Videos 4.15 and 9.45A and B)

1. Abdominals are engaged and the lumbopelvic region is supported in a neutral position.
2. Lift the leg against gravity, extending the hip and maintaining the knee in extension.

Advantages

- There is a very low load on hip joint.
- Simultaneously addresses early hip muscle activation/endurance or strengthening along with core stabilization.

Teaching tips

- Common errors to correct:
  - Avoid lumbar extension or pelvic rotation.
- Methods to address or prevent compensations:

- Ask the patient to engage the abdominals first to counteract the tendency to extend the lumbar spine while extending the hip (Video 9.45B).
- It is important that patients learn to activate hip extensors rather than substituting with lumbar extension. Demonstrating the movement can be useful to show the desired movement.
- Placing a mirror on the side of the patient allows the patient to observe the movement and correct the action after understanding the concept of proximal stability.
- The therapist can use tactile input or an image of placing an object on the spine and not allowing the pelvis to move from side to side.

Alternatives

- Four-point over a stability ball (Video 9.45C) or BOSU (Video 9.17C) provides more support if unable to hold four-point position.
- Standing with the torso supported on a table (Video 9.17D)

Progression

- Add weight or elastic resistance band around the midfoot while holding the other end of band in opposite hand (four-point kneeling).
- Hold the leg in the extended position and draw a square shape with foot, requiring the patient to hold extension for longer durations.

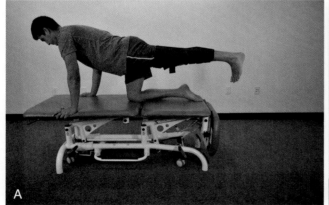
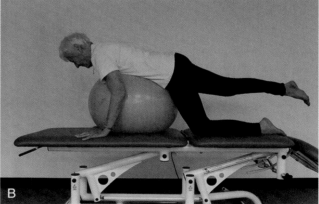

Fig. 9.45

9.46 Progressive weight-bearing (with or without loading support)

Purpose
- Increase tolerance to compressive loads
- Teach awareness of weight-bearing alignment
- Prepare for full weight-bearing.

Position
- Standing, equal weight-bearing on each leg

Action
1. Shift weight onto involved leg to take 75% of body weight, then 90% body weight, loading the forefoot and rearfoot.
2. Hold weight shift 10 seconds and then return to bearing equal weight on each leg.

Advantages
- Closed chain activity minimizes shear loads, facilitates co-contraction, and increases proprioceptive input.
- Functional position and activity
- Teaches postural awareness of lower extremity alignment before gait training or more advanced double- or single-leg-stance exercises.

Teaching tips
- Common errors to correct:
  - Excessive knee flexion, valgus or varus, hip adduction, Trendelenburg sign, trunk lateral flexion, or pelvic rotation

- Methods to address or prevent compensations:
  - Demonstrate proper alignment during the movement and have the patient reproduce using a mirror.
  - Standing with each foot on a bathroom scale can provide quantitative feedback about the amount of weight being placed on each leg.

Alternatives
- If partial weight-bearing precautions require less than 50%, add support using parallel bars, with a standard walker, unweighting harness.
- Split-stance weight shifting in the sagittal plane will prepare for gait training.
- Aquatic therapy or deweighting on a treadmill (Fig. 9.46A and B).

Progression
- Increase target percentage weight-bearing.
- Increase time held.
- Increase speed of weight shift and acceptance.
- Split-stance position to weight shift in the sagittal plane.
- Progress weight shift to single-leg stance.
- Increase speed of weight shift.
- Use weight shift followed by rapidly flexing the hip and knee and moving the rear leg forward to challenge weight acceptance and balance.
- Progress to step-ups or -downs (Exercise 9.31).

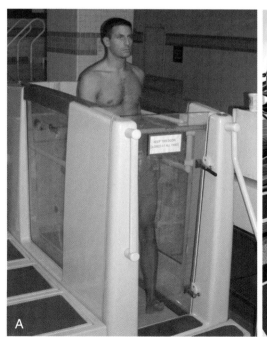
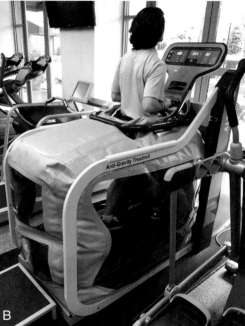

Fig. 9.46 Progressive weight-bearing with low joint loading using an underwater tank (A) or gravity deloading device (B). (From Manske RC. *Fundamental Orthopedic Management for the Physical Therapist Assistant*. 4th ed. St. Louis, MO: Elsevier; 2016.)

9.47   Supported partial sit-to-stand

See Fig. 9.47.

Purpose

- Improve generalized lower extremity activation
- Introduce weight-bearing or improve lower extremity symmetry
- Transfer training
- Improve functional ankle, knee or hip control
- Early exercise for squat reeducation

Position

- Sitting forward on the front edge of an elevated surface
- Trunk and cervical spine is supported using active trunk muscle engagement
- Knees flexed greater than 90 degrees
- Hands on the edge of the surface or on armrests

Action (Video 2.24)

1. Hinge forward at the hips to bring the center of mass over the balls of feet.
2. Bring the head and upper trunk forward together rather than only moving at the hips.
3. Stand up using the gluteus maximus, hamstrings and quads to extend the hips and knees to neutral position.
4. Use the arms to assist movement as needed.
5. Reverse the motion, hinging forward at the hips and flexing the knees, and lowering back to a seated position using eccentric control.

Advantages

- Sitting between repetitions allows the patient to rest and recover.
- The support of the plinth provides feedback and can be adjusted for postsurgical precautions (e.g., when closed chain isometrics are allowed from 90 to 45 degrees after ACL reconstruction).
- The feedback from the hands assists with equal weight-bearing.

Teaching tips

- Instruction examples:
  - "Push into the ground as you move your body over your feet."
  - "Only use your arms to push off the table as much as you need to."
  - "Use your hips and your knees to stand up."
  - "Reverse the movement by bending your hips and knees and keeping your body weight forward. Lower your pelvis down slowly to the table."
- Common errors to correct:
  - Holding the body weight behind the feet (insufficient weight shift forward)
  - Using the spine to straighten the body rather than the legs
  - Only using the quadriceps rather than using the hip extensors to drive the movement

Alternatives

- The further the patient leans forward, the less body weight the patient will need to lift because the center of mass is over the base of support with smaller resultant moment arms at the hips and knees. This movement pattern also makes it easier to use both the hip and knee extensors.
- A split-stance position with the stronger leg back and the involved leg forward increases the base of support in the sagittal plane. This position allows a forward weight shift before starting to stand and may be needed when one leg is stronger than the other or if balance is poor.

Progression

- Decrease height of surface the patient is sitting on.
- Decrease use of arm support.
- Progress to reaching forward with both arms.
- Increase time of isometric holds.
- Increase eccentric challenge by slowing down the lowering phase.
- Progress to 75% weight-bearing on the injured leg, followed by single-leg.
- Single-leg
- Increase repetitions.
- Progress to sit-to-stand from a chair.

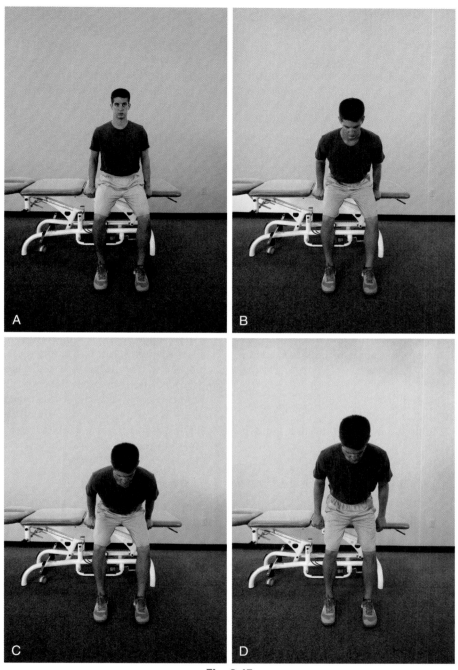

Fig. 9.47

9.48 Pre-gait and gait progression

Purpose
- Retrain correct gait mechanics
- Improve forward weight progression
- Closed chain activity to increase stability through co-contraction with lower shear forces and increased proprioceptive input
- Prepare for gait, single-leg stance, and lunge activities
- Low load introduction

Position
- Standing in split stance, surgical or injured lower extremity is forward.
- Arms placed in simulated reciprocal arm swing position.

Action
1. Shift weight onto front leg, slightly flexing the front hip and knee, moving the trunk over the center of the front foot.
2. Hold the weight shift, and lift the heel of the rear off the floor while the forefoot stays on the floor.
3. Hold position for 3–5 seconds, then shift weight back to starting position.
4. Progress to advancing the uninvolved leg forward to contact the heel in front while swinging arms in opposition with trunk and pelvic rotation.

Teaching tips
- Methods to address or prevent compensations:
  - Use a mirror to provide feedback.
  - Placing targets on the floor can help with goals for step length.

- Step width should be hip distance apart (distance is also dependent on the bony alignment, individuals with genu valgus may need a wider stance).
- Perform the movement in the parallel bars if the patient is afraid of falling or shows fear avoidance strategies/behavior.
- If the patient is avoiding weight-bearing due to history of pain, psychological approaches can be used to encourage weight acceptance.

Advantages
- Develops gait pattern in controlled manner with concentration on weight shift

Alternatives
- Walking in a pool or using an unweighting harness to decrease load

Progression
- Reach further forward with opposite arm.
- Increase repetitions.
- Increase speed.
- Increase height of knee and foot clearance.
- Treadmill or level ground gait training

Specific parameters
- Average gait speed 1.3 m/sec (3 mph) is more energy-efficient than slower or faster walking speed. Speed is the product of step length (Fig. 9.48) and cadence (steps per minute). Gait deviations or excessive vertical or sideways motion of the center of mass increases energy expenditure.[22]
- In a 20- to 30-year-old, normal gait speed requires 32% VO_2max; in a 75-year-old, energy expenditure increases to 48% VO_2max.[22]

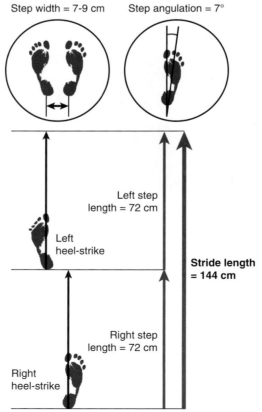

Step width = 7-9 cm   Step angulation = 7°

Left step length = 72 cm

Left heel-strike

Stride length = 144 cm

Right step length = 72 cm

Right heel-strike

Fig. 9.48 (From Neumann DA. *Kinesiology of the Musculoskeletal System*. 3rd ed. St. Louis, MO: Elsevier; 2017.)

PHASE II/III

9.49 Lunges

See Fig. 9.49.

Purpose

- Closed chain lower extremity strengthening in the sagittal plane
- Preparation for sports-specific requirements
- Strengthening through knee range with weight shift

Position

- Standing behind 6-inch step or box or a target for lunges on the floor

Action (Fig. 9.49A–C)

1. Shift weight forward to forefoot and step onto the box with involved lower extremity, contacting with the heel first or toward the target.
2. Flex the back knee and lower the front knee toward floor.
3. Press heel down onto box or from the floor and push back to standing position on the floor.

Teaching tips

- Instruction example:
  - "Shift your weight forward onto the balls of your feet, then step-up onto the box with your injured leg. Land with your heel first and feel the muscles on the back of your hip and thigh tighten up to support you. Bend your knee forward, then press through your front heel to push yourself back to your starting position."
- Common error to correct:
  - Dynamic valgus motion during the lunge
  - Not shifting weight fully to the front leg
- Methods to address or prevent compensations:
  - Visual targets can be used to keep the knee facing toward a line or an object placed in front of the leading leg or a line in the middle of the feet to encourage moving to side of the front leg.
  - A laser strapped to the thigh can be used to help with smooth coordination of the movement to avoid angulation or rotation during the movement.
  - Mirrors help with feedback and knowledge of results as well as self-correction.
  - Pressure through the heel of the front leg will help facilitate the hip extensors on the return action.

Advantages

- Closed chain activity lower shear forces, co-contraction, increases proprioceptive input.
- Functional movement
- Generalized strengthening for entire lower extremity

Alternatives

- Lunge onto BOSU

Progression

- Incrementally decrease height of step or box until lunging on the floor (Fig. 9.49D–F).
- Lunge sideways.
- Increase repetitions.
- Increase range.
- Increase depth of lunge (Fig. 9.49G).
- Lunge in a diagonal.
- Alternating lunges using a star pattern taped to the floor for different directions (Fig 9.49H and I; Video 9.49)
- In-line lunges
- Increase speed.
- Change directions or sides of the lunge.
- Add hand weights or arm motion at the same time (reciprocal).

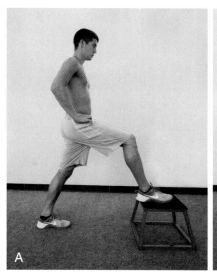 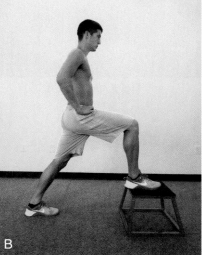 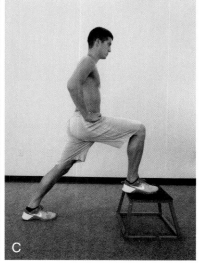

Fig. 9.49

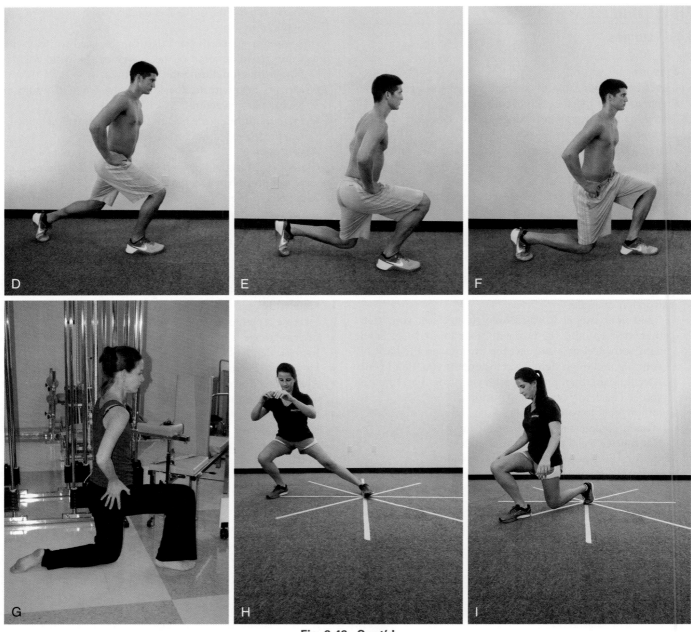

Fig. 9.49, Cont'd

9.50 Hopping, skipping

See Fig. 9.50.

Purpose
- Teach quick transition of weight-bearing from one leg to the other
- Preparatory activity for jogging
- Preparatory activity for teaching jumping mechanics
- Early-level plyometric exercise
- Facilitates proprioceptive responses

Precautions
- Only appropriate if the patient can perform squats on one leg without any compensations.
- Start with appropriate arm support nearby.
- Progress from hopping in place before moving in multiple directions.

Position
- Patient is standing with feet hip distance apart, arms slightly flexed at elbow.

Action
1. Shift weight forward and lift one knee while simultaneously rising up onto the ball of the foot of the opposite leg.
2. Hop off the supporting foot, flexing the hip to 90 degrees while simultaneously landing on ball of the other foot. This sequence is continued for prescribed distance or time.

Advantages
- This is a good preparatory activity for returning to running.

Teaching tips
- Instruction example:
  - Demonstrate, briefly describe, and then allow the patient to try to replicate the motion.

Alternatives
- Skip in the pool to decrease loading on the joints

Progression
- Increase speed.
- Hop on the same leg and increase repetitions.
- Increase height of hop.
- Add resistance or belt around waist with a posterior directed force.
- Forward progressive hops (Fig. 9.50)
- Only progress to hops for distance (Fig. 9.50A; Video 9.50A) once full range, strength, and control is demonstrated.
- Change direction sideways (Fig. 9.50B–D), diagonally (Fig. 9.50E–F and G–L; Video 9.50B), or change directions.
- Specific outcome measures:
  - Single hop (Fig. 9.50A [A]) or triple hop (Fig. 9.50A [B]) for distance (see Chapters 4 and 8)
  - Vertical jump distance (see Chapters 4 and 8)

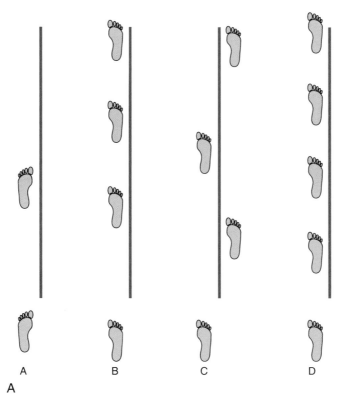

A

Fig. 9.50 (A) Hop outcome measures. (*A*) Single-leg hop for distance. (*B*) Triple hop for distance. (*C*) Crossover hop. (*D*) Progressive hop for time. (From Manske RC. *Fundamental Orthopedic Management for the Physical Therapist Assistant.* 4th ed. St. Louis, MO: Elsevier; 2016.)

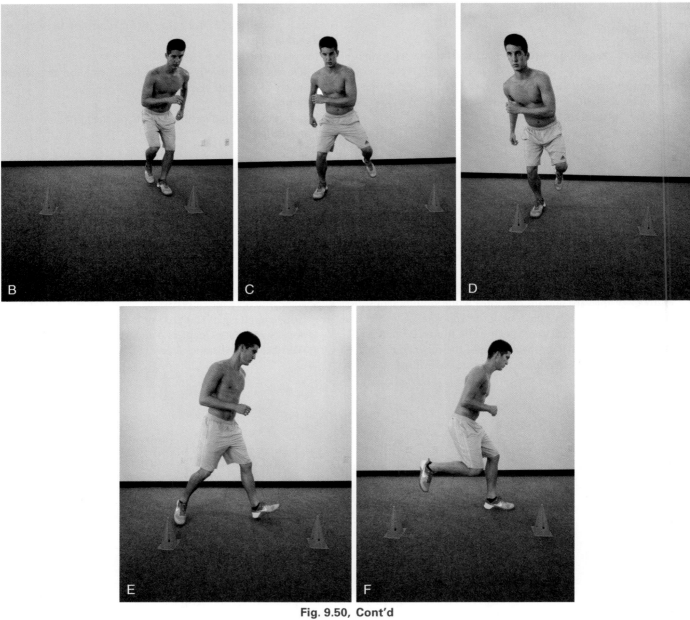

Fig. 9.50, Cont'd

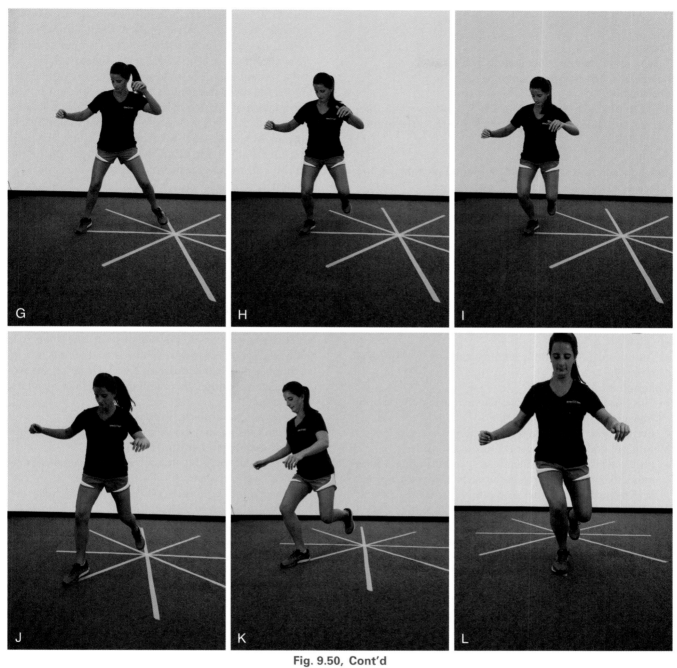

Fig. 9.50, Cont'd

9.51 Jump progressions

See Fig. 9.51.

Purpose

- Teach proper jumping and landing mechanics
- Return to sports requiring jumping

Position

- Standing behind box, knees and feet hip-distance apart
- Neutral arch pressing feet into ground, creating sensation of a big footprint

Action

1. Flex hips and knees, sitting into hips, and pressing big toes into floor maintaining alignment over the foot.
2. Reverse the motion by quickly extending hips and knees, moving weight forward and jumping onto a box landing, with soft knees, articulating through the foot, hinged forward at hips, and chest over the balls of feet.

Advantages

- Landing on a box versus the floor decreases ground reaction forces.

Teaching tips

- Instruction examples:
  - "Land softly."
  - "Jump and absorb on the landing, keeping the knees and hips soft."
- Common error to correct:
  - The knees should not roll inward during the landing (dynamic valgus; Fig. 9.51D).
  - Even weight-bearing on both legs
- Methods to address or prevent compensations:
  - People typically injure themselves while landing a jump rather than taking off or in the air, so first emphasize proper landing mechanics rather than achieving maximal height.
  - Videotape the movement and point out the desired mechanics and compensations.
  - Use visual feedback and external focus to assist with corrections for dynamic valgus (Fig. 9.51D), excessive internal rotation, or asymmetrical weight shift.

Alternatives

- Jump on a leg press, Pilates Reformer with trampoline attachment, rebounder or shuttle to decrease the chance of falling or the vertical forces.

- Introduce jumping on a mini-trampoline to assess the patient's ability to tolerate impact. Light jumping, where the feet barely leave the surface of the trampoline will help develop confidence (Fig. 9.51H and I; Video 3.23).
- If the patient can decelerate momentum, continue jumping on the mini-trampoline and softly land on both feet in a squatting position. The body should not bob up and down and the trampoline should remain still. Teaching the patient to seek feedback from the landing surface prepares the patient for using the feet as well as the knees and hips to reduce reaction forces when jumping on the ground.

Progression

- Increase the height of jump on the mini-trampoline.
- Jump off a box (Fig. 9.51A–C).
- Assess the functional strength of the involved versus the uninvolved leg by jumping off both legs and landing on one leg and sticking the landing, then the other (Fig. 9.51E and H–L).
- Decrease the height of the box.
- Jump on the floor (Fig. 9.51F, G, M–S).
- Once the patient consistently demonstrates the ability to land softly with good control, he or she is ready to begin a more traditional plyometric program in which he or she would immediately rebound after landing rather than maintaining the position.
- Parameters specific to this exercise:
  - Avoid causing an overuse injury by limiting frequency of jump training to 1–2 times/week.
  - Incorporate jumping after a warm-up, but before fatigue affects performance.
  - Repeat jumps only as tolerance and form permit.
  - Allow full recovery between sets.
- Specific outcome measures:
  - Vertical jump distance (see Chapters 4 and 8)
  - Triple hop distance (see Chapters 4 and 8)

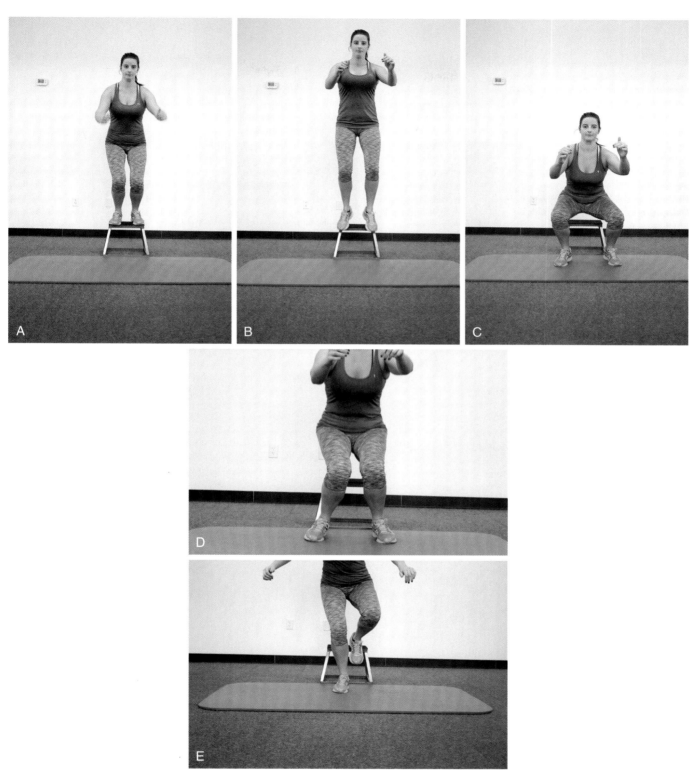

Fig. 9.51

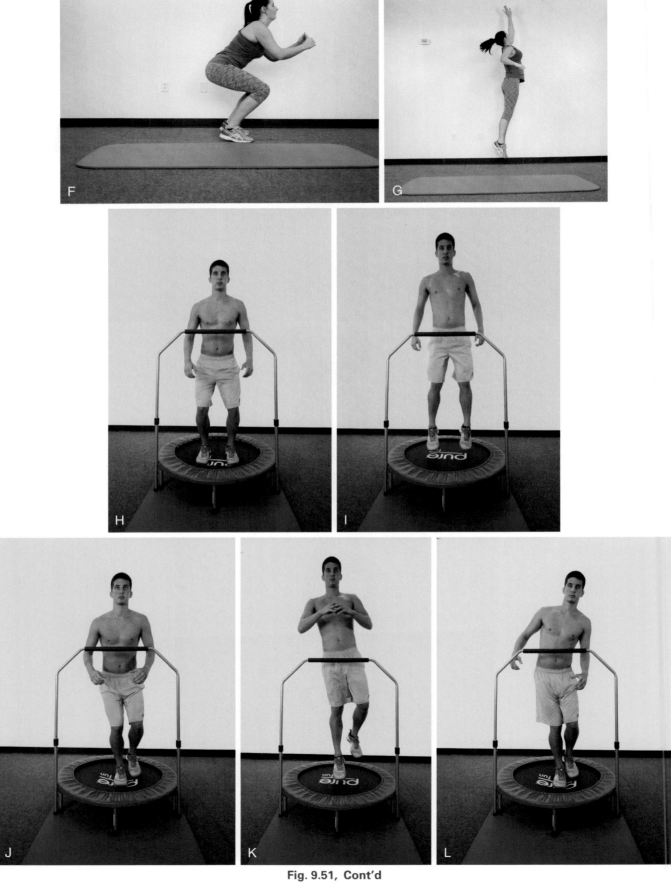

Fig. 9.51, Cont'd

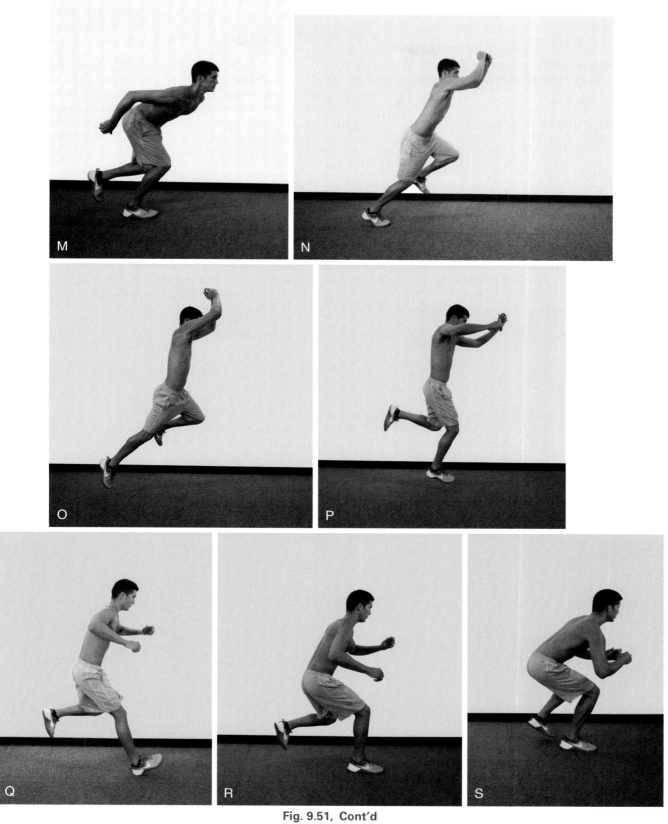

Fig. 9.51, Cont'd

9.52 Reaction time and sports-specific drills

See Fig. 9.52.

Purpose

- To train the patient on changing direction or responding to outside demands with variations in distance, speed, movement, or tasks to simulate random requirements game situation.

Position

- Athletic stance with the knees and hips flexed
- Neutral spine

Action

1. Patient begins by jogging in a 45-degree diagonal from midline. The therapist provides an auditory signal such as a bell or command, to indicate a change of direction.
2. The patient plants, spins on forefoot, and changes direction to begin jogging at 45 degrees to other side. With each signal patient has to change direction. This continues along a stretch of 40–50 feet.
3. Directions, distances, or speed can be varied.

Advantages

- Higher level integration of timing and combination of planes of movement.

Alternatives

- Change angles or targets such as ladder drills (Video 7.1).
- Use cones or tape on the floor for change of direction points (Fig. 9.51A1–A3 and C1–C8).
- Turn at point of change or use touch-and-go methods (touching the ground with one hand or both).
- Use sports-specific methods; for example, skaters may need sliding or side-stepping (Fig 9.52B1–B3) or running in a semi-crouch position, football or basketball players can be challenged by catching or throwing a ball at different intervals, soccer or basketball players can be challenged by dribbling a ball and passing at different intervals.

Progression

- Increase speed.
- Increase distance.
- Add resistance by attaching sport cords around the waist Fig 9.51A4–A7.
- Change surfaces.
- Specific outcome measures:
  - Time for one circuit with specific cues
  - Accuracy

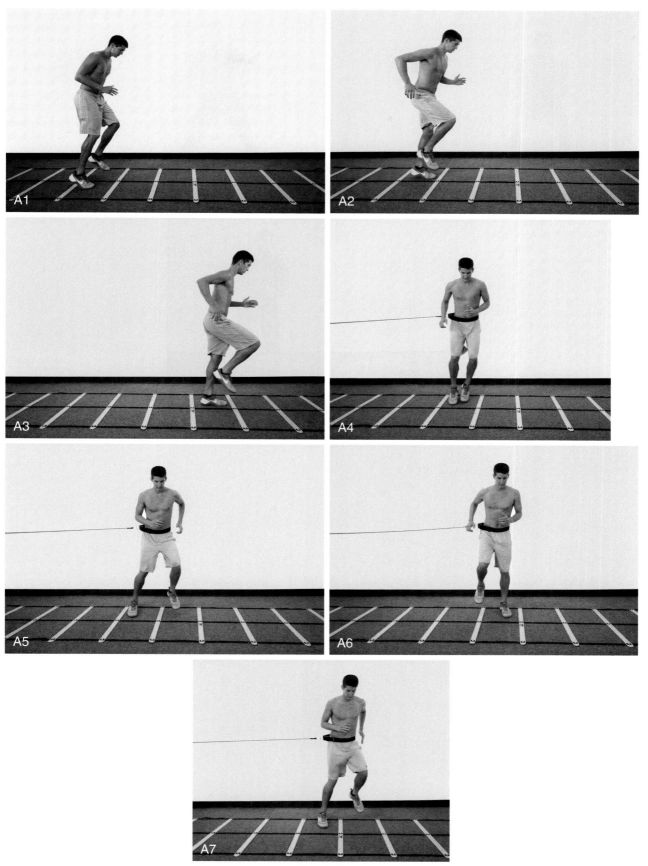

Fig. 9.52

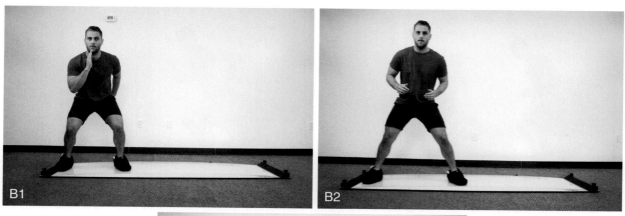

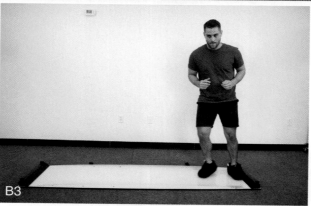

Fig. 9.52, Cont'd

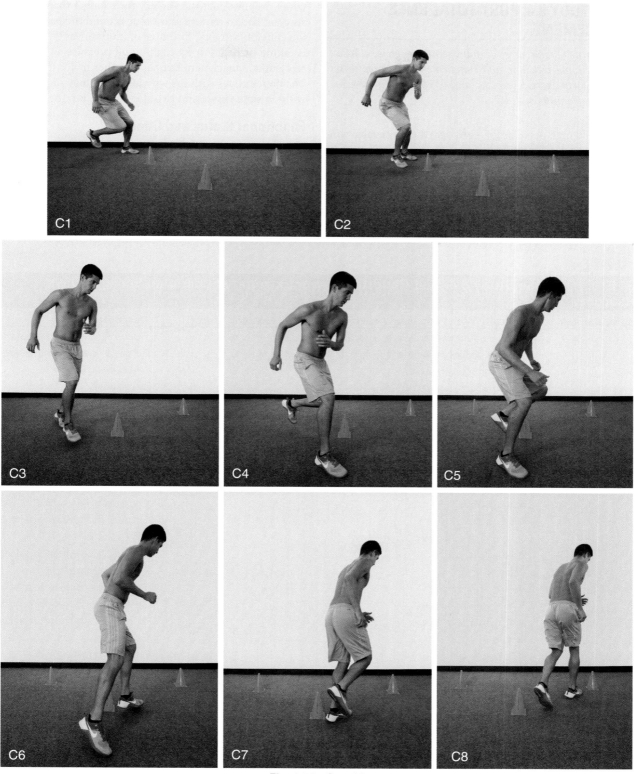

Fig. 9.52, Cont'd

CASE STUDY 9.4: POST-TOTAL KNEE REPLACEMENT

This case illustrate (1) postsurgical management exercise choices, (2) use of functional outcome and impairment measures to set goals and to inform exercise choices, and (3) postoperative exercise progression from Phase I–III.

A 68-year-old man presents for a physical therapy evaluation 10 days following a right total knee replacement (TKR) with a referral of "Evaluate and treat post total knee replacement with no complications." He has a history of meniscus damage from a high school football injury and increasing knee pain over the past 15 years. He elected to undergo a TKR when the pain had become severe (8/10) and was present throughout the day. The patient reports that the surgery took longer than expected; the surgeon had to remove scar tissue around the patella and in the knee. Before surgery, his range of motion was 0–90 degrees. He is taking medication for high blood pressure and hypercholesterolemia management but has no other major medical history. The patient lives with his wife in a one-story ranch-style home with no steps inside and two steps to get into the front door.

Functional Status and Goals

The patient is progressing well after the surgery and is walking with a walker without assistance. He is able to transfer from sit-to-stand and on/off the toilet without any assistance and in/out of the shower with minimal assistance and using a grab bar. He has moderate difficulty with transferring in and out of the car. LEFS score is 10/8 (Table 9.10).

TABLE 9.10 **Case Study 9.4: Self-Reported Lower Extremity Functional Scale 10 Days Postsurgery**

Question Number	Difficulty With Functional Activities	Numeric Score[a]	Descriptor
1.	Any of your usual work, housework, or social activities	0	Extreme difficulty/unable to perform
2.	Your usual hobbies, recreational or sporting activities	0	Extreme difficulty/unable to perform
3.	Getting into or out of the bath	2	Moderate difficulty
4.	Walking between rooms	2	Moderate difficulty
5.	Putting on your shoes and socks	0	Extreme difficulty/unable to perform
6.	Squatting	0	Extreme difficulty/unable to perform
7.	Lifting an object, like a bag of groceries from the floor	0	Extreme difficulty/unable to perform
8.	Performing light activities around your home	0	Extreme difficulty/unable to perform
9.	Performing heavy activities around your home	0	Extreme difficulty/unable to perform
10.	Getting into or out of your car	1	Quite a bit of difficulty
11.	Walking 2 blocks	0	Extreme difficulty/unable to perform
12.	Walking a mile	0	Extreme difficulty/unable to perform
13.	Going up or down 10 stairs	1	Quite a bit of difficulty
14.	Standing for 1 hour	0	Extreme difficulty/unable to perform
15.	Sitting for 1 hour	1	Quite a bit of difficulty
16.	Running on even ground	0	Extreme difficulty/unable to perform
17.	Running on uneven ground	0	Extreme difficulty/unable to perform
18.	Making sharp turns while running fast	0	Extreme difficulty/unable to perform
19.	Hopping	0	Extreme difficulty/unable to perform
20.	Rolling over in bed	2	Moderate difficulty
	Total	9/80	

Lower Extremity Functional Scale.[71]
[a]0 = Extreme difficulty/unable to perform; 4 = no difficulty.

BOX 9.12 Interpretation of Subjective Findings and Surgical History

- Early postsurgical management with the need to consider skin and tissue healing and effusion resolution.
- Knee flexion and extension active and passive range of motion will be important to assess and address early.
- Presurgical knee range of motion limitations (only 90 degrees of flexion) may impact recovery of full knee flexion. Early range of motion to promote connective tissue healing in directions to allow as much flexion as possible will need to be performed without stressing the sagittal incision or increasing inflammation. Inflammation and effusion will need to be monitored after progressing knee flexion range of motion.
- The effusion will influence pain when the limb is dependent (standing) and with inactivity.
- Although the reported severity of pain is high, this is expected in the postoperative course, and it is more important to obtain full range of motion for full function during the early treatment than to avoid pain responses completely. However, excessive force on the healing tissues will need to be avoided to limit inflammation (especially with knee flexion where the incision site is at maximum strain). Pain is monitored with movement as well as at rest.[73]

- Muscle activation and function of the muscles directly around the surgical site at the knee as well as proximal and distal joints needs to be assessed. Neuromuscular activation is likely to be impacted by postsurgical pain and/or neuromuscular inhibition related to effusion, but connective tissue limitations and muscle atrophy from before the surgery may also influence muscle function.
- As the surgeon had to spend additional time during the surgery to remove scar tissue, goals to restore range as soon as possible are important to limit further scar tissue build-up in directions that will limit function.
- The patient did not mention any other surgical complications but surgical sequelae such as deep vein thrombosis, excessive hematoma and effusion, blood loss leading to orthostatic hypotension, balance deficits, and risk of infection should be kept in mind.
- LEFS shows severe dysfunction (www.rehabmeasures.org)[71,74]; however, once the pain and effusion related to the surgical procedure decreases and range of motion and muscle function improve, rapid improvements in function are likely. Functional goals will be linked to expectations for the impairments influencing specific activities, along with evidence related to post surgical outcomes from the literature and clinical experience. The goals linked to each item in the LEFS are presented in Tables 9.13, 9.15, and 9.17.

TABLE 9.11 Range of Motion (Degrees) on Initial Evaluation and Related Goals

Active ROM	Right	Left	Goal (R Leg)	L Leg
Hip	WNL	WNL		
Knee				
Flexion	60 (passive 70)	130	110	
Extension	−10 (passive −5)	0	0	
Ankle				
Dorsiflexion	−2	5	10	10
Plantarflexion	40	45	45	

WNL, Within normal limits.

Patient's Goals

1. Sleep without disturbance from pain for 2–4 hours
2. Walk without an assistive device
3. Be able to go up and down steps without difficulty
4. Return to playing golf

Subjective Complaints

- *Severity*: Knee pain is reported to be at 6/10 and increases to 9/10 when flexing the knee to end range in a non–weight-bearing position.
- *Irritability*: Pain is worse in the morning (decreases after moving around), with sit-to-stand (decreases to baseline), and after standing for 3 minutes or more (decreases to baseline when he elevates the leg). He spends most of his day sitting in a recliner. Pain medication (Tylenol 3) decreases pain to 4/10. He is also using ice packs and ice massage after activity, which does help the pain.
- *Nature*: Postsurgical pain, postsurgical effusion from TKR
- *Stage*: Acute postoperative recovery, Phase I

See Box 9.12 for interpretation.

Objective Findings

- *Posture/alignment*: Bilateral tibial varum, supination in standing. Avoids weight-bearing on surgical leg in standing.
- *Girth*: Moderate effusion around the knee joint: 3 cm difference at the joint line, 2.5 cm immediately above the patella, and 1 cm greater on the right 5 cm below the joint line. There is also moderate atrophy of the right quadriceps with 2 cm less on the affected side 15 cm above the joint line. The patient is wearing compression stockings to decrease edema.
- *Range of motion:* See Table 9.11.
- *Muscle function:* See Table 9.12.
- *Palpation and joint play:*
  - Patella mobility is decreased in the superior/inferior direction.
  - Moderate effusion and edema around the knee and some edema in the calf.
  - Incisions are healing (anterior incision, arthroscope incisions × 3 above, below and at the joint line), covered with clear surgical tape.
  - The patient is using compression wraps (Ace bandage) in addition to compression stockings.

TABLE 9.12   Manual Muscle Testing on Initial Evaluation and Related Goals

Movement	Right	Left	Goal (R Leg)	L leg
Hip				
Flexion	3–	4	4	
Extension	3–	4–	4	4
Abduction	3–	4–	4	4
Adduction	4–	4–	4	4
IR rotation/ER rotation	NT (delayed)	4		
Knee				
Flexion	3–	4	4	
Extension	3–	4	4	
Ankle				
Dorsiflexion	4–	4	4	
Plantarflexion	4–	4	4	

ER, External rotation; *IR*, internal rotation *NT*, not tested.

Note: Reliability of manual testing for grades above a grade 3 is limited,[75,76] and goals are generalized. Specific functional requirements and exercise loads are likely to provide more specific goals for within-phase progression, and functional outcome measures are more important than judging muscle function using this form of testing. The presence of effusion and pain is likely to inhibit performance with resistive testing, and, once these impairments have improved, muscle testing (at least for the ankle and hip) may improve without major muscle hypertrophy or neuromuscular activation changes.

- *Gait and movement analysis:*
  - *Sit-to-stand*: He has difficulty with sit-to-stand related to lack of knee flexion and pain (6–7/10). He is able to perform the transfer without assistance using the walker.
  - *Gait*: The patient is able to ambulate on level surfaces using the walker partial weight-bearing. He maintains the right knee in flexion throughout the gait cycle with decreased stance time, no push off, asymmetrical gait, and slow gait speed. 10 m gait speed is 2.0 m/sec.
  - *Transfers from car*: He has difficulty clearing his right leg and uses his hands to move the surgical leg, as well as difficulty with standing, using the car door to stand up. The transfers are very painful (6–8/10).
  - *Stairs*: He is able to ascend 4 stairs leading with left leg and descend leading with right leg using a stair rail with minimal assistance. While there is minimal increase in pain, he is somewhat unsteady and slow.

Evaluation

- *Medical diagnosis*: Total knee arthroplasty
- *Physical therapy diagnosis*: Difficulty walking, functional deficits with sit-to-stand, car transfers, stairs, and sleeping
- *Contributing impairments*: Postsurgical effusion knee mobility limitations, decreased muscle function, post surgical pain
- *Prognosis*: Good prognosis for return to functional activities, hobbies, and social participation. Knee flexion limitations may be influenced by restrictions present before the surgery.[77–79] Scar tissue removal during the surgery improves the prognosis for return of flexion necessary for functional

range of motion, but range should be achieved as soon as possible after the surgery in order to shape connective tissue healing.

Precautions

- Balance precautions[80]
- Monitor for postoperative bleeding, excessive swelling, and pain in the calf (thrombosis).
- Monitor for postoperative orthostatic hypotension.
- Progress range of motion slowly to avoid excessive inflammation.

Short-Term Goals

See Table 9.13.

Impairment Goals

Within 2 weeks (four visits) the patient will be able to:
- Perform transfers independently (bed to chair, toilet) with minimal difficulty.
- Assume weight on the surgical leg in double-leg stance with upper extremity support and maintain position for 30 seconds.
- Ambulate with walker without assistance for household distances with equal weight-bearing, full knee extension.
- Reduce postoperative edema and effusion to minimal differences between legs.
- Increase range of motion to allow active flexion greater than 80 degrees in sitting, active extension to 0 degrees.
- Activate the quadriceps in terminal range (10–0 degrees) to maintain full knee extension for at least 10 seconds.
- Decrease pain with movement to 4/10, resting pain 3/10.

TABLE 9.13   Case Study 9.4: Lower Extremity Functional Scale 2-Week Goals (4 Visits)

	Initial	Goal for 2 Weeks (4 Visits)	Rationale
1. **Any of your usual work, housework, or social activities**	0	1 (quite a bit of difficulty)	Improved tolerance with standing, sitting, and gait is likely to allow some participation in household and social activities
2. Your usual hobbies, recreational or sporting activities	0		Delayed until Phase III
3. Getting into or out of the bath	2		Delayed until good standing leg balance on the surgical leg
4. **Walking between rooms***	2	3 (minimal difficulty)	Improved tolerance is a reasonable goal with decreased effusion, increased muscle activity, and ability to shift weight onto surgical leg
5. **Putting on your shoes and socks**	0	1 (quite a bit of difficulty)	Using reacher – requires increased knee flexion
6. Squatting	0		Delayed until full symmetrical weight-bearing in standing and sufficient range (>80 degrees of flexion)
7. Lifting an object, like a bag of groceries from the floor	0		Delayed until full symmetrical weight-bearing without an assistive device, sufficient flexion, and tolerance with squats
8. **Performing light activities around your home**	0	1 (quite a bit of difficulty)	Improved tolerance with standing, sitting and gait is likely to allow some participation in household activities
9. Performing heavy activities around your home	0		Delayed until minimal or no difficulty with light activity
10. **Getting into or out of your car**	1	2 (moderate difficulty)	Improved knee range and pain levels, along with teaching the patient how to perform the movement is likely to improve the transfer
11. Walking 2 blocks	0		Delayed until symmetrical gait pattern for short distances and no increase in effusion with walking household distances
12. Walking a mile	0		Delayed until minimal difficulty with walking 2 blocks
13. **Going up or down 10 stairs***	1	2 (moderate difficulty)	Improved knee range, muscle function and decreased pain is likely to impact ability to go up and down stairs. The patient is already able to negotiate 4 steps with minimal assistance.
14. **Standing for 1 hour**	0		Modified goal to stand for more than 15 minutes, this goal is potentially possible within 4 weeks.
15. **Sitting for 1 hour**	1	2 (moderate difficulty)	Decreased effusion and increased range is likely to improve sitting tolerance
16. *Running on even ground*	*0*		Not a goal secondary to personal characteristics and presurgical function
17. *Running on uneven ground*	*0*		Not a goal secondary to personal characteristics and presurgical function
18. *Making sharp turns while running fast*	*0*		Not a goal secondary to personal characteristics and presurgical function
19. *Hopping*	*0*		Not a goal secondary to personal characteristics and presurgical function
20. **Rolling over in bed***	2	3 (minimal difficulty)	If the patient's effusion and pain levels decrease, and range of motion decreases, this goal is feasible
			The total LEFS goal does not exceed the minimal detectable change or minimal clinically important difference for the 2-week time frame, but the improvements that are feasible based on possible resolution of impairments are included for this time frame. Goals for the 4-week time frame will be adjusted based on progress and will likely exceed the MDC/MCID.
Total	9/80	2-week goal: 18/80	Total feasible functional outcome measure (long term) is 58/80

Lower Extremity Functional Scale.[71]
MDC and MCID 9 points out of 80.[1,72]
*Patient identified goals: Goals set for 2 weeks (bold); goals that are not feasible at this time (italics).

Exercise Choices for Initial Treatment

See Table 9.14.

Phase II: Post Total Knee Replacement

All short-term impairment goals have been reached after 2 weeks although pain at full active flexion (80 degrees) is still moderate (5/10). Range of motion has improved to 0–90 degrees (passive) and 0–80 degrees (active). There is minimal effusion and the incision has closed and is healing well. The patient is transferring independently with minimal difficulty, and he is ambulating with a walker (weight-bearing as tolerated) with improved symmetry for household distances. He is able to activate his quadriceps in terminal range but still has difficulty holding the position for more than 10 seconds. Exercise goals are based on LEFS subscales (Table 9.15) and impairments are adjusted.

Impairment Goals. Within 4–8 weeks (8–16 visits), the patient will:

- Increase active flexion >105 degrees in sitting, active extension to 0 degrees
- Demonstrate adequate knee extensor endurance to hold a straight leg raise with the knee at 0 degrees for >20 seconds
- Demonstrate sufficient knee extensor and flexor endurance to move through full range against gravity for greater than 25 repetitions against 2 kg
- Demonstrate the ability to transfer weight onto the affected leg and stand on one leg using some arm support for greater than 30 seconds
- Demonstrate independence with a home exercise program
- Ascend a 4-inch step 10 times with minimal hand support

Exercise Choices at 2 Weeks. See Table 9.16.

TABLE 9.14	Exercise Choices After Total Knee Replacement (Initial Treatment)
Goal	**Exercise Choices**
Decrease effusion and edema (multiple repetitions, elevated positions, muscle pumping emphasis, high frequency)	• Ankle pumps (Exercise 9.37) • Isometric quadriceps and hamstring contractions: short hold, multiple repetitions (Exercises 9.39, 9.40)
Promote muscle activation (appropriate muscle recruitment, exercise limited if compensations are noted, high repetitions or time for isometric holds >10 seconds)	• Straight-leg raise with isometric quadriceps contraction (dosage set for quadriceps endurance and ability to maintain knee extension for longer than 10 seconds) (Exercise 9.42) • Isometric quadriceps and hamstring contractions (Exercises 9.39 and 9.40): holds >10 seconds for endurance, multiple repetitions (progressive hold, isometrics in new ranges once effusion decreases). Initially the leg is supported on the plinth, then progressed to resting the ankle on top of a small ball to challenge the quadriceps and hamstring isometrics as well as hip stabilization. • Isometrics in the end range to encourage activation in the range where active insufficiency is present. The therapist raises the leg to fully extend the knee. The patient performs an isometric quadriceps contraction and then the therapist slowly removes the support from the lower limb and the patient is asked to maintain the fully extended position. The patient can be taught to use a strap or the other leg to perform active-assisted extension to replicate the exercise on their own (Exercise 9.43A)
Promote muscle function in surrounding areas to distribute forces	• Bridging using left leg for general strengthening with the right leg supported on a ball (Exercise 9.21) • Hip abduction in side lying (Exercise 9.26B) • Hip extension off the edge of the table (Exercise 9.45 alternate)
Promote range of motion recovery (multiple repetitions without fatigue but to end of range, short hold or oscillations)	• Passive or active-assisted knee extension in supine with support under the ankle (Exercise 9.1A) • Prone hang (Exercise 9.1C) • Active knee flexion in sitting (focus on achieving maximum end range, multiple repetitions with progressive range) (Exercise 9.3 in sitting) • Elevate and support the patient's leg on an exercise ball while the patient rolls ball to flex to end range (multiple repetitions, progressive increase in range) (Exercise 9.4B)
Progressive return to ambulation and function	• Progressive weight-bearing on post surgical limb in parallel bars and using assistive device (Exercise 9.46) • Partial sit-to-stand (Exercise 9.47) • Progressive gait training (Exercise 9.48) • Movement reeducation transfers in and out of the car • Stair training

TABLE 9.15   Case Study 9.4: New Goals for Week 4

		Initial	Goals Set for 2 Weeks at Initial Visit	Adjusted Short-Term Goals (Week 4)
1.	**Any of your usual work, housework, or social activities**	0	1 (quite a bit of difficulty)	**2 (moderate difficulty)**
2.	Your usual hobbies, recreational, or sporting activities	0		
3.	Getting into or out of the bath	2		**3 (minimal difficulty)** Able to stand on one leg with good balance and hand support
4.	**Walking between rooms***	2	3 (minimal difficulty)	
5.	**Putting on your shoes and socks**	0	1 (quite a bit of difficulty)	**2 (moderate difficulty)**
6.	Squatting	0		1 (quite a bit of difficulty) Goal to perform double-leg squats from 0–45 degrees with minimal pain (3/10)
7.	Lifting an object, like a bag of groceries from the floor	0		
8.	**Performing light activities around your home**	0	1 (quite a bit of difficulty)	**2 (moderate difficulty)** for assistance with household chores
9.	Performing heavy activities around your home	0		
10.	**Getting into or out of your car**	1	2 (moderate difficulty)	**3 (mild difficulty)**
11.	Walking 2 blocks	0		2 (moderate difficulty) with walker
12.	Walking a mile	0		
13.	**Going up or down 10 stairs***	1	2 (moderate difficulty)	**3 (mild difficulty)**
14.	**Standing for 1 hour**	0	Able to stand for 30 minutes with quite a bit of difficulty, 15 minutes with minimal difficulty	**1 (quite a bit of difficulty)**
15.	**Sitting for 1 hour**	1	2 (moderate difficulty)	**3 (minimal difficulty)**
20.	**Rolling over in bed***	2	3 (minimal difficulty)	Goal maintained
	Total	9/80	2 week goal: 18/80	New goal week 4: 29/80 (exceeds MDC, MCID 9 points from initial evaluation)

Lower Extremity Functional Scale.[71]
MDC and MCID 9 points out of 80.[1,72]
Patient identified goals: Most important goals for week 4 (bold).

TABLE 9.16 Exercise Choices at 2 Weeks

	Home Program	Outpatient Exercise Program
Decrease effusion and edema (multiple repetitions, elevated positions, muscle pumping emphasis, high frequency)	Continue ankle pumps at home after leg is dependent for some time or if there is any distal swelling (Exercise 9.37)	
Promote muscle activation (appropriate muscle recruitment, exercise limited if compensations are noted, high repetitions or time for isometric holds >10 seconds)	Continue straight leg raise with isometric quadriceps contraction at home (increase time held) (Exercise 9.42) Hip abduction and hip extension as tolerated (Exercises 9.26B and 9.45A)	Replace isometrics in the end range with resisted short-arc quads through terminal range with holds at 0 degrees. Increasing weight (strap-on weights) as the patient is able to maintain the position for more than 10 seconds at terminal extension. Continue hip abduction in side lying with knee fully extended and increase repetitions and resistance (Exercise 9.26B) Continue hip extension in four-point kneeling, increase repetitions then resistance (Exercise 9.45A)
Promote muscle endurance through range (15–25 repetitions to fatigue, limb weight resistance against gravity)	Open chain knee extension through range, short arc quads and active knee flexion against gravity after introduced in physical therapy sessions (Exercise 9.43 and Exercise 9.44).	Add open chain knee extension through range (terminal extension short arc and long arc quads against gravity in sitting (Exercise 9.43) Add open chain knee flexion through range (terminal flexion and from midrange to end range against gravity in prone) (Exercise 9.44). Add strap-on weights once the patient is able to perform >3 sets of 30 repetitions through full range before fatigue
Promote muscle function in proximal areas and opposite limb to distribute forces	Bridging using left leg for general strengthening with the right leg supported on a cushion (Exercise 9.21)	Continue hip abduction in side lying with knee fully extended (Exercise 9.26B) Continue hip extension in four-point kneeling (Exercise 9.45A) Add multi-hip strengthening for surgical leg (Exercise 9.20) Continue bridging in supine with surgical leg supported on an exercise ball Add leg press machine (low loads) in small ranges and isometric holds at 50–0 degrees (bilateral weight-bearing) (Exercise 9.19)
Promote range of motion recovery (multiple repetitions without fatigue but to end of range, short hold, or oscillations), progress to holds at end of range as long as tolerated	Active knee extension in supine with support under the ankle (Exercise 9.1B) Prone hang (Exercise 9.1C). Increase hold or weight Active knee flexion in sitting (focus on achieving maximum end range, multiple repetitions with progressive range) (Exercise 9.3 in sitting) Add active knee flexion with self-assisted knee flexion in prone using a strap (Exercise 9.4B) after introduced in physical therapy sessions	Add ankle dorsiflexion stretch (bilaterally in sitting with a strap) Add active knee flexion in sitting with therapist assistance for prolonged stretch (Exercise 9.3 in sitting) Continue with ball-assisted knee flexion (multiple repetitions, progressive increase in range) (Exercise 9.4B) Add self-assisted knee flexion in prone using a strap (Exercise 9.4B) Add bike: half revolutions with seat height set to accommodate either flexion or extension end range (Exercise 9.7)
Improve weight-bearing acceptance and transfer	Continue progressive weight-bearing on post surgical limb using assistive device at home (Exercise 9.46)	Progress weight transfer in double-leg standing and stride standing in parallel bars to 75% weight-bearing then single-leg balance with assistive device (Exercise 9.46), then to single-leg stance in parallel bars
Progressive return to ambulation and function, movement reeducation, and strengthening	Progress gait training with increased distance and time in the home and in the community with assistive device (Exercise 9.48) Increase range for partial sit-to-stand (Exercise 9.47)	Progress gait training in the parallel bars without as much upper extremity support (Exercise 9.48) Progress step-ups and down from 2 inches to 4 inches with surgical leg and hand support (parallel bars) maintaining dynamic alignment (Exercise 9.31) Mini-squat progression with upper body support in parallel bars (Exercise 9.30) Balance activities in double-leg stance with upper extremity challenge progressing to single-leg once able to transfer onto surgical leg with appropriate alignment (Exercise 9.24)

TABLE 9.17   Case Study 9.4: New Goals for Week 16

		Initial	Goals for 2 Weeks	Goals for Week 4	New Goals for Week 16 (4–6 Visits)
1.	Any of your usual work, house-work, or social activities	0	1 (quite a bit of difficulty)	2 (moderate difficulty)	**4 (no difficulty)**
2.	Your usual hobbies, recreational, or sporting activities*	0			**2 (quite a bit of difficulty)** Resume putting and chipping
3.	Getting into or out of the bath	2		3 (minimal difficulty) (Able to stand on one leg with good balance and hand support)	**4 (no difficulty)**
4.	Walking between rooms	2	3 (minimal difficulty)		**4 (no difficulty)**
5.	Putting on your shoes and socks*	0	1 (quite a bit of difficulty)	2 (moderate difficulty)	**3 (minimal difficulty)**
6.	Squatting	0		1 (quite a bit of difficulty). Goal to perform double-leg squats from 0 to 45 degrees with minimal pain (3/10)	**2 (moderate difficulty)** Goal to perform double-leg squat to 60 degrees with minimal pain (3/10)
7.	Lifting an object, like a bag of groceries from the floor	0			**1 (quite a bit of difficulty)** Goal to be able to lift objects from surfaces slightly above floor level
8.	Performing light activities around your home*	0	1 (quite a bit of difficulty)	2 (moderate difficulty) for assistance with household chores	**4 (no difficulty)**
9.	Performing heavy activities around your home	0			
10.	Getting into or out of your car	1	2 (moderate difficulty)	3 (mild difficulty)	**4 (no difficulty)**
11.	Walking 2 blocks*	0		2 (moderate difficulty) with walker	**4 (no difficulty)**
12.	Walking a mile	0			**1 (quite a bit of difficulty)**
13.	Going up or down 10 stairs*	1	2 (moderate difficulty)	3 (mild difficulty)	**4 (no difficulty)**
14.	Standing for 1 hour	0	Able to stand for 30 minutes with quite a bit of difficulty, 15 minutes with minimal difficulty	1 (quite a bit of difficulty)	**3 (mild difficulty)**
15.	Sitting for 1 hour	1	2 (moderate difficulty)	3 (minimal difficulty)	**4 (no difficulty)**
20.	Rolling over in bed*	2	3 (minimal difficulty)	Goal maintained	**4 (no difficulty)**
	Total	9/80	2 week goal: 18/80	4–8 week goal: 28/80	Week 16 Goal: 48/80

Lower Extremity Functional Scale.[71]
MDC and MCID 9 points out of 80.[1,72]
Items in bold set as goals for week 16.
*Patient goals.

Phase III: Post Total Knee Replacement or Arthroplasty

At week 9, after starting physical therapy, the patient is walking independently without an assistive device for community distances. Range of motion has increased to 0–110 degrees in sitting and prone. Goals are advanced for week 16, and clinic visits are scheduled on a weekly and then bi-weekly basis (Table 9.17).

Impairment Goals (Weeks 9–16, 4–6 Visits). The patient will be able to:

- Ambulate independently for community distances without deviations or compensations with a gait speed of >1.2 m/sec and equal stance time
- Perform active flexion >115 degrees in sitting, active extension to 0 degrees
- Demonstrate squats through 60 degrees and sit-to-stand transfer with equal symmetry
- Demonstrate the ability to stand on one leg with some arm support for greater than 30 seconds
- Ascend and descend 8-inch steps using a reciprocal pattern for 1 flight of stairs without using the handrail
- Report minimal difficulty with functional activities
- Demonstrate the ability to monitor and challenge home exercise, including generalized aerobic endurance activities
- Start return to golf with drills

Exercise Choices at Week 8 (Phase III). See Table 9.18.

TABLE 9.18   Exercise Choices at Week 8 (Phase III)

	Home Program	Outpatient Exercise Program
Promote muscle endurance through range (15–25 repetitions to fatigue, limb, and strap-on weight resistance against gravity)	Continue open chain knee extension through range, short arc quads and active knee flexion against gravity using strap-on weights (Exercise 9.43 and Exercise 9.44).	Open chain knee extension through range (terminal extension short arc and long arc quads against gravity in sitting using strap-on weights with progressive increases as tolerated [Exercise 9.43]) Open chain knee flexion through range (terminal flexion and from midrange to end range against gravity in prone) (Exercise 9.44). Strap-on weight increased once the patient is able to perform >3 sets of 30 repetitions through full range before fatigue
Promote muscle function in proximal areas and around the knee for functional activities (higher load to fatigue with 6–10 repetitions, no lower extremity or trunk compensations)	Bridging using left leg for general strengthening with the straight leg raise (Exercise 9.21) Hip abduction in side lying with knee fully extended (Exercise 9.26B) and hip extension in four-point kneeling (Exercise 9.45)	Increase resistance for multi-hip strengthening for surgical leg (open chain) and standing on the surgical leg (closed chain) (Exercise 9.20) Leg press machine full range with loads allowing 6–10 repetitions with fatigue of the knee muscles and equal weight-bearing from mid to end range and lower loads from full flexion to mid-range. Add single-leg exercise with adjusted resistance (right leg) (Exercise 9.19) Mini-squat progression in pain free ranges with elastic resistance to promote hip abductor and external rotator use to maintain sagittal alignment and distribute forces. Progress to unstable support (Exercise 9.30)
Promote and maintain range of motion recovery 25–30 repetitions reaching end range or hold at end range, low load avoid compensations)	Discontinue active knee extension in supine with support under the ankle and prone hang Discontinue active knee flexion in sitting, continue active knee flexion with self-assisted knee flexion in prone using a strap to reach full functional requirements 110–120 degrees Continue ankle dorsiflexion stretch with a strap	Discontinue therapist-assisted and ball-assisted flexion stretches. Continue with Bike -full revolutions with seat height set to accommodate either flexion or extension end range (Exercise 9.7) Terminal extension (single-leg) or full flexion (single-leg) emphasis with all muscle function exercises to regain active control through range.
Improve weight-bearing acceptance and transfer	Continue progressive weight-bearing on post surgical limb without assistive device at home (Exercise 9.46)	Progress weight transfer in double-leg standing and stride standing in parallel bars to 75% weight-bearing then single-leg balance with assistive device (Exercise 9.46), then to single-leg stance in parallel bars
Progressive return to ambulation and function, movement re-education and strengthening	Progress walking distance and speed in the community with and without assistive device (Exercise 9.48) Substitute deeper range mini squats for partial sit-to-stand (see strengthening)	Progress speed using treadmill (Exercise 9.48) Progress stepping over objects, direction changes, dual tasks (walking drills similar to Exercise 9.52) Progress speed and repetitions of step-ups and down maintaining dynamic alignment (Exercise 9.31) Balance activities with single-leg stance (Exercise 9.27) Reaction time training in different planes Individual activity specific activities: transfers to the floor to play with grandchildren, standing hip rotation drills in preparation for return to golf

REFERENCES

Introduction

1. Magee DJ. *Orthopaedic Assessment*. 6th ed. St. Louis, MO: Saunders Elsevier; 2014.
2. Neumann DA. *Kinesiology for the Musculoskeletal System*. 3rd ed. 2017.
3. Hawkins RJ. *Musculoskeletal examination*. St. Louis, MO: Mosby; 1995.
4. Magee DJ, Sueki D. *Orthopedic Physical Assessment Atlas and Video*. St. Louis, MO: Elsevier Saunders; 2011.
5. Staheli LT, Corbett M, Wyss C, et al. Lower extremity rotational problems in children: normal values to guide management. *J Bone Joint Surg Am*. 1985;67:39–47.
6. Lee TQ, Morris G, Csintalan RP. The influence of tibial and femoral rotation on patellofemoral contact area and pressure. *J Orthop Sports Phys Ther*. 2003;33:686–693.
7. Bencke J, Christiansen D, Jensen K, et al. Measuring medial longitudinal arch deformation during gait. A reliability study. *Gait Posture*. 2012;35(3):400–404.
8. Tsai CT, Chang WD, Lee JP. Effects of short-term treatment with Kinesiotaping for plantar fasciitis. *J Musculoskelet Pain*. 2010;18: 71–80.
9. Van de Water AT, Spksnijder CM. Efficacy of taping for the treatment of plantar fasciosis: a systematic review of controlled trials. *J Am Podiatr Med Assoc*. 2010;100:41–51.
10. Martin R, Davenport TE, Reischl SF, et al. Heel pain-plantar fasciitis: revision 2014. Clinical practice guidelines linked to the International Classification of Functioning, Disability and Health from the Orthopaedic Section of the American Physical Therapy Association. *J Orthop Phys Ther*. 2014;44911:A1–A23. https://doi.org/10.2519/jospt.2014.0303.
11. Evans AM, Copper AW, Scharfbillig RW, et al. Reliability of the foot posture index and traditional measures of foot position. *J Am Podiatr Med Assoc*. 2003;93(3):203–213.
12. Redmond AC, Crosbie J, Ouvrier RA. Development and validation of a novel rating system for scoring standing foot posture: the foot posture index. *Clin Biomech*. 2006;21:89–98.

13. Malliaris P, Cook J, Purdam C, Rio E. Patellar tendinopathy: clinical diagnosis, load management and advice for challenging case presentations. *J Orthop Sports Phys Ther*. 2015;45(11):887–898.

14. Lee TQ, Anzel SH, Bennet KA, et al. The influence of fixed rotational deformities of the femur on the patellofemoral contact pressures in human cadaver knees. *Clin Orthop Relat Res*. 1994;302:69–74.

15. Pantano KJ, White SC, Gilchrist LA, Leddy J. Differences in peak knee valgus angles between individuals with high and low Q-angles during a single limb squat. *Clin Biomech (Bristol, Avon)*. 2005;20:966–972.

Case 9.1

16. Michael JWP, Schluter-Brust KU, Eysel P. The epidemiology, etiology, diagnosis, and treatment of osteoarthritis of the knee. *Dtsch Arztebl Int*. 2010;107(9):152–162. https://doi.org/10.3238/arztebl.2010.0152.

17. Messier SP, Gutekunst DJ, Davis C, Devita P. Weight loss reduces knee-joint loads in overweight and obese older adults with knee osteoarthritis. *Arthritis Rheum*. 2005;52(7):2026–2032. https://doi.org/10.1002/art.21139.

18. Gersing AS, Schwaiger BJ, Nevitt MC, Joseph GB, et al. Is weight loss associated with less progression of changes in knee articular cartilage among obese and overweight patients as assessed with MR imaging over 48 months? Data from the Osteoarthritis Initiative. *Radiology*. 2017. online ahead of print. https://doi.org/10.1148/radiol.2017161005.

19. Christensen R, Astrup A, Bliddal H. Weight loss: the treatment of choice for knee osteoarthritis? A randomized trial. *Osteoarthritis Cartilage*. 2005;13(1):20–27. https://doi.org/10.1016/j.joca.2004.10.008.

20. Christensen R, Bartels EM, Astrup A, Bliddal H. Effect of weight reduction in obese patients diagnosed with knee osteoarthritis: a systematic review and meta-analysis. *Ann Rheum Dis*. 2006;66(4):433–439. https://doi.org/10.1136/ard.2006.065904.

21. Mündermann A, Dyrby CO, Andriacchi TP. Secondary gait changes in patients with medial compartment knee osteoarthritis: increased load at the ankle, knee, and hip during walking. *Arthritis Rheum*. 2005;52(9):2835–2844. https://doi.org/10.1002/art.21262.

22. Simoneau G, Heiderscheit B. Kinesiology of walking. In: Neumann DA, ed. *Kinesiology of the Musculoskeletal System. Foundations for Rehabilitation*. 3rd ed. St. Louis, MO: Mosby Elsevier; 2017:654–705.

23. Childs JD, Sparto PJ, Fitzgerald G, Bizzini M, Irrgang JJ. Alterations in lower extremity movement and muscle activation patterns in individuals with knee osteoarthritis. *Clin Biomech*. 2004;19(1):44–49. https://doi.org/10.1016/j.clinbiomech.2003.08.007.

24. Madry H, Kohn D. Conservative treatment of knee osteoarthritis. *Der Unfallchirurg*. 2004;107(8):689–699. http://europepmc.org/abstract/med/15300328.

25. Mcalindon T, Bannuru R, Sullivan M, et al. OARSI guidelines for the non-surgical management of knee osteoarthritis. *Osteoarthritis Cartilage*. 2014;22(3):363–388. https://doi.org/10.1016/j.joca.2014.01.003.

26. Bennell KL, Hinman RS. A review of the clinical evidence for exercise in osteoarthritis of the hip and knee. *J Sci Med Sport*. 2011;14(1):4–9. https://doi.org/10.1016/j.jsams.2010.08.002.

27. Keating EM, Faris PM, Ritter MA, Kane J. Use of lateral heel and sole wedges in the treatment of medial osteoarthritis of the knee. *Orthop Rev*. 1993;22(8):921–924. http://europepmc.org/abstract/med/8265230.

28. Baker K, McAlindon T. Exercise for knee osteoarthritis. *Curr Opin Rheumatol*. 2000;12(5):456–463. http://ovidsp.tx.ovid.com.lp.hscl.ufl.edu/sp-3.25.0a/ovidweb.cgi?

29. Pelletier J-P, Raynauld J-P, Berthiaume M-J, et al. Risk factors associated with the loss of cartilage volume on weight-bearing areas in knee osteoarthritis patients assessed by quantitative magnetic resonance imaging: a longitudinal study. *Arthritis Res Ther*. 2007;9(4). https://doi.org/10.1186/ar2272.

30. Sled EA, Khoja L, Deluzio KJ, Olney SJ, Culham EG. Effect of a home program of hip abductor exercises on knee joint loading, strength, function, and pain in people with knee osteoarthritis: a clinical trial. *Physical Therapy*. 2010;90(6):895–904. https://doi.org/10.2522/ptj.20090294.

31. Hill CL, Hunter DJ, Niu J, et al. Synovitis detected on magnetic resonance imaging and its relation to pain and cartilage loss in knee osteoarthritis. *Ann Rheum Dis*. 2007;66(12):1599–1603. https://doi.org/10.1136/ard.2006.067470.

32. Sharma L. The Role of Knee Alignment in disease progression and functional decline in knee osteoarthritis. *JAMA*. 2001;286(2):188–195. https://doi.org/10.1001/jama.286.2.188.

33. Bennell KL, Hunt MA, Wrigley TV, Hunter DJ, Hinman RS. The effects of hip muscle strengthening on knee load, pain, and function in people with knee osteoarthritis: a protocol for a randomised, single-blind controlled trial. *BMC Musculoskelet Disord*. 2007;8(1). https://doi.org/10.1186/1471-2474-8-121.

34. Fransen M, McConnell S, Harmer AR, Van der Esch M, Simic M, Bennell KL. *Exercise for osteoarthritis of the knee | Cochrane*. http://www.cochrane.org/CD004376/MUSKEL_exercise-for-osteoarthritis-of-the-knee. Published January 8, 2015. Accessed May 24, 2017.

Case 9.2

35. Logerstedt DS, Synder-Mackler L, Ritter RC, Axe MJ, Godges JJ. Knee stability and movement impairment coordination impairments: knee ligament sprain. Clinical practice guidelines linked to the International Classification of Functioning, Disability, and Health from the Orthopaedic Section of the American Physical Therapy Association. *J Orthop Sports Phys Ther*. 2010;40(4):A1–A37.

36. Fitzgerald GK, Axe MJ, Snyder-Mackler L. A decision-making scheme for returning patients to high-level activity with nonoperative treatment after anterior cruciate ligament rupture. *Knee Surg Sports Traumatol Arthrosc*. 2000;8:76–82.

37. Wilk KE, et al. Recent advances in the rehabilitation of anterior cruciate ligament injuries. *J Orthop Sports Phys Ther*. 2012;42(3):153–171.

38. Escamilla RF, et al. Anterior cruciate ligament strain and tensile forces for weight-bearing and non-weight-bearing exercises: a guide to exercise selection. *J Orthop Sports Phys Ther*. 2012;42(3):208–220.

39. Dingenen B, Janssens L, Luyckx T, Claes S, Bellemans J. Staes. Lower extremity muscle activation onset times from double-leg stance to single-leg stance in anterior cruciate ligament injured subjects. *Human Movt Sc*. 2015;44:234–245.

40. Fitzgerald GK, Axe MJ, Synder-Mackler L. Proposed practice guidelines for nonoperative anterior cruciate ligament rehabilitation of physically active individuals. *J Orthop Sports Phys Ther*. 2000;30(4):194–203.

41. Fitzgerald GK, Axe MJ, Synder-Mackler L. The efficacy of perturbation training in nonoperative anterior cruciate ligament rehabilitation programs for physically active individuals. *Phys Ther*. 2000;80:128–140.

42. Mueller MJ, Maluf KS. Tissue adaptation to physical stress: a proposed "Physical Stress Theory" to guide physical therapy practice, education and research. *Phys Ther.* 2002;82(4):383–403.

43. Benjaminese A, Gokeler A, Dowling AV, et al. Optimization of the anterior cruciate ligament injury prevention paradigm: novel feedback techniques to enhance motor learning and reduce injury risk. *J Orthop Sports Phys Ther.* 2015;45(3):170–182.

44. Ageberg E, Roos EM. The association between knee confidence and muscle power, hop performance, and postural orientation in people with anterior cruciate ligament injury. *J Orthop Sports Phys Ther.* 2016;46(6):477–482.

45. Fleming BC, Beynnon BD, Renstrom PA, Peura GD, Nichols CE, Johnson RJ. The strain behavior of the anterior cruciate ligament during bicycling. An in vivo study. *Am J Sports Med.* 1998;26:109–118.

46. Escamilla RF, Zheng N, Macleod TD, et al. Cruciate ligament forces between short-step and long-step forward lunge. *Med Sci Sports Exerc.* 2010;42:1932–1942.

47. Escamilla RF, Zheng N, Macleod TD, et al. Cruciate ligament tensile forces during the forward and side lunge. *Clin Biomech (Bristol, Avon).* 2010;25:213–221.

48. Farrokhi S, Pollard CD, Souza RB, Chen YJ, Reischl S, Powers CM. Trunk position influences the kinematics, kinetics, and muscle activity of the lead lower extremity during the forward lunge exercise. *J Orthop Sports Phys Ther.* 2008;38:403–409.

Case 9.3

49. Witvrouw E, et al. Patellofemoral pain: consensus statement from the 3rd International Patellofemoral Pain Research Retreat held in Vancouver, September 2013. *Br J Sports Med.* 2014;48: 411–414.

50. Crossley KM, et al. 2016 Patellofemoral pain consensus statement from the 4th International Patellofemoral Pain Research Retreat, Manchester. Part 1: terminology, definitions, clinical examination, natural history, patellofemoral osteoarthritis and patient-reported outcome measures. *Br J Sports Med.* 2016;00:1–5.

51. Rabin A, et al. Factors associated with visually assessed quality of movement during a lateral step-down test among individuals with patellofemoral pain. *J Orthop Sports Phys Ther.* 2014;44(12):937–946.

52. Bolgla LA, et al. Hip strength and hip and knee kinematics during stair descent in females with and without patellofemoral pain syndrome. *J Orthop Sports Phys Ther.* 2008;38(1):12–18.

53. Robinson RL, Nee RJ. Analysis of hip strength in females seeking physical therapy treatment for unilateral patellofemoral pain syndrome. *J Orthop Sports Phys Ther.* 2007;37(5):232–238.

54. Salsich GB, Graci V, Maxam DE. The effects of movement pattern modification on lower extremity kinematics and pain in women with patellofemoral pain. *J Orthop Sports Phys Ther.* 2012;42(12):1017–1024.

55. Chinkulprasert C, Vachalathiti R, Powers CM. Patellofemoral joint forces and stress during forward step-up, lateral step-up, and forward step-down exercises. *J Orthop Sports Phys Ther.* 2011;41(4):241–248.

56. Barton CJ, Lack S, Malliaras P, et al. Gluteal muscle activity and patellofemoral pain syndrome: a systematic review. *Br J Sports Med.* 2013;47:207–214.

57. Fukuda TY, Melo WP, Zaffalon BM, et al. Hip posterolateral musculature strengthening in sedentary women with patellofemoral pain syndrome: a randomized controlled clinical trial with 1-year follow-up. *J Orthop Sports Phys Ther.* 2012;42:823–830.

58. Dolak KL, Silkman C, Medina McKeon J, et al. Hip strengthening before functional exercises reduces pain sooner than quadriceps strengthening in females with patellofemoral pain syndrome: a randomized clinical trial. *J Orthop Sports Phys Ther.* 2011;41:560–570.

59. Khayambashi K, Mohammadkhani Z, Ghaznavi K, et al. The effects of isolated hip abductor and external rotator muscle strengthening on pain, health status, and hip strength in females with patellofemoral pain: a randomized controlled trial. *J Orthop Sports Phys Ther.* 2012;42:22–29.

60. Willy RW, Davis IS. The effect of a hip-strengthening program on mechanics during running and during a single-leg squat. *J Orthop Sports Phys Ther.* 2011;41:625–632.

61. Aminaka N, Pietrosimone BG, Armstrong CW, et al. Patellofemoral pain syndrome alters neuromuscular control and kinetics during stair ambulation. *J Electromyogr Kinesiol.* 2011;21:551–645.

62. McKenzie K, Galea V, Wessel J, et al. Lower extremity kinematics of females with patellofemoral pain syndrome while stair stepping. *J Orthop Sports Phys Ther.* 2010;40:625–632.

63. Hofmann CL, Holyoak DT, Juris PM. Trunk and shank position influences patellofemoral joint stress in the lead and trail limbs during the forward lunge exercise. *J Orthop Sports Phys Ther.* 2017;47(1):31–40.

64. Powers CM, et al. Patellofemoral joint stress during weight-bearing and non-weight-bearing quadriceps exercises. *J Orthop Sports Phys Ther.* 2014;44(5):320–327.

65. Janssen I, Steele JR, Munro BJ, Brown NA. Predicting the patella tendon force generated when landing from a jump. *Med Sci Sports Exerc.* 2013;45:927–934.

66. Silva RS, Ferreira ALG, Nakagawa TH, Santos JEM, Serrao FV. Rehabilitation of patellar tendinopathy using hip extensor strengthening and landing-strategy modification: case report with 6-month follow-up. *J Orthop Sports Phys Ther.* 2015;45(11):899–909.

67. Zhang SN, Bates BT, Dufek JS. Contributions of lower extremity joints to energy dissipation during landings. *Med Sci Sports Exerc.* 2000;32:812–819.

68. Souza RB, et al. Femur rotation and patellofemoral joint kinematics: a weight-bearing magnetic resonance imaging analysis. *J Orthop Sports Phys Ther.* 2010;40(5):277–285.

69. Teng HL, Powers CM. Sagittal plane trunk posture influences patellofemoral joint stress during running. *J Orthop Sports Phys Ther.* 2014;44(10):785–792.

70. Cheung RT, Davis IS. Landing pattern modification to improve patellofemoral pain in runners: a case series. *J Orthop Sports Phys Ther.* 2011;41(12):914–919.

Case Study 9.4

71. Binkley JM, Stratford PW, Lott SA, Riddle DI. The Lower Extremity Functional Scale (LEFS): scale development, measurement properties, and clinical application. *Phys Ther.* 1999;79:371–383.

72. Cleland J, Cleland JA, Koppenhaver S. *Netter's Orthopaedic Clinical Examination - An Evidence-based Approach.* 2nd ed. St. Louis, MO: Saunders Elsevier; 2011.

73. Sayers A, et al. Rest pain and movement-evoked pain as unique constructs in hip and knee replacements. *Arthritis Care Res.* 2016;68(2):237–245.

74. www.rehabmeasures.org.

75. Knepler C, Bahannon RW. *Subjectivity of Forces Associated with Manual-Muscle Test Grades of 3, 4-, and 4. Perceptual and Motor Skills.* http://journals.sagepub.com/doi/abs/10.2466/pms.1998.87.3f.1123. Published December 1, 1998. Accessed May 25, 2017.

76. Bohannon RW, Corrigan D. A broad range of forces is encompassed by the maximum manual muscle test grade of five. *Percept Motor Skills*. 2000;90(3):747–750. https://doi.org/10.2466/pms.2000.90.3.747.

77. Barker KL, Jenkins C, Pandit H, Murray D. Muscle power and function two years after unicompartmental knee replacement. *Knee*. 2012;19(4):360–364. https://doi.org/10.1016/j.knee.2011.05.006.

78. Kennedy DM, Stratford PW, Riddle DL, Hanna SE, Gollish JD. Assessing recovery and establishing prognosis following total knee arthroplasty. *Phys Ther*. 2008;88(1):22–32. https://doi.org/10.2522/ptj.20070051.

79. Mizner RL, Petterson SC, Snyder-Mackler L. Quadriceps strength and the time course of functional recovery after total knee arthroplasty. *J Orthopaed Sports Phys Ther*. 2005;35(7):424–436. https://doi.org/10.2519/jospt.2005.35.7.424.

80. Cahill JB, Kosman LM. Total knee arthroplasty. In: Cioppa-Mosca J, Cahill JB, Young Tucker C, eds. *Hospital for Special Surgery. Handbook of Postsurgical Rehabilitation Guidelines for the Orthopedic Clinician*. St. Louis, MO: Mosby Elsevier; 2008:9–15.

10

Upper Extremity Workbook

Kim Dunleavy and Amy Kubo Slowik

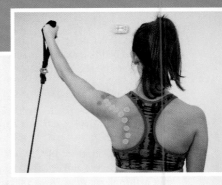

The workbook chapters are designed to provide examples of exercises for four of the categories described in Chapter 6. The general biomechanical concepts applicable for the region are provided at the beginning of the chapter. Each section includes the general exercise approaches for the category, precautions and contraindications, general parameters, tests and measures, and compensations in the beginning of the section. The purpose, position, exercise description and actions, teaching tips, advantages, alternatives, and progressions are listed for the selected exercises. The exercises have been chosen to illustrate the types of exercise to be considered and may also be suitable for other categories or for other regions. There are multiple exercise options and modifications, and the exercises in this chapter are not meant to be all-inclusive. Case studies are included at the end of each section and the concepts used for the final category

(individuals with chronic pain behaviors and psychological elements) are applied in selected case study examples.

BIOMECHANICAL CONCEPTS

The biomechanical concepts for the upper extremity are influenced by the large ranges of motion in multiple planes needed for grasping, reaching, feeding, and dressing. The linkage of the upper extremity to the trunk is mostly through muscle attachments originating on the scapular, cervical, and thoracic areas, and therefore postural position influences the muscle alignment and biomechanical efficiency. The fine-tuned motion necessary for grip activities and coordination also influences the type of functional requirements. Exercise implications are outlined in Table 10.1.

TABLE 10.1 Biomechanical Concepts and Exercise Implications for the Upper Extremity	
Biomechanical Concepts	**Exercise Implications**
1. Core Position	
Cervicothoracic and postural alignment influences scapular position, muscle alignment/length, and shoulder range of motion.[1,4,5] (See Chapter 4)	Consider cervicothoracic alignment and position with ALL upper extremity exercises.
Common spinal alignment issues that affect scapular position include:	Address upper thoracic and cervical mobility and muscle length if contributing to stress or if impacting the upper extremity range of motion.[1,2]
• Forward head (tipping) (Fig. 4.9A)	Erect posture has been found to increase the available shoulder elevation range of motion,[3–5] and the ability to actively correct seated position may diminish scapular anterior tilting (tipping) and decrease scapular upward rotation.[4]
• Thoracic kyphosis (tipping) (Fig. 4.9A)	
• Flat thoracic spine (winging) (Fig. 4.9B)	
• Scoliosis (rotation or elevation)	
• Asymmetry (leads to downward rotation of the scapula if the trunk is side-bent or a general downward slope of the shoulder regions is present [Table Fig. 10.1])	Postural corrections can be included during exercise and positions selected to maximize proprioceptive input or to target specific muscle activity to resist gravity or external load.
• Thoracolumbar lordosis (tipping or winging) and downward rotation (Table Fig. 10.1)	

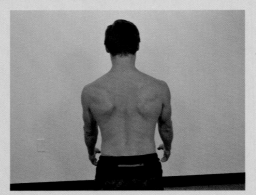

Table Fig. 10.1 Tipping, winging, and downward rotation related to thoracolumbar lordosis and downward slope of the shoulders.

Biomechanical Concepts	Exercise Implications
2. Scapulothoracic Movement and Control Scapular movement and control depends on neuromuscular control rather than passive constraints. Normal elevation in the sagittal, frontal, or scapular planes involves both scapular movement (accounting for up to one-third of the motion or 60 degrees) and glenohumeral motion (approximately two-thirds or 120 degrees).[6] There is normally 45–55 degrees of scapula upward rotation, placing the glenoid at an angle to allow upper extremity use above the shoulder.[8] During normal elevation, the scapula also tilts posteriorly (20–40 degrees) and rotates externally (15–35 degrees).[6] As a number of the shoulder muscles, including the rotator cuff, deltoid, and long head of biceps, attach to the scapula and others attach to the clavicle, the muscle alignment and ability to produce tension is also impacted by the scapula position.[6] Approximation of the scapula to the rib cage links the upper limb to the thoracic spine and provides a moving base for the glenohumeral muscles. Abnormal scapulothoracic kinematics (sometimes described as scapular dyskinesia) or poor coordination of scapular movement relative to the glenohumeral motion is a typical observation in patients with shoulder dysfunction and often observed with other upper extremity injury.[4] Along with limited muscle function and mobility, the altered movement patterns can contribute to the amount of load absorbed by the glenohumeral muscle and joint structures.[4,7] Serratus anterior, upper trapezius, and lower trapezius muscles are responsible for the force couple producing upward rotation of the scapula through elevation.[4,6,8] Serratus anterior activity contributes to all components of elevation (upward rotation, posterior tilt, and external rotation) and links the scapula to the rib cage, preventing winging, anterior tilting, and downward rotation.[8] Individuals with shoulder impingement symptoms and instability have been found to have reduced scapulothoracic upward rotation in early elevation, with reduced posterior tilting in higher ranges of elevation, although there is considerable variability in movement patterns for individuals with and without shoulder dysfunction (Table Fig. 10.2).[4,9–12] In contrast, patients with adhesive capsulitis or stiffness and rotator cuff tears typically compensate for lack of mobility or strength by excessive or early scapular motion (upward rotation and/or elevation) but also exhibit decreased posterior tilt.[4]	The emphasis of exercise for the upper extremity is to enable movement required for function rather than "stability," although scapular linkage and appropriate timing is an important component of the neuromuscular coordination. Inclusion of scapulothoracic muscle exercise in all programs is recommended, with individual programs aiming to improve the relevant impairments in flexibility, activation, coordination, or strength deficits.[9,12,13] Scapular upward rotation during initial and early elevation, taking into account the starting position of the scapula, may be important to assist with neuromuscular reeducation of scapulothoracic movement timing and coordination. Individuals with shoulder pain have been found to have decreased activation of the serratus anterior, and, as the muscle contributes to all elements required for the scapula elevation, exercises targeting the timing and function of the serratus anterior are important.[4] Limited posterior tilting can be related to anterior muscle flexibility, a flexed upper thoracic position, or inadequate posterior muscle activity in the higher ranges. Each potential cause of the abnormal mechanics will require different parameters with prolonged stretching of the anterior muscles (pectoralis major, minor or latissimus dorsi), thoracic mobility exercise or posterior muscle activation, endurance, or strengthening matched to the relevant impairments.

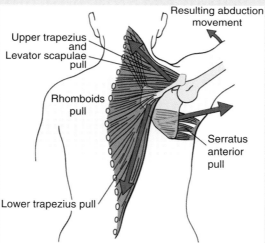

Table Fig. 10.2 Muscles responsible for scapula upward rotation. (Magee DJ, Zachazewski JE, Quillen WS, et al. *Pathology and Intervention in Musculoskeletal Rehabilitation.* 2nd. ed. St. Louis, MO: Elsevier; 2016.)

Starting positions for postural alignment contributing to increased load on the glenohumeral structures: • Downward rotation (Fig. 4.4A) • Winging (Fig. 4.4B) • Anterior tipping (Fig. 4.4C) • Scapulothoracic movement compensations • Early (or late) upward rotation • Early or excessive scapula elevation (Fig. 4.8A) • Spinal compensations (Fig. 4.8B)	The starting range for scapular movement can often be modified by placing the arm in specific starting positions (with or without support), using props, or working in ranges where the scapular muscles are in a favorable position. Compensations due to muscle imbalances, limited glenohumeral range of motion/muscle flexibility, or muscle weakness can be addressed through exercises to address the relevant impairments. Motor control concepts may be necessary to teach different movement sequences, and sensory input (closed chain or tactile feedback) can be helpful to improve muscle timing or activation. Load may need to be adjusted or range of motion improved before addressing timing. Consider the effect of gravity and arm weight when selecting positions for upper extremity exercise.

Continued

Biomechanical Concepts	**Exercise Implications**

3. Impingement

Compression of the supraspinatus and subacromial bursa between the humeral head and the acromion occurs anywhere between 34 and 72 degrees,[14] with superior glide of the head of the humerus. In patients with impingement syndromes, the subacromial space has been shown to be decreased compared to controls using magnetic resonance imaging (MRI).[15,16] Excessive or early superior glide or upward force is thought to be related to limited rotator cuff approximation of the humerus to the glenoid, while the deltoid provides an abduction force (see the section on rotator cuff mechanics).[8,17] The narrowing may also be related to effusion or from the acromion shape (Table Fig. 10.3).

Late clearance of the greater tuberosity from under the acromion is also thought to contribute to compression of the supraspinatus, subacromial bursa, long head of biceps, and the superior rotator cuff.[18,19] Shoulder internal rotation during elevation, particularly with prolonged positions or with load in the "empty can" position, increases compressive loads[20] and typically aggravates and reproduces symptoms.[8,9,21–24]

The resulting impingement manifests as pain during an arc of movement starting between 35 and 70 degrees, with decreased pain after external rotation clears the humeral head from under the acromial arch at around 120 degrees.[6,25,26] Impingement of the long head of the biceps occurs higher in the flexion range or earlier if the arm is maintained in internal rotation throughout the elevation (Table Fig. 10.4), similar to the Neer's impingement test.[26,27]

Patients can be taught to externally rotate throughout elevation (thumbs up throughout the range) to avoid impingement during exercise and activities of daily living. If external rotation clears the subacromial structures, further pain-free range of motion may be possible immediately and the painful arc avoided during exercise or function. If this is not possible, higher ranges of elevation range may need to be limited.

If it is not possible to reduce pain by modifying scapulothoracic (tipping, late upward rotation, lack of posterior tilt) or glenohumeral (internal rotation) mechanics, the painful range may need to be avoided during early management while other contributing factors are addressed.

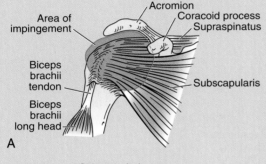

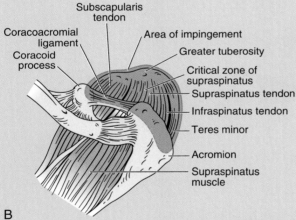

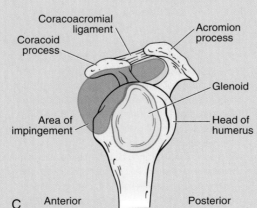

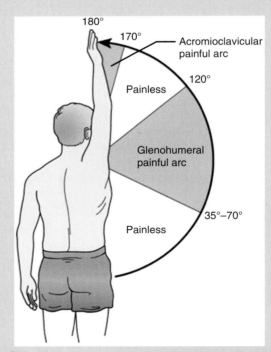

Table Fig. 10.3 Structures (A and B) and areas (A–C) involved in shoulder impingement. (From Magee DJ, Zachazewski JE, Quillen WS, et al. *Pathology and Intervention in Musculoskeletal Rehabilitation.* 2nd. ed. St. Louis, MO: Elsevier; 2016.)

Table Fig. 10.4 Shoulder abduction—painful arcs of movement related to glenohumeral joint impingement or acromioclavicular joint dysfunction. (From Magee DJ. *Orthopedic Physical Assessment.* 6th ed. St. Louis, MO: Elsevier; 2016.)

Biomechanical Concepts	Exercise Implications

4. Rotator Cuff Mechanics

The rotator cuff actively approximates the head of the humerus into the glenoid fossa and is responsible for compressing or linking the head of the humerus to the glenoid. As the scapula rotates during shoulder abduction and flexion, the glenoid faces progressively upward. Coordination of the rotator cuff muscles along with the scapula control is imperative to keep the humeral head aligned with the moving base.[7] The head of the humerus is significantly larger than the glenoid, and only 25–30% of the surface is in contact with the glenoid during motion, increasing the need for rotator cuff approximation of the joint (Table Fig. 10.5).[28]

Midrange of the rotator cuff muscles is around 60 or 70 degrees of flexion, in neutral rotation.

Position and angle of the glenoid will influence the ability of the rotator cuff to provide glenohumeral approximation, rotational control, and force couples. The "normal" position of the scapula relative to the rib cage faces approximately 30–35 degrees anteriorly from the frontal plane and is slightly upwardly rotated (±3–10 degrees) with an additional 5-degree upward direction of the glenoid.[6,22] The upward rotation of the glenoid assists with placing the joint in a position where there is less distraction than if the scapula faces downward.

Rotator cuff activation is required to maintain the axis of the glenohumeral joint and link the upper extremity to the scapula through synchronous activity.[8] The compressive forces increase with progressive elevation, reportedly reaching as high as 80–90% of body weight.[6,29] While closed chain positions provide proprioceptive input to assist with local stabilizer recruitment, the amount of joint compression and ability to support body weight also needs to be considered.[30]

In addition to controlling humeral head translation, the rotator cuff muscles also produce internal and external rotation and scapular plane abduction (especially at lower ranges of elevation; Table Figs. 10.6 and 10.7).[8]

Prepositioning the arm in optimal positions for activation in the scaption plane and midrange can be helpful when the rotator cuff muscles are weak.

Supported positions of the arm will decrease the amount of muscle support required to approximate the head of the humerus into the glenoid.

The multiple functions of the rotator cuff need to be considered when developing an exercise program for the rotator cuff. Electromyographic (EMG) studies of the relative activation of the rotator cuff muscle in different exercises can be used to assist with progression of exercises targeting specific muscles,[8] but the ability to approximate the head of the humerus and control position through range precedes control of rotation through range.

Closed chain positions can be used to promote generalized rotator cuff activation and approximation of the joint; however, the amount of load will need to be adjusted based on the rotator cuff capabilities and damage.[30] Ground reaction forces in quadruped positions are lower (19% body weight) than push-ups (34% body weight).[30]

Individuals with rotator cuff damage may not be able to tolerate compressive forces with large external moment arms, and applying forces closer to the shoulder or with flexed elbows would be preferable.[6]

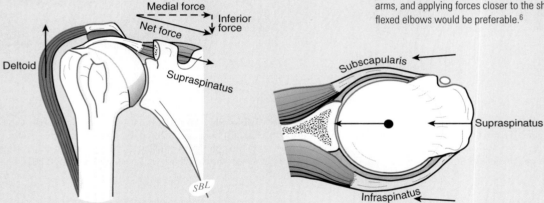

Table Fig. 10.5 Forces required from the rotator cuff muscles for abduction and approximation of the head of the humerus to the glenoid. (From Magee DJ, Zachazewski JE, Quillen WS, et al. *Pathology and Intervention in Musculoskeletal Rehabilitation*. 2nd. ed. St. Louis, MO: Elsevier; 2016.)

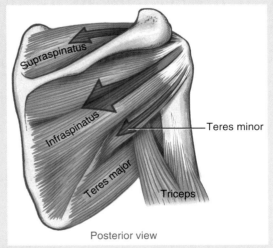

Posterior view

Table Fig. 10.6 Posterior components of the rotator cuff force couple approximating the head of the humerus relative to the scapula. (From Neumann DA. *Kinesiology of the Musculoskeletal System*. 3rd ed. St. Louis, MO: Elsevier; 2017.)

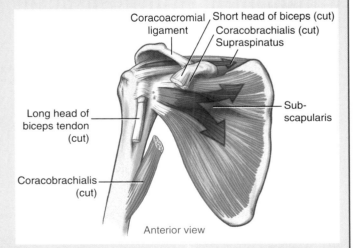

Anterior view

Table Fig. 10.7 Anterior components of the rotator cuff force couple for approximation of the head of the humerus to the scapula. (From Neumann DA. *Kinesiology of the Musculoskeletal System*. 3rd ed. St. Louis, MO: Elsevier; 2017.)

Continued

TABLE 10.1   Biomechanical Concepts and Exercise Implications for the Upper Extremity—cont'd

Biomechanical Concepts	Exercise Implications

4. Rotator Cuff Mechanics—cont'd

The supraspinatus tendon is at maximum length when the arm is next to the body in sitting or standing. The full tension (strain) on the muscle–tendon complex increases if there is downward rotation, tipping, or forward shoulders, further increasing the strain resulting from the weight of the arm (Table Fig. 10.8).[22]

Because of the angle and constant tension of the supraspinatus tendon, along with the potential for friction and compression under the acromion, it is vulnerable to fraying (Table Fig. 10.9).[6,31] The muscle needs to generate forces to resist the load of the arm weight and is subjected to high loads during abduction, especially when loads are supported at a distance from the body.[6]

The risk increases in the presence of osteophytes or an abnormally shaped acromion (Table Fig. 10.10).

Both the supraspinatus tendon and the long head of biceps are vulnerable to subacromial compression (Table Fig. 10.9), particularly with shoulder internal rotation in elevation (Fig. 4.7B).

The risk increases in the presence of osteophytes or an abnormally shaped acromion (Table Fig. 10.10).

The supraspinatus tendon also has an area of poor vascular supply in the midtendon, reducing potential for recovery (Table Fig. 10.11).

Patients with impingement or rotator cuff problems may need to be positioned with the arm supported in supine, prone, or with the arm on a table in sitting to avoid full strain of the supraspinatus if injured. Scapular upward rotation assists with positioning the glenoid.

Excessive weight in lengthened (or elevated) positions should be avoided with rotator cuff degeneration, impingement, tendon tears, or instability.

Patients with superior rotator cuff tears or degenerative changes may need to avoid high loads in extreme ranges during functional activities and specific exercise. The length of external moment arms may need to be considered as well as the amount of load.

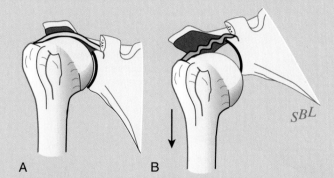

Table Fig. 10.8 Distraction forces on the glenohumeral joint resulting in strain of the supraspinatus tendon with downward rotation of the scapula can contribute to tendon overload. (From Neumann DA. *Kinesiology of the Musculoskeletal System.* 3rd ed. St. Louis, MO: Elsevier; 2017.)

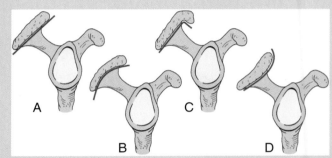

Table Fig. 10.10 Natural variation in shapes of the acromion. (A) Flat, (B) concave, (C) hooked, and (D) convex. There is a higher risk of impingement with C or D. (From Magee DJ. *Orthopedic Physical Assessment.* 6th ed. St. Louis, MO: Elsevier; 2016.)

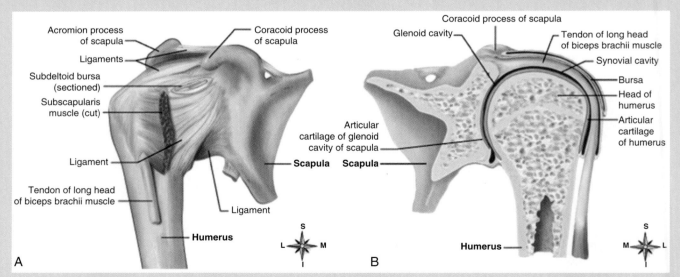

Table Fig. 10.9 Position of the long head of biceps brachii and bursa in the subacromial space. (From Magee DJ, Zachazewski JE, Quillen WS, et al. *Pathology and Intervention in Musculoskeletal Rehabilitation.* 2nd. ed. St. Louis, MO: Elsevier; 2016.)

Biomechanical Concepts | **Exercise Implications**

The supraspinatus tendon also has an area of poor vascular supply in the midtendon, reducing potential for recovery (Table Fig. 10.11).

Rotator cuff degeneration is common, with up to 30% of individuals over the age of 60 found to have defects, although tears may not be symptomatic. The degeneration over time can progress to loss of superior rotator cuff integrity, further increasing the superior migration of the humeral head and osteoarthritic changes.[31] In younger individuals macrotrauma or microtrauma is possible with partial- or full-thickness tears of any of the rotator cuff muscles.

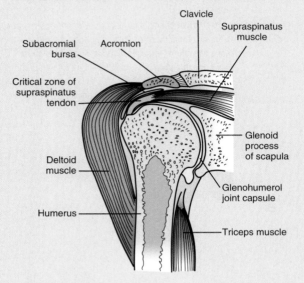

Table Fig. 10.11 The critical zone of the supraspinatus tendon in the mid-tendon has a poor blood supply, potentially reducing recovery potential for recovery with repetitive compression. (Magee DJ, Zachazewski JE, Quillen WS, et al. *Pathology and Intervention in Musculoskeletal Rehabilitation.* 2nd. ed. St. Louis, MO: Elsevier; 2016.)

5. Valgus Angle

Normal valgus angle of the upper extremity for females is 13–16 degrees and males is 11–14 degrees.[32] The valgus angle influences the elbow and wrist alignment. In the frontal plane, the natural forearm and wrist position is wider than the hips (Fig. 4.4E).

A patient with a large valgus angle is more likely to compensate at the shoulder, pronate, or increase forces on the elbow if the arm and hand position is close to the body during elevation.

A large valgus angle increases the angulation and changes the angulation of the muscles attaching around the elbow (see Clinical Example 4.5). This is particularly important for patients with tendinopathy at the elbow, wrist, and hand. Increased angulation combined with tension while holding or manipulating objects increases stress in tendons or at the insertions (Table Fig. 10.12).

The muscles providing support for the scapulothoracic and glenohumeral joints are at a relative mid-position in the scaption plane. The distance of the arm with respect to the body may need to be wider if there is a large valgus angle.

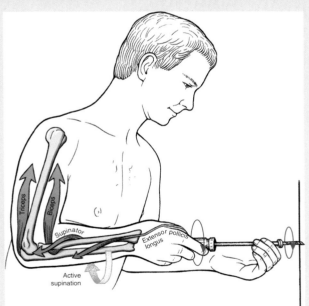

Table Fig. 10.12 Repetitive hand and forearm motion in everyday work or functional activities increases stress on the forearm, wrist, and finger muscles and tendons. (From Neumann DA. *Kinesiology of the Musculoskeletal System.* 3rd ed. St. Louis, MO: Elsevier; 2017.)

TABLE 10.1	Biomechanical Concepts and Exercise Implications for the Upper Extremity—cont'd
Biomechanical Concepts	**Exercise Implications**
6. Functional Requirements of the Upper Extremity Many upper extremity functions involve open chain movements that also require precision, ability to grip, and coordination (Table Fig. 10.13). Examples of activities of daily living requiring precision: • Dressing • Bathing • Eating • Computer work Certain occupations will require greater endurance or strength at higher ranges (e.g., construction workers, painters)	Range of motion, muscle function, and neuromuscular coordination goals should take into account the patient's age and requirements for activities of daily living, occupation, and hobbies. Restoring normal open chain function is important for upper extremity injuries and requires some focus on precision. As range of motion increases, exercises will need to be adjusted to maintain range and develop strength in the new ranges.

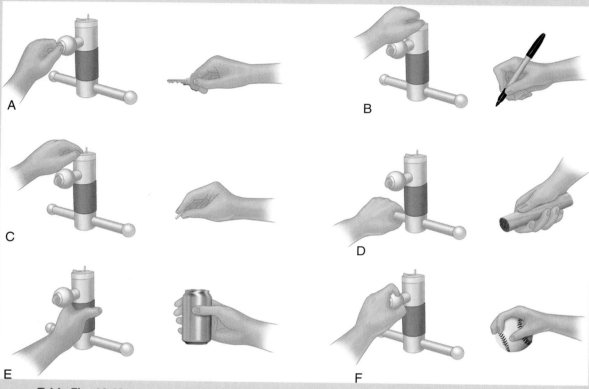

Table Fig. 10.13 Grip activities used in regular daily activities. (A) Pinch grip (holding a key). (B) Prehension grip or three-fingered grip (holding a pen). (C) Fine motor skills for placement of small objects. (D) Cylindrical grip for turning objects. (E) Cylindrical grip for holding cans. (F) Spherical grip for turning a doorknob or throwing a ball.

TABLE 10.1 Biomechanical Concepts and Exercise Implications for the Upper Extremity—cont'd

Biomechanical Concepts

7. Muscle Function (see Chapter 2)[33]

Local stabilizers (postural muscles) include:
- Rotator cuff muscles (Table Figs. 10.14 and 10.15B)
- Extensor carpi radialis brevis
- Intrinsics

Exercise Implications

The local stabilizers are activated at a lower threshold than the global stabilizers and movers; exercise intensity is therefore lower when targeting stability (see Table 2.8). Early anticipatory timing is facilitated through specific timing of cueing while proprioceptive input is used to promote postural muscles responses. Progression of exercise is guided by motor control concepts (see Chapter 7) with knowledge of results and feedback to train neuromuscular coordination. Sequencing, synchrony of activation, and endurance parameters are also integral components, especially for rotator cuff and scapulothoracic mechanics.

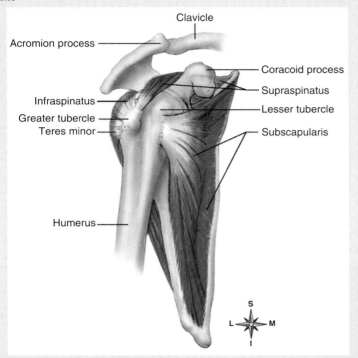

Table Fig. 10.14 Rotator cuff—local stabilizing muscles. (From Patton KT, Thibodeau GA, Douglas MM. *Essentials of Anatomy and Physiology.* St. Louis, MO: Mosby; 2012.)

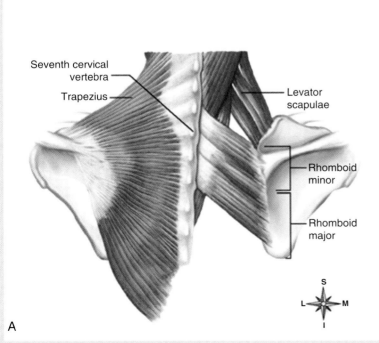

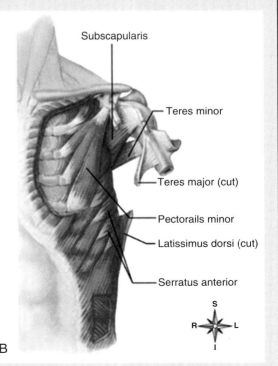

Table Fig. 10.15 Posterior view of superficial and deep global scapula stabilizers. (From Patton KT, Thibodeau GA, Douglas MM. *Essentials of Anatomy and Physiology.* St. Louis, MO: Mosby; 2012.)

Continued

TABLE 10.1   Biomechanical Concepts and Exercise Implications for the Upper Extremity—cont'd

Biomechanical Concepts	Exercise Implications
Global stabilizers include: • Scapulothoracic stabilizers (serratus anterior [Table Fig. 10.2], rhomboids, trapezius [Table Fig. 10.15], pectoralis major and minor [Table Figs. 10.15B, 10.16A]) • Deltoid (Table Fig. 10.17A) • Latissimus dorsi (Table Fig. 10.16B) • Brachialis and brachioradialis (Table Fig. 10.17A) Global movers: • Latissimus dorsi (Table Fig. 10.16B) • Pectoralis major (Table Fig. 10.16A) • Trapezius (Table Fig. 10.15A) • Brachialis (Table Fig. 10.17A) • Biceps (Table Fig. 10.17A, B) • Triceps (Table Fig. 10.17A) • Coracobrachialis (Table Fig. 10.17B) • Extensor carpi radialis longus • Extensor carpi ulnaris • Flexor carpi radialis and ulnaris • Flexor digitorum	Dosage for global stabilizers is progressed from endurance to strength loads, while dosage for global movers uses higher load and speed for strength or power. Fine motor coordination focus with high specificity is required for hand and wrist muscles.

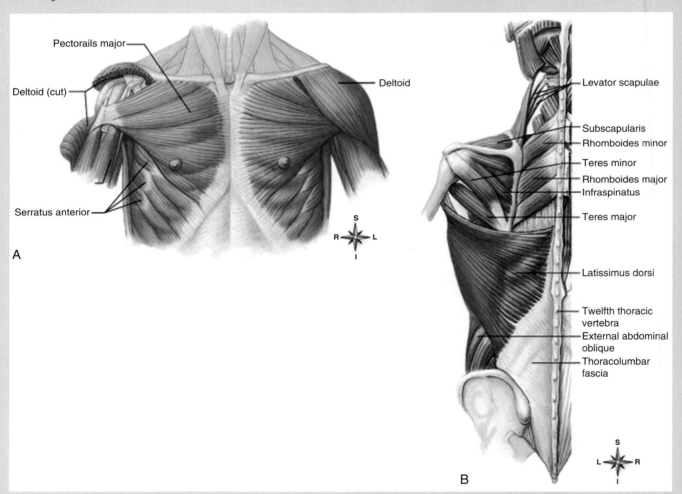

Table Fig. 10.16 (A) Anterior view of superficial global movers and global stabilizers (deltoid, serratus anterior). (B) Posterior view of superficial global movers (latissimus dorsi), mid and deep global stabilizers and movers (levator scapulae, rhomboids, teres major), and posterior rotator cuff local stabilizers or global stabilizers (teres minor, infraspinatus). (From Patton KT, Thibodeau GA, Douglas MM. *Essentials of Anatomy and Physiology.* St. Louis, MO: Mosby; 2012.)

TABLE 10.1 Biomechanical Concepts and Exercise Implications for the Upper Extremity—cont'd

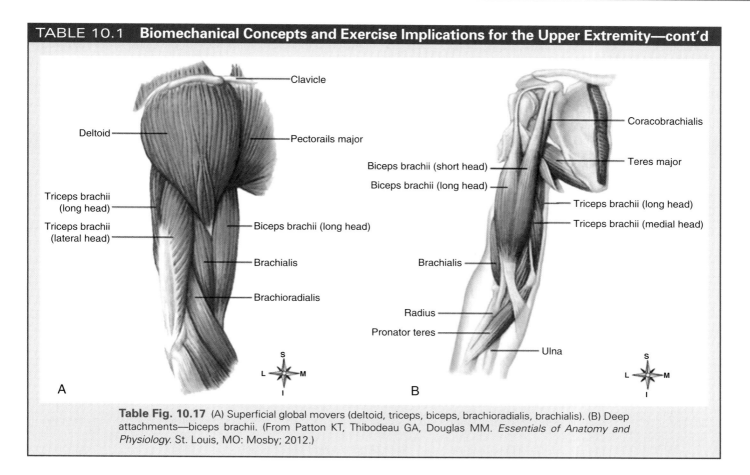

Table Fig. 10.17 (A) Superficial global movers (deltoid, triceps, biceps, brachioradialis, brachialis). (B) Deep attachments—biceps brachii. (From Patton KT, Thibodeau GA, Douglas MM. *Essentials of Anatomy and Physiology.* St. Louis, MO: Mosby; 2012.)

SECTION 1: HYPOMOBILITY

GENERAL EXERCISE APPROACHES

The types of exercise used to address hypomobility are described in Chapter 6 (see Tables 6.3 and 6.4), and the comparison between parameters used for hypo- and hypermobility are included in Table 6.4. A review of the goals, methods, parameters, and measurements are included in Table 10.2. Also refer to Boxes 10.1 and 10.2.

TABLE 10.2	Goals, Methods, Parameters, and Measurement: Hypomobility		
Goals	**Methods**	**Parameters**	**Measurement**
Decrease swelling (edema or effusion), muscle spasm, and related pain symptoms	Circulatory "pumping" exercises Moving joint actively in mid to end range (does not have to reach end range) without compensation and excessive pain Isometric contractions with adequate relaxation to create "pumping" effect	Multiple repetitions (>30) Low loads Supported positions Adequate rest periods between sets Repeat frequently throughout the day Pain should decrease with continued repetitions	Circumferential measurements in areas Pain reports (both at rest, with activity and related to movement toward end range) Goniometric measurement of range of motion (should improve as the swelling decreases)
Increase body temperature before mobility exercise to maximize improvements	General aerobic exercise	Equipment set to allow repeated motion within available range Low to moderate resistance Intensity set to achieve perceived exertion of 11–13 but no increase in pain during exercise Initially, time set for warm-up rather than aerobic endurance, progress to aerobic endurance	Perceived exertion Pain intensity during and after exercise
Increase capsule and/or connective tissue mobility	Non–weight-bearing, open chain exercise to end range (therapist-assisted, self-assisted, equipment- assisted) using: Oscillatory motion reaching end range Active, active-assisted motion or resisted movement through range to limits without compensation Passive positioning Prolonged stretch (to address connective tissue and muscle length)	High repetitions (>25) Low load allowing maximal range, progress load as tolerated Controlled speed Reach end range without excessive pain reproduction Progress to prolonged hold once patient is tolerating motion to end range without increasing symptoms excessively during or after exercise	Goniometric measurements of range of motion End feel and relative amount of motion before end feel (passive motion, joint play) Selective tissue tension evaluation; relationship between amount of active and passive range of motion Functional self-report (DASH)
Improve muscle flexibility (including two-joint muscles)	Passive positioning Prolonged stretching (performed by therapist or self-stretch by patient) at end range of joint motion reaching full length of muscle–tendon complex at one or both ends in direction of fibers Contract-relax Hold-relax	Sustained hold (15–30 seconds) *OR* multiple repetitions to end range Low loads allowing maximal range, progress load as tolerated Contract-relax or hold-relax uses maximal resistance for target muscle groups followed by immediate relaxation and motion into the maximal length of target muscle Range should increase with time held or repetitions	Goniometric range of motion (active or passive) End feel with passive movement relative to amount of range of motion Muscle flexibility special tests
Increase neural mobility with specific neural stretching techniques	Neural gliding and/or stretching techniques	Motion targeted to increase mobility of specific neural tissue with range and hold depends on severity and irritability Multiple repetitions with motion to end range or within range short of symptom reproduction *OR* starting to reproduce symptoms Prolonged hold if low severity and irritability	Neural tension tests Goniometric measurement Symptom reproduction with combined functional positions
Improve upper-quarter mobility	Generalized upper-quarter spinal mobility	Capsule or connective tissue (see connective tissue section above) Muscle flexibility (see muscle flexibility section)	Range of motion (inclinometer or goniometer) End feel with passive movement relative to amount of range of motion Muscle flexibility special tests

TABLE 10.2   Goals, Methods, Parameters, and Measurement: Hypomobility—cont'd

Goals	Methods	Parameters	Measurement
Improve upper-quarter proximal support, postural awareness, and endurance (scapulothoracic, cervicothoracic)	Generalized upper-quarter spinal postural positioning and endurance during all exercises Upper-quarter aerobic conditioning	High repetitions (>15 repetitions) *OR* prolonged hold in position (timed) before loss of position, fatigue, or compensation in order to provide support for upper extremity	Ability to maintain optimal alignment during exercise or function Time able to maintain optimal alignment before fatigue or compensations Perceived exertion/degree of specific fatigue during prolonged position or exercise
Increase muscle activation and endurance in newly available range gained from other techniques (joint mobilization, joint mobility exercise, or muscle flexibility) Improve and maintain dynamic mobility and extensibility of tissue	Muscle activation in new ranges: may be gravity-assisted, -eliminated, or -resisted positions Progressive resistive exercise for endurance and tissue stimulus in new range	High repetitions (>30) Low load Newly obtained range End range if possible Facilitate muscle activation in specific range after mobility exercises	Movement observation Ability to activate through available passive range Number of repetitions reaching end of possible range Dynamometer Ability to maintain positions (time)
Teach active methods to maintain and improve functional mobility	Functional training Self-stretching or mobility exercise	Motor control concepts: practice with specificity to use available range, training concepts for practice with precision, and monitoring	Ability to perform functional movement through range without compensations or feedback Functional mobility measures Functional movement self-reports (DASH) Ability to perform activities without compensations or home programs independently Functional mobility measures (hand behind back or hand behind head compared to opposite side, ability to perform basic grooming or dressing, reaching or carrying items)

BOX 10.1   Contraindications and Precautions

1. Mobility exercise is not indicated for severe instabilities or fractures with insufficient healing.
2. There is a need to determine if adequate healing is present after trauma (fractures, rotator cuff, tendon or ligament tears).
3. Acute inflammation requires caution (e.g., with acute inflammation related to inflammatory conditions such as rheumatoid arthritis).
4. Address swelling and edema first, avoiding excessive force.
5. Use caution with the amount of force and load in the presence of muscle spasm and guarding (e.g., in early phases of adhesive capsulitis).
6. Use caution with the amount of force if there is connective tissue disorders or in the presence of weak connective tissue after immobilization or related to aging.
7. See Section 10.4 for postsurgical precautions.
8. Monitor responses to extreme range or load and adjust if pain or spasm increases during treatment.
9. Decrease extent of load and strain the following visit if soreness is present sooner than 8 hours after mobility exercise.

BOX 10.2   Compensations and Tolerance of Mobility Exercise

- Avoid compensations in areas of relative mobility in surrounding regions.
- Stabilize proximal and distal segments.
- Use supported positions if there is any chance of loss of balance or excessive compensations.
- Ask patients to report any discomfort.
- Monitor for delayed-onset muscle soreness, increased effusion, or edema after treatment.

EXERCISE DESCRIPTIONS

GENERALIZED UPPER BODY AEROBIC EXERCISE

10.1 Upper Body Ergometry (UBE)

See Fig. 10.1.

Purpose
- Generalized upper body aerobic activity for warm-up
- Increased circulation (upper quarter)
- Promotes thoracic rotation or cervicothoracic rotation combined with upper extremity movement (this would be considered a sport-specific task for golf or other sports requiring full trunk rotation)
- Improves upper-quarter and upper-extremity muscular endurance

Precautions
- Monitor pulse/blood pressure responses pre- and post-exercise if any cardiovascular comorbidities.
- Patients with cervical or thoracic mobility limitations will benefit from this exercise but should be monitored for pain, particularly in the case of referred pain or neural symptoms. Range of motion of the exercise may need to be adjusted to avoid exacerbating pain.

Position
- Seated in front of the upper extremity ergometer
- Seat height and distance from the handles is adjusted based on available pain-free upper extremity range of motion and desired range of motion. If the seat height is too low, the patient will repetitively lift the arm above 90 degrees which could lead to impingement symptoms.
- Upright spinal posture and cervicothoracic alignment *OR* support the spine with pillows or the backrest
- Adjust the grip position with the thumb facing up to avoid shoulder internal rotation.

Action
1. Forward or backward circular motion of the handles with or without resistance.
2. Action can emphasize thoracic rotation or both thoracic rotation and upper extremity motion. Increased cervicothoracic motion can be achieved by asking the patient to keep the head level and focus the gaze on one spot in front of them while the arms and torso moves below the head. The seat should be at a distance where the maximal trunk rotation is required to achieve the full circular motion.

Teaching tips
- Instruction examples:
  - "Rotate from your body and let your arms follow the handles."
  - Emphasis can be placed on scapula protraction: "Push the handle forward as you rotate."
  - To emphasize scapula retraction: "Pull the handle toward you on the side that is moving backward."
- Common errors to correct:
  - Letting the body move side-to-side instead of rotating the trunk (Video 7.2).
  - Not stabilizing the cervical spine, but allowing the cervical spine to rotate with the arms
  - Only using the arms, not initiating movement from the proximal muscles; gripping and pulling with the elbow flexors, forearms, and hands
  - Losing the upright supportive position
  - Scapula compensations; elevating the scapula, rounding or tipping the scapula to create the movement
- Methods to address or prevent compensations:
  - Cueing for loss of scapula compensations
  - Instruct the patient to: "Only grip the handle as tightly as you need to hold onto it" to avoid overusing the hand and forearm muscles to ensure initiation from the proximal muscles.
  - Adjust visual gaze to remain forward at eye level. Suggest a target for the patient to fix the gaze.
  - Adjust the position of the seat to ensure appropriate height and distance to avoid over reaching or pulling with the arms.

Advantages
- Resistance can be easily adjusted.
- Equipment can provide concurrent feedback on energy expenditure, speed, and power.
- Useful for warm-up and for combined spinal (thoracic or cervicothoracic limitations) and upper extremity mobility
- Can be used for generalized or specific upper-quarter deconditioning or decreased aerobic capacity.

Specialized parameters
- Set time to provide a warm-up without excessive fatigue (not to exceed 11–13 on perceived exertion scale).
- Increase time based on low perceived exertion.
- Increase shoulder flexion range of motion by adjusting the seat height, or cervicothoracic rotation by adjusting the seat distance from the arm unit.
- Increase resistance once sufficient mobility has been achieved and no soreness is reported after the exercise.

Alternatives
- Airdyne bike (can be performed sitting or standing)
- Elliptical machine using arm resistance
- NuStep machine using the arms (see Fig. 10.29)

Progression
- Increase range as range of motion improves.
- Use forward *and* backward directions.
- Increase time.
- Increase resistance.
- Increase speed.
- Decrease backrest support to challenge seated postural endurance.

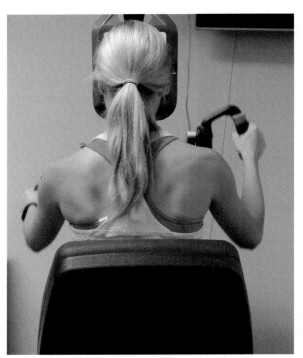

Fig. 10.1 An Upper Extremity Ergometer (UBE) can be used to address shoulder mobility and muscle function, overall aerobic endurance, or thoracic mobility.

PASSIVE OR ACTIVE ASSISTED EXERCISE

10.2 Prone Gravity-Assisted Flexion to 90 Degrees

See Fig. 10.2.

Purpose
- Increase shoulder circulation
- Provide mild traction for the glenohumeral joint
- Pain relief
- Provide gravity-assisted motion at ranges between 45 and 90 degrees (depends on angle of trunk)
- Maintain shoulder range of motion (below 90 degrees)

Position
- Prone, cervical spine in a neutral position. The patient can place his hand, palm down, on the table and rest his forehead on top of his hand. Alternatively, the patient can rest his forehead on a folded towel.
- Body toward edge of treatment table (or bed for home program)
- Arm resting at side

Action (Video 1.3)
1. Move the arm off the edge of the treatment table and allow gravity to assist the upper extremity move toward 90 degrees as the hand is lowered toward the ground.
2. Hold for 2–3 minutes if tolerated.

Teaching tips
- Instruction example:
  - "Carefully move your arm off the edge of the table and lower your hand toward the floor."

Advantages
- Useful for early Phase I management to decrease pain or increase range toward 90 degrees of flexion and can be used as a home program.
- Less risk of overuse of trapezius for elevation, trunk compensations, or impingement than in upright positions.

Alternatives
- Self-assisted
- Buoyancy-assisted
- Therapist-assisted motion.

Progression
- Add weight for additional traction.
- Progress to prone pulley-assisted movement if no contraindication (Exercise 10.3).
- Progress to supine gravity-assisted motion for additional range once 90 degrees of flexion is achieved without impingement symptoms.

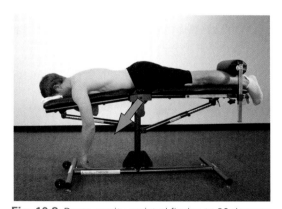

Fig. 10.2 Prone gravity-assisted flexion to 90 degrees.

10.3 Prone Pulley-Assisted Flexion

See Fig. 10.3.

Purpose
- Provide pulley assistance in available ranges between 45 and 120 degrees flexion
- Promote active inferior glide of glenohumeral joint and active initiation of posterior rotator cuff muscles
- Increase flexion mobility using gravity and pulley assistance when the patient is able to perform active extension against gravity
- Active shoulder extension followed by passive assistance is a form of contract-relax exercise

Precautions
- Use caution with the amount of weight following a rotator cuff tear or surgical repair.

Position
- Prone, body toward edge of treatment table, head toward the pulleys using the face hole or resting on towels

Action (Video 1.5)
1. Set the pulley system axis below the body to provide assistance into flexion.
2. Select sufficient weight to move the patient's arm forward without pulling too forcefully.
3. Patient uses shoulder extensors and posterior rotator cuff muscles to initiate active extension followed by passive pulley assistance into flexion (contract-relax).
4. The shoulder should remain externally rotated to avoid impingement (Fig. 10.3A).
5. Range can be set based on available shoulder flexion by either adjusting the pulley stop or distance between the bench/treatment table and the pulleys.

Advantages
- Useful in Phase I or Phase II management.
- Shoulder motion while providing support for cervical and thoracic regions.

Teaching tips
- Instruction example:
  - "Keep the front and back of your shoulders wide while you pull your hand back toward your hip. Control the return without letting the weights go."
- Common errors to correct:
  - Observe for excessive elevation or rounding forward with shoulder extension.
- Methods to address or prevent compensations:
  - Grasping the pulley handle with the forearm pronated and the shoulder joint internally rotated (Fig. 10.3B) facilitate the muscles that extend as well as internally rotate the shoulder (latissimus dorsi, teres major, pec major). If there is a need to avoid impingement or if the patient is overusing these strong global movers, the patient should grasp the pulley handle with the forearm supinated and the shoulder joint laterally rotated.
  - Muscle imbalances of the anterior and posterior shoulder musculature may also require using shoulder extensors such as the long head of the triceps and posterior deltoid.
  - Ensure scapular stabilization before initiating the movement.

Alternatives
- Free weights can be used to assist motion to 90 degrees in this position.

Progression
- Increase range, repetitions, or weight.
- Progress to isometric hold against the resistance to full relaxation and hold with stretch if no impingement symptoms.
- Progress to supine gravity-assisted motion for additional range once 90 degrees flexion is possible without impingement symptoms (Exercise 10.5).

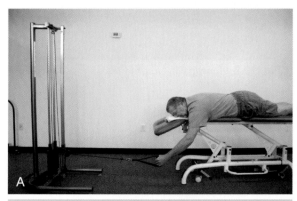
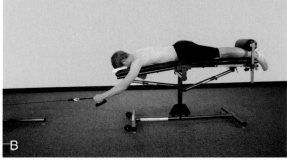

Fig. 10.3 Prone pulley-assisted flexion with external rotation (A) and internal rotation (B).

10.4 Self-Assisted Flexion

See Fig. 10.4.

Purpose
- Symmetrical shoulder flexion in the scaption plane for mobility
- Assistance to maintain range when muscle strength does not allow active movement against gravity or when rotator cuff healing precautions require limited stress on the muscle complex
- Range can be increased slightly or range obtained during therapist manual treatment can be maintained by using the unaffected arm

Precautions
- Only indicated if active motion is allowed
- Avoid moving into ranges that reproduce impingement symptoms and ensure that motion includes scapula upward rotation.

Position
- Supine, holding wooden pole (Fig. 10.4A)
- Starting with the shoulder externally rotated and moving in the scaption plane will help prevent impingement.
- The pole should be held with the thumbs up and wider than shoulder width.

Action
1. Initiate motion at the scapula by using the serratus anterior to assist with upward rotation.
2. Flex the shoulder, using both arms and keeping both ends of the pole moving at the same speed and equal range.
3. Maintain the thoracic spine and ribs on the treatment table.

Teaching tips
- Instruction example:
  - "Initiate the motion from your shoulder blade onto the rib cage and then move the pole up toward the ceiling before lifting your arms overhead."
- Common errors to correct:
  - Extending the thoracic (and sometimes the lumbar spine) in order to obtain more range.

- Allowing the unaffected arm to move beyond the available range of the shoulder with limitations causing upper body rotation or internal rotation
- Methods to address or prevent compensations:
  - Instruct the patient to keep the bottom ribs down on the mat to isolate the motion to the shoulders.

Advantages
- Range is assisted by gravity once past 90 degrees.
- Visual input assists with limiting compensations.
- The pole also provides some feedback and provides a visual target for an upward arc of motion with scapula upward rotation using the serratus anterior (rather than only using upper trapezius).
- The supine position supports the cervical and thoracic region and provides a stable base for muscles attaching the spine.

Alternatives
- Grasping the hands together is an alternative (Fig. 10.4B); however, the relative shoulder adduction may limit range and is more likely to result in compensations.
- Pulley assistance to assist the flexion. The pulley axis should be set above shoulder height (Exercise 10.5). A latissimus pull-down bar can be used to provide bilateral assistance or a single pulley can be used if the patient is able to actively extend the shoulder on the affected side against the pulley resistance (Video 5.4).
- If the patient's mobility is limited but active range is possible, self-assistance from the opposite hand under the arm can be used to increase the range (Fig. 10.4C).
- The exercise can be performed in supine or sitting.

Progression
- Increase range.
- Increase intensity of hold at full range, using unaffected arm to assist terminal range.
- Increase time held at end range.

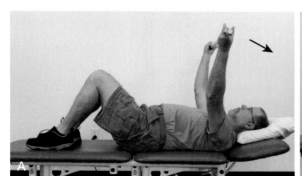
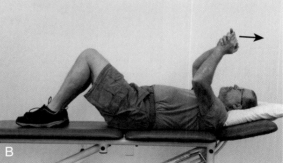
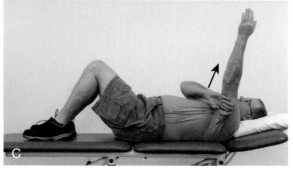

Fig. 10.4 Self-assisted flexion. (A) Bilateral assistance holding a pole. (B) Grasping with the unaffected arm. (C) Active flexion with self-assistance for additional range or overpressure.

10.5   Supine Pulley-Assisted Flexion, Abduction

See Fig. 10.5.

Purpose
- Provide pulley assistance in available ranges between 45 and 160 degrees flexion or abduction
- Promote active inferior glide of the glenohumeral joint
- Active initiation of shoulder posterior rotator cuff muscles

Position
- Supine, with the involved shoulder in line with the pulley, facing away from pulleys.

Action (Video 5.4)
1. Set pulley system to provide assistance into flexion (or abduction).
2. Select a weight that is heavy enough to lift the weight of the patient's arm without pulling too forcefully.
3. The patient uses the shoulder extensors and posterior rotator cuff muscles to actively extend the shoulder, then the pulleys passively assist movement into flexion.
4. The shoulder should remain externally rotated throughout to avoid impingement.
5. Range can be set by adjusting the pulley stop or distance of the bench/treatment table from the pulleys.

Advantages
- Useful during Phase II management.
- Allows shoulder motion while providing support for cervical and thoracic regions.

Teaching tips
- Instruction example:
  - "Keeping your thumb pointed up throughout the exercise, pull your little finger down by your hip. Allow the weight of the pulley to help you lift your arm back to the starting position."

Alternatives
- Free weights can be used to assist motion beyond 90 degrees, but often results in compensations with excessive motion of the scapula rather than glenohumeral joint.
- Bilateral shoulder extension using a lat pull-down bar provides the same motion and provides visual feedback (Video 5.4). The movement is in the scaption plane or abduction.

Progression
- Increase range, repetitions, or weight.
- Can progress to isometric hold against the resistance to full relaxation and hold with stretch if no impingement symptoms.
- Progress to sitting once 90 degrees flexion is possible without compensations and no impingement is present.

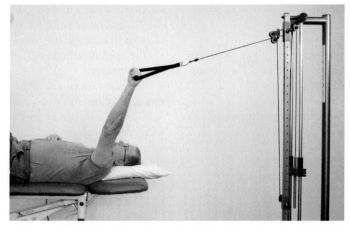

Fig. 10.5 Supine pulley-assisted flexion following resisted shoulder extension. Note that, ideally, the shoulder should be externally rotated with the thumb facing the pulleys.

OSCILLATIONS OR PROLONGED SELF-STRETCHING AND FLEXIBILITY

10.6 Supine Prolonged External or Internal Rotation Stretch

See Fig. 10.6.

Purpose

Prolonged stretch, as tolerated, for improving rotation

Position

- Supine
- The involved arm abducted 45 degrees (or higher, based on available range), supported on a pillow or foam pads if needed

Action

1. Using the weight of the arm with or without holding a light weight, allow gravity to move the shoulder into either external (Fig. 10.6A) or internal rotation. (Fig. 10.6B), reaching the end range (Video 10.6).
2. Hold for as long as tolerated.

Advantages

- Can be used as a home program.
- Prolonged stretch is used to promote connective tissue adaptations and extensibility.
- Gravity is used to provide a low-load prolonged positional stretch using the weight of the arm with or without free weights.

Teaching tips

- Common errors to correct:
  - Avoid arching or extending the spine off the treatment table to lower the hand closer to the ground (external rotation).
- Methods to address or prevent compensations:
  - Observe the patient's natural posture of the glenohumeral joint and maintain this alignment when positioning the patient for this exercise. The joint should not be allowed to move upward in response to the rotational stretch.
  - The patient can use his opposite hand to monitor the anterior shoulder position. The patient should be able to self-correct the movement and avoid lifting off the table, elevating, or moving anteriorly.

Alternatives

- The therapist can first assist the movement into the desired position, followed by the patient holding the position.
- Sleeper stretch (Exercise 10.7)
- Use oscillations in small ranges if prolonged stretch is not possible.

Progression

- Increase time in position.
- Increase sets.
- Increase weight.

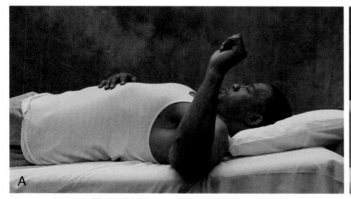 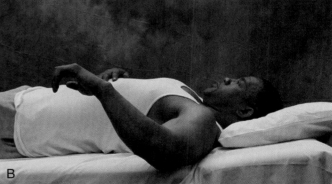

Fig. 10.6 Supine prolonged external (A) or internal rotation (B) stretch reaching available end-range (see Video 10.6).

10.7   Sleeper Stretch

See Fig. 10.7.

Purpose

Increasing external or internal rotation using oscillations or prolonged stretch.

Position

- Side-lying on the involved side with the scapula stabilized under the body, head supported on a pillow.
- Shoulder flexed (based on available flexion range)

Action (Video 5.1)

1. Shoulder external rotation (Fig. 10.7A) or internal rotation (Fig. 10.7B)
2. Patient uses the opposite hand to provide additional stretch while the scapula of the affected shoulder is anchored by the patient's body weight.

Advantages

- Side-lying position prevents compensations and generalized motion of the shoulder by stabilizing the scapula underneath the body while stretching.

- Patient is able to assist the movement.

Teaching tips

- Instruction example:
  - "Keep your shoulder blade under your body. Allow your hand to lower toward the table. Use your opposite hand to press down gently on your wrist to increase the stretch."

Alternatives

- Supine external or internal stretch using a weight (potential for more compensations)
- Use of a weight to assist with prolonged stretch
- Alternate between internal and external rotation

Progression

- Increase range.
- Progress from oscillations or active motion through range to prolonged hold.
- Increase time held.
- Add weight.

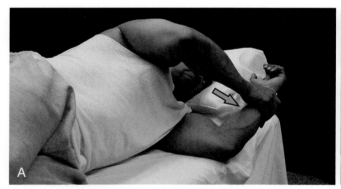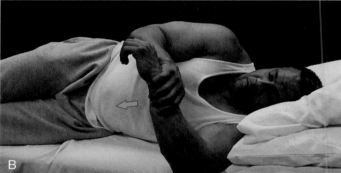

Fig. 10.7 Side-lying sleeper stretch (external [A] and internal [B] rotation). See Video 5.1.

SPECIFIC MUSCLE FLEXIBILITY EXERCISES

10.8 Pectoralis Major (Sternal Portion) and Minor Stretch

See Fig. 10.8.

Purpose
- Increase flexibility of the sternal portion of pectoralis major and the pectoralis minor

Precautions
- If anterior glenohumeral laxity or instability is present, do not stretch past the frontal plane.
- Patients with rounded or forward shoulders, cervical forward head, or thoracic kyphosis often have tight pectoralis muscles and the position may need adjusting to avoid placing excessive stress on the anterior shoulder.
- If the patient has primary postural positions influenced by thoracic or cervicothoracic mobility limitations, these impairments should be addressed before, or simultaneously with, pectoralis muscle flexibility exercises. Only using pectoralis stretching can place additional stress on the anterior shoulder if the stretching is performed in vertical positions without addressing the spinal mobility limitations.

Position
- Supine, shoulders abducted and externally rotated
- Fingertips under head (Fig. 10.8A) or arms outstretched into a V position (Fig. 10.8B, C), or, if there is limited shoulder flexion, in horizontal abduction (Fig. 10.8D; Video 4.5)

Action
1. Stabilize the rib cage and lumbar spine, using upper abdominal muscle activation to anchor the lower ribs.
2. Move through full available range of combined shoulder abduction and external rotation as allowed without thoracic spine extension.

Advantages
- Supine position limits spinal compensations (increased spinal extension)
- The supine pectoral muscle stretch is safer than the standing corner stretch, which can place stress on the anterior shoulder (Fig. 10.8E, F).

Teaching tips
- Instruction example:
  - "Leading with your thumbs, raise your arms out to the sides toward your head."

Alternatives
- Prop the shoulder with a foam pad or pillow if rounded shoulders or kyphosis are present to target the pectoralis major stretch without compensations due to the underlying position.
- Adjust the shoulder abduction range to stretch different tissue alignment and connective tissue components.
- Arms outstretched to a "T" position will target the clavicular portion of the pectoralis major.
- Prop the arm to decrease the range if unable to tolerate the full stretch.

Progression
- Combine pectoralis stretch with thoracic extension over pillows, BOSU, or foam pads to increase muscle stretch at the thoracic wall.
- Add lower trunk rotation, starting in supine, with knees and hips flexed and feet on mat in hook lying, arms positioned as described earlier. Lower the knees to one side, allowing the pelvis and rib cage on the opposite side to lift, but keeping both shoulders down. This will increase the stretch of the pectoral muscles on the side opposite of the knees.

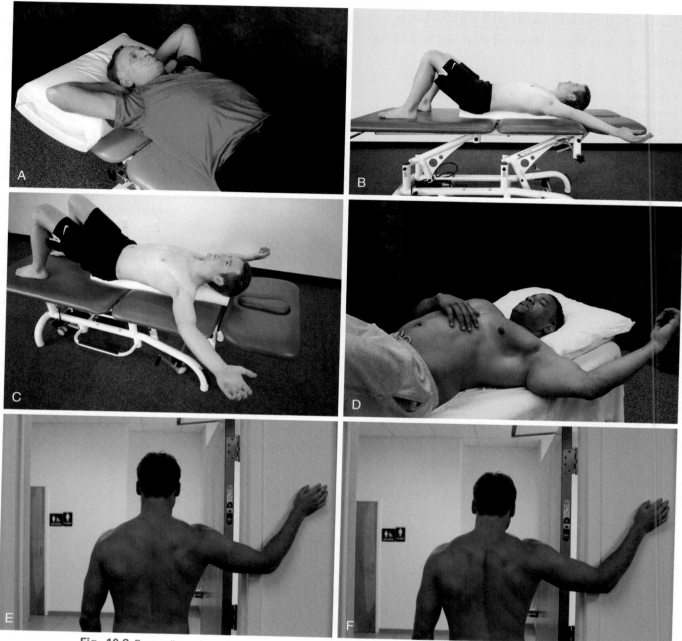

Fig. 10.8 Pectoralis major, minor stretch. (A) Hands behind head. (B and C) Arms outstretched to a V position. (D) Horizontal abduction with shoulder range limitations. (E) Pectoralis stretch in a doorway. (F) Compensations with scapula retraction can place additional strain on the anterior shoulder or cervical spine through the cervical muscle attachments.

10.9 Pectoralis Major: Clavicular Portion Stretch

See Fig. 10.9.

Purpose
- Increase flexibility of clavicular portion of the pectoralis major

Precautions
- See Exercise 10.9 for precautions listed for general pectoralis stretching.
- Monitor the corner stretch or doorway stretch closely for compensations or placing stress on the anterior shoulder by moving through too large a range.
- Contraindicated with acute bicipital tendinopathy

Position
- Standing inside an open doorway or next to a table
- Feet staggered with one foot in front of the other
- Palm of the hand on the wall with the shoulder in neutral position while maintaining external rotation.

Action
1. Precede the movement with abdominal muscle activation to anchor the distal ribs.
2. Shift weight forward slightly onto front foot to passively extend the shoulder without thoracic spine extension.
3. Maintain the shoulder position in abduction and external rotation with the palm facing the wall.
4. Hold the position to tolerance for 20–30 seconds.

Teaching tips
- Instruction examples:
  - "Leading with your chest rather than your nose, shift your weight onto your front foot and feel a stretch across the front of your chest."
  - "You should support your body weight with your front leg rather than your arms."
- Common errors to correct:
  - Compensating by moving head forward or rotating the trunk
  - Increasing cervical and/or thoracic extension during corner or doorway stretch
  - Avoid internally rotating the shoulder during the stretch.

Advantages
- This exercise can be used if there is sufficient shoulder extension past neutral.
- Exercise may be useful to assist functional activities which require reaching the hand behind the back.

Alternatives
- This stretch can be performed with one arm at a time. Resting the forearm rather than the palm of the hand on the doorway tends to maintain the shoulder rotation and decrease the stress on the anterior shoulder by avoiding excessive horizontal abduction during the stretch.
- Supine shoulder extension off the treatment table
- Hand behind the back active extension
- Arms outstretched to a "T" position with the shoulder externally rotated will target the horizontal fibers the pectoralis major (Exercise 10.8).
- Oscillations or short holds with repeated movements

Progression
- Increase range.
- Increase the time the stretch is held for.

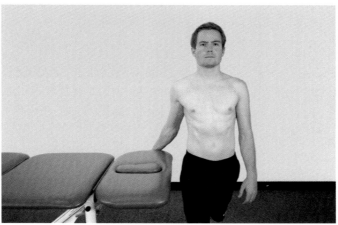

Fig. 10.9 Pectoralis major clavicular portion stretch.

10.10   Posterior Rotator Cuff Stretch

See Fig. 10.10.

Purpose

- Increase flexibility of posterior rotator cuff

Precautions

- Limit range if full stretch reproduces impingement symptoms (particularly crossover impingement).
- May need to substitute an alternative stretch if there is insufficient flexion.

Position

- Standing or sitting with shoulder flexed as range permits

Action

1. Horizontally adduct the shoulder across the body.
2. Hold the position with the opposite arm as tolerated for 20–30 seconds.

Advantages

- The posterior rotator cuff is often restricted from muscle guarding or after immobilization in a sling. Stretching the posterior rotator cuff can assist with improving flexion range of motion

Teaching tips

- Instruction example:
  - "Keep your shoulder down and back as you bring your arm across your body."
- Common errors to correct:
  - Avoid excessive scapular motion (protraction or elevation) to target posterior shoulder musculature: "Avoid shrugging or rounding the shoulder forward."

Alternatives

- Therapist-assisted posterior cuff stretching or soft tissue mobilization (Video 10.10)

Progression

- Increase range.
- Increase hold.
- Change directions of stretch to match range restrictions.

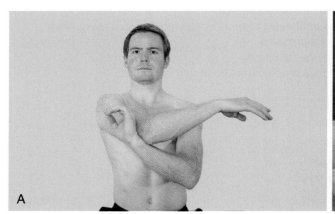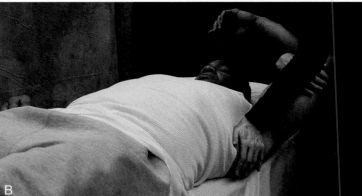

Fig. 10.10 Posterior rotator cuff stretch. (A) Crossover stretch (B) Therapist-assisted posterior rotator cuff stretch (see Video 10.10).

10.11   Latissimus Dorsi Stretch

See Fig. 10.11.

Purpose
- Increase flexibility of latissimus dorsi
- Increase flexibility of inferior rotator cuff
- Increase thoracic lateral flexion.

Precautions
- Discontinue this stretch if lumbar spine pain is experienced or neurological symptoms are reproduced.

Position
- Standing, arm fully elevated into abduction
- Opposite hand grasps wrist or forearm overhead or both arms are placed on an upright support (Fig. 10.11A)

Action
1. Precede lateral flexion with abdominal muscle activation to anchor the distal ribs.
2. Keeping the body weight equally distributed between both feet, flex the trunk away from the side being stretched (Fig. 10.11A).
3. Attain full range of combined shoulder abduction and external rotation as allowed, without allowing thoracic spine rotation.
4. Hold position to tolerance for 20–30 seconds.

Advantages
- Only used if there is sufficient shoulder abduction

- Used in Phase III for higher level athletes or if a contributing factor to repetitive strain injuries, particularly with overhead functional activities.

Teaching tips
- Instruction examples:
  - "Use your opposite hand to lengthen your arm as you bend to the side."
  - "Keep your gaze across the room as you bend to the side."
- Common error to correct:
  - Combining thoracic rotation with lateral flexion

Alternatives
- Position in side-lying over pillows, bolsters, BOSU, or exercise ball to obtain full lateral flexion position (Fig. 10.11B).
- Sitting at a table, arms extended in front of body, palms up. Slide arms forward on the table.
- Standing with both arms supported on a table or chair, hinge the body at the hips, stretching the body away from the arms (Fig. 10.11C), or place one arm on an exercise ball and hinge the hips back toward the heels (Fig. 10.11D).

Progression
- Increase range.
- Increase hold.

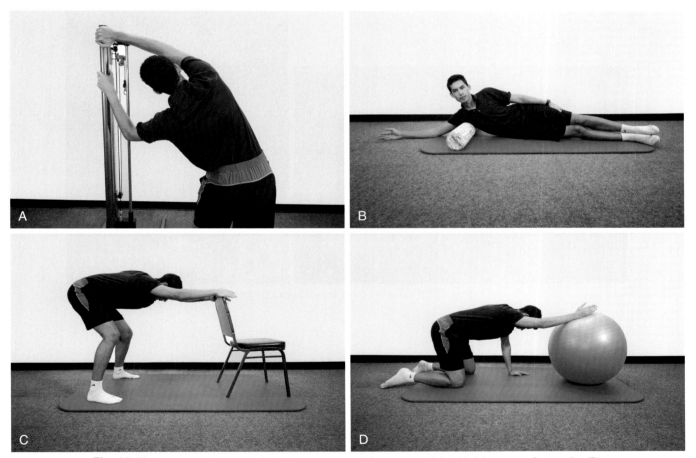

Fig. 10.11 Lattisimus dorsi stretch holding onto an upright support (A), in side-lying over a foam roller (B), standing hinge with arms on a chair (C), or one arm on an exercise ball (D).

10.12   Wrist Flexor and Extensor Stretch

See Fig. 10.12.

Purpose

- Increase flexibility of wrist and finger flexors or extensors

Position

- Standing or sitting, elbow extension.

Action

- Use opposite hand to assist with full wrist extension, finger extension and supination to stretch wrist and finger flexors (Fig. 10.12A; see arrows).
- Use opposite hand to assist with full wrist flexion, finger flexion, pronation to stretch wrist and finger extensors (Fig. 10.12B; see arrows).
- Hold position to tolerance for 20–30 seconds.

Advantages

- Used in Phase II or III if a contributing factor to repetitive strain injuries

- Decreased wrist flexor or extensor flexibility may be a causative factor for repetitive strain injuries at the elbow (golfer's elbow or tennis elbow) or following wrist or hand fractures.

Alternatives

- Therapist-assisted stretch
- Upper extremity closed chain exercises will require 90 degrees or more of wrist extension. Using the side of a table, a balance board, or a BOSU can accommodate wrist extension limitations.
- Closed chain wrist flexor stretch: palm on hand on floor, keeping heel of the hand down, rock weight forward.

Progression

- Increase range.
- Increase the time the stretch is held for.

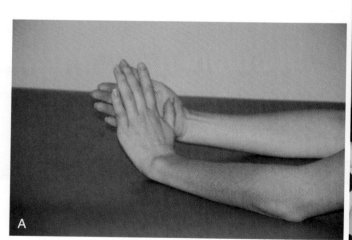
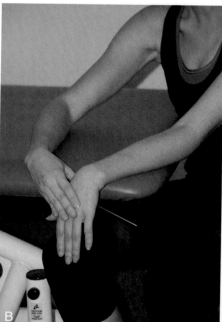

Fig. 10.12 Wrist flexor (A) and extensor (B) stretch.

10.13 Self-Assisted and Active Mobility: Elbow, Wrist, Fingers

See Fig. 10.13.

Purpose

- Improve joint mobility after immobilization or recovery from trauma or related to other conditions resulting in mobility deficits

Position

- Sitting, using opposite hand to perform passive or active assisted movement

Action

- Passive elbow flexion or extension
- Wrist flexion, extension, radial or ulnar deviation
- Pronation or supination
- Finger flexion or extension (Video 6.10)
- Finger distraction (Video 10.13)

Advantages

- Patient is usually able to perform movements passively with appropriate progression to active-assisted or active movement.

Alternatives

- Therapist-assisted mobility

Progression

- Increase range.
- Increase hold.
- Progress to active range of motion.

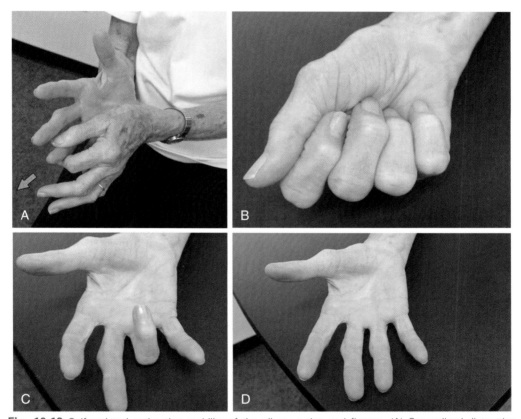

Fig. 10.13 Self-assisted and active mobility of the elbow, wrist, and fingers. (A) Generalized distraction proximal interphalangeal and metacarpalphalangeal joints. (B) Active flexion of fingers toward the palm. (C) Individual active finger flexion. (D) Generalized active extension and abduction fingers.

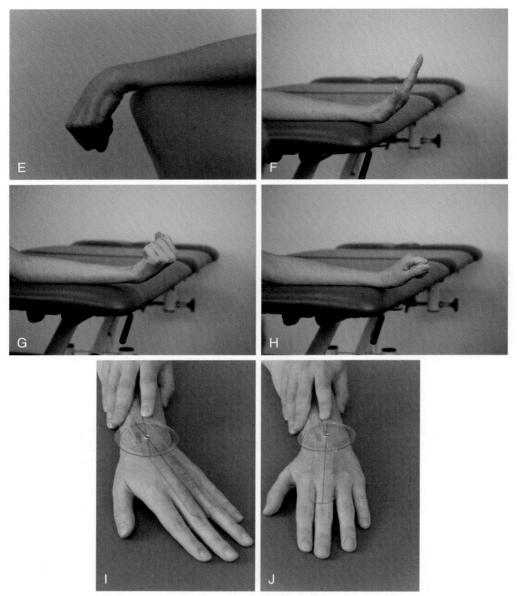

Fig. 10.13, cont'd Active mobility. (E) Wrist flexion. (F) Wrist extension. (G) Wrist flexion with finger flexion. (H) Wrist extension with finger flexion. (I) Radial deviation. (J) Ulnar deviation.

CASE STUDY 10.1: UPPER EXTREMITY ADHESIVE CAPSULITIS POST-MANIPULATION

This case illustrates concepts for primary hypomobility impairments with additional implications after manipulation (postsurgery concepts). Parameters based on seas well as the importance of the diagnosis are also illustrated for adhesive capsulitis.

A 54-year-old woman presents with a history of a gradual onset of right shoulder pain and stiffness, starting 1 year previously. She has no history of trauma, but her medical history includes hypothyroidism and previous intermittent neck and shoulder pain. Two days ago, she underwent translational manipulation under anesthesia,[34,35] and the surgeon obtained 150 degrees of right shoulder flexion, 140 degrees abduction, and 45 degrees of external rotation in neutral. She is referred to physical therapy for passive and active mobility, joint mobilization, and progressive resistive exercise. The patient is taking ibuprofen for pain.

Functional Status and Goals

Before the manipulation, she was unable to lift loads; had difficulty with any motion above shoulder level, including dressing and bathing; and had difficulty sleeping. At present, the patient is unable to perform household tasks and has difficulty carrying a purse and other small objects. She is unable to use her left arm for grooming (hair, showering) and has difficulty donning shirts and jackets. Her sleep is still interrupted by pain. She is employed as a secretary but is on sick leave since the surgery. Her DASH score is 63.3.

Patient's Goals

She would like to be able to use her left arm for self-care without pain, sleep for 6 hours, and eventually return to her hobbies: painting, cooking, and walking her dog.

Subjective Complaints

- *Severity*: She describes her pain in the anterolateral left arm as constant and aching (4/10), increasing to 6/10 with movement. She also reports some "tightness" in her neck, periscapular, and thoracic areas.
- *Irritability*: Pain increases with any movement to 6/10 but goes down to 4/10 after resting for 15 minutes. She wakes up with pain if she lies on her shoulder, and it takes 20 minutes to return to sleep.
- *Nature*: Postsurgical pain, shoulder mobility limitations (adhesive capsulitis)
- *Stage*: Chronic adhesive capsulitis but acute post surgical manipulation (Box 10.3)

Objective Findings

- Posture and alignment:
  - Forward head
  - Rounded shoulders
  - Tipped and protracted scapula
  - Thoracic kyphosis – slight
  - Increased lumbar lordosis
  - Protective shoulder position holding left arm
- *Range of motion* (Table 10.3): Cervical active ROM is within normal limits for flexion and extension, but left rotation is limited to 30 degrees with stretching pain in the right trapezius region, and left lateral flexion is limited to 30 degrees, with tightness and pain in the right trapezius region (3/10).
- *Resisted ROM*: All resisted isometrics are weaker on the right in neutral, and pain increases with resisted abduction, internal and external rotation (tested in neutral). There is some pain with resisted biceps contractions. Resisted movements are not tested higher in the range.
- *Muscle length*: Decreased extensibility of the pectoralis major and minor soft tissue mobility (full-length testing is not done at this point due to available passive range of motion). There is also limited mobility of the posterior rotator cuff including subscapularis tested below 70 degrees of flexion moving the scapula away from the humerus in an inferior direction. Upper trapezius, levator scapula, and scalenes are all restricted.

BOX 10.3 Interpretation of Subjective Complaints and History

Evaluation

The MODERATE severity is expected after the surgical manipulation, MODERATE irritability is present with movement and sleeping.[36] Symptoms will need to be monitored during and after examination and exercise. The nature and history of the condition indicate established connective tissue changes. Along with the more recent inflammation and bleeding post-manipulation, there is a high priority to limit further fibrosis and retain the motion obtained with the manipulation.

TABLE 10.3 Right Shoulder Range of Motion

Right Shoulder Motion	Active ROM Right Shoulder (Degrees)	Passive ROM Right Shoulder (Degrees)
Flexion	0–74, increased pain 60–74	0–90, with severe pain 80–90, muscle guarding
Extension	0–8, with pain moderate pain (4/10)	0–10, with pain and guarding anterior shoulder
Abduction	0–30, with severe pain (6/10)	0–50, with pain 45–51 in anterior, inferior shoulder
Adduction	0–30, without change in pain	0–35, no major increase in pain
Internal rotation	Within normal limits in neutral, without change in pain, at 60 flexion–0–30	Within normal limits in neutral, no change in pain 60 flexion–35 internal rotation, muscle spasm
External rotation	0–30 at neutral, with severe pain (6/10) Not tested in abduction	0–30, with severe pain 15–30 (6/10) in shoulder, muscle guarding 0 at 45 of abduction

BOX 10.4 Interpretation of Objective Findings and Selective Tissue Tension for the Right Shoulder

- Active range is less than passive for flexion and abduction (15 degrees less flexion, 20 degrees less abduction) limited by muscle guarding and pain.
- Current findings for active and passive range are very limited compared to range obtained during surgery (150 degrees of flexion, 140 degrees abduction, and 45 degrees of external rotation in neutral).
- The restricted movement in all directions and decreased accessory motion fits with patterns associated with adhesive capsulitis.[36]
- Muscle guarding, bruising, swelling, and tenderness are consistent with post-manipulation soreness, and soft tissue pain needs to be considered for early treatment intensity.
- Emphasis on decreasing pain and muscle guarding during initial visits will be necessary to gain as much passive range as possible. The acuity of the surgical intervention and potential for contractures and fibrosis after the surgery indicate that passive mobility should be relatively aggressive despite pain levels.
- Include cervical and thoracic mobility in the treatment plan.

BOX 10.5 Shoulder Pain with Mobility Deficits (Adhesive Capsulitis) Diagnosis

The patient's presentation fits with the diagnosis due to[36]:
- Demographics and comorbidities (between 40 and 65 years, female, hypothyroidism)
- History of gradual and progressive loss of active and passive shoulder elevation and rotation and pain
- Moderate disability
- Passive range of motion limitations in all directions, with greater loss of rotation in higher ranges of abduction, along with restricted physiological accessory motion.

Ideally, physical therapy treatment should begin as soon as possible after manipulation, with daily treatment if feasible, coupled with frequent home exercise.[34,35] In this case, the time lapse of 2 days between the surgery and onset of physical therapy is not ideal, and some of the post-manipulation range gains have not been maintained. However, therapy was initiated before the time frames for fibrosis to become established (10–14 days), and there is still potential for improvement.[42]

- *Palpation*: The right shoulder is swollen and discolored and is tender on palpation of the rotator cuff region. Soft tissue mobility is restricted for the right upper trapezius and levator scapulae and extremely limited in the right inferior rotator cuff region. The cervical paraspinal muscles are in spasm.
- *Joint play*:
  - *Shoulder*: Decreased accessory mobility in all directions with muscle guarding and pain
  - *Cervical*: Decreased joint play and pain C2–C3, C4–C5, C6–T1 and posterior anterior pressure at C6–7 and T1 with referred pain into the right shoulder
- *Neurological screening*: Normal
- *Movement patterns*: All movements are guarded, with early elevation of the shoulder girdle and slight trunk motion to the right during elevation (Box 10.4).

Evaluation

- *Medical diagnosis*: Adhesive capsulitis, post manipulation
- *Physical therapy diagnosis*: Shoulder pain and mobility deficits associated with adhesive capsulitis, post-manipulation pain and guarding (Phase I; Box 10.5)
- *Contributing factors and impairments* (Box 10.6):
  - Glenohumeral joint capsule restrictions
  - Postural alignment: Forward head, thoracic kyphosis, scapula tipping
  - Soft tissue restrictions and guarding: Decreased flexibility of pectoralis major, minor, posterior rotator cuff; subscapularis, scalenes, levator scapula
  - Recent surgical manipulation: Inflammation, edema, bruising, muscle guarding
  - Pain and related muscle guarding
  - Prolonged compensations with reinforced neuromuscular patterns (early scapula elevation, thoracic motion)

BOX 10.6 Implications for Exercise

- Early range of motion is indicated to increase range toward the limits gained during manipulation.
- Passive, active-assisted, and gravity-assisted movement are indicated for early exercise prescription with low stress while attempting to gain maximum elongation. Exercise should follow soft tissue and joint mobilization.
- Limit the amount of force initially while working toward the end of the passive range.
- Monitor pain responses during and after exercise, respecting excessive increases (more than 2 of 10), but early mobility is a priority to maximize the range as early as possible.
- Pain and muscle guarding can be addressed using oscillations within or reaching end range.
- Adjust alignment of stretch or mobility exercise to retain or increase maximal length of recently manipulated structures, especially the posterior and inferior rotator cuff and the glenohumeral joint capsule.
- Maintain proximal spinal position during treatment and isolate shoulder movement using supportive positions while attempting to regain maximum mobility.
- Promote optimal muscle balance around axis of glenohumeral joint during stretching to avoid excessive stress on weaker areas of capsule or connective tissue.
- Teach the patient to avoid early or excessive scapular motion during elevation during self-assisted, active-assisted, and active movement.
- Avoid early movement compensations by using the serratus anterior to provide adequate scapula upward rotation before activating the upper trapezius for elevation.
- Shoulder should be externally rotated during elevation (to avoid impingement).
- Cervicothoracic mobility and muscle flexibility for muscles attaching to the cervical spine are also limited, and spinal muscle flexibility and upper-quarter mobility exercises should be introduced during the exercise program.
- Manual therapy techniques should be followed with cervicothoracic mobility exercises.

Precautions

- Avoid excessive stress and strain simultaneously.
- Monitor for impingement symptoms and use positions that avoid impingement.
- Respect the patient's pain severity and irritability while attempting to increase range; avoid forceful stretching with muscle spasm.

Prognosis

Moderate for achieving mobility obtained during surgery within 6 months based on chronic history of adhesive capsulitis.[36,37] Adhesive capsulitis is often self-limiting over time (usually within 2 years), but in most cases there are still range of motion deficits that influence function.[38–40] Hypothyroidism impacts prognosis negatively.[36]

Goals (2 weeks):

- Increase passive shoulder flexion, abduction to within 10 degrees and within 5 degrees of external rotation of range obtained in surgery.
- Increase ability to reach to shoulder level with decreased pain with movement to 4/10.
- Increase cervical rotation to 45 degrees, lateral flexion to 40 degrees bilaterally.

- Improve disability score DASH 53 (minimal clinically important difference is 10.2 points).[41]
- Patient will be able to sleep for 3 hours without waking.
- The patient will report improvements (1–2 points each) for preparing a meal, washing her hair, carrying small objects, and dressing.
- Patient will be able to perform self-assisted and gravity-assisted exercise independently.

Treatment and Exercise Choices

Initial Treatment Choices

1. *Manual therapy*: Glenohumeral traction, inferior glides, posterior glides. Grade II mobilization (pain relief, muscle spasm), followed by Grade III mobilization (pain relief, regain range obtained during surgery)
2. Soft tissue mobilization to inferior and posterior rotator cuff, pectoralis major, trapezius, peri-scapular region, and cervical paraspinal muscles
3. Cervical and thoracic joint manipulation/mobilization
4. Exercise (see Table 10.4)

TABLE 10.4 Case 10.1 Phase I Exercise Choice Examples

Exercise	Goal	Parameters	Rationale and Modifications
Passive Range of Motion Flexion, abduction in scaption plane, internal and external rotation in neutral and at 70 degrees of flexion in scaption with oscillations (Exercise 10.52)	Increase range of motion to range obtained after manipulation Decrease muscle spasm and protective reactions to allow further range of motion	Mid to end of available range with oscillations High repetition	Initial repetitions are performed using easy oscillations to decrease pain and muscle guarding and followed by moving progressively toward end range. If muscle guarding increases decrease intensity of force or back off from full range. Passive movement follows joint mobilization (gentle distraction, oscillations reaching end range for accessory glides in all directions).
Active-assisted Motion Prone gravity-assisted flexion (Exercise 10.2) Supine self-assisted flexion (Exercise 10.4) Pendular exercises (Exercise 10.50) Modification for self-assisted internal and external rotation using a T-bar in sitting (Exercise 10.6)	Increase range of motion to range obtained with manipulation		Assisted motion can be performed as a home program and needs to be performed often to retain range and reduce effusion. Regular home exercises will also decrease pain and muscle guarding.
Muscle Flexibility Therapist-assisted stretching followed by active cervical range of motion Upper trapezius, scalenes and levator stretch in supine (Exercises 11.16–11.18) Therapist-assisted posterior rotator cuff stretch (Exercise 10.10)	Increase muscle flexibility of the cervical region	Supine with the shoulder supported End range; start by reaching end range without a hold, progress to 15–20 second hold Monitor for excessive increase in pain levels and decrease force or range if there is an excessive increase in pain	Cervical range can be held for longer and performed by the patient. In the first visit, the emphasis is to reach the end range but not to aggravate pain or guarding. The holds are limited initially and oscillations or gentle soft tissue mobilization may be needed before, or interspersed with reaching the end range for the shoulder.

Continued

TABLE 10.4   Upper Extremity Hypomobility: Phase I Exercise Choice Examples—cont'd

Exercise	Goal	Parameters	Rationale and Modifications
Generalized Aerobic Exercise			
UBE (Exercise 10.1)	Promote intraarticular motion to assist with resolving effusion, residual bruising and post surgical fluid removal Address pain Improve circulation and removal of waste products postsurgery	Time based on pain responses, extremely low resistance ROM adjusted by seat height and position relative to machine to allow full revolutions	Progressive range as patient becomes more comfortable Monitor pain, ease of movement Educate patient about excessive compensations but primary goal is to obtain relatively pain-free ROM
Rhythmic Initiation			
Manual resistance for internal and external rotation arm supported on table in sitting, progress to self-resisted (Exercise 10.18)	Decrease pain, promote local stabilizer activation, promote removal of inflammatory exudate, decrease muscle spasm	Very light resistance for activation rather than strengthening dosage Arm at 30 degrees of flexion in scaption, neutral rotation with the elbow flexed Multiple repetitions, relaxation between sets	Primary goal is to decrease pain, activate rotator cuff muscles to decrease spasm, and increase circulatory responses to remove postsurgical exudate and bruising
Muscle Activation and Positioning			
Scapulothoracic upward rotation, in supine with the arm supported by the therapist at 60 degrees of flexion in scaption (Exercise 10.14)	Promote motor learning of scapula connection using serratus anterior to improve scapula upward rotation	Motor learning of optimal muscle activation; awareness of spinal posture and scapular motion position with support of the arm Use passive movement and tactile cues if patient is unable to attain the connection or understand how to perform the movement	Scaption and external rotation below the active limit of shoulder flexion (70 degrees) Supine is used to minimize thoracic and cervical muscle requirements for proximal stability to allow motor learning of the scapulothoracic motion Avoid compensations: elevation, tipping, or excessive protraction and downward rotation from the pectoralis muscles
Assisted Mobility and Muscle Activation, Pain Relief			
Pulley-assisted flexion (Exercise 10.3)	Assisted flexion range of motion, contract-relax for the posterior rotator cuff muscles to decrease pain and muscle spasm	Active shoulder extension from 70 to 30 degrees against pulleys followed by assistance from the pulleys and gravity into flexion. Low resistance, no hold progressing repetitions, then time in the flexed position before increasing load	Maintain external rotation during movement

SECTION 2: HYPERMOBILITY

The types of exercise used for hypermobility are described in Chapter 6 (see Table 6.3), and the comparison between parameters used for hypomobility and hypermobility are included in Table 6.4. A review of the goals, methods, parameters, and measurements are included in Table 10.5. The overall goal is to promote force closure (neuromuscular control, muscle function) to distribute forces and initiate muscle activation. Typical diagnoses involving hypermobility in the upper extremity are:

- Specific shoulder instability (post dislocation, anterior instability, inferior instability, posterior instability)
- Generalized instability (e.g., Ehlers-Danlos syndrome, genetic hypermobility)

In situations where hypermobility and hypomobility exist together, hypermobility guidelines will take precedence in order to protect symptomatic structures, but hypomobile structures contributing to the accumulation of forces will also be addressed in the treatment plan. These conditions may fit under the repetitive strain category. The guidelines are also appropriate when addressing hypermobility following surgical intervention after the initial precautions and postoperative recovery (Phases II and III).

CONTRAINDICATIONS AND PRECAUTIONS

1. Intensity, difficulty, and level of exercise depends on severity, irritability, and acuteness of the symptoms.
2. Protect passive structures from excessive stress or strain, limit end ranges and amount of stress.
3. Avoid excessive range (may be direction-specific).
4. No stretching.

TABLE 10.5   Goals, Methods, Parameters, and Measurement: Hypomobility

Goals	Methods	Parameters	Assessment/Measurement
Improve local stabilizer muscle activation and improve neuromuscular timing (e.g., rotator cuff)	Promote neuromuscular control using motor control principles Closed chain and multiple forms of sensory input (visual, tactile including taping) Use balance responses or oscillations to promote muscle activation, alternating contractions	Supported positions, progressing to unsupported Inner-range to midrange for specific instability Midrange for generalized instability or hypermobility Timing of local stabilizers before use of global movers (anticipatory sequencing) Multiple repetitions with adequate rest *OR* alternating movement High repetition or prolonged hold with specificity of contractions Parameters progressed based on motor learning to maintain position or control of range without exacerbation of symptoms	Ability to maintain scapulothoracic connection and glenohumeral axis of motion (observation of neuromuscular coordination, or time held in position) Biomechanical analysis of distribution of forces (visual analysis of timing, axis of motion) Ability to hold isometric contractions (timed) or number of repetitions Pain responses Amount of feedback and correction needed
Improve ability to maintain midrange joint position; muscle endurance	Isometrics Small-range isotonics Promote neuromuscular control using motor control principles Closed chain and multiple forms of sensory input (visual, tactile including taping)	Progress from isometrics to multiple-angle isometrics to controlled small-range isotonics Prolonged contraction for isometrics Low load, progressing to load as tolerated High repetition for small range isotonics Use of local or global stabilizers	Ability to maintain scapulothoracic connection and glenohumeral axis of motion (observation of neuromuscular coordination, or time held in position) Biomechanics analysis of distribution of forces (visual analysis of timing, axis of motion) Ability to hold isometric contractions (timed) or number of repetitions Achieving a targeted position for a length of time Amount of feedback and correction needed Pain responses Functional tasks requiring maintaining a position DASH
Improve ability to withstand external forces and avoid reaching extremes of range	Promote neuromuscular control using motor control principles Multiple forms of sensory input (visual, tactile, including taping) Progress to eccentric control	Slow progression into controlled end-range Eccentric control to limit end range Progress to higher loads, low repetitions (isometric or isotonic)	Achievement of targets (% of successful trials) Amount of feedback and correction needed DASH
Improve neuromuscular coordination and response time for functional requirements	Promote neuromuscular control using motor control principles	Reaction time and controlled movement	Achievement of targets Amount of feedback and correction needed DASH

5. Specific precautions are listed with individual exercises.
6. Pain responses and muscle spasm can mask underlying hypermobility, and, once the pain decreases, exercise caution with active range of motion control.
7. With hypermobility, sensory input is often impaired, and patients may not be able to monitor position or range limits without additional feedback (tactile, verbal, or visual).
8. Adjust starting positions or ranges of movement to avoid impingement symptoms.
9. Active and resisted exercises are contraindicated during the protective phases of healing for rotator cuff tears/repairs or unhealed fractures.

GENERAL PARAMETERS

- Midrange (joint or muscle)
- Supported position, progressing to unsupported
- Closed chain exercises will promote centralized axis of motion
- Repeat movements with feedback until able to perform movement independently
- Dosage starts with from low-load/high-repetitions (>25) (or low-loads/prolonged holds for isometric contractions) before fatigue, with an emphasis on appropriate timing, sequencing, and targets for muscle activation and endurance.
- Dosage progresses by increasing load/lower repetitions (<15) in mid range. The patient must be able to maintain the mid-range position before attempting to increase the load.
- Neuromuscular coordination is emphasized throughout the treatment progression, challenging specificity, achievement of targets, and correction of movement patterns. Oscillations may be used to help facilitate muscle activation and firing surrounding the hypermobile joint.
- Progressing the range is the last priority, whereas the ability to control functional range is always a goal. Full range of motion is not necessarily a goal.

- Progress to challenging control through range (eccentric control or proprioceptive challenges).

TESTS AND MEASURES

See Magee,[26] and Magee and Sueki[27] for more detailed description of available tests and measures, and for interpretation and psychometric properties.
1. Pain reports
2. Functional movement outcome measures for endurance or strength
3. Ability to perform activities without compensations or home programs independently
4. DASH
5. Functional activity measures or simulated activities
6. Push up or plank timed tests

OBSERVATION FOR COMPENSATIONS AND RESPONSES

- Ensure stabilization at the area of concern as the first priority, but observe for overall alignment at proximal and distal areas that influence the forces on the joint.
- Observe for signs of fatigue: loss of position or muscle activation.
- If the joint or hypermobile region needs support, use supported positions.
- Ask patients to report any discomfort during *or* after the exercise.
- Monitor for delayed-onset muscle soreness, increased effusion, or edema after treatment.
- Monitor for impingement, pain, or discomfort when reaching impingement ranges or avoiding a painful arc by changing the plane of motion during elevation.

EXERCISES

LOCAL STABILIZER RECRUITMENT AND NEUROMUSCULAR COORDINATION TRAINING

PROGRESSIVE RESISTANCE: GLOBAL STABILIZER FUNCTION

PROGRESSIVE RESISTANCE: GLOBAL MOVER FUNCTION

FUNCTIONAL TRAINING, SPEED, AND RESPONSE TIME

EXERCISES DESCRIBED IN OTHER SECTIONS

- Progressive resistive exercise
- Neuromuscular coordination
- Functional training
- Functional training, speed and response time

EXERCISE DESCRIPTIONS

LOCAL STABILIZER RECRUITMENT AND NEUROMUSCULAR COORDINATION TRAINING

10.14   Supine Scapula Connection: Therapist-Guided

See Fig. 10.14.

Purpose
- Teach the patient how to initiate upward rotation using the serratus anterior during elevation and create a balanced force couple without allowing the upper trapezius to predominate.
- Teach the patient to recruit serratus to provide scapula connection to the thoracic region for proximal stability in the upper extremity if the patient has difficulty with scapulothoracic connection or abnormal scapulohumeral rhythm (i.e., early or excessive use of upper trapezius).

Position
- Supine, arms in scaption below 90 degrees.

Action
- Scapula protraction and upward rotation

Advantages
- The head, neck and spine are supported in a neutral starting position in supine so that the patient can focus efforts on the scapular motion rather than spinal posture.
- Supine allows visualization of arm motion and decreases use of trapezius against gravity.

Teaching tips
- Instruction examples:
  - "Keep the shoulders wide as you slide the scapula from the back and around the sides of your rib cage."
  - "Start the movement from under your shoulders scooping in a curve, finishing by reaching the arm forward through the inside of your arm."
- Common errors to correct:
  - Substituting thoracic flexion for scapula upward rotation
  - The cervical lordosis may be increased in response to anterior tipping or excessive use of the pectoralis muscles in the supine position.
- Methods to address or prevent compensations:
  - Emphasize serratus anterior (scapula upward rotation) as the target muscle as opposed to allowing the pectoralis major (shoulder horizontal adduction) to predominate.
  - Observe the pectoralis major during the movement. If a major contraction occurs, this muscle is predominating.

- Options to teach the correct movement include:
  - Tactile cueing to demonstrate the upward rotation direction
  - Tactile cueing along the ribs, just anterior to the scapula: "Lift from under your armpit, not from your chest." Demonstrate the movement or provide gentle compressive feedback through the outside of the palm to encourage an arc of movement from under the shoulder.
  - Demonstrate the motion or use passive assistance for the patient to be able to observe and feel the scapular motion.
  - Use resistance to guide scapula in upward rotation with more resistance on the palm toward the lateral border.
  - Perform the exercise one arm at a time, asking the patient to palpate the pectoralis major muscle with their other hand. "Try to keep this muscle quiet as you do this exercise."
- Emphasize scapulothoracic movement as opposed to glenohumeral horizontal adduction. Have the patient hold an object between the hands (pole, cardboard box, exercise ball) to avoid opening or closing the hands.
- Stabilize the spine to ensure scapulothoracic movement, not thoracic and cervical flexion and extension.

Alternatives
- Quadruped for closed chain protraction (Video 10.14A)
- Wrap a resistance band around thoracic spine and lower scapula with light tension created after stabilizing the band around the palms to provide tactile input.
- Use manual resistance or assistance to guide direction of motion in supine or in side-lying (Fig. 10.14B).
- Lying supine on foam roller as an unstable base to promote spinal stabilization and to allow the scapula to move freely without friction from the supporting surface.

Progression
- Hold an exercise ball for additional visual and tactile feedback.
- Use free weights (dumb bells, weighted balls or rods) for resistance (Exercise 10.15).
- Increase range of shoulder movement with upward rotation.
- Hold the position or increase repetitions.
- Perform in sitting or standing; the functional position against gravity requires synchrony of the scapulothoracic motion, and using the correct pattern in this position requires higher serratus anterior muscle activation (Exercise 10.24, Video 10.14B).[8]
- Progress to including the upward rotation in other exercises; this exercise may be discontinued once the patient is able to perform the movement consistently.

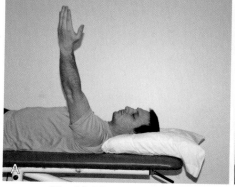
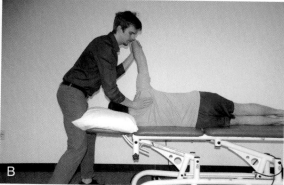

Fig. 10.14 Scapula connection initiation in supine (A) and side-lying with tactile cues (B).

10.15   Scapula Protraction/Upward Rotation With Weights

See Fig. 10.15.

Purpose
- Increase strength and neuromuscular coordination of the serratus anterior to promote scapula connection and upward rotation during elevation, assisting with a balanced force couple without allowing the upper trapezius to predominate.

Position
- Supine with arms in scaption slightly below 90 degrees
- Shoulders externally rotated
- Holding free weights

Action
- Scapula upward rotation with weights

Advantages
- Supine allows visualization of arm motion to activate the serratus anterior and decreases upper trapezius use against gravity[8,43]
- Progressive resistance for scapulothoracic motion in open chain motion is possible in supine when weight-bearing or anti-gravity shoulder elevation above 120 degrees is difficult or not indicated (precautions related to healing, range of motion limitations, pain in higher ranges of motion or rotator cuff weakness).

Teaching tips
- Methods to address or prevent compensations (see Teaching tips for Exercise 10.14):

- The therapist should take sufficient time instructing the patient in supine with guidance because this is a difficult movement to perform effectively (Exercise 10.14). Use therapist-delivered manual resistance to guide movement using a pole, if needed (Fig. 10.15B).
- Ensure that the patient is able to activate the serratus anterior to create the movement before introducing resistance or the patient will often substitute pectoralis major or minor actions with increased load.

Alternatives
- Quadruped for closed chain scapula connection
- Lying supine on foam roller to promote spinal stabilization due to unstable base and to allow the scapula to move freely without friction from the underlying or supporting surface (Fig. 10.15A–C)
- Use of ball or weighted rod to increase resistance or maintain spacing between hands

Progression
- Increase resistance.
- Increase sets.
- Increase resistance with isometric holds.
- Maintain the scapula position and challenge endurance with elbow flexion and extension (bilateral, unilateral, or reciprocal).
- Upright sitting or standing positions
- Quadruped closed chain weight shift, unstable support or extremity lifts (Exercises 10.25 and 11.28)

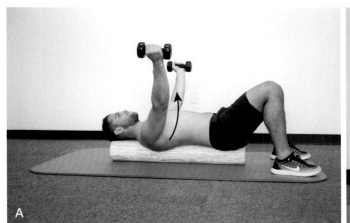
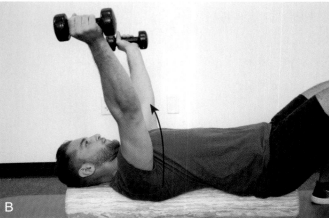

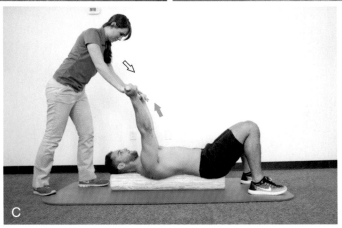

Fig. 10.15 Scapula upward rotation with weights lying on a foam roller (A and B) or manual resistance through a pole (C).

10.16   Rhythmic Oscillations, Circumduction

See Fig. 10.16.

Purpose
- Facilitate rotator cuff as local stabilizer with scapulothoracic and spinal stabilization (local stabilizer function).
- Neuromuscular coordination for glenohumeral and scapulothoracic endurance.

Position
- Supine with arms in scaption slightly below 90 degrees
- Shoulder external rotation holding free weights

Action (Video 6.25)
- Small-range oscillations or circumduction in both directions

Advantages
- Supine position allows visualization of arm motion and decreases need for trapezius to support arms against gravity
- Oscillations and small-range circumduction: high-frequency activation of rotator cuff and scapula stabilizers to maintain position and improve alternating function and endurance for motion in open chain motion (when weight bearing is not indicated).
- This exercise is helpful to patients with postural conditions that would benefit from training the scapula upward rotation: thoracic kyphosis, downwardly rotated scapula, anterior tipping.

Teaching tips
- Instruction examples:
  - "Move from your shoulder blades and shoulders rather than initiating with your hands."
  - "Shake the weights, but not your body."
- Method to address or prevent compensations:
  - Using a light grip on the weight will decrease the likelihood of overworking the distal and global mover muscles and without support from the targeted scapula and rotator cuff muscles.

Alternatives
- Do not use weights if the patient is unable to maintain position.
- Use a wooden pole to provide manual resistance, increase leverage, or provide challenge for both arms (Exercise 10.18).
- Lying supine on foam roller will promote spinal stabilization on an unstable base.
- Hold a large exercise ball to increase resistance.

Progression
- Increase repetitions.
- Increase time held in position.
- Increase speed.
- Increase resistance.
- Increase sets.

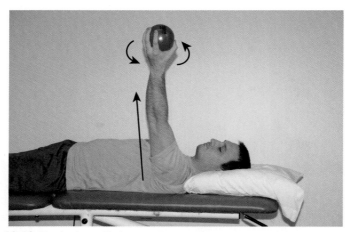

Fig. 10.16 Rhythmic oscillations or circumduction using a weighted ball in supine.

10.17 Standing, Modified Closed Chain Circumduction With Ball Against Wall

See Fig. 10.17.

Purpose
- Increase neuromuscular coordination and strength of rotator cuff
- Improve scapulothoracic neuromuscular coordination
- Improve cervicothoracic stabilization with upper extremity challenge

Position
- Standing with arm in scaption (variable range) with hand on small or large ball
- Ensure that spinal posture is in optimal alignment with active engagement of the spinal stabilizers.
- The body is facing square to the wall with hand on the ball.

Action (Video 10.17)
1. Connect the scapulohumeral muscles to the thoracic wall by initiating scapula protraction with slight upward rotation.
2. Roll the ball in small circles on the wall while maintaining the scapula position.

Advantages
- Modified closed chain activity provides sensory feedback without excessive load.
- Mid position is achieved for rotator cuff and scapulothoracic stabilizers.
- Circumduction challenges multiple muscles to promote stabilizing function.
- This exercise is helpful for patients with postural conditions that would benefit from training scapula upward rotation: thoracic kyphosis, downwardly rotated scapula, anterior tipping.

Teaching tips
- Instruction example:
  - "Moving from your shoulder blade, gently press the ball into the wall and maintain the pressure while drawing small circles with the ball."
- Common errors to correct:
  - Avoid rotating the spine while lifting the arm to place the hand on the wall.
  - Initiate the movement from the scapula rather than the hand to promote rotator cuff and scapula stabilization rather than wrist motion.

Alternatives
- Quadruped, closed chain: While the closed chain option provides additional sensory input and the support from the opposite arm limits spinal rotation, the amount of weight on the upper extremity is greater than in standing. The spinal extensor requirements to oppose gravity are also increased in the quadruped versus standing position. An exercise ball can be used under the torso to decrease the amount of weight-bearing on the upper extremities (Exercise 10.25).
- Lying supine on foam roller promotes spinal stabilization on an unstable base (see Fig. 10.15).
- Use a weighted ball or weighted rod to increase resistance.

Progression
- Increase sets.
- Increase manual resistance applied with isometric holds.
- Substitute different patterns for circumduction (e.g., alphabet or writing a word) to challenge different recruitment patterns.
- Hold and tap a small weighted ball against the wall at varying angles.

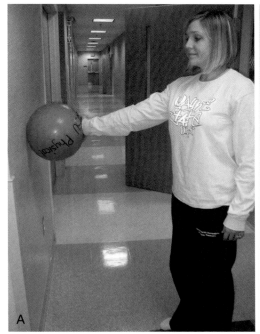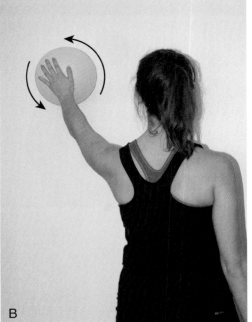

Fig. 10.17 Standing, modified closed chain circumduction with ball against a wall.

10.18   Therapist-Applied Manual Resistance

See Fig. 10.18.

Purpose

- Activate specific muscles against resistance while maintaining position.

Position

- Supine, upper extremity in desired position

Action (Video 2.20)

1. Therapist applies manual resistance in multiple directions.
2. Ask the patient to maintain the position.
3. Start gradually applying the resistance after cueing the patient to push against the resistance.
4. Allow the patient to anticipate and react to the applied pressure.

Advantages

- Manual resistance provides sensory feedback and promotes specific muscle activation.
- Isometric stabilization is useful for initiating muscle activation and stabilization without excessive stress on connective tissue.
- Starting position can be established to avoid impingement or excessive tension in the presence of hypermobility or instability (Fig. 10.18A, B).

Teaching tips

- Instruction example:
  - "Match my resistance without overpowering me."

Alternatives

- Hold an exercise ball or pole and apply resistance through the object to provide additional leverage and generalized resistance (Fig. 10.18D–F).
- Alternate rhythmic stabilization (Fig. 10.18B, C).
- Multiple angle isometrics: challenge the muscle at different lengths by progressively adjusting the starting position into more challenging ranges for the patient.
- Apply resistance through small ranges progressing to larger range functional diagonal patterns for throwing using proprioceptive neuromuscular facilitation (PNF) patterns.

Progression

- Remove visual input by having the patient close his or her eyes during the exercise to challenge responses to unanticipated stimuli.
- Progress to gravity-resisted or external resistance (Video 2.21).
- Use PNF patterns (Exercise 10.36).

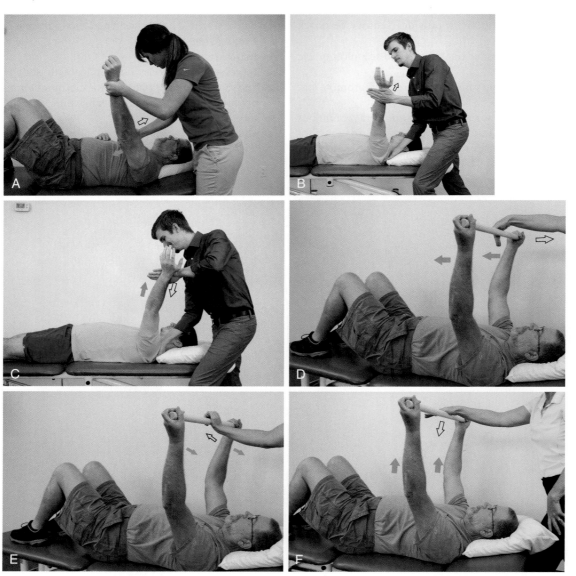

Fig. 10.18 Therapist-applied isometric or isotonic manual resistance in supine.

10.19   Rotator Cuff Activation: Therapist-Applied Alternating Isometrics

See Fig. 10.19.

Purpose
- Activation and early strengthening of the rotator cuff

Position
- Sitting, arm supported on a plinth or table in scaption
- Neutral rotation
- Elbow flexed to 90 degrees.
- Range can be adjusted by raising or lowering the table.

Action
1. The therapist asks the patient to resist against therapist-applied force that is gradually increased and released.
2. The therapist changes and alternates the direction of force while the patient resists and maintains isometric internal and external rotation.

Advantages
- Scaption plane to place glenohumeral joint in optimal alignment
- Rotator cuff in relative mid-position
- Arm weight supported
- Limits tensile stress on supraspinatus tendon and other rotator cuff muscles while activating muscle
- Easily modified starting position to avoid impingement

Teaching tips
- Instruction examples:
  - "Match my resistance without overpowering me."
  - "Hold your arm in this position; don't let me move you."

Alternatives
- Self-resisted, resistance band, or pulley resistance; isometric or isotonic
- Add an unstable surface under the elbow or upper arm (a small inflatable or weighted ball).

Progression
- Midrange isotonic rotation: start in a neutral mid-position and progress to holding at angles moving into more external or internal rotation.
- Range is increased or changed to provide multiple-angle isometrics.
- Different planes of motion are included in flexion, scaption, or abduction.
- Eliminate arm support.
- Ask the patient to close his or her eyes, requiring responses to unanticipated stimuli.
- Adjust timing (increase speed) or direction of resistance.
- Increase repetitions.
- Increase time.
- Increase speed of change of directions.
- Therapist can provide resistance through an object held in the hand. The patient must stabilize the object in his or her hand, and, depending on the shape or size of the object, can increase the challenge by increasing the lever arm.
- Progress to self-resisted movement for a home program.
- Body Blade (Exercise 10.22) or rhythmic alternating oscillations with weighted balls (Exercise 10.16).

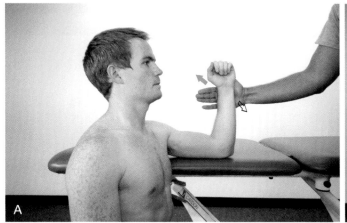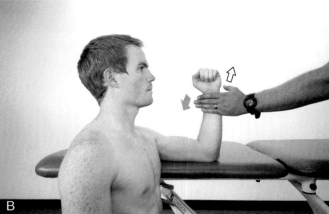

Fig. 10.19 Rotator cuff activation: therapist-applied resistance for alternating isometrics in sitting with arm support.

10.20 Supported Midrange Self-Resisted Isometrics

See Fig. 10.20.

Purpose

- Activate muscles in mid-position: scaption and glenohumeral joint position.

Position

- Sitting, arm supported on a table in scaption
- Neutral rotation
- Elbow flexed to 90 degrees.

Action

1. Opposite hand is used to provide resistance while maintaining the stationary position on the table.
2. Resistance can be applied in any direction for isometric muscle activation with slow build-up and slow release while maintaining the shoulder position.

Advantages

- Patient controls the amount of resistance and speed of application.

Alternatives

- Resistance direction is changed.
- Alternating resistance

Progression

- Increase resistance.
- Increase speed.
- Progress to external resistance isometrics with pulleys (Exercise 10.23), resistance band, or Body Blade (Exercise 10.22).

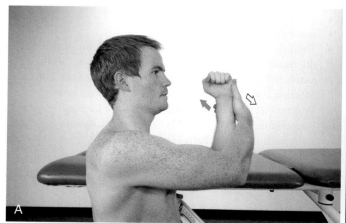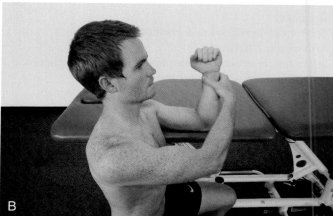

Fig. 10.20 Supported mid-range self-resisted isometrics.

10.21 Side-Lying Oscillations or Isometrics With Ball

See Fig. 10.21.

Purpose

- Activate the rotator cuff and scapulothoracic muscles with small-range, alternating movements to promote local stabilizer function at different ranges.

Precautions

- Contraindicated for unhealed fracture and protective phase of rotator cuff tear or repair

Position

- Side-lying
- Head supported

Action

- Small pulses

Advantages

- Targets rotator cuff and scapulothoracic muscles challenging muscle activation without major compressive load.

Teaching tips

- Instruction examples:
  - "Initiating the movement from your shoulder blade, pulse your arm up and down."

Alternatives

- Body blade (Exercise 10.22)
- Circumduction in modified closed chain position against wall (Exercise 10.17)
- Open chain oscillations with weights in different ranges (Fig. 10.21A,B)

Progression

- Increase speed.
- Increase time.
- Vary ranges.
- Add circumduction.
- Increase range of motion.

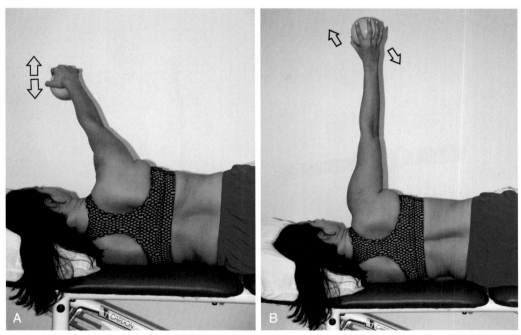

Fig. 10.21 Side-lying oscillations or isometrics.

10.22   Supine, Seated or Standing: Body Blade

See Fig. 10.22.

Purpose

- Rotator cuff and scapulothoracic muscle stabilization and generalized cervicothoracic endurance with activation of the local and global stabilizers
- Generating oscillating motion of the Body Blade while maintaining upper extremity positioning requires rotator cuff and scapulothoracic muscle stabilization, promotes neuromuscular coordination to respond to outside stimuli.
- Alternating muscle contractions are graded to match the outside stimuli and can be used to meet activation, endurance, or strength goals.

Position

- Supine, sitting (Fig. 10.22A), or standing (Fig. 10.22B–E)

Action

1. Hold the Body Blade in front of the body in scaption or different planes (Fig. 10.22B–E).
2. Shake the Body Blade to generate oscillatory resistance from the Blade while maintaining the scapulothoracic and glenohumeral position.

Advantages

- Oscillatory challenge promotes neuromuscular coordination.

Teaching tips

- It is easiest to start with the Body Blade held low, at hip level when standing,

Alternatives

- Oscillations without the Body Blade
- Starting at different points in the range or requiring different combinations of shoulder muscle range
- Oscillations using exercise ball in side-lying (Exercise 10.21)

Progression

- Increase time.
- Increase speed of oscillation.
- Moving through range; keep the Body Blade oscillating while moving it through an arc of motion.
- Vary direction of motion.
- Vary planes of movement with short repetitions in each position for functional goals such as throwing.
- Hold Body blade in one hand.
- Use a larger Body Blade to increase overall resistance.

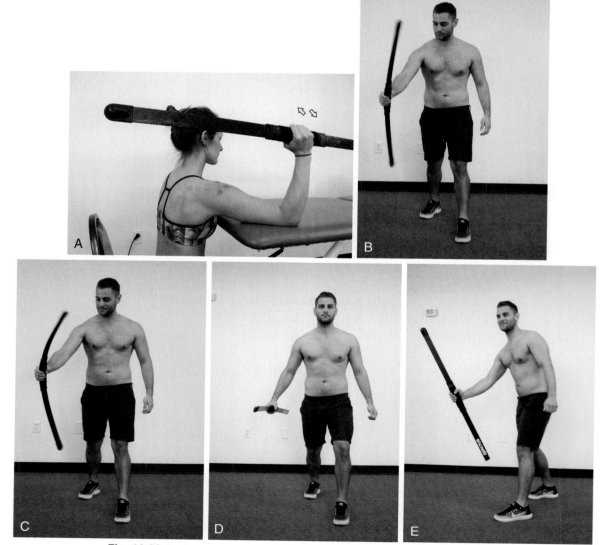

Fig. 10.22 Supine, seated (A), or standing (B–E) body blade oscillatory resistance.

PROGRESSIVE RESISTANCE: GLOBAL STABILIZER FUNCTION

10.23 Pulley Isometrics: Rotation

See Fig. 10.23.

Purpose

- Increase endurance or strength in midrange

Precautions

- Not indicated during protected phase of rotator cuff repair or tear or after fractures during early healing

Position

- Sitting, with arm supported
- Elbow flexed
- Facing diagonally away from the pulleys

Action

1. Therapist or patient uses opposite hand to pull the cable out and place handle in the affected hand to resist the load from the pulley.
2. The load from the pulley should be sufficient to challenge holding the arm in place but not enough to pull the arm toward the force. The patient needs to be aware of the potential for the force to pull the arm excessively and prepare to resist the movement.
3. The therapist should hold the rope until the patient has demonstrated the ability to resist the force.
4. The patient needs to be able to reach the rope with the opposite hand to take the weight off the symptomatic arm if needed.

Advantages

- Midrange endurance or strengthening without excessive connective tissue or joint stress

- Activate and strengthen rotator cuff without impingement forces
- Rotator cuff activation and strengthening without excessive tensile forces on rotator cuff connective tissue

Teaching tips

- Instruction examples:
  - "I am going to give you this pulley handle. The pulley weight may pull your arm toward the pulley system. Try to keep your arm still and resist the load. Brace your arm position and don't let it change."
  - "If you are starting to fatigue and cannot hold the position anymore, use your opposite hand to help control the rope and weight to let the weight stack lower toward the ground."

Alternatives

- Resistance band
- Self-resistance
- Therapist isometric resistance; rhythmic stabilization
- Oscillations

Progression

- Increase time in position.
- Increase sets.
- Increase resistance.
- Progress to small-range isotonics (Video 10.33A, B).
- Progress to eccentric control through inner ranges.
- Rest the elbow or upper arm on an unstable surface (foam, small ball).
- Remove the support and ask the patient to hold the position while resisting the pulley weight.

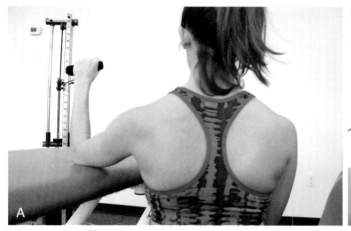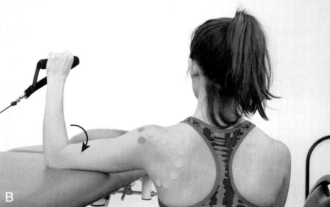

Fig. 10.23 Pulley isometrics: shoulder external rotation supported in mid-range scaption (A) or abduction (B).

10.24 Standing Upward Rotation Punches

See Fig. 10.24.

Purpose

- Improve neuromuscular coordination, including scapula upward rotation and scapulohumeral rhythm

Position

- Standing, facing away from pulleys, leaning slightly forward from the hips in a lunge position or in bilateral stance
- The patient holds the pulley handle in hand, with the forearm supinated or in neutral; the elbow is flexed.
- The pulley axis is set below shoulder to oppose shoulder flexion into elevation.

Action

1. Establish and set the scapula connection (see Exercise 10.14).
2. Move the arm starting from the scapula upward and forward in a curve, in the scaption plane (Fig. 11.24A, B).
3. Maintain shoulder external rotation to avoid impingement.

Advantages

- Muscle activation and strengthening against gravity and weight once local stabilizer function and scapulothoracic connection is achieved
- Light resistance provides sensory and visual input to promote an upward curve to facilitate scapula upward rotation early in range rather than early or excessive elevation.
- The upward rotation from the serratus anterior is important for distributing forces through shoulder elevation and to provide a platform for the rotator cuff muscles to work off during motion.
- Dynamic neuromuscular coordination of the scapulothoracic muscles and relationship to the upper quarter is important to train throughout the shoulder elevation range for functional activities.

Teaching tips

- Instruction example:
  - "Scoop from under your shoulder starting from the shoulder blade as you move your arm up and forward."
  - "Start from your shoulder blade and finish the movement through your hand."

- Common errors to correct:
  - Watch for early or excessive use of the trapezius or pectoralis muscles to create the punching motion.
  - Initiating the movement from the hand and elbow rather than starting from a proximal to distal sequence
  - Observe and correct the cervical or thoracic position as much as possible; a forward head position or thoracic kyphosis can result in scapula tipping, or excessive use of the pectoral muscles can cause anterior tipping.
  - If there is decreased muscle flexibility, limit the movement to the shoulder elevation or protraction range before the point where scapula tipping or downward rotation starts to occur.
- Methods to address or prevent compensations:
  - Ensure that the patient understands how to properly activate the serratus anterior before adding additional challenge with a more complex movement pattern and resistance (Exercises 10.14 and 10.15).
  - Limit range and load if compensations are present.
  - Only progress the load if there are no compensations and the scapulothoracic timing and mechanics is supporting the glenohumeral movement.

Alternatives

- Elevation without resistance
- Elevation against resistance band wrapped around the scapula and held in both hands
- Scapula upward rotation and protraction in different ranges with an exercise ball on the wall (Fig. 10.24C) or against equipment resistance in sitting (Fig. 10.24D and E; Video 10.24A)
- Supine if the patient is unable to correct the movement sequence or needs feedback for the spine position (Exercises 10.14, 10.15, and 10.18).

Progression

- Increase range.
- Increase resistance.
- Punches in different directions.
- Punches with trunk or hip rotation.
- Punches transferring weight in a lunge position (Video 10.24B), stepping or lunging in different directions.

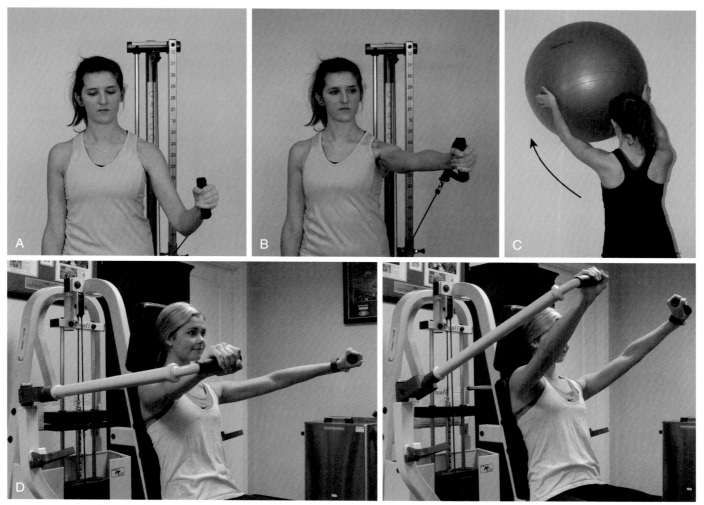

Fig. 10.24 Scapula upward rotation against pulley resistance in standing (A and B), rolling an exercise ball up the wall (C), or against machine resistance (D and E).

10.25 Four-Point Kneeling on Exercise Ball: Weight Shifting

See Fig. 10.25.

Purpose

- Supported weight shifting for early closed chain neuromuscular coordination
- Improve local stabilizer function.

Precautions

- This exercise is not indicated for patients with major rotator cuff tears, extensive arthritis, or labral tears.

Position

- Four-point kneeling with abdomen supported on an exercise ball
- Hands placed slightly wider than shoulder width
- Slight external rotation.

Action

1. Maintain cervicothoracic alignment and scapulothoracic connection.
2. Weight shift slightly to one side, taking more weight onto one arm than the other (Fig. 10.25A).

Advantages

- Exercise ball provides support for body weight.
- Ball height will determine how much support is provided relative to the patient's arm and leg length.
- Muscle activation, endurance, and neuromuscular coordination is in a closed chain position for stabilization, particularly for generalized instability or impaired proprioception.

Teaching tips

- Instruction examples:
  - "Staying lifted out of your shoulders, shift your weight toward one hand."
  - "Keep your head lifted during the shift."
  - "Shift your rib cage just enough to take the weight on your right arm. You should not be hanging on your shoulder; use your abdominal muscles and the ball to support your body weight."

Alternatives

- Use fists instead of hands flat if there is wrist discomfort.

Progression

- Time in the shifted position can be increased, based on ability to hold position without loss of core position or scapulothoracic connection.
- Movement from one arm to the next can be increased to challenge the weight acceptance and neuromuscular coordination.
- Use unstable base; hands on balance board to challenge and initiate rotator cuff and scapulothoracic muscle activity.
- Lift knees off the ground to a plank position over the ball (Fig. 10.25B and C) or roll the body forward until the lower legs are supported by the ball requiring a longer lever arm and a more unstable challenge for the upper extremities (Fig. 10.25C and D).
- Remove support from the exercise ball by deflating the ball or using a smaller ball.
- Progress to four-point kneeling without a ball.

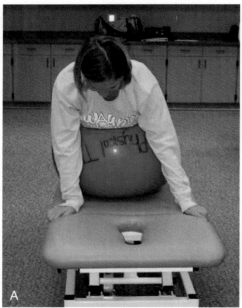
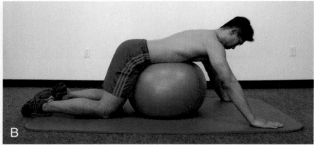
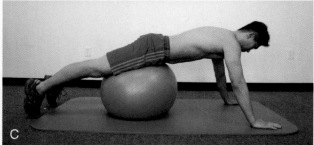
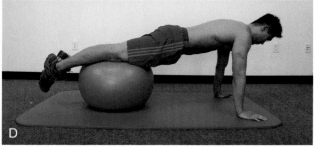

Fig. 10.25 Four-point kneeling on exercise ball: weight shifting side-to-side (A), forward lifting to a plank position (B and C), and progression without leg support (C and D).

PROGRESSIVE RESISTANCE: GLOBAL MOVER FUNCTION

10.26 Inner Range: Flys

See Fig. 10.26.

Purpose

- Increase strength of global stabilizers to protect the anterior glenohumeral joint structures
- Neuromuscular training and eccentric control for anterior instability

Precautions

- Maintain motion within the inner, or at most, middle range (not beyond neutral) to avoid placing stress on anterior capsule.

Position

- Set machine or pulley tension to limit horizontal abduction (motion behind the body) and only allow motion toward inner range of the pectoralis and deltoid muscles for horizontal adduction.
- The patient is seated with the seat height adjusted to keep shoulder range below 90 degrees, elbows flexed to 90 degrees (Fig. 10.26A).

Action

1. Set the head and upper body position alignment and establish scapulothoracic connection throughout movement.
2. Horizontally adduct shoulders using pectoralis major and anterior shoulder muscles, followed by eccentric, slow controlled movement back to starting position.

Advantages

- Equipment can be set to block motion beyond desired range.

Teaching tips

- Instruction example:
  - "Maintaining your head and spine position, bring your forearms together, then slowly and carefully control the return to the starting position."

- Common error to correct:
  - Avoid excessive shoulder elevation, forward head position, or thoracic motion to compensate or assist movement.
- Methods to address or prevent compensations:
  - Progressive load is determined by the ability to control the range and speed of the eccentric contraction.
  - Set the range to avoid the shoulder horizontal abduction.
  - Teach the patient to adjust sitting posture and set-up (distance from the body to the machine, height of the seat) to prevent "hanging" on the shoulders, arching the lumbar and thoracic spine, or forward head position.
  - Teach the patient to be aware of the amount of range desired and to control the eccentric return.

Alternatives

- Supine or incline bench position using free weights (Fig. 10.26B–D, Video 10.26)
- The floor can be used to limit the horizontal abduction movement to neutral, or pads/pillows or other props can be placed under the upper arms in the starting position to further limit horizontal abduction range.

Progression

- Build from high repetitions, low load, to less repetitions, moderate load.
- Supine on foam roller to challenge spinal stabilization; this position also requires control of the arm position to avoid the arm moving below the plane of the body.
- Supine supported by exercise ball
- Decrease speed for eccentric control component.
- Increase weight (with small range or isometrics).
- Increase range (with lower weight).
- Use closed chain positions to challenge endurance and strength (Exercise 10.25, 10.27 push-ups (limited ranges), and 10.46 planks).

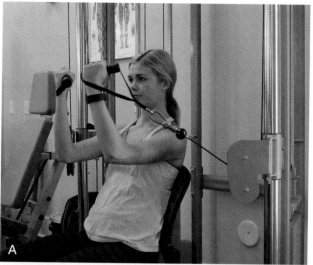

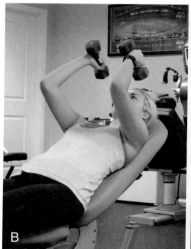

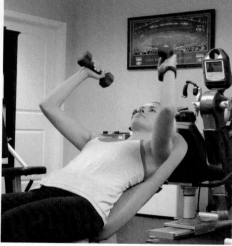

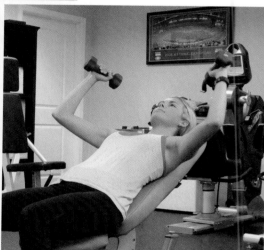

Fig. 10.26 Inner range flys against pulley resistance (A). Free weights on an incline bench (B–D).

10.27 Wall Push-Ups, Push-Up Progression

See Fig. 10.27.

Purpose
- Generalized strengthening of global glenohumeral and scapulothoracic muscles
- Neuromuscular coordination

Precautions
- Full push-ups are contraindicated for patients with anterior glenohumeral instability in the early stages of rehab and before sufficient scapulothoracic and shoulder strength has been developed.

Position
- Leaning toward wall with hands resting on the wall (or positioned on an exercise ball [Fig. 10.27 A–D])
- Hands are wider than shoulder-width apart in slight external rotation.
- The hands are positioned below shoulder level.
- The head, cervical, and thoracic spine are aligned and neutral.
- Shoulder girdle is stable on rib cage.

Action
1. Actively protract and slightly upwardly rotate scapula to link and stabilize the scapula to the rib cage.
2. Maintain the scapulothoracic connection and postural position and flex and extend the elbows, moving the chest toward the wall (Fig. 10.27B).
3. The entire body should move through space as a connected unit.

Advantages
- Position is easy to assume; however, compensations with head motion and loss of scapula connection are common.

Teaching tips
- Instruction example:
  - "Start in a plank position against the wall with your hands slightly wider than shoulder distance apart. You should be in one long line from your ears to your heels, leaning against the wall. Lower your chest toward the wall, not your nose."

- Common errors to correct:
  - Allowing the head to move forward beyond the trunk alignment (Fig. 10.27D)
  - Moving the body forward without controlling the movement from the upper body or letting the scapula retract without scapula connection to the ribcage (Fig. 10.27 E–G)
  - Avoid using a push-up "plus" position when anterior tipping or a thoracic kyphosis is present. The "plus" action causes further rounding and tipping.
- Methods to address or prevent compensations:
  - The therapist can provide tactile input to teach the patient to maintain the spine position on the patient's thoracic spine and with a hand on the back of patient's head.
  - "Keep your head up on your spine and your head in contact with my hand."
  - A wooden pole or foam roller placed on the patient's spine can assist with teaching the patient to coordinate the movement.

Alternatives
- Punches against resistance
- Assuming, then maintaining, plank position against the wall, without pressing up and down
- Four-point kneeling on exercise ball: weight shifting (Exercise 10.25)

Progression
- Slow down the eccentric component of the movement.
- Use an unstable surface for both hands (small balls, exercise ball, balance board, foam roller; Video 10.27A).
- Push up from four point kneeling position (Fig. 10.27H–J).
- Push up at an incline (Fig. 10.27K, L).
- Push up over an exercise ball using different amounts of body support (see Fig. 10.25 B–D for position).
- Full push-ups (progress by increasing repetitions or slowing downward motion for eccentric control; Fig. 10.27M–O, Video 10.27B)
- Push up with one hand on a higher surface (step or box)
- Push ups on unstable surfaces (foam roller, balance board)

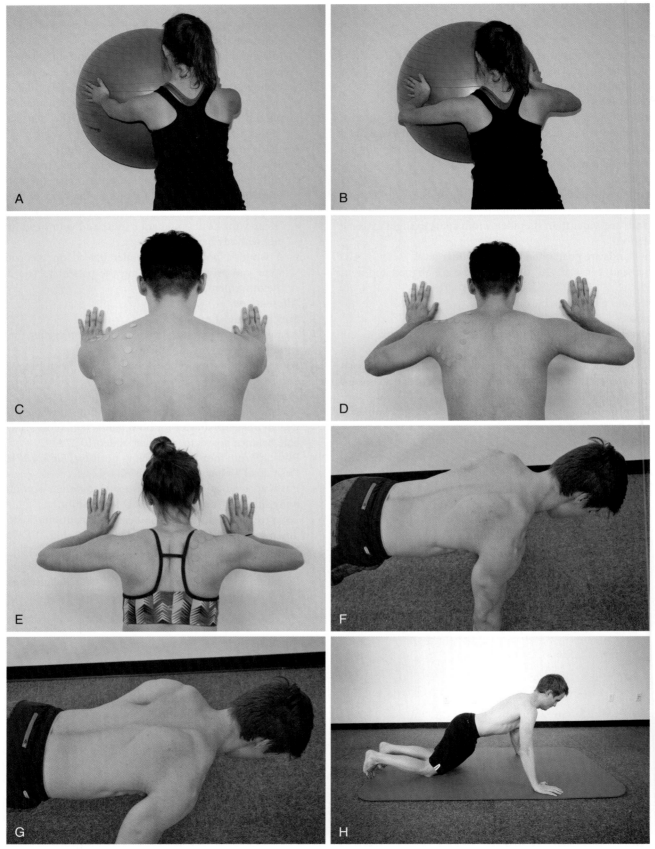

Fig. 10.27 Push-up progressions using an exercise ball on the wall (A and B), wall without a ball (C–E), compensations (D–G), four-point kneeling on the floor (H–J).

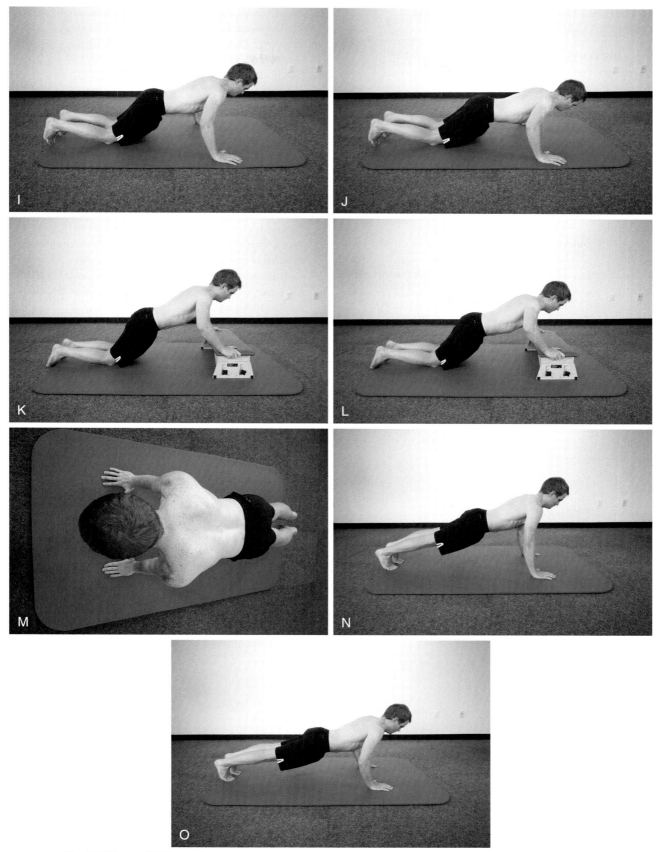

Fig. 10.27, cont'd Four-point kneeling on the floor (H–J), incline on a bench (K and L), full plank push-up (M–O).

FUNCTIONAL TRAINING, SPEED, AND RESPONSE TIME

10.28 Throwing/Catching Balls: Rebounder

See Fig. 10.28.

Purpose
- Train coordination and increase speed of neuromuscular responses to outside stimuli

Precautions
- Avoid full range with instability.
- Adjust the elevation range if there are impingement symptoms.
- Use light weight with rotator cuff tears or major instability.

Position
- Lunge standing, facing the rebounder with the arm in front of the body
- Degree of shoulder elevation is adjusted to a comfortable midrange.
- Degree of external rotation is controlled by the patient.

Action
1. Throwing and catching a weighted ball at a rebounder (Fig. 10.28A–D)
2. The patient is asked to throw toward the center point of the rebounder and track the number of repetitions with a successful catch (coordination) or to throw and catch until the shoulder fatigues (endurance), recording the time.
3. As the patient improves, speed and power can be emphasized by focusing on throwing harder and counting the successful catches in a minute.

Advantages
- Controlled responses at a short distance

- Need for neuromuscular coordination to respond to outside challenges or for proprioceptive improvement
- Improving reaction time

Teaching tips
- Methods to address or prevent compensations:
  - Avoid excessive stress on the anterior glenohumeral structures during the wind up phase of throwing by using lightweight balls.

Alternatives
- Throwing balls with a partner
- Vary the angle of the rebounder
- Different shoulder or upper extremity position or type of throwing
- Change speed
- Face sideways to the rebounder
- Use a whiffle ball instead of a weighted ball to train eccentric control of posterior cuff on follow-through.
- Throwing and catching a ball in higher ranges against a wall
- Using sports equipment (baseball mitts, tennis volleys, basketball drills against the wall)

Progression
- Increase repetitions.
- Increase range or weight of ball (Fig. 10.26).
- Increase emphasis on targets (mark a target on the rebounder).
- Vary the sequence of targets in response to outside cues.

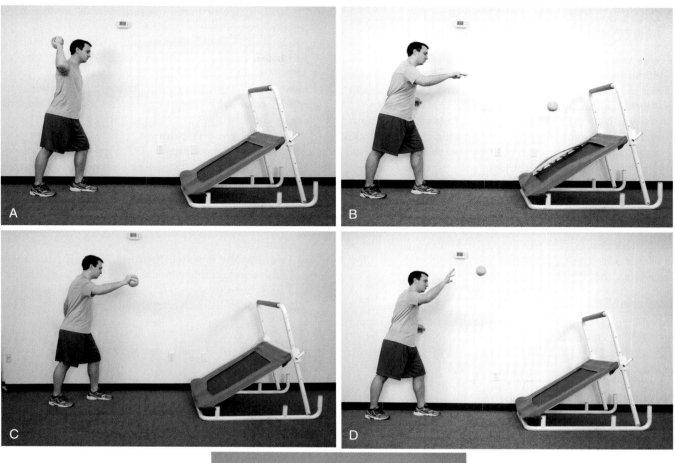

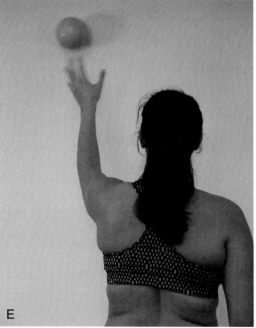

Fig. 10.28 Throwing and catching weighted balls from a rebounder (A–D) or against a wall (E).

◎ CASE STUDY 10.2: HYPERMOBILITY (ANTERIOR SHOULDER INSTABILITY)

This case presents the progression of exercise choices and methods for anterior instability with an emphasis on limiting stress on the anterior shoulder while promoting force closure. Options to limit specific stress during weight lifting techniques are also presented.

A 24-year-old female college student presents with complaints of intermittent shoulder pain usually following a gym workout. She is a former cheerleader and currently works out with weights. There is no history of trauma. The pain has been present intermittently for the past 5 years, but the painful episodes have become progressively more frequent. She has no major health conditions and is generally very flexible, but she has occasional cervical pain when she studies for exams. Her upper body workout consists of push-ups, bench press with free weights, rows with pulleys, biceps and triceps curls (free weights), flys, deltoid raises, pull-ups, dips, incline press, and elliptical machine with arm resistance.

Functional Status and Goals

She is able to perform all functional activities and only has pain after working out and sometimes after sleeping on her right shoulder. QuickDASH score is 18. She wants to be able to work out without pain.

Subjective Complaints

- *Severity*: Intermittent pain anterolateral right arm (2–4/10)
- *Irritability*: Pain usually starts 2–4 hours after working out with upper extremity weights, decreases within 24 hours
- *Nature*: Possible instability and/or tendinopathy
- *Stage*: Chronic

Objective Findings

- *Posture/alignment*: Forward head, increased lordosis, scapula winging, late scapula upward rotation
- *Range of motion*: See Table 10.6.

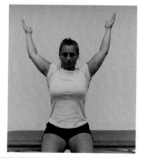

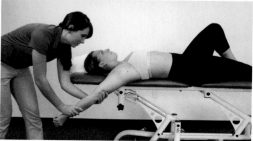

- *Cervical*: Range of motion within normal limits, no pain reproduction
- *RROM*: All isometric tests strong bilaterally in midrange, pain-free
- *Muscle length*: No limitations
- *Joint mobility*: Increased mobility in all directions, some apprehension with passive external rotation and extension, empty end feel
- *Neurological screening*: Normal
- *Special tests*: Beighton's score 4/7,[26,45] positive load and shift test,[27,46,47] positive Rockwood test for anterior instability[26]
- *Impingement tests*: Neer's negative with full range, Hawkins-Kennedy negative, empty can negative[27]
- *Movement patterns*:
  - Scapula winging during shoulder elevation (flexion and abduction)
  - Push-up: She is able to perform 30+ full push-ups but lacks scapula connection during the lowering phase

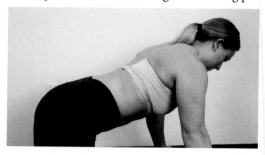

- Dips: Anterior shoulder position, forward body position placing extreme stress on anterior shoulder
- Latissimus dorsi pull downs with the bar behind head; her forward head position, shoulder tipping, and anterior shoulder position increases the more the bar is moved.
- Upright rows: No scapula connection, rounded and forward shoulder position throughout, forward head
- Bench press: She increases her lumbar lordosis and extends her lower thoracic spine before moving the bar toward the ceiling. On the downward return, her elbows move beyond the body with poor control, allowing the anterior shoulder to move forward into maximum horizontal abduction.
- Incline press and snatch lifts: Arms move overhead rapidly and position of the weights is behind her body

TABLE 10.6	**Right Shoulder Range of Motion**		
	AROM	**PROM**	**Normative Ranges for Age[44]**
Flexion	190	Same	180
Extension	40 some pain end of range	55	60
Abduction	170	Same	180
Adduction	50	Same	60
External rotation neutral	80	Same	70
External rotation at 90 degrees	100	110	80–90
Internal rotation neutral	60	Same	60
Internal rotation at 90 degrees	55	Same	60

Evaluation

- *Medical diagnosis*: Atraumatic anterior instability[7,47]
- *Physical therapy diagnosis*: Directional instability (hypermobility), neuromuscular coordination deficits,[7,48] no impingement symptoms (no painful arc, negative Hawkins Kennedy, Neer's)[49]
- *Contributing impairments*:
  - Postural alignment: Forward head, rounded shoulders, scapula winging
  - Weight lifting: Training overload without recovery
  - Movement and training patterns during weight lifting are placing excessive stress and strain on the anterior shoulder[50]
  - Difficulty with neuromuscular coordination and scapula stabilization during weight lifting activities
  - Some generalized laxity

Precautions

- Avoid excessive stress on the anterior shoulder in positions where the head of the humerus is translating anteriorly or the capsule is stretched (horizontal abduction, external rotation in higher ranges of abduction in the frontal plane or posterior to the frontal plane, and extension). Perform exercises in the scaption plane or sagittal plane to limit anterior shoulder stretch
- Monitor and adjust upper-quarter posture (kyphosis, forward head posture) to avoid scapula positions that increase stress on shoulder capsule (tipping, rounded shoulders).
- Impingement precautions:
  - Externally rotate the shoulder during elevation.
  - Avoid shoulder internal rotation in elevated positions

Prognosis

The patient has low levels of pain and irritability with the major factors influencing her symptoms related to weight-lifting patterns. If she is able to adjust the mechanics and training patterns, the prognosis to reduce symptoms is good to excellent. Burkhead and Rockwood[51] suggest that 80% of patients with atraumatic instability respond well if rehabilitation is appropriate. She will need to continue avoid placing stress on the anterior shoulder (Boxes 10.7, 10.8, and 10.9, and Table 10.7).

BOX 10.7 Implications for Exercise

- The symptomatic instability is related to uncontrolled forward translation of the head of the humerus into the anterior capsule and rotator cuff. Coordination of the rotator cuff firing and balance to promote force closure to ensure optimal muscle balance around a central axis of the glenohumeral joint is therefore important.[7]
- Scapula linkage and proximal upper-quarter positioning are also essential to support the glenohumeral mechanics.[22] An emphasis on proximal scapula control early in the rehabilitation sequence, before glenohumeral muscle emphasis, is recommended by a number of authors.[4,7,52,53] Promoting an active scapula force couple using serratus anterior to provide adequate upward rotation and scapulothoracic connection during the early scapulohumeral rhythm will be followed by progressive coordination and strengthening throughout the range once the sequencing has been reinforced.[4,54]

- Exercise parameters will need to address coordination and sequencing as well as proprioception, followed by endurance and then strength training within inner to midranges of the anterior shoulder muscles (pectoralis major, anterior deltoid) and the scapula stabilizers.
- Use unstable surfaces to promote stabilizing muscle activity.[55]
- Mid-position local and global stabilizer (scapulothoracic and glenohumeral) neuromuscular coordination training is recommended.
- Proprioceptive input and closed chain positions using motor control concepts are used to adjust neuromuscular coordination.
- Eccentric control is important while training the proprioceptive awareness to limit movement behind the body or when approaching the frontal plane when the loads may stress the anterior shoulder passive restraints.
- Adjusting weight-lifting training mechanics will be essential for transfer of movement strategies and to address contributing forces to the microtrauma. Weight-lifting mechanics will need to be adjusted, including limiting range and stress in the extreme ranges of shoulder extension. The position and range for exercises stressing the anterior shoulder can be adjusted for some exercises while others will need to be replaced.[50]
- Observe for scapula winging and loss of active control of cervicothoracic position during exercise. Correct and cue for position or stop the exercise even if the patient is not experiencing fatigue.
- Exercise should be pain-free, and pain responses is monitored after the exercise session as an indicator of excessive stress/strain. However, initial exercise loads and challenge is relatively aggressive based on limited severity and irritability, the patient's overall fitness levels, and the need to challenge neuromuscular coordination and muscle function without placing excessive strain on the glenohumeral restraints. Progression is based on the ability to coordinate the movement without compensations and once she is able to control the anterior shoulder position, scapulothoracic, and cervicothoracic coordination.

BOX 10.8 Modification of Weight-Lifting Mechanics

Review and modify mechanics for push-ups, bench press with free weights, biceps and triceps curls (free weights), flys, deltoid raises, elliptical with arm resistance, latissimus dorsi pull-downs.[50]

- Modify:
  - Change starting position for rows with pulleys from upright sitting to recline sitting and maintaining the arms in front of body) to limit shoulder extension and anterior translation.
  - Limit push-ups to small range (before the elbows move past the level of the body) by placing a box under her body at the limit.
  - Limit shoulder extension for triceps by performing with her arms in front of the body against pulleys from behind.
  - Avoid tipping or winging (cueing and using a mirror) and perform in front of the body in midrange rather than in neutral. Initial training is with the arm supported on a table and on an unstable surface to challenge proprioception and stabilization.
  - Control the range of horizontal abduction for flys by setting the equipment so that the range is limited to the scaption plane.
  - Bench press: Perform on the floor with free weights and limit the range of horizontal abduction.
  - Latissimus dorsi pull-downs: Change to arms in front of body and decrease range[50] (see Exercise 10.32).
- Discontinue dips and pull-ups

BOX 10.9 Examples of Methods to Avoid Stretch of the Anterior Shoulder

- Use visual feedback for exercises where the patient can observe her shoulder position (e.g., flys, deltoid raises, elliptical).
- Use positioning to limit the elbows going behind the body and shoulder extension for rows with support for the thoracic spine and a reclined position to limit range.
- Place an object on the ground, under her torso, to limit range for push-ups.
- Set machines to limit horizontal shoulder extension for flys.
- Use positioning to limit range of shoulder extension for bench press with dumbbells rather than a narrow bench and a rack. Educate the patient on amount of weight, range, and the use of a spotter to avoid the anterior shoulder position.

Treatment Choices

Exercise choices take into account the need to limit combined stress and strain on the anterior shoulder structures and build force closure and neuromuscular coordination to support and disperse forces (see Boxes 10.7, 10.8, and 10.9, and Table 10.7).

TABLE 10.7 Exercise Choices

Treatment	1	2	3	4	5	6	7	8	9	10
Scapula connection activation with therapist feedback and isometric challenge on a foam roller (Exercises 10.14 and 10.15)	X	X	X Add dumbbells for scapula protraction	X						
Manual resistance scapula upward rotation on a foam roller and a pole to increase lever arm (Exercise 10.18)	X	X	Multiple angle isometrics ↑ time held	X						
Scapulothoracic endurance using weighted balls (Exercises 10.14 and 10.15), circumduction (Exercise 10.16)	X	X	↑ time	X						
Closed chain circumduction in scaption (Exercise 10.17)			X	X	X	↑ range	X			
Body Blade perturbations in standing in scaption at different ranges of flexion with scapula connection (Exercise 10.22)	X	X	↑ to 3 sets	X	↑ to 4 sets	X	X			
Standing upward rotation punches against pulley resistance (Exercise 10.24)		X	X	↑ resistance	X	X Multiple ranges	↑ resistance	X	X Multiple diagonals	X
Closed chain weight shift on a balance board (Exercise 10.25)		X	X	X	X↑ hold	X				
Inner-range flys (machine resistance) (Exercise 10.26)		X		X	X	↑ resistance	X	X	↑ resistance	X
Inner-range flys (free weight, horizontal adduction 45 to 0 degrees, eccentric control) supine on foam roller (Exercise 10.26)				X	X	X	↑ resistance	X	Slower speed	X
Shoulder internal rotation and external rotation against pulley resistance (midrange rotation in scaption) (Exercise 10.23)					Isometrics X		X↑ Hold	X	↑ resistance	Small- range isotonics
Inner range flys in reclined sitting with free weights (Exercise 10.26)					X	X	X	↑ resistance	X	X
Push ups (small range, four-point, then plank; Exercise 10.27)						Small range X		↑ reps	X	X Slower speed on downward movement
Latissimus dorsi pull-downs (Exercise 10.32)	X						X	↑ resistance	X	X
Kettle bell lunges (Exercise 10.37)							X	X	X	↑ resistance
Planks on unstable surface (BOSU) (Exercise 10.46)							X	X	↑ time	X

SECTION 3: REPETITIVE STRAIN

GENERAL TREATMENT APPROACHES

The types of exercise used for repetitive strain injuries are described in Chapter 6 (see Table 6.6). A review of the goals, methods, parameters, and measurements are included in Table 10.8. The priority for repetitive strain injuries is to improve the movement biomechanics while allowing tissue recovery. The overall goals are to distribute forces to avoid excessive force on inflamed, irritated, or degenerated tissue; to promote proper alignment; and to optimize biomechanical efficiency, as well as to promote symmetrical and efficient muscle function. In order to address other contributing factors, improving flexibility and length of restricted soft tissue or joint motion and promoting overall endurance are also key intervention strategies. If hypermobility is present, the goals for hypermobility take precedence over those for hypomobility, and additional care is warranted to avoid stresses on the area of concern.

Typical diagnoses in this category include:
- Tendinopathy (bicipital, supraspinatus, lateral or medial epicondylitis, De Quervain's syndrome)
- Impingement syndrome (shoulder impingement, carpal tunnel, nerve entrapments)
- Degenerative conditions (osteoarthritis, rotator cuff degeneration)

TABLE 10.8 Goals, Methods, Parameters, and Measurement: Repetitive Strain

Goals		Methods	Parameters	Assessment/Measurement
Distribute forces to avoid excessive forces on inflamed, irritated, or degenerated structures		Muscle activation and endurance exercise for proximal areas surrounding the affected region including scapulothoracic connection, cervicothoracic support	Open chain or closed chain, isometric activity around affected area Apply resistance, avoiding stress on affected region Apply resistance in planes of motion or other joint motion other than affected region Specificity of activation and timing before motion Low load, high repetitions without pain responses from affected area Range is dependent on the requirements for functional activity and the ranges where stress is likely to be placed on other structures Isometric or isotonic	Pain responses after exercise (delayed-onset muscle soreness) Specific muscle function capabilities (amount of load and repetitions before fatigue) Movement patterns during exercise and functional tests Functional tests
Address causative factors increasing forces on structures and impairments resulting from compensations	Decreased joint mobility or muscle flexibility	Muscle flexibility (stretching) Joint mobility focus	End range (joint or muscle) Low loads with sustained holds Maximal length of affected tissue Progress time of hold or load Allow some time to accommodate to new lengths before progressing load Goals to achieve functional range	Pain responses during and after exercise (delayed-onset muscle soreness) Range of motion (goniometric or functional tests) End feel (especially for muscle guarding)
	Address muscle imbalances (decreased muscle activation, endurance, or strength) (especially related to scapulothoracic connection, rotator cuff stabilization)	See section on distributing forces to avoid excessive forces on inflamed, irritated, or degenerated structures; applied to surrounding regions and to affected area		
	Training factors	Adjust training intensity, frequency, or type to decrease local stress while maintaining conditioning Select alternate exercise (cross-training) Cardiovascular or muscle endurance exercise	Deloaded positions RPE 11–13 if possible without increasing symptoms Multiple repetitions, low load if possible without increasing symptoms	Pain responses during, and after exercise (delayed-onset muscle soreness) Time before onset of symptoms Functional measures DASH Time or intensity for endurance exercise

Continued

TABLE 10.8 · Goals, Methods, Parameters, and Measurement: Repetitive Strain—cont'd

Goals	Methods	Parameters	Assessment/Measurement
Adjust dynamic biomechanical alignment (scapulothoracic connection, elevation mechanics without impingement)	Promote neuromuscular control using motor control principles Multiple forms of sensory input (visual, tactile, including taping) Progress to eccentric control Progress to dynamic motion and balance	Slow progression into ranges where increased biomechanical stress is more likely Lower loads than required for functional activities with high repetition (supported or unsupported) Progress to higher loads, low repetitions (isometric or isotonic) in pain-free ranges	Achievement of targets (% of successful trials) Amount of feedback and correction needed Pain responses or movement quality through range or with repetitions Dynamic movement assessment
Promote tissue healing and optimal regeneration	Tendon: slow progression of isotonic exercise and eccentric loading	Progress from low-load/high-repetition to higher load/low-repetition Midrange, progressing to end range	Monitor symptoms Functional tests Resistive or special tests DASH
	Bone: slowly progress loading forces	Progress from low-load/high-repetition to higher load/low-repetition Use intermittent loading, then slowly increase in duration of sustained loading (without additional angulation or rotational forces)	Monitor symptoms (pain, edema) Functional tests Resistive or special tests DASH
	Cartilage: slowly progress gliding and intermittent compression and decompression with decreased weight bearing	Low-load/high-repetition, adequate rest periods	Monitor symptoms (pain, edema, effusion) Functional tests Resistive or special tests DASH
Improve neuromuscular coordination and response time for functional requirements (elevation mechanics, responses to external loads, requirements for prolonged upper extremity motion)	Promote neuromuscular control using motor control principles Closed chain or open chain, depending on functional requirements and stage of recovery Feedback for adjusting movement strategies (auditory, visual, tactile, including taping)	Supported positions progressing to unsupported, movements depend on functional requirements Multiple repetitions after desired movement strategy has been achieved Parameters progressed based on motor learning to maintain position or control through range without exacerbating symptoms	Analysis of biomechanics (visual analysis of timing, axis of motion) Ability to perform movement correctly (timed) or % of repetitions performed before fatigue or compensation Amount of feedback and correction needed % of targets reached Functional tests DASH

CONTRAINDICATIONS AND PRECAUTIONS

- Avoid combined forces resulting in microfailure (specific directions, or type of forces, ranges, specific movements or adjusting biomechanical factors).
- Avoid angulation or rotation in extreme ranges combined with high loads (see stress-strain curve in Chapter 2).
- When introducing forces to the damaged tissue, do so slowly.
- Avoid impingement ranges and combinations of movements by using shoulder external rotation through elevation into flexion and abduction, promoting proximal scapulothoracic connection and upward rotation.
- Specific precautions for:
  - Bone (stress fractures): Avoid rotational and high impact forces.
  - Tendinopathy: Avoid high loads in extreme ranges.
  - Cartilage damage (osteoarthritis): Avoid high weight-bearing forces.
  - Muscle (rotator cuff tears): Only use low-load, midrange for mild rotator cuff tears.
  - Avoid specific directions of force for directional instabilities.

GENERAL PARAMETERS

- Correcting biomechanical alignment and force distribution is a priority.
- The ability to achieve optimal position, signs of fatigue, and exacerbation of symptoms will influence the dosage.
- Supported position is progressed to unsupported.
- Closed chain activities will promote a centralized axis of motion.
- Open chain will emphasize moving through a larger range or addressing flexibility limitations.
- Initial dosages start with low-load/high-repetitions (>25) or low loads/prolonged holds for isometric contractions before fatigue with an emphasis on appropriate timing, sequencing, and targets for muscle activation and endurance.
- Dosage progresses to higher load/lower repetitions (<15) with the ability to maintain the position as a requirement before increasing the load.
- Neuromuscular coordination focus is emphasized throughout the treatment progression with high specificity, achievement of targets, and correcting movement patterns.
- Progressing range is based on functional requirements or correcting contributing factors without increasing symptoms.

TESTS AND MEASURES

See Magee[26], Magee and Sueki[27], and Cleland[56] for more detailed description of available tests and measures, interpretation, and psychometric properties.

1. Pain reports
2. Range of motion tolerated without reproducing impingement symptoms
3. Functional movement outcome measures for endurance or strength
4. Movement observation (qualitative)
5. Functional outcome measures for symmetry, repetition, or functional requirements
6. Ability to perform activities without compensations or home programs independently; specific items related to shoulder elevation, reaching, dressing, bathing, lifting, grip strength, repeated movement
7. DASH, Patient Specific Functional Scale

OBSERVING FOR COMPENSATIONS AND RESPONSES

- Maintaining proper position and alignment in the area of concern is the first priority, but observe for overall alignment at proximal and distal regions (e.g., if the primary area of dysfunction is the elbow, monitor the scapulothoracic and glenohumeral alignment and the wrist position).
- Observe for and establish proper proximal postural position and correct alignment *before* exercise.
- Evaluate scapulothoracic upward rotation and facilitate correct mechanics if contributing to repetitive strain.
- Monitor proximal areas and correct position and muscle activation to address moment arms, excessive angulation, or rotational movements.
- Observe for signs of fatigue (loss of position, substitutions or muscle activation) and monitor symptom reproduction.
- Use supported positions as needed.
- Ask patients to report any discomfort during or after the exercise.
- Monitor for delayed-onset muscle soreness, increased effusion, or edema after treatment.

EXERCISE DESCRIPTIONS

GENERALIZED AEROBIC EXERCISE

10.29 Airdyne Bike

Purpose
- Generalized thoracic rotation for upper-quarter mobility while using entire scapulothoracic and glenohumeral muscle complexes
- Exercise can be used for aerobic endurance or strengthening through range.

Precautions
- If the patient has moderate levels of pain intensity or irritability, the UBE may be more appropriate than the Airdyne Bike for a warm-up or aerobic upper-quarter conditioning as the resistance provided by the opposite arm handle with the Airdyne bike or similar equipment can be difficult to control.
- Patients with neural tension or cervical dysfunction should start at slow speeds and in small ranges.
- Avoid internal rotation by placing the hands on the handles with the thumbs facing toward the ceiling.
- Limit higher ranges of shoulder flexion in the presence of impingement symptoms or if there are range of motion deficits by increasing the seat height.
- Monitor pulse/blood pressure responses pre- and post-exercise if any cardiovascular comorbidities exist.

Position
- Seated with seat height set to accommodate available shoulder flexion range of motion.
- Ensure upright supported spinal posture
- Shoulders externally rotated (thumbs up) with hands below impingement range

Action
1. Scapula protraction and retraction are combined with thoracic rotation to move upper extremity handles forward and backward, with or without leg movement.
2. Upper body resistance is created by momentum from the opposite arm and leg action, which needs to be matched on the affected limb.

Advantages
- Generalized upper extremity and upper-quarter conditioning or decreased aerobic capacity
- Useful to address overall upper-quarter muscle activation and endurance for postural support
- Also useful for scapula protraction and retraction, aerobic conditioning, or strengthening
- Useful for warm-up

Teaching tips
- Instruction examples:
  - "Initiating from your shoulder blade, pull back with one handle and feel your rib cage move back with your elbow."
  - "At the same time, glide your opposite shoulder blade forward as that arm reaches and pushes forward."

- Common errors to correct:
  - If there is no thoracic rotation, the cervical region and scapulothoracic muscles may fatigue early.
  - Correct the starting position of the upper body and spinal alignment at the beginning of the exercise and observe for fatigue during the exercise. Brief rest periods can assist with overall fatigue while still addressing endurance.
  - Fatigue of the spinal muscles is possible and should also be monitored.
  - Observe the patient for overuse of the upper trapezius and levator scapula muscles as the arm muscles fatigue.
  - Avoid overusing the biceps and underutilizing the scapulothoracic muscles.
- Methods to address or prevent compensations:
  - Monitor for loss of postural position and cue for proximal support.
  - The upper body position is important to correct before starting the exercise and to maintain throughout the activity. The distance from the seat to the handles can influence upper body posture.
  - Maintaining the gaze forward (stabilizing the cervical spine) will result in relative cervical rotation with the shoulders moving under the head and neck. This is useful in activities involving swinging the arms while targeting an object such as golf or baseball.
  - Ensure that thoracic motion is initiated along with scapula protraction and retraction.
  - "Keep your shoulders from creeping up toward your ears."
  - Cue the patient to initiate the movements from the shoulder blade rather than the hands and to only grip the handle as tightly as necessary.

Parameters
- Time and intensity selected for generalized warm-up will not result in excessive fatigue (usually does not exceed 11–13 on perceived exertion scale).
- Initial goals for muscle activation and mobility can be progressed to endurance parameters with progressive increases in time and intensity based on time to fatigue (perceived exertion) or cardiovascular responses.
- Increase shoulder flexion range of motion by adjusting the seat height, or cervicothoracic rotation by adjusting the seat distance from the arm unit.
- Increase resistance once sufficient mobility has been achieved and no soreness is reported after the exercise. Intensity can be increased by using the opposite arm or the leg action.

Alternatives
- UBE (Exercise 10.1) or NuStep (Fig. 10.29)
- Standing, facing the handles of the Airdyne bike moving upper extremity handles

Progression
- Increase range.
- Increase speed (generates more resistance).
- Increase time.

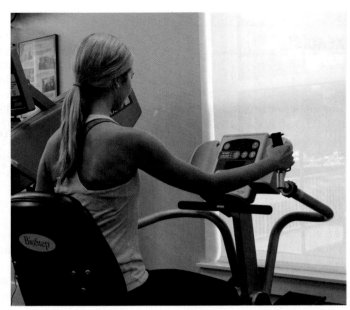

Fig. 10.29 NuStep upper body protraction and retraction along with thoracic rotation provides upper body aerobic, mobility, and strengthening challenge.

PROGRESSIVE RESISTIVE EXERCISE ADDRESSING BIOMECHANICS AND NEUROMUSCULAR COORDINATION WITHOUT EXACERBATING IMPINGEMENT

10.30 Shoulder Extension: Pulleys

See Fig. 10.30.

Purpose

- Neuromuscular coordination
- Train active inferior gliding accessory movement in the glenohumeral joint during the downward motion and eccentric control during the return.
- Promote scapulothoracic mechanics without impingement.
- Muscle strengthening or aerobic conditioning dependent on dosage

Precautions

- May need to limit the shoulder extension range to midrange for patients with downward sloping shoulders and impingement to avoid further tipping of the shoulders and superior rotator cuff tension.

Position

- Standing or sitting in a forward incline or upright position, facing pulleys, holding handle with shoulder in mid-position and scaption plane, externally rotated (thumb up).
- Starting position is set with the shoulder flexed to 80 degrees or to the range that does not reproduce impingement symptoms.
- Set the pulley stopper to block shoulder flexion beyond 80 degrees or the patient's impingement range.

Action

1. Ensure an upright supported proximal spine and cervical region.
2. Stabilize the trunk.
3. Extend shoulder toward neutral while maintaining upper-quarter position.
4. Actively control motion on the return.

Advantages

- Range can be set to avoid impingement
- Shoulder extension is less likely to result in impingement and the exercise helps train neuromuscular coordination to limit impingement.
- Active inferior glide away from the acromion provides a circulatory effect to assist with removal of subacromial bursa effusion and gliding of the shoulder joint.

- Proprioceptive and visual input assists with neuromuscular coordination.

Teaching tips

- Instruction examples:
  - "Start the movement using the muscles under the shoulder and bring the handle down toward your hip."
  - "Control the return of the weight without losing the tension on the rope or letting the weight go quickly."
- Common errors to correct:
  - Observe for tipping, increased forward head position, shifting the body weight toward the pulleys, and rotating the body.
  - Watch for allowing the weights to move quickly without controlling the speed of the return or uncontrolled jerky movement.
  - Avoid shoulder hiking or uncontrolled flexion motion resulting from unopposed motion from the weight on the return.
- Methods to address or prevent compensations:
  - Keep the shoulder externally rotated throughout the movement.
  - Limit the range or adjust the resistance if the patient is unable to control the scapula stability with cueing.
  - Instruct the patient to "Keep your shoulders wide and your body facing forward as you pull your arm down toward your hip" if the patient is hiking or rotating the body.
  - "Try not to let the weights rest at the end of the movement by stopping short of the end point (stopper)."

Alternatives

- A resistance band can be substituted for the pulley system, but must move through smaller ranges because the band tension continuously increases as it is stretched contributing to compensations.
- Exercise can be performed in supine or prone to limit spinal compensations or stress.
- Add an isometric hold at the end of the movement once there are no compensations.

Progression

- Increase resistance.
- Increase range.

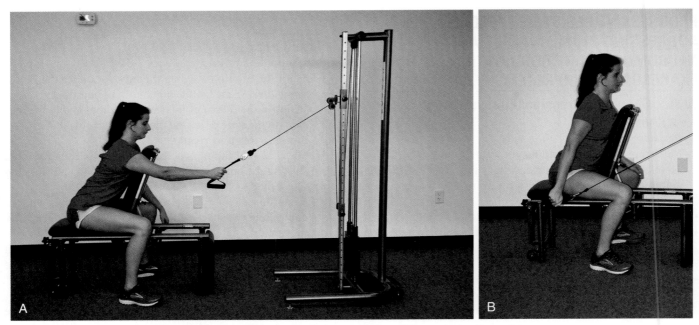

Fig. 10.30 Shoulder extension in forward incline sitting against pulley resistance.

10.31 Shoulder Adduction: Elastic Resistance or Pulleys

See Fig. 10.31.

Purpose
- Neuromuscular coordination
- Increase strength or aerobic conditioning, depending on dosage

Precautions
- Limit the shoulder adduction range to midrange for patients with downward sloping shoulders and impingement or tendonitis to avoid further depressing the shoulder and placing undue tension on the superior rotator cuff.

Position
- Standing or sitting, perpendicular to band's anchor point, with shoulder and body aligned in the frontal plane (or slightly in front of the body).
- Holding the end of the band, the shoulder is externally rotated (thumb up) and abducted to 80 degrees or less. If impingement symptoms are reported, decrease the starting position so that there are no symptoms.

Action
1. Stabilize the trunk by activating the core and abdominal muscles.
2. Adduct the shoulder toward neutral (hands at the side in anatomical position) while maintaining the upper-quarter position.
3. If elastic resistance is used, set the tension so that there is no slack at the starting point and only move through range where no compensations occur.
4. If pulleys are used, the range can be larger than with elastic resistance; the relative load is distributed through the pulley mechanism. Elastic resistance is the largest with the full stretch of the band.
5. Actively control the motion on the return.

Advantages
- Resistance bands can be used as a home program.

- Adduction activates inferior rotator cuff muscles and position limits the likelihood of impingement.

Teaching tips
- Instruction examples:
  "Keeping both sides of your waist long, pull the band down toward your side."
    - "Initiate the movement from underneath your armpit and pull downward."
    - "Stand tall as you pull down on the band."
    - "Keep your shoulders quiet as you pull down on the band."
- Common errors to correct:
    - Side bending the trunk while pulling the band
    - Rounding the shoulder forward as the band is pulled down to side
    - Increasing forward head during adduction motion
    - Not controlling the weight return to starting position or allowing the scapula to lift arm returns to the starting position

Alternatives
- Vary the ranges of motion by adjusting the starting position set-up with the resistance band
- Supine position: trunk compensations or exacerbating cervical or thoracic pain are less likely to occur.
- Multi-angle isometrics
- Change the plane of movement to target different portions of the rotator cuff and glenohumeral complex.

Progression
- Use a higher resistance band.
- Increase sets.
- Add isometric holds at different points of the range.
- Decrease speed of return.

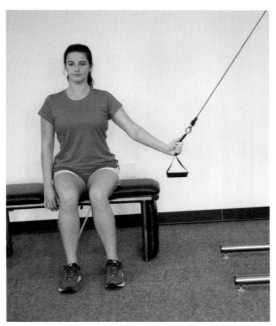

Fig. 10.31 Shoulder adduction: pulley resistance in sitting.

10.32   Bilateral Shoulder Extension or Adduction: Latissimus Dorsi Pull-Down

See Fig. 10.32.

Purpose

- Improve upper extremity neuromuscular coordination with proximal spinal alignment
- Increase strength or aerobic conditioning depending on dosage
- Challenges ability to maintain scapulothoracic connection without tipping or rounding the scapula

Position

- Standing or sitting, with hands on latissimus dorsi pull-down bar placed wider than shoulder width
- The position of the bar is established based on the available pain-free flexion range, with the weight stack resting at the starting position.
- Pressure is placed on the outside of the hands, and thumbs are wrapped over the top of the bar to avoid excessive internal rotation.
- Patients with a greater shoulder width may need to increase the distance between the hands in scaption position to accommodate the natural bony alignment.

Action (Video 10.32)

1. Set the scapulothoracic connection.
2. Establish spinal alignment and abdominal engagement before starting the movement.
3. Use the latissimus dorsi and posterior shoulder muscles to bring the bar down toward the floor. Elbows can flex during the movement (Fig. 10.32) or remain extended.
4. Keep the wrists in a neutral position.
5. Control the return of the bar.

Advantages

- Most gyms have latissimus dorsi pull-down options (equipment may require sitting or standing), and the exercise is often used for fitness purposes.
- Bilateral motion establishes spinal alignment and limits asymmetrical compensations.
- Eccentric control on the return can be used to train activation of the inferior rotator cuff to avoid excessive or early superior glide of the humeral head.

Teaching tips

- Instruction examples:
  - "Initiating from underneath your armpits, press through the outside of your hand to press the bar downward."
  - "Only hold the bar as much as you need to avoid the bar slipping."
  - "Lengthen through your spine as you pull the bar toward the floor."
  - "Keep your chest upright as you pull down the bar."
- Common errors to correct:
  - Starting with the hands placed too close together will increase the risk of shoulder compensations such as tipping or early shoulder hiking.
  - Gripping the bar excessively and initiating the movement with the hands rather than from the proximal shoulder extensors leads to shoulder internal rotation or scapula tipping.
  - Increased lordosis or rocking forward or backwards on the heels.
  - Scapula tipping, scapula elevation, or increased forward head position during the shoulder motion
  - Allowing the wrists to extend at the end of the movement
  - Flexing the elbows, retracting excessively, and allowing shoulder internal rotation
- Methods to address or prevent compensations:
  - Maintain the core activation and postural position throughout the movement without letting the lumbar spine extend or the weight tip backward.
  - The direction of the movement should be toward the floor in front of the body, not directed toward the body, which is more likely to result in anterior shoulder tipping.
  - Changing the grip so that the thumb is free and the pressure is on the outside of the hands for most of the movement can help decrease the tendency to internally rotate.

Alternatives

- Bilateral extension with individual pulleys connected with pole between handles to challenge arm symmetry
- Single-arm extension against pulleys or a resistance band (Exercise 10.30)
- Latissimus pull-downs in sitting (may be a progression if range is limited due to pain)

Progression

- Increase repetitions.
- Increase weight.
- Increase range.

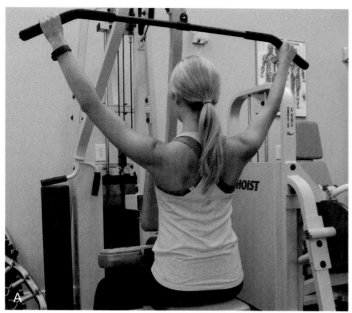
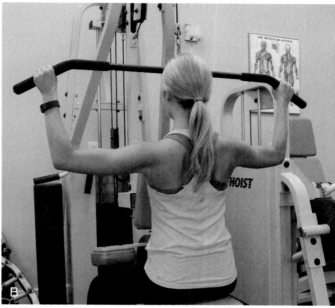

Fig. 10.32 Lattisimus dorsi pull-down with the bar in front of the body.

RESISTIVE EXERCISE TO PROVIDE OPTIMAL STIMULUS FOR TISSUE REGENERATION

10.33 Shoulder External or Internal Rotation: Pulleys or Free Weights

See Fig. 10.33.

Purpose

- Increase strength or endurance of the rotators
- Promote rotator cuff stabilization
- Provide optimal stimulus for rotator cuff muscles or tendons

Precautions

- In the presence of a rotator cuff tear, use care when prescribing resisted isotonic contractions during early exercise management. If the patient is able to demonstrate isometric stabilization of the glenohumeral joint, introduce this exercise using light resistance and small ranges as tolerated. Support for the arm and using midrange resting position is advisable in Phase I and early Phase II.
- External rotation is painful with supraspinatus tendinopathy and often with impingement. Scapular plane, midrange of rotation and limiting the amount of elevation is advisable in Phase I and early Phase II.

Position

- Sitting with the pulley system is flexed.

Action (Video 10.33A and B)

1. Establish an upright supported postural alignment.
2. Externally or internally rotate against the pulley resistance.

Advantages

- Arm is supported against gravity.
- External rotation provides stimulus for supraspinatus, teres minor, and infraspinatus muscle and tendon regeneration without excessive tension.

- Internal rotation provides stimulus for subscapularis regeneration.

Teaching tips

- Common errors to correct:
  - Loss of proximal support from the scapula: winging, downward rotation or tipping, elevation
  - Loss of proximal support from the cervicothoracic region
  - Trunk rotation to compensate for difficulty with external rotation
- Methods to address or prevent compensations:
  - If the patient has forward shoulders or the scapula is downwardly rotated, the cervical and thoracic spine starting position should be carefully observed and corrected in the starting position and during the exercise.
  - Observe for loss of scapula control (elevation, forward rotation).
  - Correct a forward slumped position by adjusting the table height and the distance the patient is positioned from the table.

Alternatives

- Side-lying supine or prone external or internal rotation against gravity, with or without weight (Fig. 10.33C–H)
- Sitting or standing external or internal rotation without arm support
- Isometrics

Progression

- Add an unstable base for arm.
- Increase repetitions.
- Increase range.
- Increase weight.
- Unsupported exercises

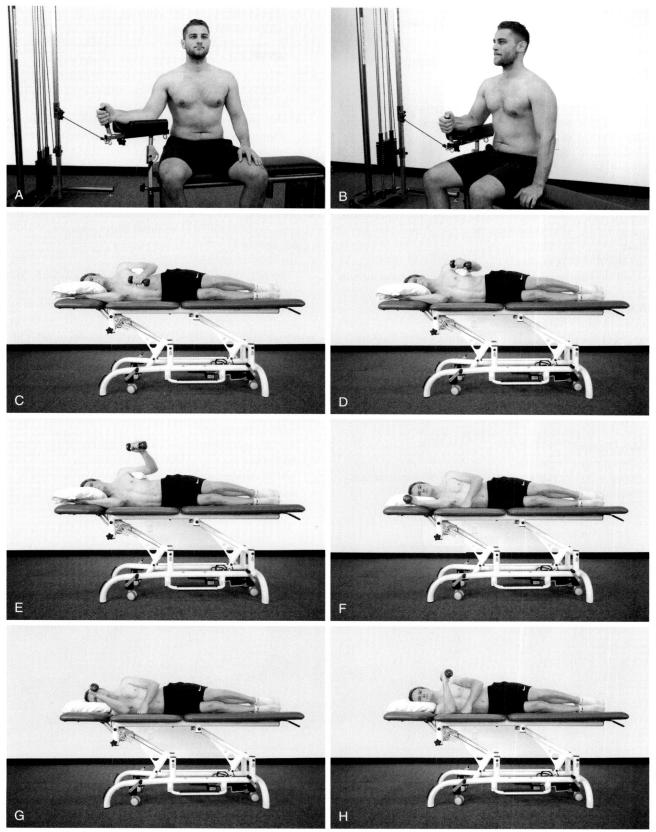

Fig. 10.33 Shoulder external (A) or internal rotation (B) in sitting with the arm weight supported against pulley resistance, side-lying using free weights against gravity, external rotation (C–E), and internal rotation (F–H).

10.34   Wrist Flexion or Extension: Free Weights

See Fig. 10.34.

Purpose
- Eccentric stimulus for wrist flexors or extensors (at the origin or insertions)
- Strengthening for wrist flexors or extensors
- Useful for repetitive strain conditions affecting the wrist and elbow flexors or extensors (golfer's, elbow, tennis elbow, finger or thumb tenosynovitis)

Position
- Sitting, holding a dumbbell or weighted ball with forearm supported on table, wrist at the edge of table
- Forearm is supinated for flexion, pronated for extension.
- Allow natural elbow valgus angle, but set proximal trunk alignment to limit rotational forces at the elbow.

Action
1. Flex (Fig. 10.34A) or extend (Fig. 10.34B) wrist.
2. Control the return movement against gravity, emphasizing eccentric lowering.

Advantages
- Upper extremity is supported.
- Alignment is easier to correct and maintain with support.

Teaching tips
- Instruction examples:
  - "Only grip as much as you need to hold the weight."
  - "Lift your knuckles toward the ceiling" (for wrist extension).
  - Lift the weight toward the ceiling, using your wrist" (for wrist flexion).
- Common errors to correct:
  - Avoid excessive radial/ulnar deviation or pronation/supination during the movement.

- Correct upper-quarter alignment is important to encourage proximal support.
- Do not allow the elbow to flex, substituting elbow flexion for wrist flexion or extension to lift the weight.
- Methods to address or prevent compensations:
  - Monitor the range of motion, angulation, and grip intensity, especially if pain is reproduced.
  - Adjust the proximal support position and alignment of the upper extremity to the natural valgus angle rather than placing the hand directly in front of the body.

Specific parameters
- Resistance is determined by fatigue of the wrist flexors or extensors *and* the ability to control the movement.
- Increasing resistance is only indicated if there are no compensations and pain is minimal with resistance.

Alternatives
- Therapist resistance
- Isometric wrist muscle and grip activities with shoulder exercise
- Self-resistance
- Resistance band
- Wrist rolling: affix a rope attached to a weight to a dowel. Raise the weight by rolling the dowel: palms up to target the wrist flexors, palms down to target the wrist extensors.

Progression
- Slower speeds for eccentric control
- Increase repetitions.
- Use unstable support (ball under forearm or upper arm).
- Add pronation or supination to wrist motion.
- Add elbow motion.
- Increase resistance.

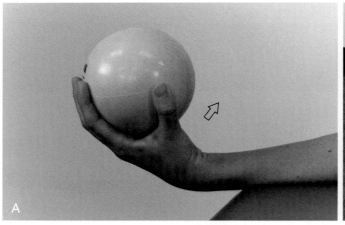 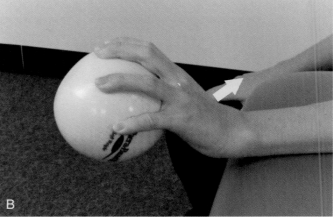

Fig. 10.34 Wrist flexion (A) or extension (B) with weighted balls.

10.35 Grip Strengthening

See Fig. 10.35.

Purpose

- Isometric strengthening of hand, wrist, and elbow muscles

Position

- Sitting, forearm in a neutral position (midway between pronation and supination) with the arm supported on a table
- Elbow flexed
- Holding dynamometer

Action

1. Test the maximum grip strength.
2. Set target resistance and monitor amount of resistance during repetitions.

Advantages

- Improves general grip strength for functional activities
- Allows visual feedback of amount of resistance
- Allows objective measurement of resistance, which simplifies documenting or modifying the exercise

Teaching tips

- Instruction examples:
  - For endurance: "Watch the dial and squeeze the handle, gradually building up your resistance until the needle hits X pounds and then hold the needle still as long as you can."
  - For strength: "Squeeze the handle until the needle reaches X pounds and hold the needle still for 6 (up to 10) seconds."
  - For power: "Squeeze the handle as hard as you can and then release. See how high you can get the needle. Rest completely and then try to match or beat that reading."
- Common error to correct:
  - Loss of proximal alignment and support (shoulder tipping, rounding)
- Method to address or prevent compensations:
  - Observe and correct proximal alignment in the starting position and during movement.

Alternatives

- Squeezing foam or tennis balls
- Target coordination and fine motor skills using pinch, prehension, cylindrical or spherical grip activities.

Progression

- Increase length of time held.
- Increase repetitions.
- Increase resistance target.
- Decrease forearm support; elbow flexion with or without support of upper arm.
- Include grip activities with upper extremity strengthening or functional activities (see Exercise 10.48). Include resistance while simulating sports-specific activities. For example, the therapist applies resistance while the patient holds a tennis racquet for shoulder internal and external rotation.

Parameters

- For endurance:
  - Determine the percentage of maximum resistance desired for endurance.
  - Squeeze the handle to achieve the target (40–60% maximum) and hold for as long as possible.
  - Rest for 1–2 minutes, repeat 3–5 times.
- For strengthening:
  - 60–80% maximum grip strength and hold for 6–10 seconds or until unable to maintain 60% of maximum.

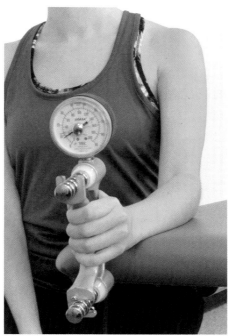

Fig. 10.35 Grip strengthening using a handheld dynamometer.

PROGRESSIVE RESISTIVE EXERCISE: GLOBAL STABILIZER OR GLOBAL MOVER STRENGTHENING

10.36 Proprioceptive Neuromuscular Facilitation (PNF) Diagonals: Elastic Resistance or Pulleys

See Fig. 10.36.

Purpose
- Combined multijoint, triplanar motion
- Neuromuscular coordination in diagonal planes (functional movements typically occur in diagonal planes)
- Increases strength or aerobic conditioning, depending on dosage

Position
- Standing facing away from the anchor point/pulleys with the resistance band or ropes above or below the shoulder, depending on diagonal plane
- Resistance band is tied or wrapped around the hand or forearm (or holding the pulley handle).
- Elastic resistance bands provide the most resistance at the fully stretched position. Check the pain-free range of motion and start the movement without stretch on the band, limiting the range to avoid increasing force. Small-range motion below impingement positions may be necessary until mechanics have improved.

Action
1. D2 flexion pattern: flexion, abduction, external rotation, supination, wrist, and finger extension (Fig. 10.36A, B)
2. Modified D1 extension pattern: extension, adduction, small-range, or no internal rotation until below impingement position (Fig. 10.36C, D)

Advantages
- Used in preparation for sports or functional activities requiring upward (D2 flexion) or downward (modified D1 extension) motion against resistance or to develop force (Phase II or progressing into Phase III)
- Racquet sports such as tennis, lacrosse, or golf and throwing sports such as baseball or softball all require diagonal movement patterns.

Teaching tips
- Instruction examples:
  - D2 flexion: "Leading with your thumb, lift your arm up and out to the side in a diagonal."
  - Modified D1 extension: "Leading with your pinky finger or palm, pull the handle down and across your body toward your opposite hip."
- Common errors to correct:
  - Using the hand and wrist to create the majority of the movement rather than using the shoulder and body
- Methods to address or prevent compensations:
  - Pulleys can be set to allow a larger range of motion with less resistance at the end of the movement.

Alternatives
- Hands-on resistance can be used to teach the pattern or to make multiple adjustments to the pattern, range, or resistance to avoid impingement or to limit compensations (Fig. 10.36E and F).
- Multiangle isometrics throughout the diagonal pattern
- Strengthening through small ranges
- Focus on timing and motor control can be integrated into movement, along with achievement of a specific target.
- Feedback can be provided using mirrors, videotaping.
- Sports-specific equipment can be added to the activity (balls, tennis racquets).

Progression
- Increase repetitions once movement coordination and timing are properly sequenced from proximal to distal without excessive compensations.
- Increase sets.
- Increase resistance within range.
- Increase available range or multiple small-range sets at different points in the range.
- Progress to sports-specific activities with external targets.

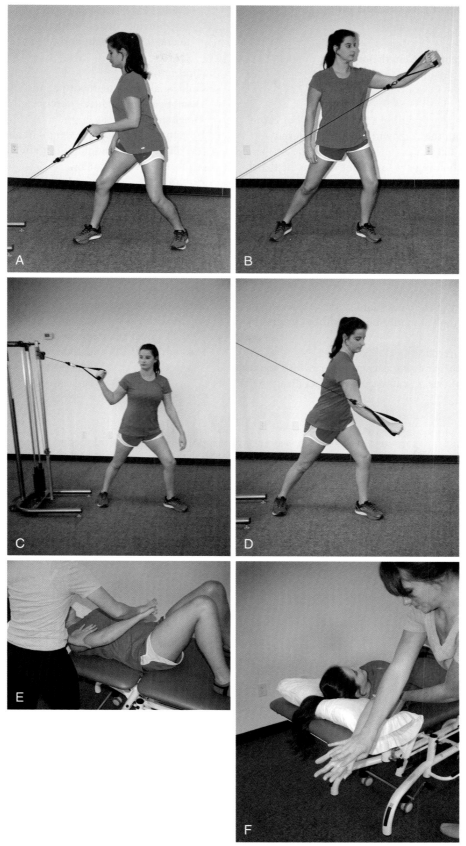

Fig. 10.36 PNF diagonals in standing D2 flexion (A and B), D1 extension (C and D) against pulley resistance, supine therapist-resistance D2 flexion (E), and D1 extension starting position (F).

10.37 Medicine Ball or Kettlebell Lifts

See Fig. 10.37.

Purpose

- Increase upper extremity strength for lifting during functional squat

Position

- Standing
- Feet are hip distance apart holding a medicine ball or kettlebell slightly away from the body with the elbows flexed

Action

- Squat toward floor holding the medicine ball or kettlebell with both hands (Fig. 10.37A, B).

Advantages

- Bilateral upper extremity activity challenges the core and proximal stabilizers symmetrically.
- Helpful preparatory activity for lifting large objects or to use arms to pull objects in close to the body.

Teaching tips

- Instruction examples:
  - "Hold the ball in your hands and squat, then lift the weight in higher than shoulder height without extending your spine."
- Common error to correct:
  - In addition to errors in lower extremity form with squats (see Exercise 9.30), watch scapula and core stabilization. If there is excessive spinal extension or if the patient is having difficulty maintaining the scapulothoracic mechanics, decrease the weight and reinforce the shoulder mechanics.

Alternatives

- Hold small weights in both hands.
- Dumbbells or weighted exercise ball
- Weighted pole
- Isometric squat, holding weight in outstretched arms at various ranges of the shoulder; flex and extend the elbows, moving through small ranges.

Progression

- Hold weights further from body with the elbows extended (increase leverage for shoulder and core muscle challenge).
- Increase weight.
- Increase repetitions.
- Add isometric holds at different ranges.
- Change squat position to lunge position in preparation for lifting.
- Add trunk and hip movement to mimic sport-specific or lifting requirements (Fig. 10.37C–H).
- Add diagonal lift patterns to challenge rotational stability through the trunk and upper extremity stability.

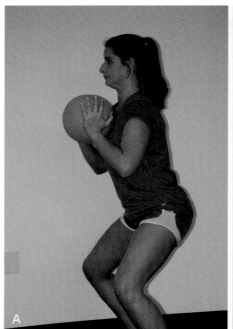 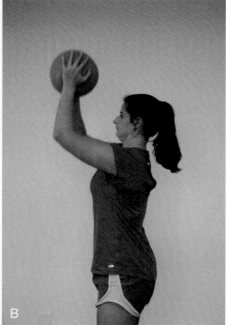

Fig. 10.37 Medicine ball lifts.

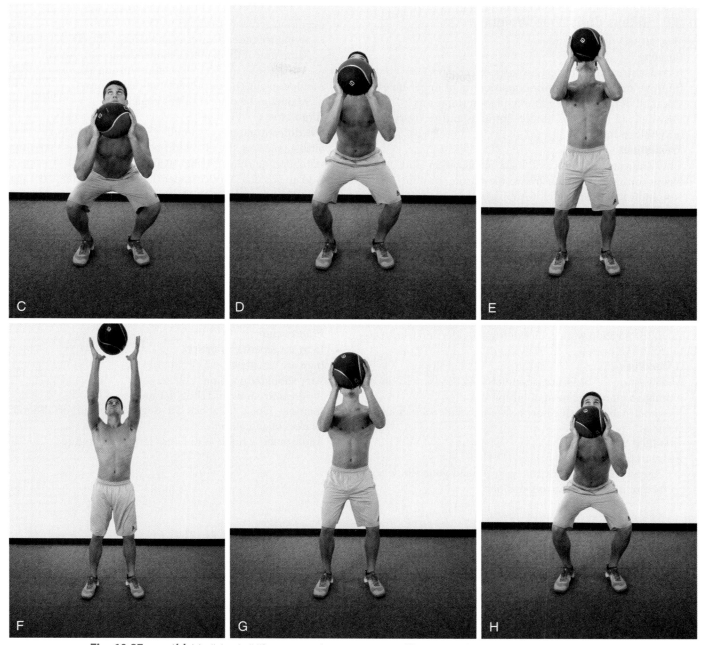

Fig. 10.37, cont'd Medicine ball lifts: progression to sports-specific squats with throwing and catching (C–H).

10.38 Biceps Curls: Free Weights

See Fig. 10.38.

Purpose

- Increase strength of biceps (isotonic or eccentric)
- Improve strength or aerobic conditioning of upper quarter, scapulothoracic, and glenohumeral joint stabilizers.
- Provide load for biceps tendon stimulus and recovery after bicipital tendinopathy

Precautions

- Only indicated if sufficient local stabilization and active biceps contraction is pain-free in the starting position
- Not indicated (especially with higher range flexion) for patients with SLAP lesions

Position

- Standing, shoulder flexed to 60–80 degrees
- Elbow extended, forearm supinated, maintaining natural valgus angle

Action

1. Flex elbow.
2. Eccentrically control the elbow movement returning to fully extended position while maintaining shoulder and trunk stability.

Advantages

- Mid-position of biceps at shoulder joint limits tension or impingement of long head of biceps.
- Proximal stability with elbow resistance challenges shoulder stability.

Teaching tips

- Instruction examples:
  - "Keep your upper arm still as you bend your elbow and then return to the starting position."

- Common errors to prevent:
  - Avoid shoulder flexion or shoulder girdle elevation at the same time if there is bicipital tendinopathy present.
  - Avoid shoulder internal rotation through the movement.
- Method to address or prevent compensations:
  - Maintain the natural valgus angle.

Alternatives

- Use different ranges of shoulder flexion (Fig. 10.38A).
- Sitting, support the elbow on a table to decrease proximal stability requirements (Fig. 10.38B, C).
- Add an unstable surface under the elbow to increase the scapulothoracic and glenohumeral muscle stabilization requirements (Fig. 10.38C, D).
- Use other forms of resistance: pulleys, resistance band.
- Start with forearm in pronation followed by supination to challenge proximal stability with distal multiplanar motion and introduce diagonal stresses to the biceps tendon.
- Place forearm in mid-pronation and supination to target brachialis and brachioradialis (elbow or wrist impairments)

Progression

- Increase repetitions or sets.
- Increase resistance.
- Vary shoulder position.
- Progress to elbow and shoulder motion.
- Increase range to above 90 degrees flexion or different degrees of abduction.
- Add isometric holds at different ranges to fatigue.

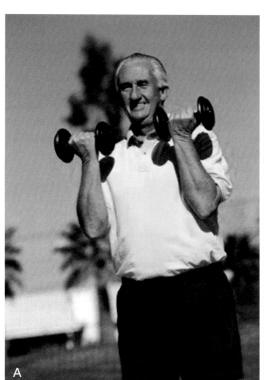

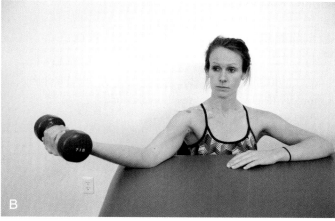

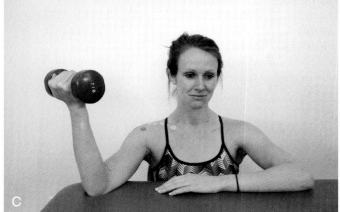

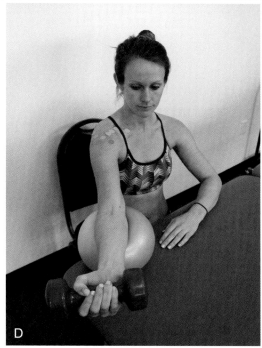

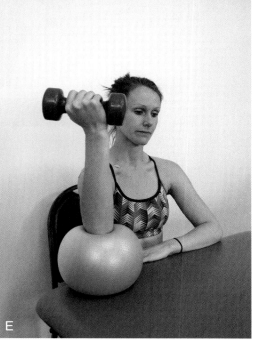

Fig. 10.38 Biceps curls with free weights in standing (A), sitting with arm support (B and C), and unstable surface (D and E). ([A] From Patton KT, Thibodeau GA, Douglas MM. *Essentials of Anatomy and Physiology.* St. Louis, MO: Mosby; 2012.)

10.39 Triceps Extension

Purpose
- Increase strength of triceps in midrange

Position
- Sitting
- Upper arm is supported on a table or machine platform at 90 degrees shoulder flexion, 90 degree elbow flexion.
- Machine is set to provide extension force.
- Resistance band or pulleys are set behind the patient.

Action
1. Extend elbow against resistance from a machine, resistance band, or pulley system.
2. The forearm is kept in supination or midposition.

Advantages
- Upper arm support allows greater resistance without excessive force on the glenohumeral joint.

Teaching tips
- Common error to correct:
  - Observe and correct anterior shoulder or shoulder girdle translation during the movement.

- Methods to address or prevent compensations:
  - Avoid using forearm pronation if the patient is losing shoulder girdle stability, rounding the shoulders, or tipping.
  - Ensure proximal thoracic and cervical support during the movement.
  - A wider starting position is preferable to avoid shoulder internal rotation to accommodate the valgus angle of the arms.

Alternatives
- Dumbbell resistance in supine, elbow extension with the shoulder in varying degrees of flexion
- Four-point kneeling with arm at side or standing with shoulder extended beyond neutral (Fig. 10.39); elbow extension is performed against gravity resistance.

Progression
- Increase resistance.
- Increase range of shoulder flexion.
- Remove support from the table.

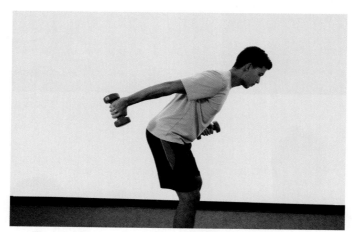

Fig. 10.39 Triceps extension using free weights in standing.

10.40   Shoulder External Rotation in Prone: Free Weights

See Fig. 10.40.

Purpose

- Increase shoulder external rotator strength in higher ranges of elevation, from mid to end range

Position

- Prone, arm supported at 90 degrees abduction on the plinth, elbow flexed, with the hand dangling toward the floor downward
- Head supported using a breathing hole in the plinth or forehead resting on a towel
- Cervical and thoracic spine position may require support over a pillow if there are fixed postural curvatures (kyphosis, forward head).

Action

1. Externally rotate against gravity using dumbbell for resistance.
2. Slowly control the movement on the return for eccentric control from the rotator cuff.

Advantages

- Prone position stabilizes the proximal upper quarter and limits compensations at the shoulder girdle.
- Prone places the upper extremity in a position requiring rotation against gravity.
- Upper arm support allows greater resistance without forces on the glenohumeral joint.

Teaching tips

- Instruction example:
  - "Keeping your shoulder stable and the arm on the table, lift the weight toward the ceiling."
- Common error to correct:
  - Lifting upper body (extending thoracic spine) to substitute for lifting with arm

Alternatives

- Use small range of motion or isometric hold at different points in the range if there is difficulty moving through full range.
- Side-lying external rotation with a small towel between the arm and the body (Exercise 10.33, Fig. 10.33C–E)
- Sitting; external rotation against pulley resistance with the arm supported in varying degrees of shoulder flexion or abduction (Exercise 10.23)
- Isometric holds

Progression

- Increase resistance.
- Increase range.
- Decrease arm support; four-point kneeling or hinge position (more challenging for overall trunk and shoulder girdle stability)
- Standing external rotation against pulleys or sports cord in lunge position

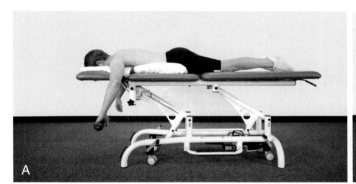
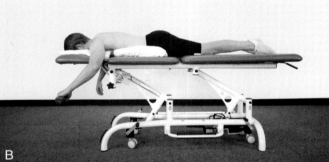
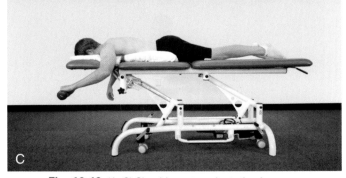

Fig. 10.40 (A–C) Shoulder external rotation in prone.

10.41   Shoulder Internal Rotation in Lunge Standing: Elastic Resistance or Pulleys

See Fig. 10.41.

Purpose

- Increase strength of shoulder rotators in higher ranges
- Challenge scapulothoracic and upper-quarter stability with less support
- Strengthening in a functional position for throwing preparation
- Challenge rotator cuff stabilization with rotation
- Neuromuscular coordination

Position

- Lunge stride standing facing away from pulleys or anchor point of a resistance band for internal rotation, facing toward the pulleys for external rotation
- Shoulder is abducted approximately 90 degrees with arm slightly in front of body or in scaption.
- Grasp the pulley handle or tie the resistance band around the palm of the hand.

Action

1. Proximal scapulothoracic and core muscle engagement before rotating the shoulder
2. Rotate the shoulder against a pulley or resistance band, maintaining the scapulothoracic connection and trunk position.

Advantages

- Mimics the position for throwing or overhead sports activities.

- Unsupported position requires greater scapulothoracic and glenohumeral stabilization.

Teaching tips

- Instruction examples:
  - "Keep your elbow lifted in space and rotate your shoulder against the resistance to finish with your palm down (for internal rotation) or rotating the shoulder so that the handle moves toward the ceiling (for external rotation)."
  - "Stabilize your core and set your shoulder blade before you rotate your arm."

Alternatives

- Sitting, upper arm supported at 90 degrees in slight scaption, with the elbow flexed and the hand on the table holding a dumbbell; externally rotate to 90 or 100 degrees (Exercise 10.23)
- Internal rotation against dumbbell resistance in supine from 90 degrees external rotation to neutral (less core stability required)

Progression

- Increase resistance.
- Isometric shoulder stabilization with forward stepping in lunge position to challenge ability to maintain shoulder position, followed by internal rotation.
- Increase range.
- Increase repetitions or sets.
- Progress to throwing drills or response time activities using the rebounder.

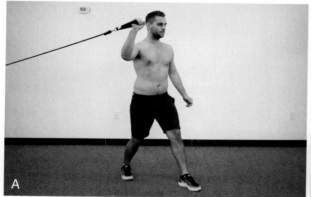
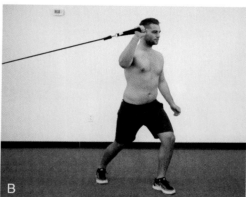
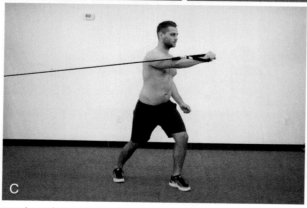

Fig. 10.41 Shoulder internal rotation against pulley resistance in lunge stride standing for throwing preparation.

10.42   Shoulder Flexion in Standing: Elastic Resistance or Pulleys

See Fig. 10.42.

Purpose
- Increase shoulder flexion strength in mid to higher ranges

Position
- Standing, facing away from the anchor point
- Arm is at the side with shoulder externally rotated, holding sports cord

Action
- Flex shoulder against sports cord, resistance band or pulley system.

Advantages
- Sports cord can be set to limit shoulder flexion range.
- Sports cord or elastic resistance can be used for a home program.

Teaching tips
- Instruction example:
  - "Brace with your core and set your shoulder blade, then lift your hand."

- Methods to address or prevent compensations:
  - Set spinal alignment and stability along with the scapulothoracic connection before flexion (anticipatory control).
  - Maintain external rotation leading with the thumbs up and establish alignment to accommodate elbow/forearm angulation due to the upper extremity valgus angle.
  - Sports cord or elastic resistance stretch is set to allow the available flexion range.

Alternatives
- Dumbbell resistance in sitting or standing
- Four-point kneeling shoulder flexion against gravity with dumbbell
- Standing in a lunge position, with the cord stabilized under the front foot to challenge core stability and scapulothoracic connection

Progression
- Increase range.
- Increase repetitions.

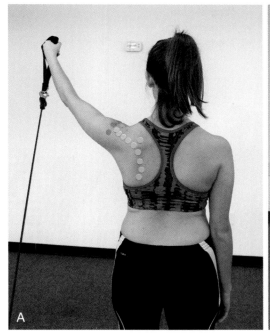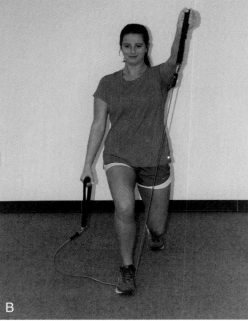

Fig. 10.42 Standing shoulder flexion against pulley resistance (A) and against sports cord in a lunge position (B).

10.43   Shoulder Abduction in Standing: Elastic Resistance or Free Weights

See Fig. 10.43.

Purpose
- Increase shoulder abduction strength in mid to higher ranges

Position
- Standing, with sports cord, tubing, or elastic resistance secured under feet
- Arm slightly in front of body.
- Scaption plane movement

Action
- Abduct arm against sports cord, resistance band, or pulley system (Fig. 10.43A, B).

Advantages
- Sports cord can be set to limit shoulder flexion range.
- Can be performed as part of home program

Teaching tips
- Instruction example:
  - "Stabilize your core and shoulder blade, then lift your arm out to the side, leading with your thumb."
- Common error to correct:
  - Initiating the movement or lifting excessively using shoulder girdle elevation, shifting weight, extending or laterally flexing the spine
- Methods to address or prevent compensations:

- Maintain external rotation and establish alignment to accommodate elbow/forearm angulation due to the upper extremity valgus angle.
- Set spinal alignment and stability along with scapulothoracic connection before flexion (anticipatory control).
- Observe and cue patient to avoid early shoulder elevation using a mirror if necessary.
- Cue the patient to reach away from the body from under the arm in a wide arc of movement rather than trying to lift the arm as high as possible.
- Check the amount of stretch and resistance on the band if the patient is compensating. Sports cord or elastic resistance stretch is set to allow the available abduction range.

Alternatives
- Dumbbell resistance in sitting or standing in upright position or forward hinge for horizontal shoulder abduction (Fig. 10.43C)
- Four-point kneeling shoulder abduction against gravity with dumbbell
- Standing in lunge position with sports cord stabilized under the front foot to challenge core stability and scapulothoracic connection (Exercise 10.43F, G)

Progression
- Increase range.
- Increase repetitions.

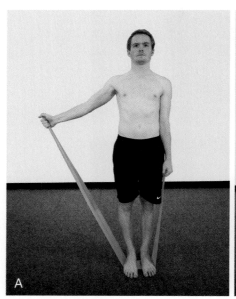 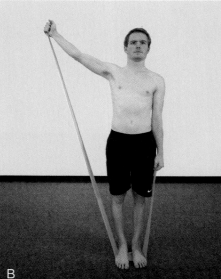 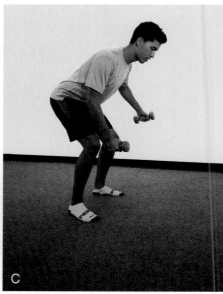

Fig. 10.43 Shoulder abduction in standing against elastic resistance (A and B) and horizontal abduction using free weights (C).

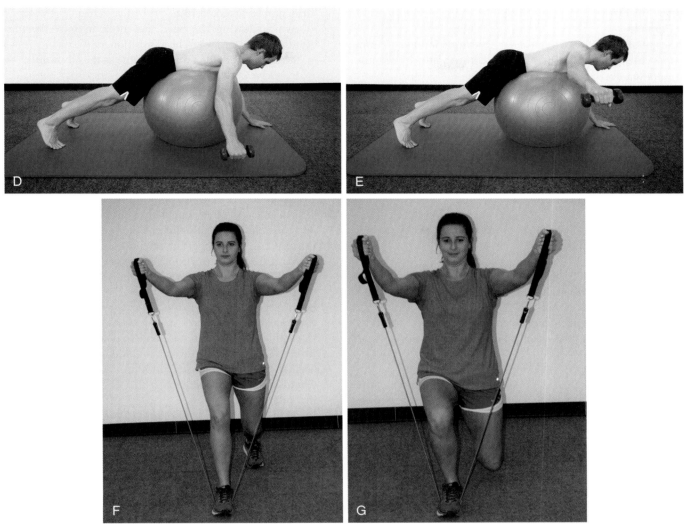

Fig. 10.43, cont'd Shoulder horizontal abduction using free weights in prone over an exercise ball (D and E) and bilateral shoulder abduction using sports cord with a lunge (F and G).

10.44 Rows

Purpose

- Scapulothoracic neuromuscular coordination to retrain movement patterns when patient compensates by scapula elevation, forward shoulders, or tipping
- Cervical endurance against gravity

Position

- Reclined seated position with both arms in front of the body using separate pulleys or resistance band
- Hands positioned lower than shoulders (below range where impingement could occur or where symptoms are reported)
- Cervical spine aligned with thoracic spine
- Scapular plane
- Shoulders externally rotated, forearms and wrists neutral (vertical grip, thumbs up)

Action

- Depress the scapulae, extend the shoulders while flexing the elbows to bring the handles toward the body (Fig. 10.44A, B).

Advantages

- Trains anterior cervical muscle endurance
- Reclined position is less likely to result in scapula tipping.

Teaching tips

- Instruction example:
  - "Keeping your head stable and lengthened as you pull the handles toward you, leaving some space between your elbows and your body."

- Common errors to correct:
  - Avoid allowing the head and neck to move forward, resulting in a forward head position.
  - Shrugging shoulder, rotating spine as the elbow lifts
  - Excessive cervical extension

Alternatives

- Seated rows with hands below shoulders (more likely to result in tipping or forward head position)
- Bent-over rows; one knee and hand on the same side supported on bench, flex and lift elbow out to the side, retracting the scapula to lift weight.
- Rowing machine (useful for Phase III, athletes requiring rowing action, or aerobic conditioning; Video 10.44)
- This exercise is often taught in a prone position, with W or T positioning. While the position and the movement of this exercise does target the retractors, the range of motion required for most functional movement is in front of the body. The W or T exercises should also be started in mid-range (below the level of the table) to avoid excessive stress on the cervical spine.

Progression

- Upright seated position once able to control spinal position with upper extremity movement (Video 10.44)
- Change direction or angle of motion.
- Control return of movement.
- Increase range.
- Increase resistance.

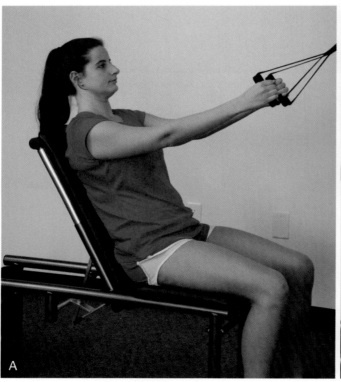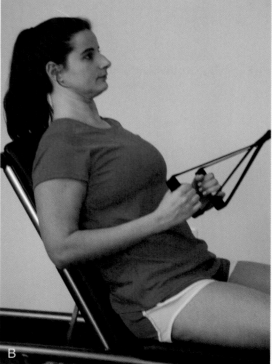

Fig. 10.44 (A and B) Rows in reclined seated position using a double-handled pulley.

10.45 Overhead Incline Press

See Fig. 10.45.

Purpose

- Increase strength to resume gym workouts or return to sports

Position

- Reclined at 45 degrees from upright, leaning back and supported by a bench
- Use a bar or dumbbells for resistance.
- Shoulders are in scaption, and hands are wider than the shoulders to accommodate the valgus angle.

Action

1. Stabilize the trunk and cervical spine (Fig. 10.45).
2. Press the bar or dumbbells toward the ceiling at an angle using scapulothoracic upward rotation and flexion into elevation.
3. Maintain shoulder scaption and external rotation throughout the motion.

Advantages

- Trains biomechanics to avoid repetitive strain related to overhead activities
- Return to weight-lifting activities

Teaching tips

- Instruction example:
  - "Press your hands up at an angle toward the ceiling."
  - The therapist can use his or her hands to provide a visual cue for the target plane or height of the movement.
- Common errors to correct:
  - Avoid lifting the weights or the bar directly over the head or behind the head.
  - Observe for loss of trunk and cervical spine stability as well as early shoulder elevation without scapula upward rotation.

Progression

- Increase repetitions.
- Increase range.
- Increase resistance.

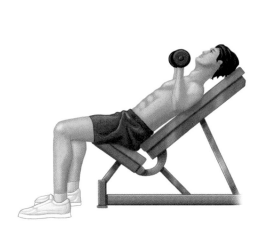 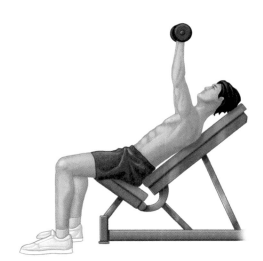

Fig. 10.45 Overhead incline press in reclined sitting position.

10.46   Planks

See Fig. 10.46.

Purpose

- Increase core, scapulothoracic, and shoulder strength and endurance in closed chain position

Position

- Start in four-point kneeling with hands slightly wider than shoulder width, shoulders slightly externally rotated, feet hip distance apart.
- Move the feet away from the body to allow the full length of the body to be used in the plank position.
- The back of the head should be higher than the line of the body.

Action

1. Set scapulothoracic connection, cervical and lumbar neutral position.
2. Lift and extend knees and hips, maintaining plank position until unable to maintain alignment (Fig. 10.45A, B).

Advantages

- Higher level core strengthening for stability
- A plank, performed with correct form and core stabilization, is a prerequisite for a full push-up.

Teaching tips

- Instruction examples:
  - "Your body should be in one long line."
  - "Lift your abdominal muscles up and keep your hips in line with your body."
- Common errors to correct:
  - Sagging or "hanging" without scapula connection or abdominal support
  - Allowing the head to drop below the bod; this results in the head weight pulling the scapula into a tipped position.
  - The arm length results in the body being at an angle to the ground, necessitating a visual focus in front of the body for cervical alignment.

Alternatives

- Forearm support instead of full elbow extension (Fig. 10.46A, B)
- Start on BOSU or smaller exercise ball and lift body off support (Fig. 10.46A).
- If the patient has wrist discomfort, a fist position can be used. Alternatively positioning the hands on dumbbells or a BOSU does not require full wrist extension (Fig. 10.46C, D).

Progression

- Increase time held.
- Add weight shift side to side or forward and backward.
- Add lifting one leg or one arm (Fig. 10.46G).
- Use an unstable surface and move one arm while the supporting arm endurance is challenged (Fig. 10.44C–M).
- Side planks partial with support under the hips or full without support (Exercise 11.32).

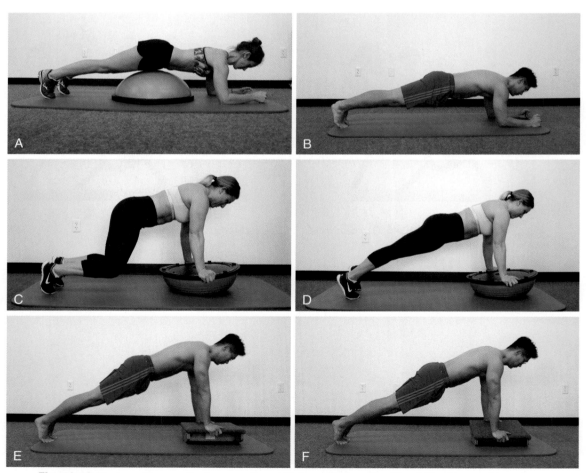

Fig. 10.46 Plank positions on the forearms (A and B), four-point kneeling (C and D), with unstable surfaces (C–F), and full plank (D–F).

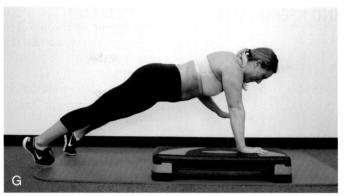

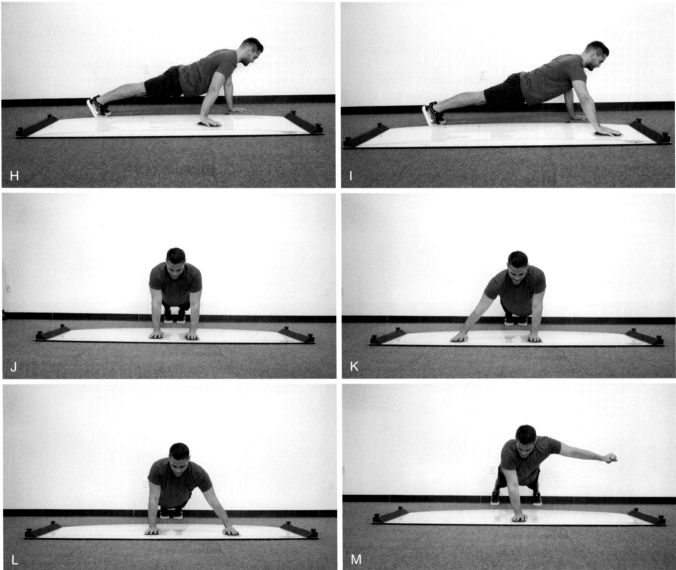

Fig. 10.46, cont'd Plank positions with one arm lift (G) and using a sliding board to challenge supporting arm stability with the shoulder at 90 degree of flexion and inner range abduction (H–M).

FUNCTIONAL TRAINING AND REEDUCATION

10.47 Throwing Drills

See Fig. 10.47.

Purpose

- Progressive neuromuscular coordination training for return to throwing (Fig. 10.47A)

Precautions

- In the presence of anterior instability, the arm range of motion for cock-up phase of throwing should be limited until the motion is pain-free with good eccentric control during single-plane exercises against gravity (see Exercise 10.26 precautions).

Position

- Stride standing
- Shoulder abducted to 90 degrees, elbow bent, holding a ball

Action

1. Throw a small ball toward the wall or a partner with one arm.
2. Begin with transferring weight from back to front foot while maintaining arm position without releasing the ball and progress to slow throwing action.
3. The emphasis of the drill can be directed toward catching in early phases (Fig. 10.47B), with progressive drills to simulate the phases and components of throwing requirements (Fig. 10.47C, D).

Advantages

- Training in parts can assist with recovery and correction of movement patterns before full return to throwing.

Teaching tips

- A patient can throw a lightweight ball into a closed treatment booth (empty) curtain if a rebounder or throwing partner is not available.

Position

- Using video or mirrors is helpful for providing visual feedback to the patient.
- Instruction example:
  - "Throw using your entire body, from your feet up, not just your arm."

Alternatives

- Using a weighted ball will train the throwing action concentrically but is more stressful to the anterior shoulder during the cock-up phase of throwing.
- Using a whiffle ball will train the eccentric control of the shoulder external rotators during the release phase of throwing.
- Throw against a rebounder for quick response time.
- Use single-plane strengthening exercises to prepare for this more advanced activity.

Progression

- Increase distance.
- Focus on accuracy.
- Blocked versus random sequences for target position, type of throw, direction
- Increase time throwing or number of repetitions.
- Increase speed.
- Increase range of shoulder motion.

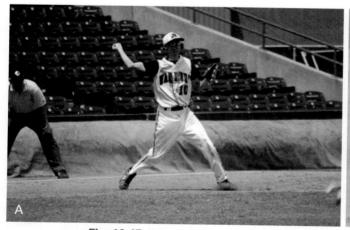
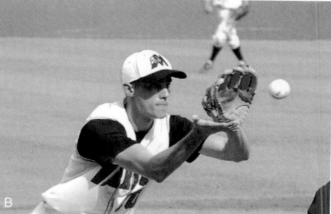

Fig. 10.47 Throwing (A) and catching (B) can be emphasized with drills using progressive parameters starting with smaller ranges, slower speeds, and shorter distances. (Photographs A and B courtesy of David Cox and Derek Drake.)

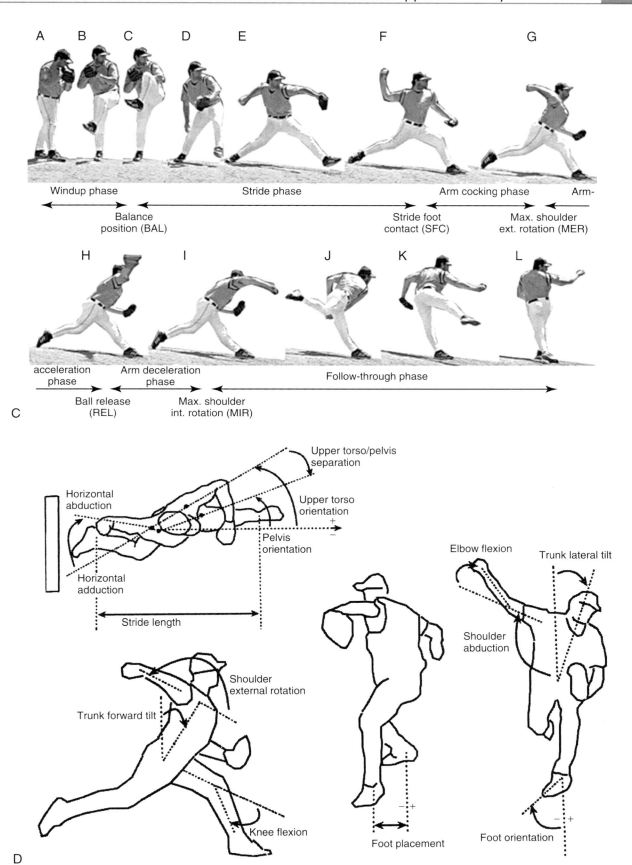

A B C D E F G

Windup phase

Stride phase

Arm cocking phase Arm-

Balance
position (BAL)

Stride foot
contact (SFC)

Max. shoulder
ext. rotation (MER)

H I J K L

acceleration
phase

Arm deceleration
phase

Follow-through phase

Ball release
(REL)

Max. shoulder
int. rotation (MIR)

C

Upper torso/pelvis
separation

Horizontal
abduction

Upper torso
orientation
+
−

Pelvis
orientation

Horizontal
adduction

Stride length

Elbow flexion

Trunk lateral tilt

Shoulder
abduction

Shoulder
external rotation

Trunk forward tilt

Knee flexion

Foot placement
− +

Foot orientation
− +

D

Fig. 10.47, cont'd Throwing drills require targeting the different phases of throwing (C) without the extremes of range, speed, or other parameters while restoring normal movement coordination required for full return to sports (D).

10.48   Overhead Sports Training

See Fig. 10.48.

Purpose

- Phase III functional training for return to sport
- Neuromuscular coordination or endurance capacity dependent on dosage or instructions
- Aerobic conditioning and to apply the principle of specific adaptation to imposed demands to prepare athlete for return to play

Precautions

- Indicated only if sufficient local stabilization and patient is able to move through desired range without impingement
- Requires sufficient scapulothoracic and glenohumeral stability
- Not indicated in early Phase II or if healing precautions are still present.
- Care with extreme ranges of motion if thoracic kyphosis, forward head position, or scapula tipping is contributing to shoulder repetitive strain
- Care with full overhead range in the presence of bicipital tendonitis or SLAP lesions

Position

- Standing or semi-squat position

Action

- Use smaller controlled versions of sports-specific overhead actions such as serving, blocking, overhead shots, swimming strokes, gymnastic skills requiring full shoulder strength and extreme flexibility, pole vaulting or other sports requirements (Fig. 10.48 A–I).
- Analyze the biomechanics and break down the movements required to prepare the patient for return to the activity.
- Build confidence through slow progression of components of movement before full reproduction of drills.
- The biomechanical analysis should include the entire body; contributing factors may include insufficient or inefficient motion related to neuromuscular coordination, mobility, or muscle function deficits in the trunk or lower extremities.
- Ask the patient what he or she needs to work on in order to return to chosen sport. The patient usually understands the movement patterns involved in the sport. The therapist can break down the movement and prescribe exercises that will safely retrain the movements needed for that sport.

Advantages

- Mimics functional activities before returning to play
- Reduce compensations for impairments before returning to faster paced drills or return to sport
- Allows the patient to develop confidence before returning to play
- Allows the patient to self-identify and correct movement deficits or patterns and encourages patient control
- Provides a mechanism to compare and contrast movement with other athletes or for progress

Alternatives

- Single-plane strengthening or aerobic capacity exercises.
- Swimming dry land drills could mimic activity and can be performed over a ball or modified training drills in the water.

Progression

- Increase repetitions.
- Increase range.
- Increase speed of movement.
- Random versus blocked practice
- Increase distance or height of transfer of object.
- Change directions.
- Include complex coordination and timing challenges.
- Add drills, including jumping, running, or cutting followed by overhead activity. (Running, jumping and agility drills involve the upper extremity.)

Parameters

- Consider the physiological needs of the replicated movements. Does this patient need to develop power (as in swinging a baseball bat) or endurance (as in swimming a 1200-meter event)? The parameters will be matched to these needs.
- Gymnastics skills require extreme range of motion, ability to stabilize the shoulder and the strength to support the body in beam, floor, vault and bar events.
- Difficulty, speed, and distance of sports-specific activities are determined by shoulder or upper extremity/proximal trunk fatigue and ability to control movement.

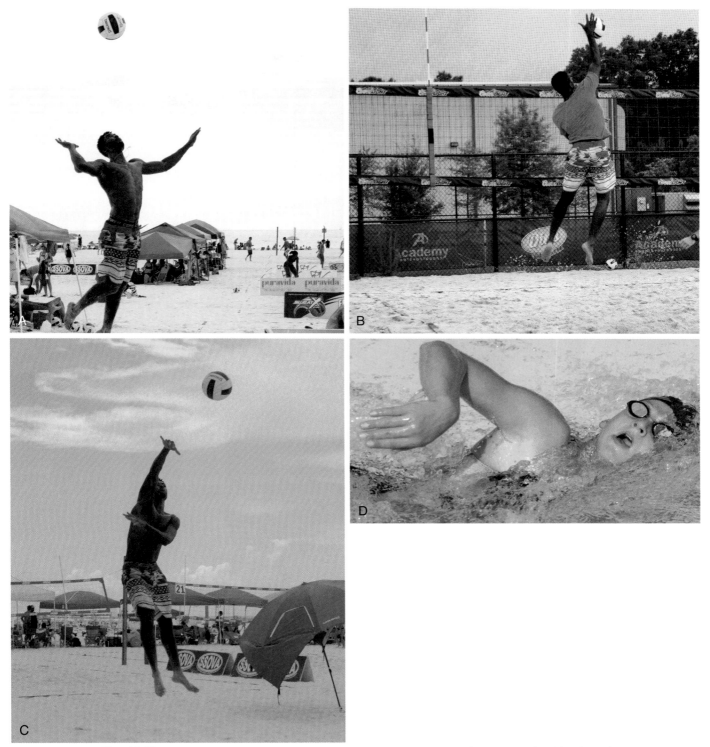

Fig. 10.48 Overhead sports training will differ based on the sport, competitive or recreational levels, and individual form. Evaluation of the requirements for the sports and the individual athlete's movement patterns will be necessary to determine return to sport programs. (A–C courtesy of Joshua Cooper and Zari Whittake; D–G courtesy of Anna Heinzman.)

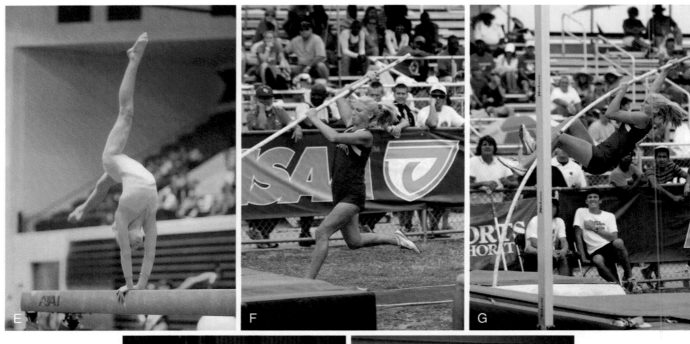

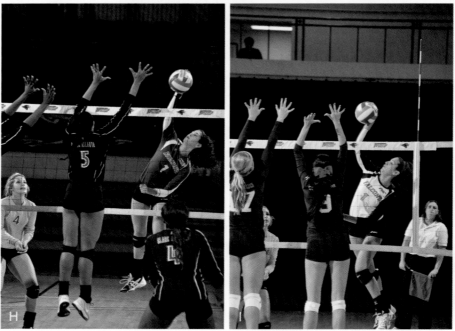

Fig. 10.48, cont'd Sports-specific requirements. (D–G Courtesy of Anna Heinzman; H and I Sarah Guidry ©, photograph courtesy of and University of Montevallo, Montevallo, Alabama.)

10.49 Grip Activities With Reaching

See Fig. 10.49.

Purpose
- Phase III functional training for activities of daily living or work-related requirements
- Improve neuromuscular coordination or improve endurance depending on dosage or instructions
- Useful for repetitive strain conditions affecting the wrist and elbow flexors or extensors (golfer's elbow, tennis elbow, finger or thumb tenosynovitis/tendonitis)

Position
- Standing
- Holding objects related to functional requirements (e.g., tennis racquet, golf clubs, keys, kitchen items, a laundry basket, or milk containers)

Action
- Reach to place objects or toward a target to match functional requirements (Fig. 10.49A, B).

Advantages
- Mimics problematic functional activities

Teaching tips
- Common error to correct:
  - Gripping with greater intensity than necessary can contribute to forearm repetitive strain disorders.
- Method to address or prevent compensations:
  - "Grip only as much as you need to hold (or manipulate) the object."

Alternatives
- Single-plane strengthening or aerobic activities
- Coordination, fine motor, and precision functional tasks (Videos 10.49A–D and 5.15–5.17)

Progression
- Increase repetitions.
- Increase range.
- Increase speed of movement.
- Random versus blocked practice
- Increase weight or size of object or distance/height of transfer.
- Set progressive goals for achievement of coordination and precision targets.

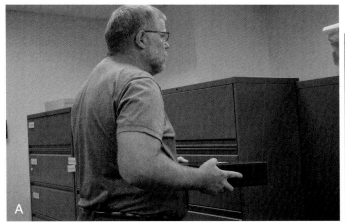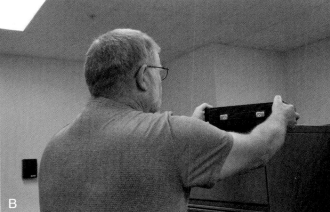

Fig. 10.49 Gripping activities with reaching: functional activity requirements are mimicked with activities.

◎ CASE STUDY 10.3: REPETITIVE STRAIN DISORDER: SHOULDER IMPINGEMENT

This case illustrates exercise choices to address contributing factors for repetitive strain microtrauma with specific focus on (1) the complex biomechanics of the scapulothoracic and glenohumeral joints and (2) biomechanical considerations to limit stress for impingement.

A 45-year-old male electrician is referred with complaints of a gradual onset of intermittent right shoulder pain with movement that has increased over the past 3 months. He is right-hand dominant and spends more than 50% of his day working overhead. He is slightly overweight, relatively inactive, and likes to do home repairs and carpentry. He has no other medical problems or history of shoulder trauma or dysfunction.

Functional Status and Goals

He is having difficulty with his work activities and is unable to perform overhead activities for more than a minute at a time due to pain. He is concerned that he will not be able to continue his occupation. He also wants to be able to do more around the house and return to his carpentry hobby. His QuickDASH score is 43.2, with the work module rated as 75.

Subjective Complaints

See Box 10.10.
- *Severity*: Pain in the shoulder is localized (2/10) but increases with work activities involving overhead tasks (4/10). There is occasional clicking and popping when he lifts his shoulder above 90 degrees. He has some stiffness in the upper back and neck but no neurological symptoms.
- *Irritability*: The pain decreases immediately when his arm is next to his side.
- *Nature*: Mechanical pain with overhead movement exacerbation
- *Stage*: Chronic, increasing pain and functional difficulty

Objective Findings

- *Posture*: Forward head, thoracic kyphosis, anterior tipping (tilting), and slight winging of the scapula
- *Cervical range of motion*: Pain-free; slight restrictions in rotation in both directions, flexion (especially combined with rotation), and sidebending
- *Thoracic range of motion*: Rotation, lateral flexion, flexion limited 25% compared to normative values. Only 5 degrees of active

thoracic extension (inclinometer). No pain, but he reports stiffness through the midback and upper thoracic region.
- *Shoulder range of motion*: See Table 10.9.
- *Muscle length*: Tight pectoralis major and minor, upper trapezius, levator scapula, posterior rotator cuff on right
- *Resisted isometrics*: Pain on resisted abduction and external rotation on the right (some weakness with pain)
- *Palpation*:
  - Normal scapular mobility
  - Tender around acromion and supraspinatus insertion, tenderness over biceps and supraspinatus tendons
- *Joint play right*:
  - Posterior glide decreased 25% with a springy end feel
  - Anterior glide within normal limits
  - Inferior glide decreased 25% with a springy end feel
  - Lateral traction decreased 50%
- *Special tests*:
  - Negative apprehension sign
  - Positive Neer's, Hawkins-Kennedy, and empty can impingement tests[27,56]

Movement observation: Late right scapula upward rotation with slight shoulder elevation, painful arc with late shoulder external rotation

Evaluation

- *Medical diagnosis*: Subacromial impingement
- *Physical therapy diagnosis*: Subacromial impingement, neuromuscular coordination deficits
- *Contributing impairments*:
  - Postural alignment: Forward head, thoracic kyphosis,[57] scapula tipping[58]
  - Decreased flexibility in right pectoralis major and minor, upper trapezius, levator scapula, posterior rotator cuff
  - Decreased joint mobility in posterior rotator cuff, posterior and inferior capsule
  - Scapular movement and scapulohumeral rhythm asymmetry/inefficiency: Early elevation, late upward rotation, prolonged internal rotation through range
  - Repetitive overhead work requiring internal and external rotation

---

BOX 10.10 Interpretation of Subjective Findings

- Severity is MILD with no irritability, allowing more aggressive examination to identify contributing factors.
- Nature of the subjective findings leads toward the most likely early hypothesis of subacromial impingement (biceps, supraspinatus, subacromial bursitis) or rotator cuff tears that need to be confirmed or denied during the objective testing.
- Other diagnoses to consider as part of the general hypotheses list are early adhesive capsulitis and contributions from the cervical spine dysfunction.
- No history of trauma and the slow onset of symptoms decreases the likelihood of labral tears.

TABLE 10.9 Shoulder Range of Motion for Case 10.3

| | RIGHT | | LEFT |
	Active	Passive	Active
Flexion	130 pain 90–130	150 pain 100–130	165
Extension	30	40	52
Abduction	100 pain 70–100	120 pain 70–120	155
Adduction	No pain with horizontal adduction	50	50
Internal rotation In neutral	30	30	65
External rotation in neutral	40 slight pain	45	80

Precautions

- Avoid impingement ranges (painful arc) with the shoulder internally rotated.

Prognosis

Prognosis is good for reduction in disability and to reduce pain in 6 weeks[59]

Treatment and Exercise Choices

- *Manual therapy*: Shoulder mobilization traction, inferior glides, posterior glides Grade III–IV below 70 degrees of flexion, posterior rotator cuff stretching, and soft tissue mobilization
- Thoracic spine thrust manipulation
- Exercise follows manual treatment (Table 10.10 and Box 10.11)

TABLE 10.10	Shoulder Impingement: Initial Exercise Choice Examples	
Exercise and Goals	**Parameters**	**Biomechanical Adjustments to Limit Stress**
Upper-quarter mobility Warm-up Increase thoracic mobility Pain reduction UBE (Exercise 10.1)	Moderate intensity but emphasis is achieving thoracic rotation range Range is set by adjusting seat height to place the shoulder below 80 degrees of flexion with no pain 8 minutes as a warm-up (no major fatigue or increase in pain)	Hand position is set to place the arm in external rotation (thumb up) to avoid compression of the subacromial structures. Emphasis is on maintaining supported spinal position without leaning against the seat and using thoracic rotation with the cervical spine stabilized. Progress to endurance focus to promote upper-quarter postural endurance.
Thoracic spine mobility exercises Increase thoracic spine mobility to assist proximal positioning and scapula posterior tilt Supine thoracic extension over BOSU with arms supporting head, Shoulder flexion below 70 degrees (Exercise 11.5) Thoracic rotation in sitting arms crossed (Exercise 11.7)	End range Short holds, progressing to longer stretch No increase in shoulder pain	Individuals with impingement have been found to have thoracic kyphosis, forward head position, and less thoracic mobility compared to matched individuals without impingement.[57] Increasing thoracic spine mobility is therefore a goal to improve the mechanics of the scapulohumeral position through range and increase available shoulder range before stress on subacromial structures.
Muscle flexibility exercises Increase muscle flexibility to allow optimal shoulder elevation without excessive upwardly directed pressure on acromion Pectoralis major stretch on BOSU below 70 degrees in ER (Exercise 10.8) Pectoralis major clavicular portion stretch (Exercise 10. 9) Upper trapezius stretch in sitting (Exercise 11.16) Sleeper stretch (Exercise 10.7)	End range Hold for 15–20 seconds Monitor for impingement pain	Avoid impingement position while stretching; pectoralis major stretch should be modified by decreasing the degree of elevation to below 70 degrees and gradually increasing diagonal stretch as the impingement symptoms improve over sessions. Avoid cervical motion, anterior tilting, and lower thoracic extension compensations while stretching. Latissimus dorsi stretching requires full elevation; delay stretching until full pain-free range is available.
Muscle activation and positioning Promote motor learning of scapula connection using serratus anterior to improve upward rotation from scapula, avoid early scapula elevation or anterior tipping Scapula connection in supine below impingement position (Exercises 10.14 and 10.15) Scapula upward rotation in standing against pulleys (Exercise 10.24)	Motor learning: optimal muscle activation; awareness of position with feedback Use resistance band or manual contact if patient is unable to elicit proper muscle activation	Scapula upward rotation is typically late in individuals with impingement and serratus anterior support is recommended to promote early upward rotation, and connection to the rib cage.[4,6,9,13]
Muscle activation of the posterior and inferior rotator cuff to facilitate the rotator force couple with limited superior translation Shoulder internal rotation and external rotation in sitting with arm supported against pulley resistance (Exercise 10.33) Shoulder external rotation in side-lying (Exercise 10.33)	Controlled range, avoid excessive upward, uncontrolled motion Multiple repetitions with low load	Pulley exercises with the arm supported are chosen to decrease the upper extremity moment arm during early exercise for open chain muscle endurance and tissue stimulus. No pain should be experienced during movement. Muscle activation and endurance dosage is chosen for early exercise. The side-lying external rotation exercise in slight abduction (with a towel roll) is chosen rather than the prone external rotation to avoid the impingement range. This exercise also requires activation of the posterior rotator cuff muscles (infraspinatus and teres minor) with less supraspinatus activation.[8,60]

BOX 10.11 **Biomechanical Choices and Adjustments to Avoid Impingement and to Address Optimal Loading**

- Teach the patient to externally rotate shoulder early during elevation, use external rotation with exercise throughout elevation, and work in the scaption plane.
- Avoid painful arc ranges.
- Exercise starting positions should place shoulder below impingement range (painful arc) or adjust the plane/rotation to avoid pain reproduction.
  - Adjust postural position through active spinal posture to minimize anterior tipping.
  - Address contributing impairments without compression of subacromial structures.
  - The emphasis on addressing proximal spinal postures and scapulothoracic movement synchrony has been discussed in the introduction and has been proposed to be an important part of management for individuals with impingement. The complexity of the scapulohumeral relationships and limitations of the available randomized controlled trials do not allow conclusive recommendations to emphasize scapular "stabilization" exercise or any one set of exercises as the only or a primary approach. However, there is evidence supporting the benefit of approaches emphasizing scapulothoracic muscle exercise as part of an integrated approach.[4,8,61–63]
- Although eccentric training has been advocated for tendon regeneration in the lower extremity, the use of eccentric exercise has only recently been investigated for the shoulder without conclusive support.[64–69] While research is ongoing, the complex mechanics of the shoulder may impact outcomes. Eccentric exercise is not recommended for early exercise management at this point in the exercise program. Progressive resistance training in positions where impingement is less likely and to target the multiple muscle groups to assist with scapulothoracic and rotator cuff function is preferred.[4,8,59,62,63,70]

SECTION 4: POSTSURGICAL MANAGEMENT

GENERAL TREATMENT APPROACHES

The major priorities after surgery or trauma are to protect the injured or surgically repaired structures from excessive force and tension, with slow progressive introduction of forces suitable to stimulate new tissue regeneration over the course of treatment. Treatment follows principles for phases of management, with different timelines based on the type of tissue, surgical incisions, and type of surgery. While the damaged tissue recovers, early exercise will focus on preventing loss of range of motion and minimizing atrophy during weight-bearing or movement restrictions. Postsurgical management will progress from protective management and resolving range of motion in the healing phase, to restoring motion, strength, and function as the healing constraints and postsurgical protocol allows. Principles outlined in the preceding sections may be appropriate to regain sufficient range of motion or flexibility (Section 10.1); promote muscle activation, endurance, and strength related to limited structural stability (Section 10.2); and address contributing factors such as biomechanical alignment and neuromuscular coordination or impairments related to prolonged immobilization (Section 10.3).

Typical postsurgical diagnoses in this category for the upper extremity include:

- Joint arthroplasty (shoulder, wrist, or finger joint replacement)
- Rotator cuff repair
- Shoulder labral repair
- Shoulder capsule adjustment or tightening (e.g., Bankart repair)
- Ligament repair or reconstruction (medial or lateral collateral ligaments elbow, thumb collateral ligaments)
- Fracture internal or external fixation
- Fusion (wrist)
- Tendon repairs (supraspinatus, finger flexor or extensor tendons)
- Trauma diagnoses
  - Ligament and capsule tears (elbow collateral ligaments, wrist ligaments, thumb ligaments)
  - Dislocation (shoulder, scapholunate)
  - Fractures (nonsurgical management of humerus, scapula, radius/ulnar, scaphoid, metacarpal, or phalangeal)

CONTRAINDICATIONS AND PRECAUTIONS

During the early healing time frames, weight-bearing or specific range of motion may be avoided completely or limited (see Chapter 2). Forces are introduced slowly after early healing is present.

Precautions are specific for the tissue properties, including the type of force, direction, length of tissue:

- Bone: Avoid rotation, angulation, or shear specific to type of fracture and internal fixation; avoid high impact forces.
- Tendon: Avoid high loads with extreme ranges (stress and strain), especially combined with angulation or rotation; avoid rapid contraction or movement away from a fixed distal segment in closed chain positions.
- Ligament/capsule: Avoid extreme strain (angulation, rotation).
- Specific precautions are applicable for joint replacements (e.g., shoulder replacements)

GOALS

- Promote force closure around surgical site to distribute forces and allow healing
- Address any possible causative factors (impairments and movement patterns) that were related to presurgical dysfunction
- Restore functional range of motion
- Restore muscle activation, endurance, strength, and power after muscle and neuromuscular adaptations related to weight-bearing or movement precautions
- Promote functional return and neuromuscular coordination while following healing precautions
- Address psychological components (fear avoidance beliefs and pain behavior)

TESTS AND MEASURES

See Magee[26] and Magee and Sueki[27] for more detailed description of available tests and measures, interpretation, and psychometric properties.

1. Pain reports (with movement, functional activity, or positions)
2. Movement observation (qualitative)
3. Ability to perform activities without compensations or home programs independently
4. DASH, patient-specific functional scale, region-specific outcome measures
5. Functional tests for dexterity and coordination (e.g., nine-hole peg test)

OBSERVATION FOR COMPENSATIONS AND RESPONSES

- Monitor the plane, specific ranges, and directions involving the injured or surgically repaired structure.
- Limit motion resulting in accumulation of force or high stress/strain on the injured structures while allowing motion in other planes.
- Keep the area of concern supported with active neuromuscular control as the first priority, but observe for overall alignment at proximal and distal areas influencing the forces on the joint.
- Monitor proximal areas and adjust position and muscle activation to address moment arms as well as excessive angulation or rotation.
- Observe for loss of position or muscle activation with fatigue and monitor symptom reproduction.
- Use supported positions when needed.
- Ask patients to report any discomfort during or after the exercise.
- Monitor for delayed-onset muscle soreness, increased effusion, or edema after treatment.

DOSAGE

Specific dosage for impairments as well as by phase.

- Phase I: Circulation and edema, restoration of functional mobility and muscle function prevention of deconditioning
- Phase II: Dosage for impairments with slower progression for surgically incised tissues

- Phase III: Continued progression of loads for injured tissue to provide optimal stimulus
- Progress toward functional activities while adhering to healing time frames and surgical protocols.
- Timelines to enter Phase III will differ based on healing status of surgically incised or healing tissue.

EXERCISES

PHASE I: RANGE OF MOTION MAINTENANCE WHEN ACTIVE MOVEMENT IS CONTRAINDICATED, PAIN RELIEF

EXERCISES INCLUDED IN OTHER SECTIONS

- Active-assisted mobility
- Generalized upper extremity aerobic capacity and mobility
- UBE
- Airdyne bike

GENERAL EXERCISE GOALS AS APPROPRIATE FOR PHASES OF HEALING

- Neuromuscular coordination: local stabilizer activation
- Progressive resistive exercise
- Neuromuscular coordination: preventing impingement and facilitating scapulothoracic connection
- Proximal core stability and endurance
- Functional training

PHASE I: MAINTAIN RANGE OF MOTION WHEN ACTIVE MOVEMENT IS CONTRAINDICATED, PAIN RELIEF

10.50   Pendular Exercises

See Fig. 10.50.

Purpose
- Increase shoulder circulation and decrease effusion
- Provide mild traction of the glenohumeral joint
- Provide gravity-assisted motion at ranges between 45 and 90 degrees (depending on angle of trunk)
- Maintain shoulder range of motion (below 90 degrees)
- Decrease pain
- Maintain passive range of motion during immediate post-operative phase, especially if active movement is contraindicated (see specific precautions)

Precautions
- Pendular exercises are intended to be relatively passive. If there is hypermobility or recently repaired structures where strain (tension) should be limited, pendular exercises may not be appropriate (contraindicated) during the early protection phases. For example, after a supraspinatus tendon repair, pendular exercises may place excessive tension on the healing structure if the shoulder is suspended and allowed to hang without muscle contraction from the rotator cuff, and adduction across the body places further strain on the structure.
- Pendular (and other exercises/movements) are contraindicated for some fractures of the upper extremity until early callus formation is present. Conversely, passive mobility may be indicated for stable fractures in the humeral head region to shape the joint surface during healing.
- As for all postsurgical patients, contraindications and precautions are determined by the surgeon. The tissue strength, extent of damage, and surgical methods will all influence the length of time needed for sufficient scar tissue formation and tissue repair, as well as the type of forces that are likely to place excess force on the tissue.
- Patients who have downward sloping shoulders, inferior subluxation, or instability should not perform this exercise unless the arm is supported using a sling.
- Cautious use of the exercise with acute tendinopathy (high severity, irritability)

Position
- Standing in a staggered stance, supporting the upper body on the unaffected arm placed in front of the body on a table or plinth below the level of the shoulder.

- The trunk is hinged forward at the hips without any rotation.
- The affected arm hangs passively using gravity to provide movement with as little upper extremity muscle activity as possible.

Action
1. Shift the body weight forward and backward, creating momentum for the arm to passively swing forward and backward, driving the movement from hip and knee flexion and extension and the weight shift, not the arm.
2. Shift the body weight side to side, creating momentum for the arm to passively swing side to side.
3. Move the body in a circular motion to create clockwise and counterclockwise circular motion of the arm.
4. Relaxation is necessary for the pain-relieving effects of traction from the weight of the dangling arm. The body should be perpendicular to the ground to allow the arm to be vertical and use gravity to provide some distraction.

Teaching tips
- Instruction example:
  - "Rock your body forward and backward until your arm starts to move. Let your arm relax and try not to fight the movement."
- Common error to correct:
  - Patients will often actively move their arm while it is dangling. Emphasize that the shoulder is moving *passively.*
- Methods to address or prevent compensations:
  - Ensure muscle relaxation before initiating movement.
  - Start with slow motion and small movement.
  - Demonstrate the movement, emphasizing that the movement comes from the weight transference.

Advantages
- Useful for early Phase I management to decrease pain or maintain passive range when active movement is contraindicated.
- Can be performed in a sling to maintain shoulder range.

Alternatives
- Self-assisted, buoyancy-assisted motion
- Therapist-assisted motion or oscillations

Progression
- Increase range.
- Increase repetitions.
- Progress to active-assisted or active movement against gravity.

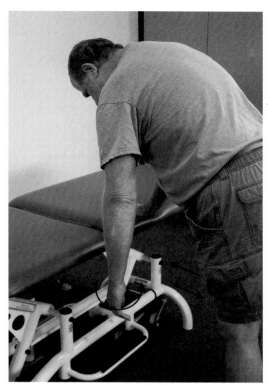

Fig. 10.50 Pendular exercise in standing.

10.51 Aquatic Therapy: Buoyancy-Assisted Movement

See Fig. 10.51.

Purpose

- Maintain or increase range of motion without active muscular contraction or excessive stress on the shoulder

Precautions

- Unstable fractures
- Active infection, open wounds, or incisions
- Allergies to chlorine or other antiseptic agents used in pool
- Fear of water
- Seizures

Position

- Standing in the water
- Greater depth increases support.
- Arm is placed on the flotation device (in front of the body to assist flexion, to the side to assist abduction).

Action

1. Squat or walk into deeper water to allow buoyancy to assist shoulder flexion or abduction.
2. Use the flotation device to support the limb for horizontal abduction or adduction.

Advantages

- If the pool is heated, there is an additional benefit of the heat for pain relief.
- Buoyancy assists with passive motion and supports the arm while allowing the patient to control the amount of range obtained.
- Use for maintaining range of motion when surgical precautions do not allow active movement (e.g., post rotator cuff repair).

Alternatives

- Therapist-assisted passive movement
- Pendular exercises
- Supine, using proper buoyancy devices to support the body

Progression

- Increase range as tolerated by adjusting the depth of the body in the water to increase shoulder elevation.
- Progress to active, then resisted movements against buoyancy with flotation devices when healing time frames allow.
- The faster the patient moves the limb through the water, the greater the resistance provided by the water.

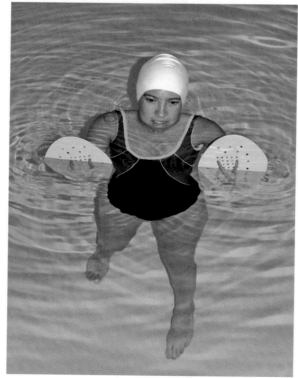

Fig. 10.51 Aquatic therapy: buoyancy-assisted flexion using paddles. The floats can also provide additional resistance for shoulder extension if the arm is moved toward the body. (From Cameron M. *Physical Agents in Rehabilitation.* 4th ed. St. Louis, MO: Elsevier; 2013.)

10.52 Passive Movement

See Fig. 10.52.

Purpose
- Maintain range of motion while respecting healing precautions

Precautions
- Range of motion may be restricted based on the postsurgical protocols.
- Passive movement after upper extremity fractures requires knowledge of the fracture location and directions of force to be limited. The therapist's hand placement should be adjusted to avoid long lever forces or forces directed toward the susceptible regions (angulation or rotational forces).

Position
- Supine, therapist holding patient's arm.

Action
- Therapist moves the arm in a plane of movement as allowed by surgical or posttrauma precautions (Fig. 10.52A, B).

Advantages
- Therapist is able to evaluate the extent of mobility limitations due to muscle flexibility or joint range of motion limitations.

Teaching tips
- Methods to address or prevent compensations:
  - It is often difficult for patients to adequately relax the arm to allow the therapist to effectively move the joint through the desired passive range of motion, especially following surgery. Support the arm fully between your hands and your body. Pause, asking the patient to "give their arm to you," and wait for the patient to relax before moving the arm.
  - Start with small, oscillatory movements and transition to small-range movements. Gradually increase the range of movement while maintaining firm, confident support to the arm.
  - A small amount of traction before moving the shoulder in different planes helps decrease pain.

Alternatives
- Oscillations within the range can be used to decrease pain and assist with increasing circulation and removal of effusion.

Progression
- Progress range.
- Progress to self-assisted movement.
- Progress to the next postsurgical phase, guided by specific tissue healing time frames and the surgeon's recommendations.

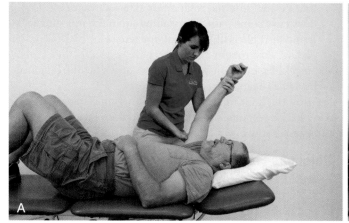
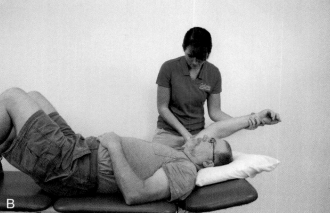

Fig. 10.52 Passive shoulder flexion provided by the therapist.

◎ CASE STUDY 10.4: ARTHROSCOPIC ROTATOR CUFF REPAIR

This case emphasizes the methods used to test for appropriate exercise dosage and to address muscle function impairments with progressive exercise after a surgical repair. Appropriate progression at 12 weeks postsurgery emphasizes the need to monitor and adjust exercises based on the patient's subjective and objective findings while taking into account healing status, rather than only considering a postsurgical protocol.

A 62-year-old man injured his right shoulder while trying to start a chain saw to cut down a tree in his yard. He was diagnosed with a moderate tear of the rotator cuff (infraspinatus [IS] and supraspinatus [SS]) after ultrasound imaging and MRI, and arthroscopic surgical repair was performed 4 weeks later. He is right-hand dominant and has a previous left shoulder injury limiting his full overhead use on the left.

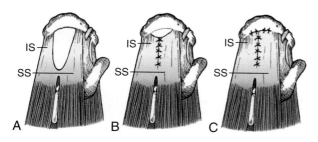

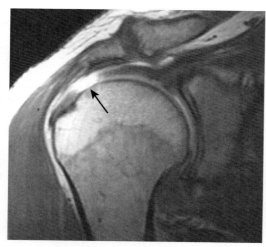

(A–C and radiograph from Rynders SD, Hart JA. *Orthopaedics for Physicians Assistants.* Philadelphia: Elsevier; 2013.)

Post-surgical Phase I Management (Week 0-6)

His shoulder was immobilized in a sling for 2 weeks after surgery. He was referred to physical therapy for passive and self-assisted range of motion, which was slowly progressed from weeks 2 to 6 (Exercise 10.52). Active range of motion below 90 degrees of flexion and less than 30 degrees of external rotation was also introduced during this time period.[71]

Phase II (Weeks 6-12)

During week 6 through week 12, active range of motion was slowly progressed with aquatic therapy (Exercise 10.51), self-assisted movement and mobility exercises seated with the arm supported, and supine and side-lying exercises without additional resistance and using short lever arms. Exercises have included (1) flexion against gravity in scaption with external rotation in supine (with and without a bar; Exercise 10.4), (2) aquatic squats to assist flexion and abduction with floats (Exercise 10.51), (3) side-lying external rotation (Exercise 10.33; alternative; no weight), (4) pulley-assisted flexion into elevation (Exercise 10.5), (5) upward rotation scapula connection progressing from therapist-guided to active movement with a light wooden pole (Exercise 10.14), and (6) internal rotation, external rotation at neutral with arm supported midrange against pulley resistance (Exercise 10.23).

He has tolerated the treatment progression well, with progressive improvements in function and decreased pain.

At week 12, he saw his surgeon who requested a slow introduction of loads, mobility, endurance, and strengthening exercise with precautions to limit load to no more than 1 kg (2.2 lb) for resisted abduction and external and internal rotation exercises and no lifting objects weighing more than 1 kg (2.2 lb).[71,72]

Functional Status and Goals

At week 12 postsurgery, he has difficulty donning and doffing t-shirts. He has stiffness in his upper back and neck with movement and sitting for long periods. He has no difficulty sleeping or using the arm for light functional activities. QuickDASH score is 65.

Subjective Complaints

- *Severity*: Shoulder feels stiff, only painful when stretching into flexion, internal rotation or external rotation (2/10). He does have some pain after waking up in the morning (3/10).
- *Irritability*: No lasting pain after exercise
- *Nature*: Post rotator cuff surgery
- *Stage*: Phase II, controlled motion and slow introduction of loads has been cleared.

See Box 10.12 for interpretation of functional status, subjective complaints, responses to treatment, and implications for objective examination.

Objective Findings

- *Posture and alignment*: Forward head, rounded shoulders, slight tipping of the scapula, arthroscopic scars over anterior and lateral right shoulder
- *Range of motion*: See Table 10.11.
- *Cervical*: Within normal limits for age, no pain

BOX 10.12   Functional Status and Responses to Treatment, Implications for Objective Examination

- The patient is progressing well after the surgery with minimal pain, good functional improvements, and no major postoperative complications.
- The surgeon has cleared the patient to start progressive resistive exercise, and range of motion (active and passive) findings will provide information related to his ability to activate muscle through available range. Maximum strength testing and special tests are still not indicated because the sutured muscle–tendon complexes are still in the protective phase of healing.[71]

- *Muscle function testing*: Comparing active range against gravity to the passive range will provide information about muscle activation, while repetitions until fatigue will reflect endurance. He has a 10-degree flexion lag and 14 degrees of abduction lag into elevation. The patient is able to maintain the position after the therapist places the arm at the terminal range, indicating neuromuscular coordination impairments[71] possibly related to limited use in the extreme ranges. He is only able to repeat shoulder flexion into elevation 9 times and into abduction 5 times before showing signs of fatigue.

  He has difficulty with scapula protraction and upward rotation in supine.
- *Movement observation*: He elevates his scapula early during elevation without late upward rotation. He also leans his body to the right during abduction and extends his spine or leans backward to assist with flexion.

Evaluation

- *Medical diagnosis*: Rotator cuff tear 12 weeks after surgical repair

TABLE 10.11	Shoulder Range of Motion		
	R AROM	**R PROM**	**L AROM**
	Right	**Right**	**Left**
Flexion	140	150	160
Extension	10	15	25
Abduction	132	146	155
Adduction	20	20	20
External rotation (neutral)	30	32	63
Internal rotation (neutral)	65	66	70
External rotation at 90 (scaption)	38	40	72
Internal rotation at 90 (scaption)	25	38	55

AROM, Active range of motion; *PROM,* passive range of motion.

- *Physical therapy diagnosis*: Shoulder mobility, muscle function deficits (activation, endurance), and neuromuscular coordination deficits after rotator cuff surgery
- *Contributing impairments*:
  - Active range of motion deficits compared to the uninvolved side (flexion 20 degrees, extension 15 degrees, abduction 23 degrees, external rotation 33 degrees in neutral, 34 degrees at 90 degrees, internal rotation 30 degrees at 90 degrees), although range is within ranges required for most functional activities.
  - Passive range of motion deficits are minimal (<10 degrees) compared to the uninvolved side for flexion, extension, abduction, and internal rotation at neutral. Passive deficits for external rotation in neutral and at 90 degrees (31/32 degrees) and internal rotation at 90 degrees (17 degrees) are larger.
  - Muscle activation deficits present for flexion and abduction into elevation (10 degree of flexion lag and 14 degrees of abduction lag)
  - Muscle endurance deficits for repeated flexion and abduction
  - Neuromuscular coordination deficits for shoulder elevation (compensatory movements)
  - Functional difficulty with dressing
  - See Box 10.13 for evaluation implications for exercise dosage and choices

Precautions

- Protect the sutured rotator cuff and avoid sudden increases in load, rapid stretching or movement, or positions where it is difficult to control the position of the shoulder. Internal and external range of motion goals are conservative and emphasis is on muscle activation, endurance, and neuromuscular coordination rather than aggressive mobility goals.

Prognosis

The rate of tendon healing decreases with age, with a 76% chance of tendon healing for his age range.[73] As a male, the chance of postoperative physical recovery is higher than

BOX 10.13 Evaluation Implications for Exercise Dosage and Choices

- The patient's age, moderate tear, and multiple tendon involvement indicate a moderate prognosis for tissue healing, and care should be taken to avoid high stress or strain (combined or separately).
- One of the major considerations is to protect the repair from excessive loading (and strain), especially as the most common time for failure is between 3 and 6 months after surgery, when the patient's pain levels are decreasing and function starts to improve.[71]
- Muscle function dosage is based on comfort (no pain with contraction), high repetitions, and very low load without reaching end range.[71,80] In a recent consensus statement from the American Society of Shoulder and Elbow Therapists, the suggested limit for muscle activity between 12 and 20 weeks is 30–49% of maximum electromyographic (EMG) levels.[71] As the patient has three factors for lower prognosis for tendon healing, lower resistance is preferred.
- In the same consensus paper, recommendations for this phase are to continue with exercise below 90 degrees (introduced earlier) with shoulder external rotation during elevation. They also recommend using a maximum of 2 lb (1 kg) for shoulder flexion or abduction against gravity with the elbow extended (long lever arm).

- Building muscle endurance with low loads and functional muscle performance will be the priority rather than parameters aiming to improve maximal muscle strength to limit overall stress on the connective tissue during healing.
- The active muscle activation in terminal ranges (flexion and abduction lag) will be addressed separately from full-range activation. Active assisted movement in supported positions will be used with low loads in the terminal ranges. Impingement mechanics need to be considered, especially as the potential for rotator cuff compression and degeneration results from uncontrolled upward motion of the humerus into the acromion. Without sufficient rotator cuff stabilization of the axis of glenohumeral motion, early scapula elevation without upward rotation increases the upward displacement.
- Goals will be set using functional improvements and pain scores, along with improvements in the muscle lag and ability to perform range actively rather than achieving range equivalent to the opposite side. Goals will be to report an improvement in the QuickDASH from 65 to 55 exceeding the MCID (8 points) and an average resting pain of 2/10 (MCID 1.1 points).[81,82]

for a female.[74] He does not have a history of diabetes, problems with bone density, preoperative shoulder stiffness, or a body mass index (BMI) of greater than 20 kg/m², which are factors that predict a poor prognosis.[74–78] However, the size of the tear (moderate) and the multiple tendon involvement are both negative prognostic factors.[73,75,78,79] Based on all of these factors, his prognosis is moderate, and some loss of function in higher degrees of elevation is possible. However, postoperative functional recovery for most activities of daily living and pain relief are still possible. Further damage is also possible if there is insufficient muscle strength and endurance, and long-term goals would need to address

slow but progressive strengthening while respecting tissue healing.[79,80]

Treatment and Exercise Choices

At 12 weeks, active self-assisted range is progressed to include planes other than scaption. As the major range of motion deficits are rotation in higher degrees of abduction, these movements are included in the home program using a T bar in supine without prolonged holds. Muscle function exercise choices are progressed from activation to endurance with progressive loads (Table 10.12).

TABLE 10.12   Case Study 10.4: Exercise Dosage for Muscle Function

	Dosage	Progression
Scapula upward rotation (pulleys) (Exercise 10.24)	Resistance is added to the exercise with the movement starting at 70 degrees of shoulder flexion in the scaption plane. An arc of movement starting with scapula upward rotation is performed after ensuring that he is able to initiate the movement. He is able to perform 18 repetitions against 1 lb before starting to compensate with excessive scapula hiking.	Increase repetitions Increase sets Punches with elbow extension Use as a home program with elastic resistance once able to perform without compensations.
Isometric and small range isotonic external and internal rotation at 45 degrees of scaption with arm supported on a table (pulleys; Exercise 10.23)	The dosage test resulted in fatigue after 15 repetitions at 45 degrees, 10 repetitions at 90 degrees with 1 lb resistance. The resistance is dropped to 0.5 lb at 90 degrees and he is able to complete 18 repetitions before fatigue.	No pain after the exercise Options for progression are to add additional sets and increase resistance for the 90-degree position
Active-assisted terminal range shoulder flexion into elevation sitting against gravity (scaption; Exercise 10.4)	Full range in scaption with external rotation assisted by the therapist followed by holding the position actively. The patient is able to hold the position for 10 seconds before fatigue. The patient is encouraged to use scapula upward rotation while maintaining upright posture.	Emphasis is on the activation and neuromuscular coordination with progressive time until fatigue, once active range is the same as passive the exercise is discontinued.
Shoulder flexion against pulleys (prone) (modification of Exercise 10.3: pulleys in the opposite direction to resist shoulder flexion)	Prone with the arm off the table resisting flexion (maintaining external rotation) from 70 to 120 degrees. He is able to complete 25 repetitions against 1 lb without pain or fatigue.	Increase resistance Increase sets Progress to kneeling then to incline lunge standing focusing on scapula upward rotation rather than early elevation (Exercise 10.42). Start without weight and only add weight once pain-free through full range.
Isotonic shoulder flexion (Exercise 10.42)	The patient is able to complete 22 repetitions from 0 to 90 degrees without pain and no weight, indicating this is an appropriate starting point to develop endurance.	Dumbbells are added once the patient can demonstrate efficient scapulohumeral rhythm
Isotonic shoulder abduction in scaption (Exercise 10.43)	The patient is able to complete 35 repetitions from 0 to 90 degrees without pain and no weight. Abduction in scaption is tested with 1 lb. The patient is only able to perform 12 repetitions before he starts complaining of mild discomfort and is unable to reach 90 degrees. The load is adjusted to 0.5 lb and he is able to reach 90 degrees without any difficulty and complete 20 repetitions.	
Elbow flexion (Exercise 10.38)	Free weights are used to challenge elbow flexion endurance conditioning while promoting rotator cuff endurance. The upper arm is supported on a table at 60 degrees of shoulder flexion to support the humerus and limit stress on the rotator cuff. The 1-kg weight limit does not apply to this exercise if the shoulder is supported, but pain, fatigue and shoulder compensations are monitored throughout. The patient is able to resist 4 lb for 18 repetitions before having difficulty maintaining the position.	Once the patient is able to maintain the shoulder position for the exercise and the patient is able to perform 15 repetitions, lighter weights can be attempted without the upper arm support.

TABLE 10.12 Case Study 10.4: Exercise Dosage for Muscle Function—cont'd		
	Dosage	**Progression**
Scapula retraction rows (reclined position) (Exercise 10.44)	The reclined position is used to assist upward motion to higher ranges above 120 degrees while controlling the movement eccentrically using the lower trapezius and concentric scapula retraction toward the body. The inclined position to limit tipping and rounded shoulders. The range is limited to avoid the elbows reaching the body.	Increase resistance and watch for control through range of motion.

◎ CASE STUDY 10.5: WRIST LIGAMENT SPRAIN

This case illustrates (1) the consideration of ligament healing following trauma, (2) slow progression of optimal forces for regeneration, and (3) force distribution.

A 24-year-old female college student fell on an outstretched arm while roller blading. Radiographs were negative for fractures, but she sprained a ligament in the midcarpal region with the possibility of subluxation of the lunate. Radiographs were negative for scapholunate dislocation. She has been wearing a wrist splint for the past 6 weeks and is now able to start active range of motion of the wrist.

Functional Status and Goals

She has difficulty with heavy household chores (mild) and carrying bags (moderate) and is unable to participate in yoga. She is able to use her computer but she is left-handed and has difficulty writing for long periods. She would like to return to all activities of daily living, including household chores, lifting, and personal care using both hands. She is a Physical Therapy student and needs to be able to use her hands for manual therapy, examination, and intervention techniques. She is scheduled for her first internship in 2 months and would like to be able to use her hand without thinking about it before this time. Her QuickDASH score is 25.[83]

Subjective Complaints

- *Severity*: Her pain level at rest is 0/10 with mild pain with wrist extension and moderate pain (6/10) with weight-bearing (pushing off a chair) or lifting.
- *Irritability*: Her pain subsides immediately after discontinuing movement. After sustained positions, such as writing for more than an hour, it takes 5 minutes for the pain to subside.
- *Nature*: Palmar wrist ligament damage with potential for instability
- *Stage*: Phase II
- See Box 10.14 for interpretation of subjective complaints.

Objective Findings

- *Posture/alignment*: She has a flat thoracic spine, slight forward head, and upper extremity valgus angle is 19 degrees
- *Range of motion*: See Table 10.13
- *Muscle length*: Wrist flexor and extensor length testing delayed
- *Palpation*: Mild pain at the ulnar aspect of the palmar wrist region. No specific pain with palpation of the scaphoid or triquetrum, some pain over the lunate region. No major pain on palpation of the ulnar collateral ligament.

BOX 10.14 Interpretation of Subjective Information

MILD severity that is exacerbated by movement (extreme extension, closed chain stress, and lifting) and prolonged writing (less severe pain). LOW irritability. The traumatic nature of the injury requires testing for instability and protection of healing structures during objective examination and intervention.

Precautions

No weight-bearing, cautious increase in force for range of motion and joint play testing. Limit range of motion testing if there is pain exacerbation above 4/10, and test without overpressure. Delay assessing functional activities placing excessive force or angulation on the wrist or requiring extreme range. Wrist ligament integrity, joint play of the wrist joints, and stability tests are indicated. Evaluation of the scaphoid, lunate, and pisiform structures is also indicated to ensure there is no damage that was not obvious in the initial post injury radiographic and physical examination.

- *Joint play*: No major increase in joint play but some pain on palpation of the central joints around the lunate and with anterior-posterior glide of the proximal radiocarpal and midcarpal joints.[27]
- *Special tests*: Some pain (2/10) with motion of the lunate on the lunotriquetral ballottement and shear tests (positive tests for instability or ligamentous damage.[27] Negative scaphoid shift test (Watson's test).[27] No major difference in gapping with passive radial or ulnar deviation or pain on palpation of the ulnar collateral ligament. Some tightness with Finkelstein's test.[27]
- *Movement observation*: She has winging in abduction and flexion on the left throughout shoulder range.

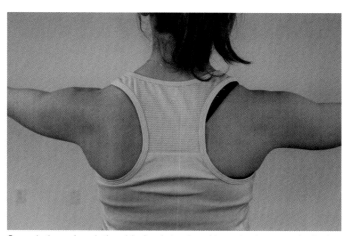

Scapulothoracic relationship in abduction. Note the increased winging on the left in abduction.

TABLE 10.13 **Range of Motion and Grip Strength on Initial Evaluation at 6 Weeks Post Injury**

	Right	Left	Resisted Isometric Midrange Testing Left	Requirements for Light ADLs[86]
Ulnar deviation	38	15	Slight pain	20 degrees
Radial deviation	27 degrees	15	No pain	20 degrees
Wrist flexion	54 degrees	48 degrees no pain	No pain	40 degrees
Wrist extension	70 degrees	36 degrees slight pain ulnar aspect palmar aspect	Slight pain	40 degrees
Pronation	Within normal limits	Within normal limits	Pain	50 degrees
Supination	Within normal limits	Within normal limits	No pain	60 degrees
Grip dynamometer: Middle setting, neutral pronation and supination, 90 degrees elbow flexion	28, 24, 20 kg	17, 14, 14 kg	No pain	

ADLs, Activities of daily living.

BOX 10.15 **Implications of Subjective and Objective Examination for Exercise Choices**

Severity and irritability of symptoms is relatively mild. The nature of the problem (palmar wrist ligament sprain with the possibility of lunate instability) indicates the need to protect the healing ligaments from excessive stress and strain. The stage (6 weeks post-injury, incomplete healing, starting point for restoration of mobility), requires slow progression within pain tolerance. Exercises to address wrist mobility will reach end range but avoid high forces or prolonged holds. Exercises to address grip strength and upper extremity function should be performed in pain-free mid-position of the available wrist range, with goals to achieve the functional position of the wrist (15–20 degrees of extension) to maximize grip, but without radial or ulnar deviation. Once she has sufficient wrist extension for the functional position, open chain exercise can be added to target shoulder endurance and strength for functional tasks while incorporating isometric wrist and hand grip. Exercises to promote proximal strength and endurance are also indicated to address her functional requirements and decreased use of the dominant arm over the past 6 weeks. Her left scapula wings in higher ranges of motion, so the exercise program to address proximal linkage should not place stress on the wrist and should involve open chain exercise.

Evaluation

- *Medical diagnosis*: Palmar ligament sprain, instability[84,85]
- *Physical therapy diagnosis*: The patient's primary impairments are limited wrist mobility secondary to pain (all directions compared with the right), pain with pronation, decreased grip strength, decreased scapulothoracic endurance, and difficulty with functional activities.

Precautions

Respect range of wrist extension limits with slow increase in stress as the range is restored. Limit stress on palmar ligaments and avoid combined angulation with wrist extension. No closed chain exercise until extension range is greater than 70 degrees, and limit stress in closed chain when the position is possible. No combined wrist extension and pronation.[86] Scaphunate subluxation or severe ligament laxity may result in chronic carpal instability and degenerative changes. It is imperative to respect the healing time frames and limit full stretch to avoid healing in lengthened positions or further damage.

Prognosis

The patient is highly motivated, young, has good body awareness, and understands why forces on her wrist should be limited. There is no evidence of subluxation or dislocation,[87–89] although consistent evaluation of progress is still important. A good prognosis is likely if she is able to limit forces during the healing process.

Treatment and Exercise Choices

See Table 10.14 and Boxes 10.15 and 10.16.

TABLE 10.14   Exercise Choices for Case 10.5: Palmar Wrist Ligament Sprain/Instability

Goal and Exercise Choice	Parameters and Dosage	Methods to Ensure Limited Stress and Strain on Wrist Ligaments	
Improve Wrist Mobility			
Active wrist extension Active wrist flexion Active wrist radial deviation Active wrist ulnar deviation	Supported position on plinth End of range, no hold active range Multiple repetitions, multiple sets, frequently during the day	Single plane movement No hold	The forearm is supported on the table to limit compensations and the patient is asked to watch the wrist and limit radial or ulnar deviation. 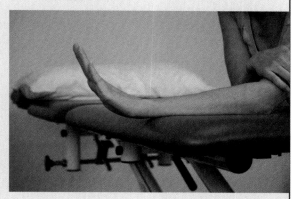 The active anti-gravity movement is repeated multiple times reaching end range without a hold (mobility dosage). Fatigue is not expected; this is a low-load exercise.
Improve Wrist Muscle Activation and Endurance in Midrange			
Isometric wrist extension, flexion (Exercise 10.34)	Isometric wrist extension at 20 degrees (functional grip position – wrist synergistic function for grip), wrist flexion against gravity neutral extension using 1.5 kg weighted ball, flexion using 1 kg ball for 30 seconds to fatigue	Support of the forearm on the plinth No radial or ulnar deviation Larger ball used for grip to limit angulation	
Improve Grip Strength			
Active grip exercises with large to moderate grip and isometric wrist activation (Exercise 10.35)	Grip dynamometer with forearm support Midposition pronation and supination, middle setting 9 kg: 60% average 1 RM (average of 3 max repetitions = 15 kg), 15 repetitions, 3 sets	No radial or ulnar deviation 15–20 degrees wrist extension	

Continued

TABLE 10.14   Exercise Choices for Case 10.5: Palmar Wrist Ligament Sprain/Instability—cont'd

Goal and Exercise Choice	Parameters and Dosage	Methods to Ensure Limited Stress and Strain on Wrist Ligaments	
Improve Proximal Shoulder and Scapulothoracic Muscle Function (Sequencing, Endurance), Along With Grip Strength and Wrist Muscle Endurance			
Open chain exercise: pulley resistance Isolated scapula upward rotation against pulleys (no elbow movement) (Exercise 10.24)	4 kg 16–18 repetition maximum before fatigue (scapula and shoulder fatigue)	Scaption plane Open chain Neutral wrist position, avoid angulation at the wrist	Scapular protraction and upward rotation 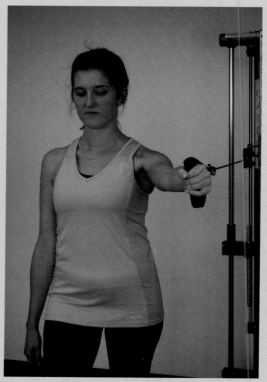 Upward rotation and scapulothoracic connection is taught without weight before movement against resistance. The arm is maintained in scaption with the wrist in neutral to slight extension.
Elbow extension with punches (Exercise 10.24)	2 kg 15 repetition maximum without wrist angulation	Scaption: wrist is maintained in slight extension.	The movement finishes with the hand wider than the body to accommodate the valgus angle and limit upper extremity rotation.
Shoulder external rotation and internal rotation (Exercise 10.33)	1 kg set based on ability to maintain the wrist position during the shoulder rotation	Isometric wrist extensor isometric endurance	No wrist motion during the rotation. Resistance is low and the exercise is stopped if there is any loss of the wrist position.

BOX 10.16   Rationale for Avoiding Closed Chain Exercise

The patient's wrist mobility is limited, and closed chain positions for the upper extremity require 60–90 degrees of wrist extension depending on the hand support and shoulder rotation. The palmar wrist ligaments are fully stretched in this position, and, during early ligament healing, the ligaments need to be protected from full strain to avoid healing in lengthened positions.

Progression for shoulder strengthening and scapulothoracic linkage to provide proximal support:

1. As the patient starts to improve her scapulothoracic connection and her scapulothoracic mechanics, shoulder movement is challenged in higher ranges. The forearms are resting lightly on the wall to provide input rather than support the body weight.

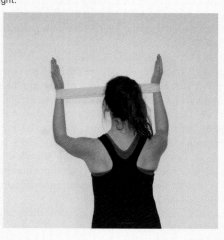

The elastic resistance provides feedback to activate the scapula stabilizers and rotator cuff while keeping the arms in scaption and maintaining shoulder external rotation. The band is placed above the wrist to limit stress on the wrist.

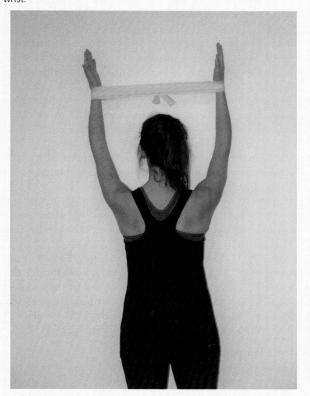

2. Proprioceptive input and upper extremity control with modified closed chain without higher compression.
   - As she starts to improve her wrist mobility and pain decreases, closed chain circular shoulder motion without body weight and modified wrist range are possible in standing (Exercise 10.17 [Fig. 10.17B]).
   - There is very limited compression through the wrist while promoting upper extremity endurance. One of the objectives of the exercise is to teach the patient to use the proximal upper extremity control to avoid excess force on the wrist.

3. Progressive shoulder and scapula control to distribute forces and provide proximal support are added using Exercise 10.24 (Fig. 10.24C) and increased challenge for proximal control (Exercise 10.23 [Fig 10.23 A, B]) while maintaining a stable neutral wrist. Grip activities are added slowly (Exercise 10.35).

REFERENCES

Introduction

1. Bullock MP, Foster NE, Wright CC. Shoulder impingement: the effect of sitting posture on shoulder pain and range of motion. *Man Ther.* 2005;10:28–37.
2. Lewis JS, Wright C, Green A. Subacromial impingement syndrome: the effect of changing posture on shoulder range of movement. *J Orthop Sports Phys Ther.* 2005;35(2):72–87.
3. Barrett E, O'Keeffe M, O'Sullivan K, Lewis J, McCreesh K. Is thoracic spine posture associated with shoulder pain, range of motion and function? A systematic review. *Man Ther.* 2016;26: 38–46.
4. Ludewig PM, Reynolds JF. The association of scapula kinematics and glenohumeral joint pathologies. *J Orthop Sports Phys Ther.* 2009;39(2):90–104.
5. Kebaetse M, McClure P, Pratt NA. Thoracic position effect on shoulder range of motion, strength, and three-dimensional scapular kinematics. *Arch Phys Med Rehab.* 1999;80(8):945–950.
6. Neumann DA. *Kinesiology for the Musculoskeletal System.* 3rd ed. 2017.
7. Mattison RR, Bouliane MJ, Magee DJ. Shoulder instability. In: Magee DJ, Quillen WS, Manske R, eds. *Pathology and Intervention in Musculoskeletal Rehabilitation.* 2nd ed. St. Louis, MO: Saunders Elsevier; 2016:188–235.
8. Escamilla RF, Yamashiro K, Paulos L, Andrews JR. Shoulder muscle activity and function in common shoulder rehabilitation exercise. *Sports Med.* 2009;39(8):663–685.
9. Michenor LA, McClure PW, Karduna AR. Anatomical and biomechanical mechanisms of subacromial impingement syndrome. *Clin Biomech.* 2003;18(5):369–379.
10. Lawrence RL, Braman JP, Laprade RF, Ludewig PM. Comparison of 3-dimensional shoulder complex kinematics in individuals with and without shoulder pain, part 1: sternoclavicular, acromioclavicular, and scapulothoracic joints. *J Orthop Sports Phys Ther.* 2014;44(9):636–645.
11. Lukasiewicz AC, McClure P, Michener L, Pratt N, Sennett B. Comparison of 3-dimensional scapular position and orientation between subjects with and without shoulder impingement. *J Orthop Sports Phys Ther.* 1999;29:574–586.
12. Ludewig PM, Cook TM. Alterations in shoulder kinematics and associated muscle activity in people with symptoms of shoulder impingement. *Phys Ther.* 2000;80(3):276–291.
13. Moezy A, Sepehrifar S, Solaymani Dodaran M. The effects of scapular stabilization based exercise therapy on pain, posture, flexibility and shoulder mobility in patients with shoulder impingement syndrome: a controlled randomized clinical trial. *Med J Islam Repub Iran.* 2014;28:87.
14. Giphart JE, van der Meijden OA, Millett PJ. The effects of arm elevation on the 3-dimensional acromiohumeral distance: a biplane fluoroscopy study with normative data. *J Shoulder Elbow Surg.* 2012;21:1593–1600.
15. Graichen H, Bonel H, Stammberger T, et al. Three-dimensional analysis of the width of the subacromial space in healthy subjects and patients with impingement syndrome. *AJR Am J Roentgenol.* 1999;172:1081–1086.
16. Hebert LJ, Moffet H, Dufour M, Moisan C. Acromiohumeral distance in a seated position in persons with impingement syndrome. *J Magn Reson Imaging.* 2003;72–79.
17. Alpert SW, Pink MM, Jobe FW, et al. Electromyographic analysis of deltoid and rotator cuff function under varying loads and speeds. *J Shoulder Elb Surg.* 2000;9(1):47–58.
18. Flatow EL, Soslowsky Lj, Ticker JB, et al. Excursion of the rotator cuff under the acromion. Patterns of subacromial contact. *Am J Sports Med.* 1994;22:779–788.
19. Michenor LA, Subasi Yesilyaprak SS, Seitz AL, Timmons MK, Walsworth MK. Supraspinatus tendon and subacromial space parameters measured in ultrasonographic imaging in subacromial impingement syndrome. *Knee Surg Sports Traumatol Arthrosc.* 2015;23:363–369.
20. Yanai T, Fuss FK, Fukunaga T. In vivo measurement of subacromial impingement: substantial compression develops in abduction and internal rotation. *Clin Biomech (Bristol, Avon).* 2006;21:692–700.
21. Timmons MK, Ericksen JJ, Yesilyaprak SS, Michener LA. Empty can exercise provokes more pain and has undesirable biomechanics compared with the full can exercise. *J Shoulder Elb Surg.* 2016;25:548–556.
22. Magee DJ, Mattison R, Reid DC. Shoulder instability and impingement syndrome. In: Magee DJ, Zachazeweski JE, Quillen WS, eds. *Pathology and Intervention in Musculoskeletal Rehabilitation.* St. Louis, MO: Saunders Elsevier; 2009:125–160.
23. Roberts CS, Davila JN, Hushke SG, et al. Magnetic resonance imaging analysis of the subacromial space in the impingement sign positions. *J Shoulder Elb Surg.* 2002;11(6):595–599.
24. Thigpen CA, Padua DA, Morgan N, et al. Scapula kinematics during supraspinatus rehabilitation exercise: a comparison of the full-can versus empty-can techniques. *Am J Sports Med.* 2006;34(4):644–652.
25. Stokdijk M, Eilers PH, Nagels J, Rozing PM. External rotation in the glenohumeral joint during elevation of the arm. *Clin Biomech (Bristol, Avon).* 2003;18:296–302.
26. Magee DJ. *Orthopaedic Assessment.* 6th ed. St. Louis, MO: Saunders Elsevier; 2014.
27. Magee DJ, Sueki D. *Orthopedic Physical Assessment Atlas and Video: Selected Special Tests and Movements.* 6th ed. St. Louis, MO: Elsevier Saunders; 2011.
28. Lew WD, Lewis JL, Craig EV. Stabilization by capsule, ligaments and labrum: stability at the extremes of motion. In: Matsen FA, Fu FH, Hawkins RJ, eds. *The Shoulder: A Balance of Mobility and Stability.* Rosemont: American Academy of Orthopedic Surgeons; 1993.
29. Terrier A, Reist A, Vogel A, Farron A. Effect of supraspinatus deficiency on humerus translation and glenohumeral contact force during abduction. *Clin Biomech (Bristol, Avon).* 2007;22: 645–651.
30. Uhl TL, Carver TJ, Mattacola CG, et al. Shoulder musculature activity during upper extremity weight bearing exercise. *J Orthop Sports Phys Ther.* 2003;33(3):109–117.
31. Chepeha JC. Shoulder trauma and hypomobility. In: Magee DJ, Quillen WS, Manske R, eds. *Pathology and Intervention in Musculoskeletal Rehabilitation.* 2nd ed. St. Louis, MO: Saunders Elsevier; 2016:157–187.
32. Dutton M. *Dutton's Orthopeadic Examination, Evaluation and Intervention.* 3rd ed. New York: McGraw Hill Medical; 2012.
33. Magee DJ, Zachazewski JE. Principles of stabilization training. In: Magee DJ, Zachazewski JE, Quillen WS, eds. *Scientific Foundations and Principles of Practice in Musculoskeletal Rehabilitation.* St. Louis, MO: Saunders Elsevier; 2007:388–413.

Section 1 Hypomobility

34. Roubal PJ, Dobritt D, Placzek JD. Glenohumeral gliding manipulation following interscalen brachial plexus block in patients with adhesive capsulitis. *J Orthop Sports Phys Ther.* 1996;24:66–77.

35. Boyles RE, Flynn TW, Whitman JM. Manipulation following regional interscalene anesthetic block for shoulder adhesive capsulitis: a case series. *Man Ther*. 2005;10:164–171.

36. Kelley MJ, Shaffer MA, Kuhn JE, et al. Shoulder pain and mobility deficits: adhesive capsulitis. *JOSPT*. 2013;43(5):A1–A31.

37. Binder AI, Bulgen DY, Hazleman BL, Roberts S. Frozen shoulder: a long term prospective study. *Ann Rheum Dis*. 1984;43:361–364.

38. Griggs S, Ahn A, Green A. Idiopathic adhesive capsulitis. A prospective functional outcome study of nonoperative treatment. *J Bone Joint Surg Am*. 2000;82-A:1398–1407.

39. Shaffer B, Tibone JE, Kerlan RK. Frozen shoulder. A long term follow up. *J Bone Joint Surg Am*. 1992;74:738–746.

40. Levine WN, Kashyap CP, Bak SF, Ahmad CS, Blane TA, Biliani LU. Nonoperative management of idiopathic adhesive capsulitis. *J Shoulder Elbow Surg*. 2007;40:145–150.

41. Roy JS, MacDermid JC, Woodhouse LJ. Measuring shoulder function: a systematic review of four questionnaires. *Arthritis Rheum*. 2009;61:623–632.

42. Lee AC, Quillen WS, Magee DJ, Zachazewski JE. Injury, inflammation and repair: tissue mechanics, the healing process and their impact on the musculoskeletal system. In: Magee DJ, Zachazewski JE, Quillen WS, eds. *Scientific Foundations and Principles of Practice in Musculoskeletal Rehabilitation*. St. Louis, MO: Saunders Elsevier; 2007:1–22.

Section 2 Hypermobility

43. Ekstrom RA, Donatelli RA, Soderberg GL. Surface electromyographic analysis of exercises for the trapezius and serratus anterior muscles. *J Orthop Sports Phys Ther*. 2003;33(5):247–258.

44. Reese NB, Bandy WD. *Joint Range of Motion and Muscle Length Testing*. 2nd ed. St. Louis, MO: Elsevier Saunders; 2010.

45. Van der Giessen LJ, Liekens D, Rutgers KJ, Hartman A, Mulder PG, Oranje AP. Validation of Beighton score and prevalence of connective tissue signs in 773 Dutch children. *J Rheumatol*. 2001;28(12):2726–2730.

46. Borsa PA, Sauers EL, Herling DE. Patterns of glenohumeral joint laxity and stiffness in healthy men and women. *Med Sci Sports Exerc*. 2000;32:1685–1690.

47. Silliman JF, Hawkins FJ. Classification and physical diagnosis of instability of the shoulder. *Clin Orthop*. 1993;291:7–19.

48. Hayes K, Callanan M, Walton J, Paxinos A, Murrell GA. Shoulder instability: management and rehabilitation. *J Orthop Sports Phys Ther*. 2002;32(10):497–502.

49. Kolber MJ, Cheatham SW, Salamh PA, Hanney WJ. Characteristics of shoulder impingement in the recreational weight-training population. *J Strength Cond Res*. 2013;27(5):1333–13339.

50. Kolber MJ, Corrao M, Hanney WJ. Characteristics of anterior shoulder instability and hyperlaxity in the weight-training population. *J Strength Cond Res*. 2014;28(4):1081–1089.

51. Burkhead W, Rockwood C. Treatment of instability of the shoulder with an exercise program. *J Bone Joint Surg Am*. 1992;70:890–896.

52. Watson L, Warby SA, Balster S, et al. The treatment of multidirectional instability with an exercise program part 1. *Shoulder Elbow*. 2016:1–8.

53. Watson L, Warby SA, Balster S, et al. The treatment of multidirectional instability with an exercise program part 2. *Shoulder Elbow*. 2016:1–8.

54. Ogston JB, Ludewig PM. Differences in 3-dimensional shoulder kinematics between persons with multidirectional instability and asymptomatic controls. *Am J Sports Med*. 2007;35(8):1361–1370.

55. Nascimento V, Torres R, Beltrao N, et al. Shoulder muscle activations levels during exercises with axial and rotational load on stable and unstable surfaces. *J Appl Biom*. 2017;33:118–123.

Section 3 Repetitive Strain

56. Cleland JA, Koppenhaver S. *Netter's Orthopaedic Clinical Examination: An Evidence-based Approach*. 2nd ed. St Louis, MO: Saunders Elsevier; 2011.

57. Land H, Gordon S, Watt K. Clinical assessment of subacromial shoulder impingement: which factors differ from the asymptomatic population? *Musc Sc Pract*. 2017;27:49–56.

58. Turgut E, Duzgun I, Baltaci G. Scapular asymmetry in participants with and without shoulder impingement syndrome; a three-dimensional motion analysis. *Clin Biomech*. 2016;38:1–8.

59. Heron SR, Woby SR, Thompson DP. Comparison of three types of exercise in the treatment of rotator cuff tendinopathy/shoulder impingement syndrome: a randomized controlled trial. *Physiotherapy*. 2017;103(2):167–173.

60. Townsend H, Jobe FW, Pink M, et al. Electromyographic analysis of the glenohumeral muscles during a baseball rehabilitation program. *Am J Sports Med*. 1991;19(3):264–272.

61. Lewis J, Mccreesh K, Roy J, Ginn K. Rotator cuff tendinopathy: navigating the diagnosis-management conundrum. *J Orthop Sports Phys Ther*. 2015;45(11):923–937.

62. Bury J, West M, Chamarro-Moriana G, Littlewood C. Effectiveness of scapula-focused approaches in patients with rotator cuff related shoulder pain: a systematic review and meta-analysis. *Man Ther*. 2016;25:35–42.

63. Struyf F, Nijs J, Mollekens S, et al. Scapular-focused treatment in patients with shoulder impingement syndrome: a randomized clinical trial. *Clin Rheumatol*. 2013;32:73–85.

64. Ortega-Castillo M, Medina-Porqueres I. Effectiveness of the eccentric exercise therapy in physically active adults with symptomatic shoulder impingement or lateral epicondylar tendinopathy: a systematic review. *J Science Med Sport*. 2016;19(6):438–453.

65. Wang JH, Iosifidis MI, Fu FH. Biomechanical basis for tendinopathy. *Clin Orthop Rel Res*. 2006;443:320–332.

66. Camargo PR, Alburquerquer-Serndin F, Slavini TF. Eccentric training as a new approach for rotator cuff tendinopathy: review and perspectives. *World J Orthop*. 2014;5(5):634–644.

67. Jonsson P, Wahlstrom P, Ohberg L, Alfredson H. Eccentric training in chronic painful impingement syndrome of the shoulder: results of a pilot study. *Knee Surg Sports Traumatol Arthrosc*. 2006;14:76–81.

68. Camargo PR, Avila MA, Alburquerquer-Serndin F, Asso NA, Hashimoto LH, Salvini TF. Eccentric training for shoulder abductors improves pain, function and isokinetic performance in subjects with shoulder impingement syndrome: a case series. *Rev Bras Fisioter*. 2012;16:74–83.

69. Maenhout AG, Mahieu NN, De Muynck M, De Wilde LF, Cools AM. Does adding heavy load eccentric training to rehabilitation of patients with unilateral subacromial impingement result in better outcome? A randomized clinical trial. *Knee Surg Sports Traumatol Arthrosc*. 2013;21:1158–1167.

70. Lombardi Jr I, Magri AG, Gleury Am, et al. Progressive resistance training in patients with shoulder impingement syndrome: a randomized controlled trial. *Arthritis Rheum*. 2008;59:615–622.

Case 10.4

71. Thigpen CA, Shaffer MA, Gaunt BW, Leggin BG, Williams GR, Wilcox RB. The American Society of Shoulder and Elbow Therapist's consensus statement on rehabilitation following arthroscopic rotator cuff repair. *J Sh Elb Surg*. 2016;25(4):521–553.

72. Maschi RA, Fives G. Rotator cuff repair: arthroscopic and open. In: Cioppa-Mosca J, Cahill JB, Cavanaugh JT, Corradi-Scalise D, Rudnick H, Wolff A. eds. *Handbook of Postsurgical Rehabilitation Guidelines for the Orthopaedic Clinician*. St. Louis, MO: Mosby Elsevier; 2008, 383–392.

73. Boileau P, Brassart N, Watkinson DJ, Carles M, Hatzidakis AM, Krishnan SG. Arthroscopic repair of full thickness tears of the supraspinatus: does the tendon really heal. *J Bone Joint Surg Am.* 2005;87:1229–1240.

74. Chung SW, Park JS, Kim SH, Shin SH, Oh JH. Quality of life after arthroscopic rotator cuff repair: evaluation using SF36 and an analysis of affecting clinical factors. *Am J Sports Med.* 2012;40:631–639.

75. Fermont AJ, Wolterbeek N, Wessel RN, et al. Prognostic factors for successful recovery after arthroscopic rotator cuff repair: a systematic literature review. *J Orthop Sports Phys Ther.* 2014;44(3):153–163.

76. Manaka T, Ito Y, Matsumoto I, Takaoka K, Nakamura H. Functional recovery period after arthroscopic cuff repair: is it predictable before surgery. *Clin Orthop Relat Res.* 2011;469:1660–1666.

77. Warrender WJ, Brown OL, Abboud JA. Outcomes of arthroscopic rotator cuff repairs in obese patients. *J Shoulder Elbow Surg.* 2011;20:961–967.

78. Gulotta LV, Nho SJ, Dodson CC, Adler RS, Altchek DW, MacGilliray JD. Prospective evaluation of arthroscopic rotator cuff repairs at 5 years: part II – prognostic factors for clinical and radiographic outcomes. *J Shoulder Elbow Surg.* 2011;20:941–946.

79. Cho NS, Rhee YG. The factors affecting the clinical outcome and integrity of arthroscopically repaired rotator cuff tears of the shoulder. *Clin Orthop Surg.* 2009;1:96–104.

80. MacCarron JA, Derwin KA, Bey MJ, et al. Failure with continuity in rotator cuff repair "healing". *Am J Sports Med.* 2013;41:134141.

81. DASH. http://dash.iwh.on.ca/. *Institute for Work & Health* 2006–2013. Toronto.

82. Mintken PE, Glynn P, Cleland JA. Psychometric properties of the shortened disabilities of the Arm, Shoulder, and Hand Questionnaire (QuickDASH) and numeric pain rating scale in patients with shoulder pain. *J Shoulder Elb Surg.* 2000;18:920–926.

Case 10.5

83. Wong JYP, Fung BK, Chu MM, Chan RK. The use of Disabilities of the Arm, Shoulder and Hand Questionnaire in rehabilitation after acute traumatic hand injuries. *J Hand Ther.* 2007;20(1):49–56.

84. Shin AY, Battalgia MJ, Bishop AT. Lunotriquetral instability: diagnosis and treatment. *J Am Acad Orthop Surg.* 2000;8:170–179.

85. Taleisnik J. Carpal instability. *J Bone Joint Surg Am.* 1988;70:1262–1268.

86. Green JB, Ranger HE, Draghetti JG, Groat LC, Schumer ED, Leslie BM. Hand, wrist and digit injuries. In: Magee DJ, Zachazewski JE, Quillen WS, eds. *Pathology and Intervention in Musculoskeletal Rehabilitation.* St. Louis, MO: Saunders Elsevier; 2009:213–305.

87. Perron AD, Brady WJ, Keats TE, Hersh RE. Orthopedic pitfalls in the ED: Lunate and perilunate injuries. *Am J Emerg Med.* 2001;19(2):157–297.

88. Watson HK, Ashmead D, Makhlouf MV. Examination of the scaphoid. *J Hand Surg Am.* 1988;13:657–660.

89. Melsom DS, Leslie IJ. Carpal dislocations. *Current Orthop.* 2007;21:288–297.

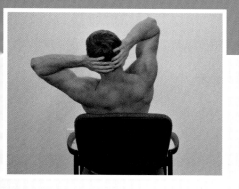

11

Spine Workbook

Kim Dunleavy and Amy Kubo Slowik

BIOMECHANICAL CONCEPTS

The numerous spinal joints and their complex movement combinations are impacted by loads applied through the extremity muscle linkages. Exercise choice and delivery should therefore consider the spine in its entirety and how the weight or movement of the patient's limbs will impact the spine. Limb movement can be used to challenge spinal stabilization and provide endurance exercise. Balance responses, gaze direction, and postural adjustments related to gravity are also used to challenge or facilitate spinal stabilization or neuromuscular coordination. Sufficient mobility, in addition to stability, is necessary for all functional movements and activities of daily living exercise implications are outlined in Table 11.1.

TABLE 11.1 Biomechanical Concepts for Spine Exercises	
Biomechanical Concepts	**Exercise Implications**
1. Spinal Structure and Function	
Large number of joints with functions for both support and mobility	Complex movement requires observation and consideration of the entire spinal complex during movement
Proximal support (Table Figs. 11.1 to 11.3)	Exercise choice and delivery must take into account: The cervical region has the most mobility of all spinal regions to meet functional requirements for vision and vestibular reflexes, but it also requires muscular support for prolonged activities with upper extremity tasks. The thoracic region is relatively stable in comparison to other spinal regions. There are numerous muscle attachments impacting the thoracic and cervical or thoracic and lumbar regions. The scapulothoracic connection is also considered part of the proximal support (see Chapter 10). The lumbar spine support includes abdominal muscle support for the anterior abdominal contents, pelvic floor for the inferior component, diaphragm for the superior aspect, and lateral and dorsal musculature.

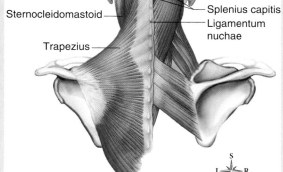

Table Fig. 11.1 (From Patton KT, Thibodeau GA, Douglas MM. *Essentials of Anatomy and Physiology.* St. Louis, MO: Mosby; 2012.)

Continued

TABLE 11.1   Biomechanical Concepts for Spine Exercises—cont'd

Biomechanical Concepts   **Exercise Implications**

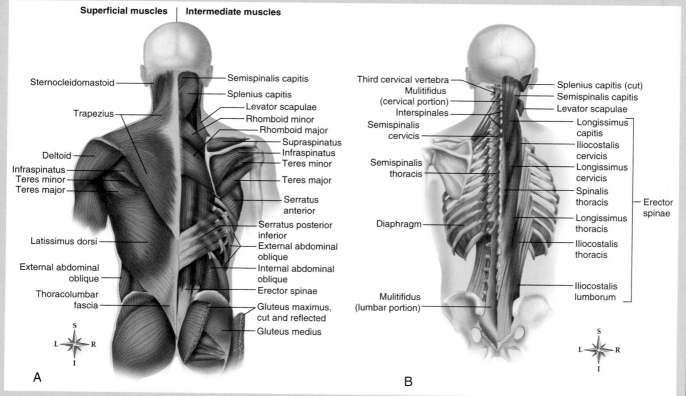

Table Fig. 11.2 (From Patton KT, Thibodeau GA, Douglas MM. *Essentials of Anatomy and Physiology.* St. Louis, MO: Mosby; 2012.)

Table Fig. 11.3 (From Patton KT, Thibodeau GA, Douglas MM. *Essentials of Anatomy and Physiology.* St. Louis, MO: Mosby; 2012.)

TABLE 11.1 Biomechanical Concepts for Spine Exercises—cont'd

Biomechanical Concepts	Exercise Implications
Specific regional functional requirements	Exercise choice and delivery must take into account: The cervical region has the most mobility requirements, and movement is impacted by the linkage with visual requirements for function. Vestibular and balance systems require fine-tuned and immediate cervical responses. The cervical region has multiple muscle attachments from the scapulothoracic region and is influenced by upper extremity motion and loads. The rib cage lends stability to the thoracic region, which has less mobility than cervical or lumbar regions. Respiration mechanics require movement of the costovertebral joints. Diaphragmatic, lateral costal, and upper accessory breathing patterns all impact the position and amount of motion available in the thoracic spine. The lumbopelvic region is influenced by forces transmitted through muscle attachments from the lower extremity and leg weight.
2. Spinal Alignment	
Cervical lordosis	Increased cervical lordosis can be supported with a towel under the curve or, if combined with a kyphosis, a pillow or foam pad propping up the head (Table Fig. 11.4)
Increased thoracic kyphosis (slight kyphosis is normal) of greater than 40 degrees is considered hyperkyphosis.[1,2]	Increased kyphosis that cannot be corrected with active extension requires props for the head (pillows, foam pads) and shoulders to limit scapula tipping or rounded shoulder positions.
Excessive curvatures contribute to soft tissue tension (kyphosis) or joint compression (lordosis)[1,2]	Establish active spinal muscle support prior to exercise to distribute forces. Observe for movement or position increasing stress at maximum curvatures. Use mobility and flexibility emphasis if there is excessive curvature Aim to promote spinal muscle activation and endurance to support curvatures on both sides and to distribute forces.
Scoliosis[1,2] (Table Figs. 11.5 to 11.8)	Promote midline alignment as much as possible, including rotation, while respecting fixed bony deformity if present. Choose non–weight-bearing or sitting positions if scoliosis results in apparent leg length discrepancies.

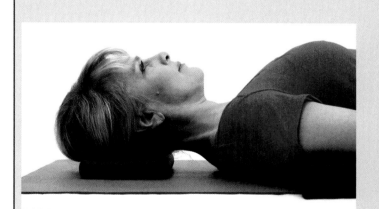

Table Fig. 11.4

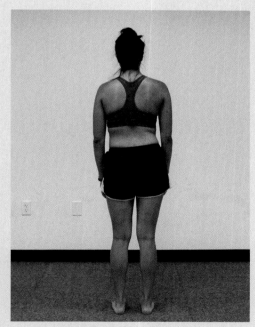

Table Fig. 11.5

Continued

TABLE 11.1   Biomechanical Concepts for Spine Exercises—cont'd

Biomechanical Concepts	Exercise Implications

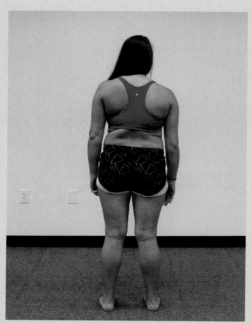

Table Fig. 11.6 Scoliosis with leg length discrepancy. Note the high pelvis and shoulder on the left.

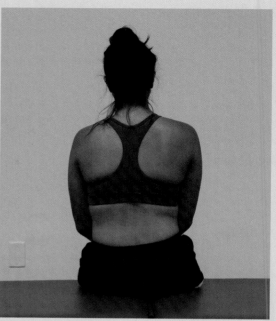

Table Fig. 11.7 Contributions from leg length discrepancies can be ruled out from evaluating alignment in sitting.

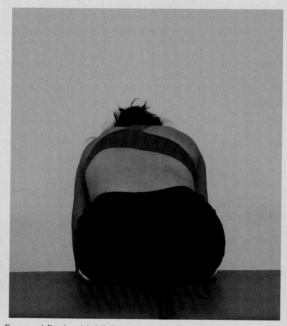

Table Fig. 11.8 Forward flexion highlights the curvatures and the left rib convexity (rib hump).

TABLE 11.1 Biomechanical Concepts for Spine Exercises—cont'd

Biomechanical Concepts	Exercise Implications
3. Axis of Motion and Distribution of Forces	
Changes in direction of curvature are often an axis of motion.	Monitor change points for excessive or localized motion. Aim to distribute forces over multiple joints and regions.
Three-dimensional spine motion occurs during gait and running to allow pelvic rotation for leg swing while still supporting the spinal alignment.[3–6] (Table Fig. 11.9)	Observe for early or excessive motion during gait or running in any specific axis in the spine, often at the lumbosacral junction or lumbothoracic junction[3,5,6]
	Limited hip mobility and pelvis rotation may result in increased mobility in the lumbar spine during gait or running, while lack of spine motion increases the energy expenditure (as much as 10% for walking).[3,7]
4. Spinal Stabilizer, Mover Muscle Function (see Table 2.4)[8,9]	
Local stabilizers provide postural support for individual joints in midrange, global stabilizers provide support for regional segments or joints throughout range (stability focus).	Timing and coordination of stabilizing muscles and primary movers impact exercise parameter choices.
	Instructions must be provided prior to movement to promote anticipatory control and attention during exercise if stability is needed. Spinal muscle stability is required to maintain trunk position for balance and to oppose forces resulting from limb motion. Unilateral limb motion with or without additional external load requires early muscle activation to oppose the distal limb motion on the opposite side. Reciprocal motion of limbs (especially with rapid movement) promotes alternating activity of the spinal stabilizers (Table Fig 11.10).
Global movers are used to create motion, power, speed, and precision (mobility focus).	Range is chosen to target stability (midrange) or mobility (through range to end range).
	Local and global stabilizers require multiple repetitions or longer time with selected load to enable endurance goal.
	Global movers require higher load, lower repetitions, with speed and precision for functional requirements. Global movers attaching to spinal segments can result in transmission of high loads (Table Fig. 11.11). If these muscles are used frequently, hypertrophy and connective tissue changes can result in decreased flexibility and create muscle imbalances.
	Choice of whether to focus on local stabilizers, global stabilizers, or global movers is based on the type of category, phase, and functional requirements.

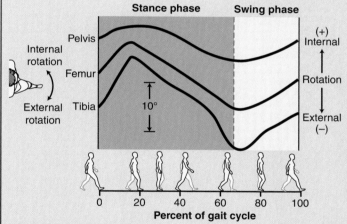

Table Fig. 11.9 (From Neumann DA. *Kinesiology of the Musculoskeletal System.* 3rd ed. St. Louis, MO: Elsevier; 2017.)

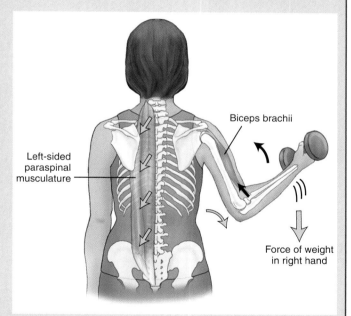

Table Fig. 11.10 (From Muscolino JE. *Kinesiology.* 2nd ed. St. Louis, MO: Mosby; 2011.)

Continued

TABLE 11.1   Biomechanical Concepts for Spine Exercises—cont'd

Biomechanical Concepts   **Exercise Implications**

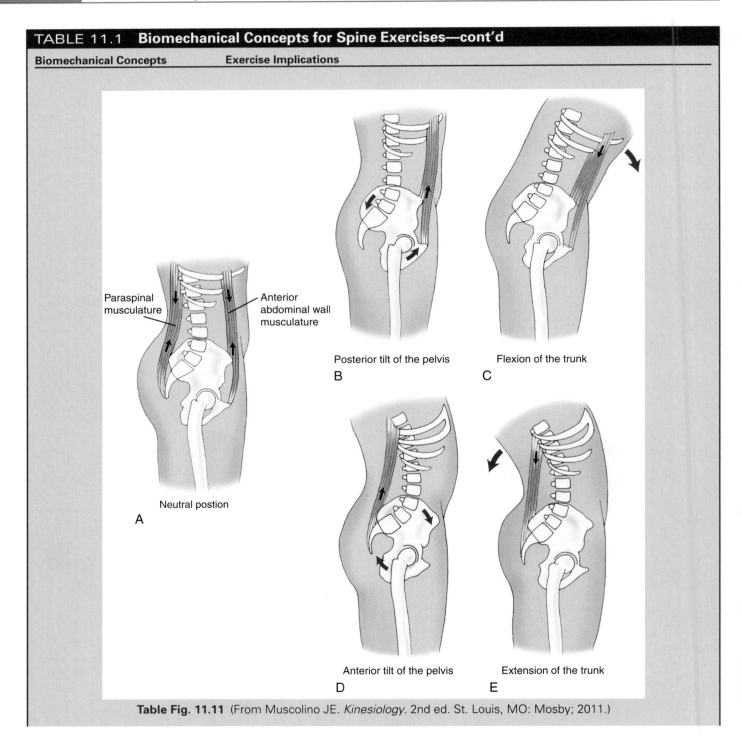

Table Fig. 11.11 (From Muscolino JE. *Kinesiology.* 2nd ed. St. Louis, MO: Mosby; 2011.)

TABLE 11.1   Biomechanical Concepts for Spine Exercises—cont'd

Biomechanical Concepts	Exercise Implications
5. Functional Requirements Functional endurance is required for prolonged positions (sitting, standing) and should be integrated into exercise parameters and home programs. Certain occupations will require greater strength or ability to support the spine with upper or lower extremity functional challenges (e.g., laborers, construction workers, firefighters, factory workers with lifting requirements, postal workers, baggage handlers). See Table Figs. 11.12 to 11.14.	Endurance focus for prolonged postural requirements If endurance for specific activities is needed, exercises should integrate these movements and positions. Strength requirements for specific functional movements Excessive motion, early motion, or lack of muscle support in the lumbar spine may contribute to increased lumbar spine forces during any closed chain activity such as step-up or -down movements, squats, lifting, or single-leg stance. Lack of trunk or pelvic motion can also increase forces higher up in the spine.

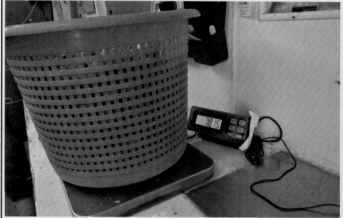

Table Fig. 11.12 High loads (especially repetitive) require greater physical strength in the extremities and trunk.

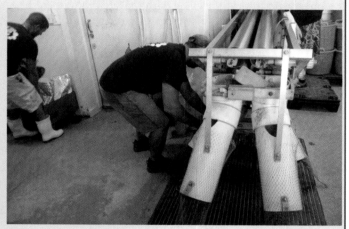

Table Fig. 11.13 Repeated bending with low loads can cause repetitive stress.

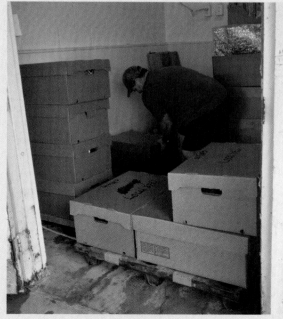

Table Fig. 11.14 Awkward positions, size of loads, and distances that objects need to be moved will impact the exercise prescription for return to work.

SECTION 11.1: HYPOMOBILITY

GENERAL EXERCISE APPROACHES

Mobility approaches are used to address specific regional mobility deficits, generalized hypomobility, or combinations of hypermobility and hypomobility. In the case of combined hypomobility and hypermobility, caution should be taken to avoid excessive force being distributed to the axis of motion in the hypermobile regions. Addressing hypomobility impairments may also be appropriate after surgical intervention (particularly after the initial protective phase) in areas other than the surgical region, with appropriate precautions related to healing or excessive force immediately surrounding the surgical site. Exercises addressing hypomobility are also appropriate for patients who present with directional preferences (decreased pain or centralization of pain toward the spine with repeated movement in a particular direction).[10-13] The types of exercise used for hypomobility are described in Chapter 6 (see Tables 6.3 and 6.4), and a comparison between parameters used for hypomobility and hypermobility is included in Table 6.4. A review of the goals, methods, parameters, and measurements for the spine is found in Table 11.2.

Manual therapy and aerobic exercise typically precede mobility exercises in the same session. In the cervical region, there is moderate support for thoracic manipulation and neck range of motion exercise accompanied by scapulothoracic and upper extremity exercise for acute neck pain with mobility deficits, and moderate support for neck and shoulder girdle endurance exercise in subacute pain classifications.[14] For patients with chronic neck pain with mobility deficits, there is moderate support for a multimodal approach using thoracic and cervical manipulation or mobilization along with exercise for the cervical and scapulothoracic regions (including parameters to address neuromuscular coordination, muscle flexibility, strengthening, and muscle or aerobic endurance).[14] As with all chronic conditions, affective or psychological factors should also be addressed.[14]

In the lumbar spine, there is strong evidence of support for manipulative therapy for patients with acute low back pain (with or without pain in the buttocks or thighs) with mobility deficits. There is evidence for using specific directional exercise for patients with acute, subacute, or chronic pain who respond positively to repeated movements with centralization of symptoms.[15] There is weak evidence of efficacy of lower extremity nerve mobility exercise to decrease pain with subacute or chronic low back pain patients who are experiencing radiating pain.[15]

TABLE 11.2	Goals, Methods, Parameters, and Measurement: Hypomobility		
Goals	**Methods**	**Parameters**	**Measurement**
Decrease muscle spasm and related pain symptoms	Circulatory-type active exercises (small-range, multiple repetitions without load) in midrange to end range (does not have to reach end range) without excessive pain Isometric contractions with adequate relaxation to create "pumping" effect Oscillations	Multiple repetitions (>30) Low loads Supported or unloaded positions Adequate rest periods between sets Repeat frequently throughout the day Existing pain should centralize or decrease with continued repetitions.	Pain reports (at rest, with activity, and related to movement toward end range) Pain responses relative to degree of range of motion or centralization of pain toward the spine with repeated movement Measurement of range of motion (goniometer/inclinometer/tape measure) Self-reported measures (Oswestry, Neck Disability Index [NDI], Patient Specific Functional Scale, Roland-Morris) Observation of movement coordination and compensations
Increase body temperature prior to mobility exercise to maximize mobility improvements or decrease pain. Improve generalized aerobic endurance	General aerobic exercise	Existing pain should centralize or decrease with continued repetitions.	Perceived exertion Pain intensity during and after exercise Pulse and respiratory rate changes as well as return to normal if progressing to aerobic endurance
Increase connective tissue mobility	Non–weight-bearing, open chain exercise to end range Oscillatory motion reaching end range Active, active-assisted motion or resisted movement through available end range without compensation Passive positioning Prolonged stretch (to address connective tissue and muscle length)	High repetitions (>25) Low load Controlled speed Reach end range Oscillations are used if severity or irritability is high. Prolonged hold once patient is tolerating active end range motion Stretching sensation should be tolerable, and existing pain should centralize or decrease with continued repetitions	Range of motion (goniometer/inclinometer/tape measure) End feel and relative amount of motion prior to end feel (passive motion, joint play) Selective tissue tension evaluation; relationship between amount of active and passive range of motion Pain responses relative to degree of range of motion or centralization of pain toward the spine with repeated movement

TABLE 11.2 Goals, Methods, Parameters, and Measurement: Hypomobility—cont'd

Goals	Methods	Parameters	Measurement
Improve muscle flexibility (including two joint muscles)	Passive positioning Prolonged stretching (performed by therapist or self-stretch by patient) at end range of joint motion reaching full length of muscle–tendon complex at one or both ends in direction of fibers Contract-relax Hold-relax	Sustained hold (15–30 seconds) *OR* short hold with short break and repeated for longer time periods (3–5 minutes) *OR* multiple repetitions to end range Low loads Contract-relax or hold-relax uses maximal resistance for target muscle groups followed by immediate relaxation and motion into the maximal length of target muscle. Range should increase with time held or repetitions. Stretching sensation should be tolerable, and existing pain should centralize or decrease with continued repetitions.	Pain reports (at rest, with activity, and related to movement toward end range) and responses relative to degree of range of motion Range of motion (goniometer/inclinometer/tape measure) End feel with passive movement relative to amount of range of motion Muscle flexibility special tests
Increase neural mobility with specific neural mobility techniques	Neural gliding and/or stretching techniques	Motion targeted to increase mobility of specific neural tissue with range and hold dependent on severity and irritability Multiple repetitions with motion to end range or within range short of symptom reproduction *OR* starting to reproduce symptoms Prolonged hold only if low severity and irritability Stretching sensation should be tolerable, and existing pain or other sensations (tingling, numbness) should centralize or decrease with continued repetitions.	Neural tension tests Range of motion (goniometer/inclinometer/tape measure) Pain reports (at rest, with activity, and related to movement toward end range) and responses relative to degree of range of motion Symptom reproduction with combined functional positions
Increase muscle activation and endurance in newly available range gained from other techniques (joint mobilization, joint mobility exercise, or muscle flexibility) Improve and maintain dynamic mobility and extensibility of tissue	Muscle activation in new ranges; may be gravity-assisted, -eliminated, or -resisted positions Progressive resistive exercise for endurance and tissue stimulus in new range	High repetitions (>30) Low load Newly obtained range End range if possible Facilitate muscle activation in specific range after mobility exercises No exacerbation of existing pain	Movement observation Ability to activate through available passive range Number of repetitions reaching end of possible range Ability to perform movement in a smooth controlled manner Functional movement observation Ability to control range of motion without excessive localization at individual areas (especially at regions of change of direction of curves)
Teach active methods to maintain and improve functional mobility	Functional training Self-stretching or mobility exercise	Motor control concepts; practice with specificity to use available range, training concepts for practice with precision and monitoring No exacerbation of existing pain	Ability to perform functional movement through range without compensations or feedback Ability to perform movement in a smooth controlled manner Functional movement observation Ability to control range of motion without excessive localization at individual areas (especially at regions of change of direction of curves) Functional mobility measures (sit-to-stand, reaching, single-leg standing balance, gait, lifting, rolling, bed mobility, seated postural position with upper extremity tasks) Functional movement self-reports (Neck Disability Index, Oswestry)

Early exercise goals address muscle spasm and movement restrictions related to pain through oscillatory or general motion, while more established connective tissue restrictions are targeted with passive positioning or prolonged stretch. Muscle flexibility is addressed using stretching exercises, with short or prolonged hold, contract-relax, or hold-relax. The muscle fiber direction and locations of the origin and insertion are taken into account in order to obtain the full length of the muscle–tendon complex. Prolonged mobility restrictions with more established connective tissue adaptations will require more aggressive mobility exercise reaching end range with prolonged holds and progressive increase in force without causing inflammation and protective reactions. Neural mobility is treated using active motion ("flossing") toward the restricted range or with longer holds in the maximum length. Once mobility starts to improve, muscle activation, neuromuscular coordination, and endurance exercises are incorporated to assist with supporting the region, maintaining the new range, and distributing forces. The loads are progressed to strength dosage, and the complexity is increased to meet functional demands as the patient progresses through Phase II and into Phase III rehabilitation.

CONTRAINDICATIONS AND PRECAUTIONS FOR MOBILITY EXERCISES

1. Not indicated for severe instabilities or fractures without early healing or surgical fixation. Self-stretching is contraindicated in early stages after surgical fixation. Mobility exercises need to be adjusted to avoid stress after a fusion.

2. Acute inflammation requires caution (e.g., with acute inflammation and osteoarthritis of the knee).
3. Intensity, difficulty, and level of exercise depends on severity, irritability, and if the symptoms are acute.
4. Combinations of hypermobility and hypomobility occurring simultaneously are common and require some caution with the degree of range in the areas of hypomobility. Ensure distributed and/or symmetrical movement with a centralized axis of motion.
5. Use caution with the amounts of force and load in the presence of muscle spasm and guarding.
6. Avoid excessive strain with inflammatory conditions.
7. Monitor responses to extreme range or load and adjust if pain or spasm increases during treatment.
8. Decrease extent of load and strain at the following visit if soreness is present sooner than 8 hours after mobility exercise.

OBSERVATION FOR COMPENSATIONS AND TOLERANCE

- Avoid compensations in areas of relative mobility in surrounding regions.
- Stabilize proximal and distal segments.
- Use supported positions if there is any chance of loss of balance or excessive compensations.
- Ask patients to report any discomfort.
- Monitor for delayed-onset muscle soreness, increased effusion, or edema after treatment.

EXERCISES

CERVICAL MOBILITY EXERCISES

THORACIC MOBILITY EXERCISES

LUMBAR MOBILITY EXERCISES

SELF-MOBILIZATION

STRETCHING

EXERCISES INCLUDED IN OTHER SECTIONS

- Latissimus dorsi stretch
- Pectoralis major stretch
- Hip flexor stretch

NEURAL MOBILITY

- Neural mobility upper extremity
- Neural mobility lower extremity

EXERCISE DESCRIPTIONS

CERVICAL MOBILITY EXERCISES

Purpose

- Increase or maintain mobility related to decreased joint mobility and muscle flexibility
- Decrease pain
- Redistribute motion

Position

- Supine
- Use foam pads or towels to support the head if forward head position, kyphosis, or rounded shoulders result in stress on the neck.
- Support the shoulders on towels or pillows if flexibility in the shoulders and thoracic region is causing stress in the cervical region.
- Use a towel under the head on a surface that allows fluid motion to decrease friction and make the movement smoother.
- The patient can place his or her hand under the cervical spine to provide feedback to ensure movement occurs in lower cervical spine region.

Contraindications and precautions

- Mobility exercises are not indicated for patients with acute whiplash or trauma. Muscle spasm may contribute to observed mobility deficits, and possible underlying damage or instability (vertebral artery damage, ligamentous instability, and fractures) needs to be cleared prior to using mobility exercise.
- If symptoms indicate high irritability or neural compression, mobility exercises may be delayed or only performed in the supine position with supervision.

General parameters

- Multiple repetitions
- End of range
- Oscillations or prolonged hold

11.1. Cervical Retraction

See Fig. 11.1.

Action (Video 11.1)

1. Activate the deep neck flexors to gently decrease the cervical lordosis
2. Avoid excessive flattening or only using the upper cervical region

Teaching tips

- Instruction examples:
  - "Nod your chin gently, flattening the back of your neck slightly."
  - "Place your hand behind your neck. Gently lengthen your neck and feel the curve flatten slightly in the lower part of your neck."
  - "Keeping your face level, lengthen out through the top of your head."

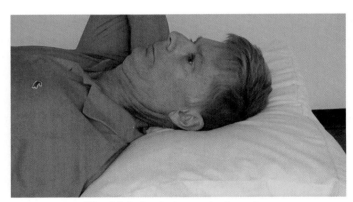

Fig. 11.1 Cervical retraction in supine.

11.2.   Lateral Flexion

See Fig. 11.2.

Action (Video 11.2A–C)

1. Laterally flex the cervical spine in the supported position while maintaining a centralized axis of motion (Fig. 11.2A).
2. To distribute forces, the motion should occur at all regions of the cervical spine and include the upper thoracic regions.

Teaching tips

- Instruction examples:
  - "Lengthen your neck slightly then tip your ear toward your shoulder." (The lengthening helps distribute motion throughout the region rather than concentrating in one or two segments.)
  - "Keep your chin level while tipping your ear toward your shoulder." (The motion should be in the frontal plane without combining rotation with lateral flexion.)

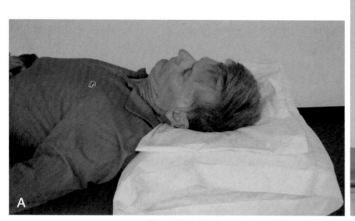
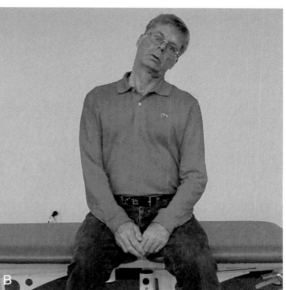

Fig. 11.2 Active cervical lateral flexion in supine (A) and sitting (B).

11.3. Rotation

See Fig. 11.3.

Action (Video 11.3A, B)

1. Rotate the cervical spine while maintaining a centralized axis of motion.
2. To distribute forces, the motion should occur throughout all regions of the cervical spine and include the upper thoracic regions.

Teaching tips for cervical mobility (Exercises 11.1–11.3)

- Instruction examples:
  - "Keep your focus moving at the same speed as your neck movement while turning your head to the side."
  - "Keep your neck lengthened as you rotate from the base of your neck to your skull" (helps avoid combining lateral flexion with rotation and distributes rotation throughout the cervical spine).
- Common error to correct:
  - Observe for multidirectional motion. If tissue resistance or restrictions are reached, a common compensation is to use other planes of motion or to allow motion at segments that have the most motion.
- Method to address or prevent compensations:
  - Limiting the motion to desired plane will be more effective to achieve full stretch of the restricted tissues.

Advantages (Exercises 11.1–11.3)

- Supported position decreases joint compression and allows distribution of forces.
- Supported position decreases need for muscle support to hold the head up against gravity.

Alternatives (Exercises 11.1–11.3)

- Active-assisted movement with the therapist guiding the motion
- Active-assisted segmental movement with the therapist blocking specific areas to localize motion
- Use a sheet under the patient's head to decrease friction.
- The patient places his or her hand in the region where more range is desired (Fig. 11.1 and Fig. 11.3A, B).

Progression (Exercises 11.1–11.3)

- Increase range.
- Increase hold at end of range.
- Decrease head support if the postural position and mobility improves.
- Active cervical retraction, rotation, or lateral flexion in sitting (upright supported position) (Fig. 11.2B and Fig. 11.3C; Video 4.31)

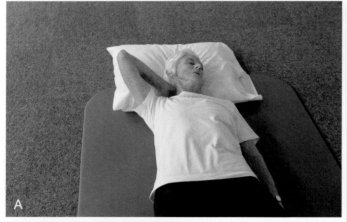
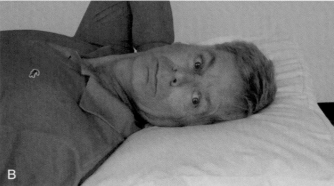
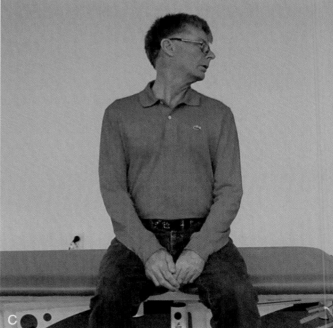

Fig. 11.3 Cervical rotation in supine (A and B) and sitting (C).

THORACIC MOBILITY EXERCISES

11.4. Thoracic Flexion in Four-Point Kneeling

See Fig. 11.4.

Purpose

- Promote thoracic flexion
- Encourage active upper thoracic and cervical extensor muscle activity on returning to the start position
- Promote awareness of thoracic and cervical spinal alignment

Position (Fig. 11.4A)

- Four-point kneeling
- Cervical, thoracic, lumbar spine, and pelvis are in a neutral alignment: the cervical position is usually slightly higher than the pelvis due to the arm length (humerus and forearm) being longer than the femur length in the four-point kneeling position.
- Arms are slightly wider than shoulder width
- Knees are aligned with hip joints
- If the patient complains of wrist discomfort with weight on the upper extremities, bearing weight on the fists, blocks, dumbbells, or small balls to keep the wrist neutral or to decrease the amount of wrist extension will often help resolve or reduce the discomfort.

Action (Fig. 11.4B; Video 11.4)

- Flex the thoracic spine, then actively control the return to a neutral position without passively (or sagging) into extension.

Advantages

- The thoracic spine region is the least mobile area of the spine due to the rib cage anatomy.
- Increasing thoracic mobility may assist with distributing forces throughout the spine and alleviating stress on either the cervical or lumbar region.
- Thoracic flexion is often needed when individuals have a flat upper back or generalized stiffness.

Teaching tips

- Instruction example:
  - "Engage your abdominals by flattening your stomach. Tip your pelvis toward your ribs and round your lower, middle, and then your upper back. Reverse the action, controlling the movement back to the starting position."
- Common errors to correct:
  - Patients often overuse the pectoralis major to flex the thoracic spine by horizontally adducting the shoulders.
  - Dropping the head below the level of the thoracic spine in the starting position or not returning the spine to the fully supported position. Typically, the spine is at an oblique angle, with the shoulders higher than the hips in four-point kneeling. If the head is parallel to the ground, the cervicothoracic region is in a flexed position.
- Methods to address or correct compensations:
  - Emphasize using the abdominals to flex the spine by starting from the lumbar spine, rather than overusing the pectoralis major.
  - An elastic resistance band wrapped across the restricted area of thoracic spine and secured under the hands can be used to provide feedback to guide movement to the desired area of the spine. Instruct the patient to move his or her spine into the band.

Alternatives

- Reverse into full thoracic extension if no lumbar or cervical spine pain is present
- Can be used to promote mobility in the lumbar spine by modifying the cueing ("Pull your abdominals into your body to help round your lower spine.")
- If the emphasis is on active upper thoracic and cervical spinal extensor activation and mobility, Exercise 11.6 can be used to isolate this area.

Progression

- Seated thoracic extension (Exercise 11.14)

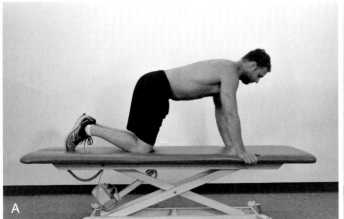
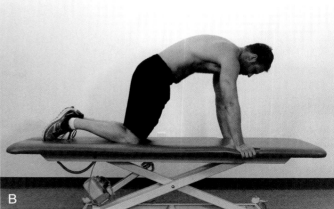

Fig. 11.4 Thoracic flexion in four-point kneeling.

11.5.   Supine Thoracic Extension Over BOSU

See Fig. 11.5.

Purpose
- Promote mobility of the upper and middle thoracic spine into extension.

Position
- Lying with the thoracic spine supported by a Both Sides Up (BOSU) balance trainer (dome side up) or a stability ball
- Neutral lumbar spine position
- Legs are hip-width apart.
- The head and neck are supported with the hands.
- If there is a large kyphosis that results in excessive forces on the cervical spine in overextended position, use a pillow or ball under the head (between the head and the dome of the BOSU).

Action (Video 11.5A)
1. Release the upper back over the BOSU to a point where the thoracic and cervical spine are supported.
2. Use the arms to support the head weight; the elbows can point forward (Fig. 11.5A) or be opened to emphasize a pectoralis stretch (Fig. 11.5B).

Teaching tips
- Instruction examples:
  - "Deepen your abdominal muscles before you lower your body down onto the BOSU."
  - "Support your head with your hands as if you were supporting the weight of a bowling ball."
  - "Use your hands to support your head and neck, only allowing your upper body to release onto the BOSU once your upper back is in contact with the BOSU."
- Common error to correct:
  - If the abdominals are not engaged to stabilize the lumbar spine, watch for lumbar or lower thoracic extension rather than upper to middle thoracic mobility.

- Methods to address or avoid compensations:
  - Observe for the lower ribs lifting with increased lower thoracic and lumbar extension. If motion is occurring in the lumbar spine, there is less mobility obtained higher up in the thoracic spine. Asking the patient to engage the upper abdominals to limit the motion will provide a stable base to stretch in the cranial direction (Video 11.5A).
  - Slide further down the BOSU if the abdominal control does not prevent excessive rib popping (Fig. 11.5B).
  - Emphasize slowly releasing onto the surface rather than collapsing without control.

Advantages
- The spine is supported while stretching, and the soft surface is comfortable for individuals with sensitivity or established kyphosis.
- The patient is able to control degree and range of the stretch by positioning the body closer to or further away from the apex of the curve of the BOSU (Fig. 11.5B).
- The exercise promotes thoracic extension with passive support and can be used even if the patient has cervical or lumbar pain.

Alternatives
- Extending the thoracic spine over a foam roller or pool noodle (placed perpendicular to the area of major restriction) increases localized stretching and mobilization and is an affordable home program option (Exercise 11.12).
- Use an exercise ball instead of the BOSU (Video 11.5B).
- Using small equipment to assist with self-mobilization (massage balls, tennis balls, mobilization wedges).

Progression
- Increase range.
- Increase duration of hold.
- Progress to active extension in prone.

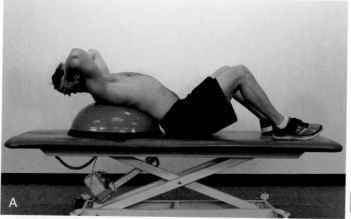
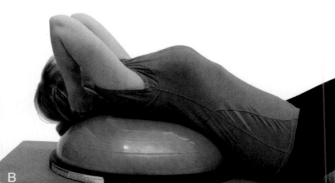

Fig. 11.5 (A and B) Thoracic extension over a BOSU with the arms supporting the head. Note that the position of the body relative to the apex of the BOSU in B allows more support of the head and upper back.

11.6. Prone Cervical and Upper Thoracic Extension Over BOSU

See Fig. 11.6.

Purpose

- Active mobility of upper thoracic region into extension against gravity
- Focus on upper thoracic and lower cervical extensors with deep neck flexor support to maintain cervical lordosis

Position

- Prone on the BOSU (Fig. 11.6A)
- Forearms and head on the ground for the starting position, head supported on a ball or foam block if needed (Fig. 11.6B)

Action (Video 11.6 A)

- Active cervical and upper thoracic extension to a neutral position (Fig. 11.6C)

Teaching tips

- Instruction examples:
  - "Lift the back of your head toward the ceiling."
  - "Reach your ears away from your shoulders as you lift up into one long line."
  - "Keep your neck in a lengthened position as you lift your head and neck."
- Common errors to correct:
  - Extending the upper cervical spine without using the lower cervical and upper thoracic extensors. (The upper cervical spine will appear hyperextended and the patient will gaze forward instead of downward [Video 11.6B].)
  - Overextending the cervical or lumbar spine
- Methods to address or prevent compensations:
  - Tactile input (therapist's hand placed on the back of the head or tapping the upper thoracic and lower cervical extensors) may be useful to assist with activation of the lower extensors (Video 11.6C). A pole or half foam roller can also be useful to provide tactile feedback for the synchronization of the cervical and upper thoracic extension.

- Activation of the deep cervical flexors is needed to counterbalance the extension and provide support for the mid-cervical lordosis. Teach activation of the deep neck flexors to support the lordosis. If needed, include exercises in supine focusing on a gentle head nod and elongation prior to the prone extension or demonstrating the movement first (see Exercise 11.1).
- The direction of the patient's visual focus is likely to influence the position of the head. During the movement, the patient will need to continue to look toward the floor rather than forward in order to avoid over extending the upper cervical spine.

Advantages

- Allows localization of extension motion to cervical and thoracic regions without extending the lumbar spine
- This exercise can be used to promote active extensor control against gravity after joint mobilization or passive stretching.
- The BOSU provides support and is more stable than an exercise ball.
- Teaches the patient proper alignment of the head and cervical spine relative to the thoracic spine.
- Prone position challenges neck stabilizer muscles to work against gravity.

Alternatives

- If the patient is unable to lift the head actively against gravity, use supported isometric stabilization of the cervical region in supine on an unstable surface such as a partially deflated ball or foam roller.
- Use an exercise ball to support the body in four-point kneeling (Fig. 11.6D–E; Video 11.6D).

Progression

- Increase range.
- Increase hold.
- Progress endurance by increasing repetitions or holding position and adding leg movement.

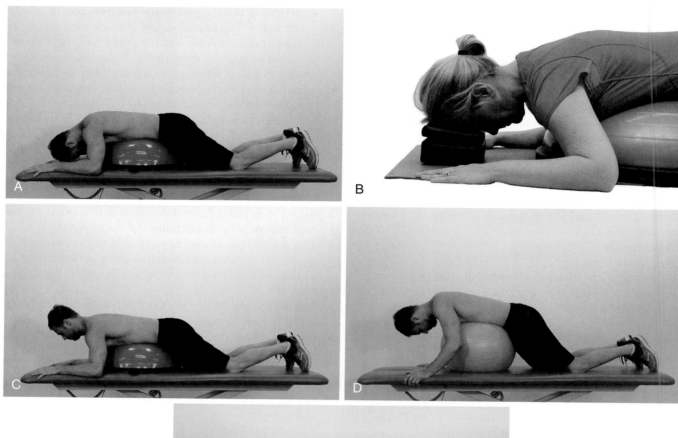

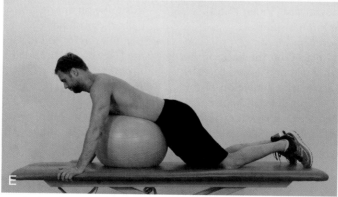

Fig. 11.6 Prone cervical and upper thoracic extension, starting position over BOSU (A) with head support if needed (B), followed by active cervical and upper thoracic extension counterbalanced by deep neck flexor activation (C). Alternative in four point kneeling over exercise ball (D and E).

11.7. Thoracic Rotation Side-Lying

See Fig. 11.7.

Purpose
- Increase or promote thoracic rotation mobility with synchronous cervical rotation and scapulothoracic connection

Position
- Side-lying, spine and pelvis neutral
- Head supported on ball, pillows, or foam pads (to maintain head and neck aligned with thoracic spine rather than laterally flexed toward the supporting surface) (Fig. 11.7A).
- Lifting the lumbar spine using the quadratus and abdominal muscles places the lumbar and thoracic spine in an active supported position (Exercise 11.29).
- Arms reaching forward, top arm lifted and parallel to the supporting surface.

Precautions
- Limit range if the patient has excessive mobility at the lumbothoracic junction and ensure that the axis of motion is occurring throughout the spine rather than concentrated in one area.
- Avoid early or excessive shoulder hyperextension.

Action (Video 11.7A)
1. Maintain the gaze on the top hand and allow the cervical spine to follow the motion while rotating the thoracic spine (Fig. 11.7B).
2. Keep the shoulder moving with the thoracic spine, synchronizing the timing and the amount of movement.
3. Maintain the scapulothoracic connection throughout the movement.

Advantages
- Limited stress on the lumbar spine region
- Gravity assistance for thoracic rotation

Teaching tips
- Position options:
  - A foam pad or small towel can be placed under the lower rib cage to help maintain a centralized axis of motion and support the spine in neutral rather than dropping toward the surface (to lift the waist). This is particularly helpful in cases where a patient has a small waist relative to wider shoulders.
- Instruction example:
  - "Open your arms and upper body like a book. Follow your top hand with your eyes."
- Common errors to correct:
  - Avoid concentrating the rotation primarily at the thoracolumbar junction.
  - Avoid localizing the movement to the shoulder by sliding the scapula back into retraction without rotating the spine or after the spinal rotation limit has been reached (Video 11.7B). If there is no spinal rotation, the exercise does not achieve the goal and can place excessive stress on the anterior shoulder.

- Methods to address or prevent compensations:
  - Placing a foam roller behind the spine can provide feedback to the patient to distribute the rotation across multiple segments rather than concentrating the rotation at just a few segments.
  - Instructing the patient to initiate the motion from the shoulder rather than initiating the movement from the hand will help ensure a proximal to distal movement sequence. If the motion is distributed throughout the spinal segments there is less chance of concentrating the motion at the thoracolumbar junction:
    - "Float your hand toward the ceiling, starting the movement from your spine rather than leading with your hand."
    - "You should feel motion throughout your spine rather than only at one point."
    - "You should be able to see your hand at all times."

Alternatives
- Seated rotation (Fig. 11.7C, D): rotating the thoracic spine with the cervical spine stabilized in space can be used to promote mobility in the upper thoracic and lower cervical regions. The patient should sit upright with good postural alignment and be asked to keep looking forward while rotating the torso, creating relative cervicothoracic rotation. Place the hands across the body on the shoulders. The lumbar spine should be in neutral, especially if the patient has an exaggerated lumbar lordosis or a combination of lumbar lordosis and thoracic kyphosis. Some lumbar rotation is expected (Fig. 11.7C).
- Seated rotation with the cervical spine rotating along with the thoracic and lumbar spine. Keeping the gaze moving on the horizon at the same speed as the thoracic rotation will help distribute the movement without leading only from the cervical region (Fig. 11.7D, E).

Progression
- Increase range.
- Increase hold.
- Progress to mobility exercises in unsupported positions requiring postural control (sitting, standing).
- Use seated thoracic rotation with an elastic resistance band wrapped around the body and under the arms. The patient holds the band with light stretch to provide sensory feedback for arm support (Fig. 11.7F). The addition of the arm weight increases the challenge but provides a relevant position for functional reeducation and additional support for the upper quarter.

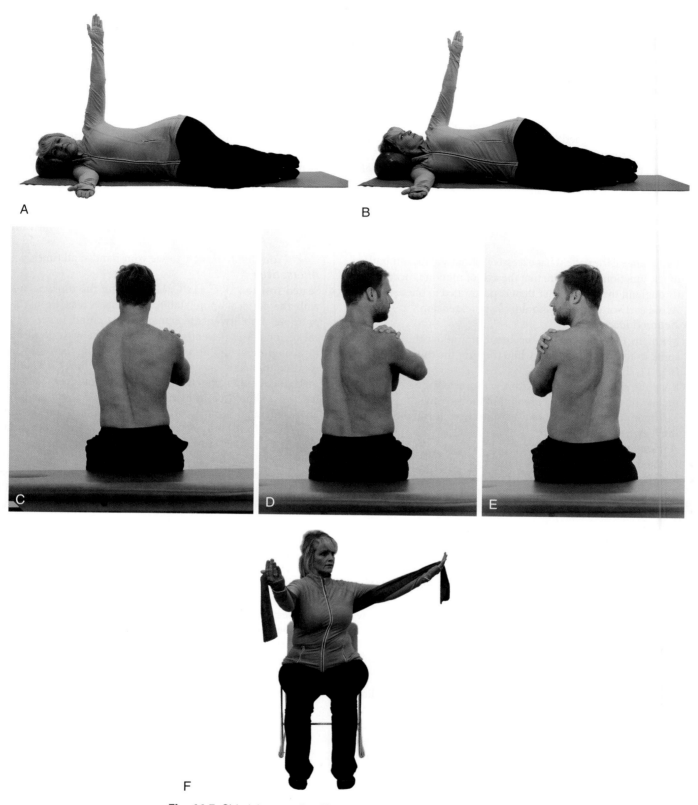

Fig. 11.7 Side-lying rotation (A,B) and progression to sitting (C–F).

LUMBAR MOBILITY EXERCISES

11.8. Pelvic Tilts

See Fig. 11.8.

Purpose
- Controlled lumbar flexion mobility

Position (Fig. 11.8A)
- Supine with the lumbar spine and pelvis in neutral
- Knees and hips flexed to 45 degrees

Action (Fig. 11.8A–C; Video 11.8)
1. Engage the deep abdominal muscles and pelvic floor using low-intensity isometric contraction.
2. Tilt the pelvis posteriorly using the abdominal muscles, then slowly return the pelvis and lumbar spine back to the neutral starting position.

Advantages
- Limited joint compression and loading
- Ability to control the lumbar spine without excessive compensations elsewhere
- Gravity-assisted motion assists with lumbar mobility and pain relief.
- Early Phase I exercise to promote gentle motion for pain relief or reversal of lumbar lordosis
- Mobility exercise with a flexion bias
- Can be used as a warm-up home exercise after sleeping for individuals who complain of early morning stiffness.

Teaching tips
- Instruction example:
  - "Engage your abdominals to tip your pelvis toward your ribs, then control the return to neutral."
- Common error to correct:
  - Watch for the hip flexors or the gluteals compensating for the abdominal muscles to tilt the pelvis.
- Method to address or prevent compensations:
  - Ask the patient to place the thumb and index finger on the rib cage and the pelvis. Instruct the patient to shorten the distance between the fingers.

Alternatives
- Rest the pelvis on a thin foam cushion or pillow if patient is sensitive to pressure on the sacrum.
- Patient-assisted passive lumbar flexion with the hands around both knees (Fig. 11.8D)

Progression
- Continue to flex spine into the thoracic region.
- Controlled eccentric abdominal control on the return by slowing the movement
- Increase the emphasis on the lower thoracic and upper lumbar region by starting with the feet on the top of a BOSU, foam blocks, or step, or with the legs supported on an exercise ball to raise the legs relative to the body (see Exercise 11.9).

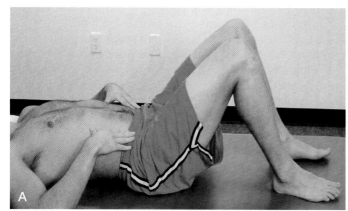
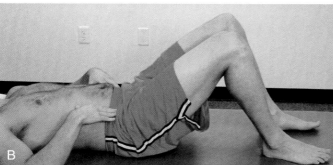
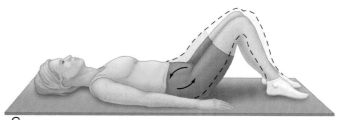
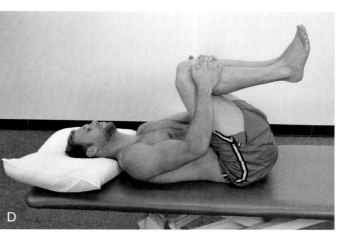

Fig. 11.8 Posterior pelvic tilt (A–C) and passive lumbar flexion (D).

11.9. Segmental Flexion with Legs Supported on a Ball

See Fig. 11.9.

Purpose
- Progression from pelvic tilt
- Increased mobility of the lower thoracic region

Position
- Supine
- Knees and hips flexed to 45 degrees
- Lower legs are placed on an exercise ball. The size of the ball is chosen to allow active spinal flexion to the desired region of the spine (Fig. 11.9A).
- The size of the ball may need to be adjusted to support the patient's lower leg length.
- If the ball is too far from the body, the patient may extend the spine or overuse the hamstrings.

Action (Video 11.9)
1. Engage the abdominals to posteriorly tilt the pelvis, then use the legs (especially gluteus maximus and hamstrings) to continue to segmentally flex the spine and lift the pelvis off the floor (Fig. 11.9B).
2. Ensure that abdominal contraction occurs prior to using the legs.
3. Once the thoracic spine is off the surface, slowly control the return movement using the abdominal muscles.
4. Spend more time flexing through areas of restriction.

Advantages
- Elevating the lower limb on top of the ball increases potential for flexion of the mid to upper lumbar region and the lower thoracic region.
- The ball provides an unstable base requiring symmetry of movement with immediate concurrent feedback about the symmetry, as well as promoting additional proximal lower limb muscle activity.
- The position of the legs decreases stress on the knee (if needed) and provides a favorable length–tension relationship for hamstrings and gluteal muscles.
- The flexion bias of the exercise is useful for patients who have limited spinal flexion mobility, when repeated flexion assists with pain centralization and when extension increases pain.

Teaching tips
- Instruction example:
  - "Engage your abdominals to tip your pelvis toward your ribs. Continue the movement by engaging your gluteal muscles and hamstrings to lift your pelvis off the mat. Then return to the floor from the top down, rolling through your ribs, lower back, then sacrum, slowly controlling the return to the table."
  - "Your spine should lift off the mat one vertebra at a time."
- Common errors to correct:
  - Avoid hyperextending the spine or initiating the movement through lumbar extension.
  - Avoid rotating or laterally flexing the spine during the movement.
- Methods to address or prevent compensations:
  - Start with small controlled ranges before progressing to higher ranges.
  - Hold the ball for the patient if he or she is having difficulty keeping the ball in place.
  - Instruct the patient to "Roll up and down the center of your spine, keeping the ball from rolling side to side."

Alternatives
- A foam roller can be used, but hamstring cramping is a common issue with this variation
- Use a larger ball or place the feet on a high bolster to concentrate the movement in the thoracic region.
- A stable surface (steps or bolster) can be used if there is difficulty maintaining symmetry or if the patient is unable to control the movement on the unstable support.
- Feet placed on a BOSU provides a smaller range but requires more ankle and hip stability in the frontal plane.

Progression
- Decrease speed on the return for greater eccentric control.
- Focus on specific ranges.

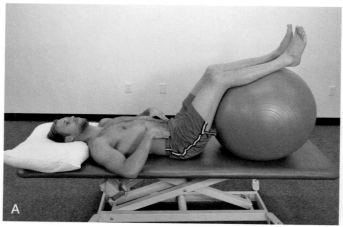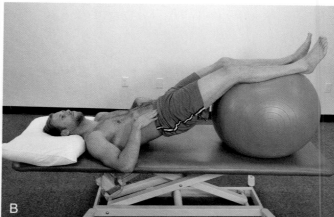

Fig. 11.9 Segmental lumbar flexion with legs supported.

11.10.   Thoracic and Lumbar Extension Over BOSU (Prone Press-up)

See Fig. 11.10.

Purpose

- Improve active thoracic and lumbar extension range of motion
- Can be used for repeated extension if there is a directional extension preference

Position

- Prone, with apex of the BOSU (dome side up) under the sternum and lower ribs (Fig. 11.6A, B)
- Thoracic spine flexed over the BOSU
- Lumbar spine in neutral
- Arms wider than the body, head facing down

Precautions

- Ensure segmental, even extension throughout the spine and observe for hinge points.
- If movement results in compression type pain, reduce the range or limit motion to above the area causing symptoms.

Action (Video 11.10)

1. Stabilize the cervical spine by gently nodding the chin and engage the abdominal muscles.
2. Use arms to push through the forearms and assist a partial push-up.
3. Extend the thoracic spine to look forward in front of the body, bringing the head up in line with the body.
4. Allow the pelvis and legs to angle back on the BOSU to lift the upper body and look forward, extending into the lumbar spine if tolerated (Fig. 11.10A).

Teaching tips

- Position the body further back from the apex for more lumbar extension and further forward for less extension.
- Instruction example:
  - "After you have lifted the head and upper body, use the arms to further lift the upper body from the BOSU. Rock back on the BOSU, extending your spine to your comfort level."
  - "Lift from your head and neck, then your upper back, then lower back."
- Common errors to correct:
  - Pushing up from the arms without achieving lumbar or thoracic extension. "The movement should come from your spine rather than only using your arms."

- Extending one area rather than throughout the spine
- Methods to address or prevent compensations:
  - If the movement and forces are concentrated in one area, slow down the movement and teach the patient to isolate the movement to the area above the hinge point.
  - Ask the patient to engage ("lift") the deep abdominals off the BOSU prior to lifting the body and keep the abdominals engaged. This is especially important if there is a need to distribute the forces throughout the thoracic region or to teach the patient how to provide support for athletic requirements requiring extreme spinal extension (e.g., gymnastics, dance, throwing sports, tennis serves, volleyball).

Advantages

- If a patient presents with a thoracic kyphosis combined with a lumbar lordosis, using the BOSU allows reversal of the thoracic kyphosis (if flexible) while avoiding excessive lumbar extension.
- Early spinal extension exercise for mobility purposes
- Indicated if repeated extension centralizes pain responses or if thoracic or lumbar spine extension range is needed, such as with postural syndromes.

Alternatives

- Range of motion can be varied.
- Exercise can be limited to pushing up onto the forearms or the elbows fully extended to gain further range (Fig. 11.10B).
- The exercise can be performed without the BOSU (Fig. 11.10C).
- Repeated movement or sustained movement can be used if there is centralization of symptoms with repeated movement.

Progression

- Progress to prone passive extension on the forearms without the BOSU support (Fig. 11.10B).
- Increase range by extending the elbows into a full "cobra" position (Fig. 11.10C).
- Hold the full position for any of the exercise options or increase repetitions.
- Slow down the movement to focus on specific regions.
- Use manual blocking to enhance use of a specific region or limit motion to upper thoracic regions.

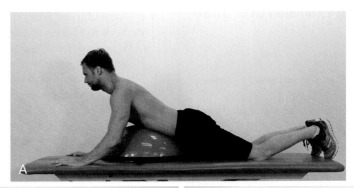

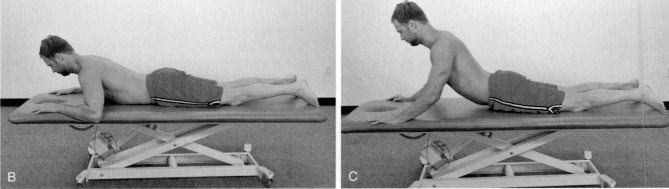

Fig. 11.10 Thoracic and lumbar extension over BOSU (A) and prone press-up (B and C).

11.11. Lumbar Rotation Active Range of Motion

See Fig. 11.11.

Purpose
- Promote spinal rotation mobility
- Midrange motion can be used for pain relief.
- Maintain rotation range obtained with mobilization

Position
- Supine, arms slightly abducted from sides
- Legs supported on an exercise ball (Fig. 11.11A)

Action (Video 11.11)
1. Engage the deep transverse abdominis muscle.
2. After stabilizing the lumbar spine in a neutral position, use the obliques to actively rotate the spine by rolling the ball to the point when the pelvis is about to lift off the floor on the opposite side (Fig. 11.11B).
3. Maintain a centralized axis of motion.

Advantages
- The ball supports the legs and allows spinal rotation without using the leg muscles or altering the axis of motion due to the leg contact with the floor.
- The gravity-eliminated supine position decreases the impact of lower extremity alignment or excessive spinal curves contributing to localized forces at the junctions between curvatures.
- Controlling the amount of range activates the obliques and spinal rotators to create controlled motion, allowing the patient to actively control the range.

Teaching tips
- Instruction example:
  - "Gently press your arms into the ground, then roll the ball to one side up to the point when your pelvis just starts to lift off the ground on the opposite side. Use your abdominal muscles to control the movement and return to the other side."
- Common error to correct:
  - If the opposite ribs and shoulder are allowed to lift off the ground, the rotation is also occurring in the thoracic and possibly the cervical spine.
- Methods to address or prevent compensations:
  - Engage the deep abdominals prior to rotating.
  - Instructing the patient to focus on keeping the shoulders and ribs in contact with the ground on both sides provides feedback for the patient to monitor the amount of rotation.

Alternatives
- Lying supine with one hip and knee flexed, the foot flat on the floor, without the exercise ball. Engage the obliques to rotate the spine and then move the bent knee across the midline toward the extended leg. This variation will limit the range but may concentrate rotation in the mid lumbar region (Fig. 11.11C).

Progression
- Increase range.
- Single-leg version; add passive overpressure with the opposite hand to provide prolonged stretch (Fig. 11.11D).

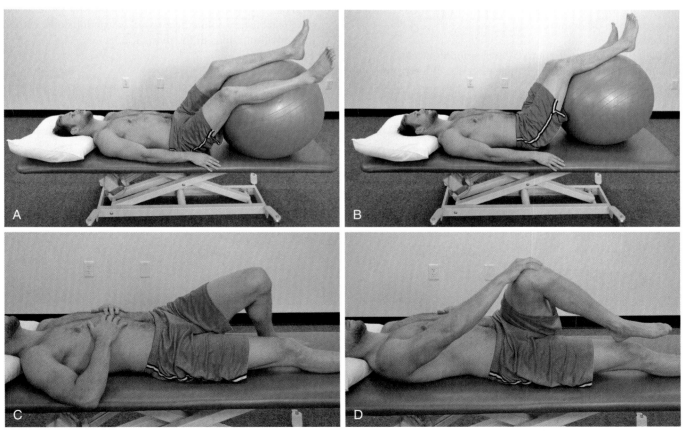

Fig. 11.11 Lumbar rotation active range of motion with legs supported (A and B), single leg bent (C), and with self-assistance for passive overpressure (D).

SELF-MOBILIZATION

Self-mobilization techniques are useful for home programs for patients with mobility restrictions who have low severity and irritability. Techniques may be indicated after mobilization to maintain range or to prevent recurrence of mobility deficits. Self-mobilization is only indicated if neural symptoms have decreased and patient is able to actively control and sequence movement. Techniques are used with caution when a patient has combinations of hypomobility and hypermobility.

11.12.   Foam Roller Self-Mobilization

See Fig. 11.12.

Purpose
- Increase or maintain thoracic extension

Position (Fig. 11.12A)
- Supine, over a foam roller or pool noodle placed perpendicular to the spine, under the area to be stretched
- Hands supporting the head

Action (Fig. 11.12B)
1. Engage the abdominal muscles to control the lumbar spine position.
2. Slowly release the thoracic region into extension over the foam roller, supporting the head with the hands.
3. Hold the position if tolerated.
4. Return to sitting by engaging the abdominals and flexing from the lumbar spine.
5. Move the foam roller to a different position to concentrate the stretch in different regions.

Advantages
- Self-stretch allows patient to control amount of range.
- Foam roller or pool noodle can be placed at different areas to concentrate mobility.

Teaching tips
- Instruction examples:
  1. To lower into the starting position: "Sit in front of the foam roller. Carefully roll back until your back touches the roller. Adjust your position on the roller by lifting your hips and moving your spine until the roller is under the area that you are trying to stretch. Lower your hips back down to the floor and begin the exercise."
  2. "Engage your abdominal muscles to prevent your low back from arching. Slowly release your spine onto the foam roller. Once you reach a position where you are feeling a stretch in your spine, hold the position and release your spine softly over the foam roller."
  3. On the return: "Deepen your abdominal muscles and support your head with your hands. Reverse your spine using your abdominal muscles without pulling on your head."

Alternatives
- Use two tennis balls in a sock or massage balls in place of a foam roller to provide more localized stretching.
- Pool noodles are smaller in diameter and offer more specificity than a typical foam roller, but are also less dense so will provide less force to the targeted area.
- A less aggressive alternative is to lie on the foam roller with the spine supported longitudinally. The head can be supported using a pillow or a foam pad. The patient uses deep breathing to increase thoracic mobility instead of extending over the roller. The arms can support the head or be placed next to the side. This alternative is more suitable for a patient who has high pain severity or irritability or for patients who have established connective tissue restrictions and extreme mobility limitations in the thoracic area.

Progression
- Increase range.
- Progress through different regions in the spine to access areas with limited mobility.

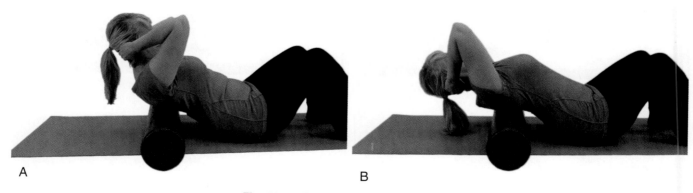

A   B

Fig. 11.12 Foam roller self-mobilization.

11.13. Supported Lateral Flexion: Exercise Ball or BOSU

See Fig. 11.13.

Purpose

- Lateral flexion self-mobilization and stretch (including latissimus dorsi and quadratus lumborum)

Position

- Using the exercise ball: kneeling or side-sitting next to the ball with the upper body partially resting on the ball. The arm closest to the ball is draped over ball so that it supports the body along the ribs (Fig. 11.13A).
- Using the BOSU: side-lying over with the upper body supported on the BOSU resting on the forearm closest to the BOSU (Fig. 11.13C)

Action

1. Using the exercise ball: The patient uses the legs to roll the body over the ball and allows the ball to assist with laterally flexing the spine (Fig. 11.13B).
2. Using the BOSU: The unsupported arm is abducted to laterally flex the trunk over the BOSU (Fig. 11.13D; Video 11.13).

Advantages

- Generalized lateral flexion stretch with the body supported allows thoracic and lumbar motion
- The equipment provides a soft surface and encourages distributed mobility, with the BOSU providing more stability than the exercise ball.
- The exercise can be used to teach distributed spinal mobility, especially for individuals with combined hypomobility and hypermobility.

Teaching tips

- Instruction examples:
  - "Curve your body to create a semi-circle over the ball (or BOSU)."
  - "Reach your top arm in a curve and go over the BOSU (or ball)."

- "Reach over the ball, taking your head and shoulders with you over the ball."
- Common errors to correct:
  - Combining thoracic rotation with lateral flexion is common and may need to be corrected using demonstration, hands-on tactile correction, or limiting the range once the combination of movement occurs.
  - If the patient has restricted shoulder mobility or limited flexibility of the latissimus dorsi, pectoralis muscles, or posterior shoulder muscles there is a chance of concentrated forces at the shoulder or at the lumbothoracic junction.
- Methods to limit or correct compensations:
  - Maintain the motion in the frontal plane by keeping the gaze across the room rather than looking at the floor (which will add rotation).
  - If there is limited shoulder mobility or muscle flexibility limiting full shoulder elevation, limit the shoulder movement short of the maximum range and keep the arm in front of the body.

Alternatives

- Laterally flexing over pillows or cushions provides a more stable support, but less range.
- A pillow or foam cushion can be used under the head and cervical spine for support when using a BOSU, or the lower arm can be used to support the head weight (Fig. 11.13E).
- Allowing the patient start with his feet staggered but against a wall provides a stable surface to push against to roll over the ball.
- Abducting the top arm overhead provides additional latissimus dorsi stretch.

Progression

- Increase range.

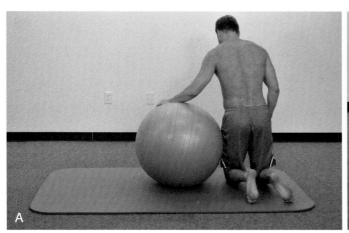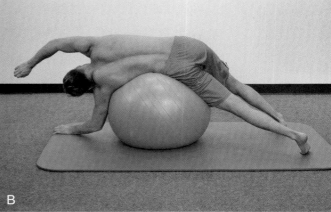

Fig. 11.13 (A and B) Supported lateral flexion over an exercise ball.

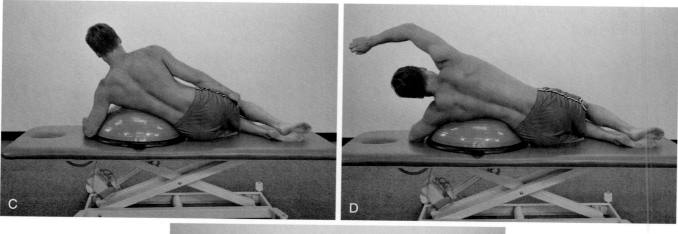

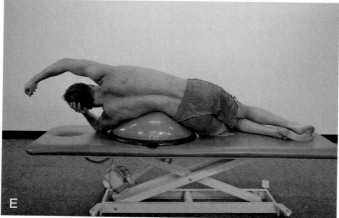

Fig. 11.13, Cont'd Supported lateral flexion over BOSU (C–E) with head support (E) or without (C and D).

11.14.   Seated Self-Mobilization: Upper Thoracic Extension

See Fig. 11.14.

Purpose

- Mobilize and stretch the upper thoracic spine into extension

Position

- Sitting in a stable chair without wheels, arms crossed across the front of the chest or behind head for support (Fig. 11.14A)
- The back of the chair should support the patient's thoracic spine up to the hypomobile segment.
- The chair back must be stable enough to support the patient's body weight when leaning over the back.
- The height of the chair back needs to support the spine without limiting the thoracic motion or causing discomfort.

Action

- Extend the upper spine with control over the chair back. Use the chair to provide an axis where motion is needed (Fig. 11.14B)

Advantages

- Convenient stretch to reverse flexed, seated postures for patients with desk jobs
- Support from chair increases localization to the upper thoracic area

Teaching tips

- Common errors to correct:
  - Early or excessive lumbar extension rather than sequential and distributed thoracic mobility
  - Avoid excessive cervical extension
- Methods to correct compensations:
  - Place interlaced fingers behind the neck if the patient is hyperextending. This will block excessive cervical spine extension.
  - To decrease the likelihood of extending into the lumbar spine during the movement, the patient's feet must contact the floor, and the thighs should be fully supported by the chair seat.

Alternatives

- Supine thoracic extension using a foam roller, balls or BOSU (Exercises 11.5 and 11.12)
- Prone active extension (Exercise 11.10)

Progression

- Increase range or increase hold.
- Active extension without the chair
- Add rotation with extension (Exercise 11.15).

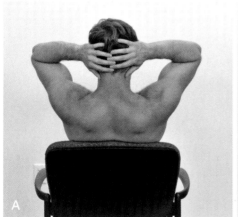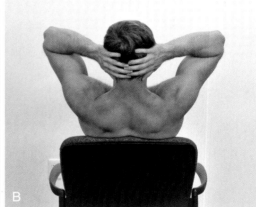

Fig. 11.14 Seated upper thoracic self-mobilization in sitting.

11.15. Seated Self-Mobilization: Rotation and Extension

See Fig. 11.15.

Purpose

- Mobilize unilateral restrictions or as a progression from extension only (Exercise 11.14)

Position

- Sitting in a stable chair without wheels, arms crossed across thoracic spine or hands supporting head
- The back of the chair should support the patient's thoracic spine up to the point where mobility is needed.
- The chair back must be stable enough to support the patient's body weight when leaning back.

Action

- Rotate, then extend the upper spine, controlling the movement over the chair back.

Advantages

- Convenient stretch to periodically reverse flexed, seated postures for patients with desk jobs
- Support from chair increases localization to upper thoracic area

Teaching tips

- Instruction example:
  - "Spiral up from the bottom to the top of your spine, then lift your sternum or front of your chest slightly to extend your upper spine against the chair back."
- Common errors to correct:
  - Shifting weight to one side instead of rotating through the spine
  - Avoid overextending the cervical spine rather than extending the thoracic spine.
- Methods to address or prevent compensations:
  - Initiate the rotation from the lumbar spine and continue to the top of the spine with the head and neck following the amount of thoracic rotation.
  - Interlaced fingers behind the neck will block excessive cervical extension.

Alternatives

- Extension and rotation using foam roller, balls, or BOSU (similar to Exercise 11.5 or 11.10 with rotation)

Progression

- Increase range or increase hold.
- Rotate and extend without the chair back as an axis.

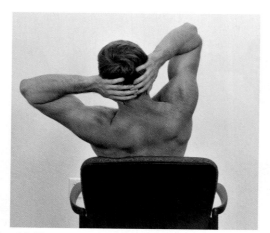

Fig. 11.15 Seated self-mobilization: rotation and extension.

STRETCHING

Muscle flexibility limitations require lengthening of the muscle in the direction of fiber alignment. Stretching may follow soft tissue mobilization, joint mobilization, or generalized aerobic warm-up. Spinal muscles require lengthening across multiple joints, and therefore flexibility exercise accompanies or follows generalized mobility techniques. Supported positions are less likely to place excessive force on symptomatic areas.

11.16.   Upper Trapezius Stretch

See Fig. 11.16.

Purpose
- Increase upper trapezius flexibility

Precautions
- This exercise is not suitable for individuals with upper cervical spine hypermobility or acute pain along with trapezius tightness as the pull from the trapezius can place excessive stress on the upper cervical joints.
- Manual stretch may be required prior to providing the exercise as a home program for individuals with headaches or upper cervical pain.
- Ensure patient comfort with stretch before adding overpressure to increase the stretch.
- Supine alternative may be suitable for individuals with upper cervical pain or headaches.

Position
- Sitting, using the hand on the side to be stretched to grasp the edge of the chair seat or tucked under thigh to stabilize the scapula from elevating and the torso from laterally flexing (Fig. 11.16A, B).

Action (Video 11.16)
1. Laterally flex the cervical spine cervical spine away from arm that is stabilized under leg or chair (Fig. 11.16A).
2. The free hand can be used to assist the stretch (Fig. 11.16B).

Advantages
- Can be performed as a home exercise in multiple settings, including breaks from desk work.

Teaching tips
- Position options:
  - Sitting against a high-backed chair provides support for the spine and limits compensation with other spinal areas.
  - Depending on the patient's arm length, the hand can be placed under the chair or placed under the thigh.
- Instruction example:
  - "Hold onto the side of your chair or tuck your hand under your thigh. Keeping your gaze straight in front of you, tilt your head away from the hand on the chair, your ear moving toward your shoulder. To increase the stretch, use your opposite hand to assist the stretch."
- Common error to correct:
  - Avoid using the hand to provide the stretch before the movement has been started in the cervical spine.

Alternatives
- Stretch in a supported position: lying down with the head supported, flex the head to the opposite side using the hand to assist with reaching end range (Fig. 11.16C).
- Support the head in slight flexion and depress both scapulae by reaching toward the feet with both arms (Fig. 11.16D).

Progression
- Increase time held or range

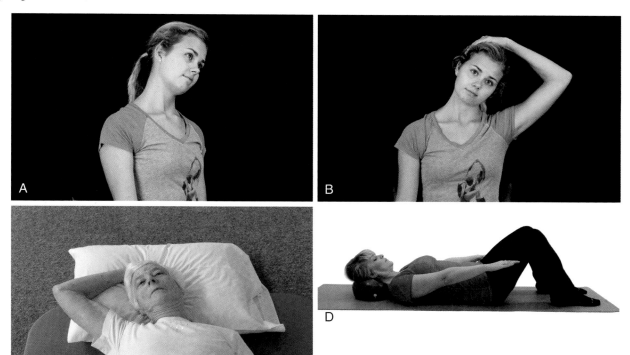

Fig. 11.16 Trapezius stretch in sitting (A and B), supine with head support (C), and modification in supine with head support and scapula depression (D).

11.17. Scalene Stretch

See Fig. 11.17.

Purpose
- Increase scalene flexibility

Position
- Sitting, opposite hand stabilized by holding onto the side of the treatment table or reaching toward the feet

Action (Video 11.17)
1. Laterally flex cervical spine to the opposite side (Fig. 11.17A) of the hand stabilizing the body
2. Rotate the upper cervical spine toward the side holding onto the chair to stretch the anterior scalenes, looking up toward the ceiling (Fig. 11.17B).

Advantages
- Supine position provides support for the weight of the head

Teaching tips
- Instruction example:
  - To stretch the right scalenes: "Hold onto the chair with your right hand and tip your head toward your left shoulder. Turn your head to look up and to the right."

- Common error to correct:
  - Allowing the chin to protrude forward into a forward head position.
- Methods to address or prevent compensations:
  - The therapist may need to guide the movement initially to show the patient how to maintain the plane of movement.

Alternatives
- Supine, therapist-assisted stretch with the head supported or in slight extension
- Contrac-relax or hold-relax after self-resistance

Progression
- Increase time or range.

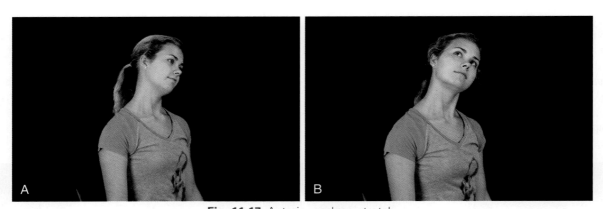

Fig. 11.17 Anterior scalene stretch.

11.18. Levator Scapula Stretch

See Fig. 11.18.

Purpose
- Increase levator scapula flexibility

Precautions
- This stretch is concentrated on the upper and middle cervical region and may aggravate upper or mid-cervical pain if a cervical lordosis is excessive or not stabilized prior to the stretch. Symptoms should be monitored carefully, along with observation of movement. Avoid over-flexing, especially in the upper cervical region. Manual stretching may be more appropriate prior to home exercise prescription.

Position
- Sitting, hand grasping the edge of the chair seat or tucked under thigh to stabilize the scapula from elevating and the torso from laterally flexing (Fig. 11.18)
- Sitting against a high-backed chair provides support for the spine and limits compensation with other spinal areas.
- Depending on the patient's arm length, the hand can be placed under the chair or placed under the thigh.

Action (Video 11.18)
1. Upper and middle cervical flexion, slight lateral flexion, and rotation away from the side being stretched. (Fig. 11.18A)

2. The opposite hand can be placed on the head and used to assist with attaining full range (Fig. 11.18B).

Advantages
- Can be performed as a home exercise in multiple settings, including breaks from desk jobs.

Teaching tips
- Instruction example:
  - "Hold onto the side of your chair or tuck your hand under your thigh. Turn your head away from the side being stretched and gently nod your chin, dropping your nose toward your knee. Your opposite hand can be used to increase the stretch."
- Common error to correct:
  - Flexing the thoracic spine instead of the cervical region

Alternatives
- Therapist-assisted stretch in supine
- Contract-relax or hold-relax

Progression
- Increase time.
- Increase range.

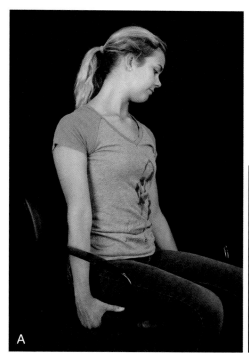
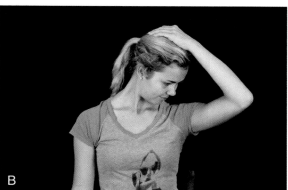

Fig. 11.18 Levator scapula stretch: the stretch can be performed with a strap or towel over upper trapezius region to limit rib elevation.

◎ CASE STUDY 11.1: CERVICAL MOBILITY DEFICITS WITH HEADACHES

This case illustrates the use of mobility exercises to address mobility impairments for a patient with headaches. Given symptoms that are moderately to highly severe, and highly irritable, this case study also presents the rationale behind the initial parameters and subsequent modifications to the parameters.

A 57-year-old man with a history of neck pain, stiffness, and headaches for more than 15 years is referred for treatment. His headaches are intermittent but can be debilitating. His work as an accountant requires sitting for long periods in front of the computer, which aggravates his neck pain. Driving for longer than an hour also results in increased neck pain. His hobbies include golf and cooking. There is no history of whiplash or other cervical trauma, and he has been cleared for other sources of headaches. Comorbidities include hypercholesterolemia and mild hypertension (without medication), but no other major medical history.

Functional Status and Goals

His neck pain is affecting his ability to work through the day, he is unable to play golf for more than nine holes, and the pain is affecting his social life. The headaches cause extreme pain and nausea, and he has had to miss work on at least 1 day a month in the past 6 months. Any unusual physical activity or prolonged sitting, particularly when looking down, increases neck pain and, at times, headaches. Neck Disability Index is 22/50. His goals are to return to playing golf, to be able to drive, and to tolerate sitting for longer than an hour at a time without the increased pain.

BOX 11.1   Interpretation of Subjective Information

The patient's symptoms are consistent with chronic neck pain with headaches.[14] His MODERATE TO SEVERE neck pain along with HIGHLY IRRITABLE and SEVERE headaches with nausea lasting for up to 24 hours require extreme caution with examination and treatment intensity.[16] His disability is also severe when he has headaches.[16,17] Prolonged sitting and computer work is a contributing factor[18] and indicate the need for evaluation of seated posture and any postural, range of motion, or muscle flexibility contributions.[18,19] Because lifting weights and overhead activities both increase his pain, exercises involving the upper extremity will be used with caution. Sustained flexion (and sitting) will be avoided for exercises early in the treatment process. Exercises will be discontinued or immediately adjusted with any increase in headaches during treatment. Pain and headache responses will be monitored after treatment and exercises progressed slowly until the irritability and frequency of headaches decreases.

Subjective Complaints

- *Severity*: He is unable to sit for more than 1 hour driving or at work without neck pain increasing to 3/10. He is unable to lift more than 5 pounds or use arms for prolonged periods without increasing pain to 5/10 (delayed onset 2–4 hours later). He is currently only sleeping for 3 hours without waking up; pain is worse when sleeping on side. Headaches vary; behind eyes or back of head with severity ranging from a dull ache (3/10) to severe (8/10) and are associated with nausea and inability to concentrate or function. He also reports muscle aching and stiffness in his upper back (Box 11.1).
- *Irritability*: Headaches are reproduced by lifting objects, using the upper extremity for overhead activities (prolonged or with weight), or prolonged seated activities and during periods of high work stress (computer, reading, writing). Although he is able to associate the increase in pain with lifting incidents, he cannot identify what causes his severe headaches. Pain and headaches typically present within 4–6 hours after lifting, while driving or prolonged overhead activities increases pain within 8 hours. His intermittent headaches will last up to 24 hours, limiting his ability to concentrate, work, or function. Tylenol or ice decrease the intensity of his neck pain, but not consistently.
- *Nature*: Cervical pain with headaches, no upper extremity symptoms
- *Stage*: Chronic, Phase II, worsening

Objective Findings

- *Posture and alignment*: Forward head, increased cervical lordosis, step-off at cervicothoracic junction, increased kyphosis, rounded shoulders
- *Range of motion*: See Table 11.3. Cervical range of motion is measured with a CROM device in erect sitting. Range of motion values differ when measured in erect compared to habitual postures, and measurement instructions should be consistent for re-evaluation.[20] Thoracic range of motion is measured with inclinometers. Active range of motion is measured with no overpressure due to severity and irritability of symptoms. Improvements (minimal detectable change [MDC]95: 95% certainty of real change) need to exceed 8 degrees for cervical rotation and lateral flexion, 10 degrees for flexion, and 8 degrees for extension.[20]
- *Muscle length*: Decreased flexibility of upper trapezius, scalenes, levator scapulae, and pectoralis major
- *Muscle function*: Activation: difficulty activating the deep neck flexors, craniocervical flexion test; only able to maintain 10 seconds at 22 mm Hg.[21,22]

TABLE 11.3   Range of Motion

	Cervical ROM (CROM)	Pain	Lumbothoracic ROM (Inclinometer)
Flex	0–45	Slight pulling pain	24 degrees, tight
Extension	0–15	Increases pain in the neck and head 3/10	10 degrees, stiff, tight
Lateral flex R	0–15	Tight on L, pain back of head and neck R	8 degrees, axis of motion at thoracolumbar junction
Lateral flex L	0–22	Tight on R	12 degrees, axis of motion at thoracolumbar junction
Rotation R	0–30	Pain on R	16 degrees, very limited if the head is stabilized
Rotation L	0–40	Tight on R	10 degrees, very limited if the head is stabilized

- *Special tests*: Upper cervical ligament stability tests, vertebral artery tests were negative (some increase in pain with full range.[23,24]
- *Palpation and joint play*: Upper to mid-thoracic joint mobility extremely limited in all directions, including costovertebral joints and first rib. Mid to lower cervical joint play decreased with soft tissue end feel in all directions. Cervical extension reproduced pain in the upper cervical area, occiput, and eyes (3/10). Cervical rotation and lateral flexion cause pain and tightness on the opposite side of the neck. Upper cervical region (C0–C1, C1–C2) relatively more mobile than all other cervical joints. Very restricted soft tissue mobility trapezius, scalenes, levator scalenes. Upper cervical muscle spasm and pain with palpation of soft tissue.

Evaluation

- *Medical diagnosis*: Chronic mechanical neck pain, neck pain with headaches[14,25–27]
- *Physical therapy diagnosis*: Chronic cervical pain with headaches and mobility deficits[14,25–27]
- *Contributing impairments*:
  - Increased thoracic kyphosis and cervical lordosis
  - Decreased joint range of motion (cervical and thoracic)
  - Muscle flexibility restrictions
  - Decreased joint mobility mid-cervical, lower cervical, upper thoracic, mid-thoracic, and costovertebral joints
  - Prolonged soft tissue restrictions related to desk work and driving
  - Limited cervical and thoracic extensor endurance, deep neck flexor activation and endurance
  - Relative increased mobility in upper cervical region

- *Other contributing factors:*
  - Prolonged work activities in sitting and computer work
  - Potential for aggravation of symptoms with movement toward the end of range, higher loads or other repetitive upper limb activities (see Box 11.2 for implications of evaluation for exercise choices).[28]

Precautions

- Care with prolonged stretching or high loads in upper cervical region (due to headaches with moderate to severe severity and irritability)
- Limit upper extremity load to less than 5 lb due to exacerbation of symptoms with upper extremity use.
- Avoid prolonged overhead upper extremity activity.
- Avoid sustained seated flexion or flexion exercises until severity and irritability has decreased.
- Stop and/or adjust exercise if any exacerbation of headaches.
- Monitor responses after treatment and exercise, especially headaches (Box 11.3).

Prognosis

Based on his age,[14,25,29] chronic neck pain history,[14,29] moderate to severe self-reported disability (30–50% is regarded as the range for severe disability[14,16]), and work requirements, the patient's prognosis for completely resolving pain and disability is only moderate. There is moderate evidence that mobility deficit impairments respond well to the combination of manual therapy and exercise,[14,25] with goals to exceed minimal detectable change of 6–10 degrees (see Table 11.3)[20] The patient's prognosis is negatively impacted by the presence of severe headaches[29]; while decreasing the intensity and frequency of

---

BOX 11.2 Implications of Evaluation for Exercise Choices

Generalized cervical and thoracic hypomobility and muscle flexibility limitations are the primary impairments. Exercise will be combined with joint mobilization because the combination of manual therapy and exercise has been found to be superior to either intervention alone.[26,30–34] In patients with chronic neck pain and headaches,[31] there is low-quality evidence of greater long-term pain reduction and function for combined management compared to no treatment, and high-quality evidence of superior short-term pain relief than for exercise alone, along with similar patient satisfaction, long-term pain relief, function, and patient-perceived effect and quality of life[26] compared to manipulative therapy, exercise, combined treatment, and no treatment. Both manipulative therapy and exercise resulted in a decreased frequency of headaches and reduced intensity of pain with moderate and clinically relevant effect sizes which lasted for 12 months. Approximately 10% of patients in the combined group gained more relief than either intervention alone, although the differences were not significant compared to the individual intervention groups.[26] In a systematic review and meta-analysis of seven randomized controlled trials, therapeutic exercise was found to have significant medium-sized effects on pain in the short and medium term, and medium effects on disability that were not significant.[35] In a systematic review that examined the parameters used for different studies using the FITT descriptors (frequency, intensity, time and type), the authors concluded that multimodal approaches were more beneficial for strength, function, and quality of life improvements.[36] In an update for the Bone and Joint Decade Task Force on Neck Pain, low-load endurance exercise for the craniocervical and cervicoscapular regions was recommended for episodic and chronic tension-type

or cervicogenic headaches, along with relaxation training or multimodal care including spinal mobilization, exercise, and postural correction.[34]

Excessive or localized force in the upper cervical region could exacerbate headaches and therefore should be avoided. Supportive positions are preferred initially, and manual therapy should be followed by active mobility exercises to reinforce joint mobility improvements. Postural position is likely to impact the overall forces concentrating in the upper cervical region, and improvements in thoracic spine[37] and mid-cervical mobility[38] may assist with distribution of forces. After range has improved, muscle function will need to be retrained to support the cervicothoracic spinal segments and absorb some of the forces required for both prolonged positional tasks and to withstand load from upper extremity movements for golf and other activities of daily living.[28]

Specific muscle activation of the deep neck flexors and extensors will be included in the exercise program, with early exercise parameters including support and midrange positions to limit stress and pain.[28] The exercises will start with head props to accommodate his forward head position and a towel under the neck to support cervical lordosis. Soft tissue mobilization will precede gentle stretching, which should begin with the therapist providing the stretch while supporting the cervical spine and proximal origins of the muscle. Stretching exercises will start in supine to support the head weight and avoid excessive shear forces in the upper cervical region. While endurance and strength are required for the cervical muscles,[39] these goals will be delayed until the neuromuscular coordination and sequencing has improved, range has increased, and pain severity/irritability (especially headaches) has improved.

headaches is feasible, complete resolution is not necessarily expected. He does have a positive outlook and is motivated to return to work. Changes of between 5 and 10 points in the Neck Disability Index (NDI) are needed to exceed the minimum clinically important difference.[14,16]

Treatment and Exercise Choices

1. *Manual therapy*: Mobilization: mid- and upper thoracic region and costovertebral joints (posterior-anterior glides), lower and mid-cervical mobilization (manual traction-gapping, anterior-posterior and lateral glides), first and second rib mobilization (see Box 11.3).

2. *Soft tissue mobilization*: Lower cervical and lateral soft tissue mobilization, trapezius, scalenes, and rhomboids (proximal origins are stabilized by the therapist's hands and distal insertions are stretched by the therapist to avoid excessive force on the cervical region, specifically the upper cervical region).

3. Initial exercise choices following soft tissue and joint mobilization are presented in Table 11.4, and modifications and choices affected by the severity and irritability are presented in Box 11.3.

BOX 11.3   Modifications and Choices Due to Moderate to High Severity and Irritability

- Perform exercises in supine to limit forces on the cervical region.
- While the mobility exercises are intended to increase range in the lower cervical region, avoid sustained holds and excessive forces, especially in the upper cervical region. Closely monitor the upper cervical spine position to avoid excessive stress that may provoke headaches.
- Monitor pain severity during (and after) treatment.
- Delay introducing the following exercises until after headache intensity and irritability has decreased:
  - *Upper trapezius stretch*: Muscle attachments in the upper cervical region may cause stress and exacerbate headaches.
  - *Rhomboid strengthening*: Address thoracic spine hypomobility and forward head position first. Scapula retraction does not correct a kyphotic position if there is insufficient thoracic spine mobility. A forward head posture and thoracic kyphosis places levator scapulae and trapezius in relatively stretched position, and retracting the scapula without correcting the head position is likely to further increase the tension and stress on the cervical

region. Once mobility and postural position has improved, thoracic and cervical extension muscle endurance can be challenged using scapulothoracic and upper extremity exercise using mechanics described in Chapter 10.
  - *Prone cervical extension*: Lacking as the patient lacks adequate thoracic mobility, prone lower cervical extension is likely to place excessive force on the upper cervical region. The cervical extensor muscle activation will be introduced after some mobility has been restored.[28]
- Evaluation of functional activities and impairments is delayed until severity and irritability has decreased:[28]
- Dynamic postural control (prolonged seated activities, prolonged upper extremity activities)
- Prolonged specific muscle endurance (cervical flexors and extensors) against gravity or with load[28,39]
- Scapulothoracic function during upper extremity elevation
- Scapulothoracic function during functional tasks involving load
- Functional activities mimicking golf or lifting

TABLE 11.4   Exercise Choices, Positions, Parameters, and Modifications: Cervical Mobility Deficits and Headaches

Exercise	Position	Parameters	Monitoring During Exercise, Modifications	Rationale and Goals
Cervical retraction (Exercise 11.1)	Supine	Gentle, mid to end range, multiple (15+ repetitions)	Avoid any reproduction of headaches, upper or mid-cervical pain Localize motion to lower cervical region Avoid excessive flexion in upper cervical region and monitor for stress	Supported position limits pressure on cervical joints. Improve lower cervical mobility.
Cervical lateral flexion (Exercise 11.2)	Supine	Reach end range, multiple reps	Towel roll under cervical lordosis, small flat pillow, initially to support head Establish deep neck flexor activation prior to laterally flexing the mid to lower region Therapist provides hands-on feedback	Promote joint mobility without joint compression in a supported position.
Cervical rotation (Exercise 11.3)	Supine	Toward end range, multiple reps	Towel roll under lordosis, small flat pillow to support head Deep neck flexor activation prior to rotation of mid to lower region Therapist assists with localizing movement until the patient is able to monitor the exercise independently	Promote joint mobility without joint compression in supported position. Activate deep neck flexors to promote rotation around a supported axis of motion and distribute forces throughout multiple areas.

TABLE 11.4 Exercise Choices, Positions, Parameters, and Modifications: Cervical Mobility Deficits and Headaches—cont'd

Exercise	Position	Parameters	Monitoring During Exercise, Modifications	Rationale and Goals
Thoracic extension (Exercise 11.5)	Supine	Reach end range but short hold, to tolerance, multiple breaks	Supine over the BOSU with the head supported with both hands, extension Pillow support for the head Adjust the positioning to avoid any discomfort in cervical region Adjust the range if patient reports discomfort or pain within 6 hours of treatment	The supine supported position provides gravity assistance for relatively passive mobility and decreases need for adjustments in multiple regions. Pillow support for the head is used until soft tissue and joint mobility improves enough to allow head to rest on floor without tension.
Pectoralis stretching (Exercise 10.8)	Supine	To limit of flexibility without thoracic or cervical motion or stress from hands	No pressure on head	Supine, supported position decreases need for adjustments in multiple regions and limits compensations in head and neck often observed in sitting or standing.
Deep cervical neck flexor activation (Exercise 11.19)	Supine, using a blood pressure cuff	Only to point of pain exacerbation	Watch for excessive retraction and overuse of superficial muscles.	Activate the deep neck flexors to initiate neuromuscular training.

SECTION 11.2: HYPERMOBILITY

GENERAL EXERCISE APPROACHES

The description of hypermobility is used as a comparison to the hypomobility impairments to assist with the understanding of exercise concepts to provide active neuromuscular control in the midrange and toward end range when the ligamentous or structural restraint systems are not providing sufficient support. The ICD diagnosis classifications using the description of "instability" fall into this category, as do those with generalized and specific laxity.[14,15] The Low Back Pain Clinical Guidelines describe management for individuals with instability or hypermobility for patients with acute, subacute, or chronic low back pain with movement coordination impairments.[15] In the 2017 Neck Pain guidelines, neck pain with movement coordination impairments also encompasses whiplash injuries.[14] A comparison of the symptoms and examination findings for individuals with neck or back pain for the mobility categories is presented in Table 11.5.

The classification systems also include neck pain with headaches, neck pain or low back pain with radiating (radicular) pain, low back pain with related cognitive and affective tendencies. The low back pain guidelines are expanded to include the stage of recovery. The neck pain guidelines do not include a separate category for the cognitive and affective tendencies, while neck pain with headaches can overlap the mobility category and the neuromuscular coordination category.

The overall exercise goal for individuals with regional or general hypermobility is to promote force closure (neuromuscular control and muscle function) to distribute forces by initiating muscle activation in a coordinated manner, thus developing muscle endurance and strength. Neuromuscular coordination requires addressing appropriate muscle imbalances. In the spine, hypermobility can be related to generalized connective tissue laxity (e.g., Ehlers-Danlos syndrome, genetic hypermobility) or as a secondary consequence of degenerative disc disease with disc space narrowing. However, specific or relative hypermobility is also possible when there are regions of hypermobility related to concentration of forces such as at the transition between major curvatures or from repeated movement patterns with high loads and strain at the axis of motion or when other regional impairments such as decreased flexibility of global muscles may also concentrate forces in the hypermobile region. In situations where hypermobility and hypomobility exist together, hypermobility guidelines will take precedence to protect symptomatic structures during exercise. However, impairments in other regions contributing

TABLE 11.5   Comparison of Examination Findings for Hypomobility/Mobility Deficits and Hypermobility/Neuromuscular Coordination Deficits

Neck[14]	Low Back[15]
Hypomobility/Mobility Deficits	
Subjective Symptoms	
• Central/unilateral neck pain often associated with referred pain in the shoulder girdle or upper extremity • Range of motion limitations and reports of stiffness (reproduce symptoms)	• Central/unilateral low back pain often associated with referred pain in the lower extremity • Range of motion limitations and reports of stiffness (reproduce symptoms)
Objective Examination	
• Limited cervical range of motion • Neck and/or referred pain reproduced at end of active and passive range and with segmental provocation tests • Decreased cervical and thoracic segmental mobility • Decreased cervicoscapulothoracic endurance, strength, diminished neuromotor coordination	• Limited lumbar range of motion • Lumbar pain and/or referred pain reproduced at end of active and passive range and with segmental provocation tests • Decreased lumbar and low thoracic segmental mobility • Decreased lumbar endurance, strength, diminished neuromotor coordination
Hypermobility/Neuromuscular Coordination Deficits	
Subjective Symptoms	
• Acute, subacute, or chronic neck pain often associated with referred pain in the upper extremity (no neurological symptoms) • Possibility of dizziness/nausea • Possibility of headaches, difficulty concentrating, hypersensitivity to stimuli • Possible mechanism related to trauma	• Acute, subacute or chronic low back pain often associated with referred pain in the lower extremity (no neurological symptoms) • Symptoms reproduced or increased with end range movement
Objective Examination	
• Symptoms reproduced or increased with end range movement • Symptoms reproduced with provocation of spinal segments • Segmental instability may be present • Decreased neck flexor or extensor or muscle endurance or strength • Movement coordination impairments • Sensorimotor impairment (including proprioceptive deficits and hypersensitivity reproduced with pressure algometry)	• Symptoms reproduced or increased with end range movement • Symptoms reproduced with provocation of spinal segments • Segmental instability may be present • Decreased trunk or pelvic muscle endurance or strength • Movement coordination impairments

Data from Gross AR, et al.[14] and Delitto A, et al.[15]

to the accumulation of forces are also included in the treatment plan, and often joint mobilization or specific mobility exercises that do not stress the hypermobile areas are important. Hypermobility impairments may be present with repetitive strain category or after surgical intervention has occurred. The types of exercise used for hypermobility are described in

Chapter 6, and the comparison between parameters used for hypomobility and hypermobility is included in Table 6.4. A review of the goals, methods, parameters, and measurements is shown in Table 11.6.

In the cervical region there is moderate evidence that patients with acute movement coordination impairments may benefit

TABLE 11.6 Goals, Methods, Parameters, and Measurement: Hypermobility

Goals	Methods	Parameters	Assessment/Measurement
Initiate muscle activation of local stabilizers and improve neuromuscular timing	Promote muscle activation, early timing of stabilizing muscles, and neuromuscular control using motor control principles[40–45] Closed chain Multiple forms of sensory input (visual, tactile, verbal cueing) Use balance responses or oscillations to promote muscle activation and alternating contractions	Supported positions progressing to unsupported Inner to midrange for specific instability, midrange for generalized instability or hypermobility[14,15] Anticipatory sequencing muscle activation: local stabilizers precede global movers[41,44] Multiple repetitions with adequate rest *OR* alternating movement High repetition or prolonged hold with specificity of contractions Parameters progressed based on motor learning to maintain position or control of range without exacerbation of symptoms	Ability to maintain position and axis of motion (observation of neuromuscular coordination or time held in position) Analysis of biomechanics for distribution of forces (visual analysis of timing, axis of motion) Ability to hold isometric contractions (timed) or number of repetitions Pain responses Amount of feedback and correction needed
Improve ability to maintain midrange joint position; muscle endurance	Isometrics Small range isotonics Promote neuromuscular control using motor control principles Closed chain and multiple forms of sensory input (visual, tactile, balance))	Progression from isometrics to multiple-angle isometrics to controlled small-range isotonics Prolonged contraction for isometrics Low load, progressing to load as tolerated High repetition for small range isotonics Use of local or global stabilizers	Ability to maintain scapulothoracic connection and glenohumeral axis of motion (observation of neuromuscular coordination or time held in position) Analysis of biomechanics for distribution of forces (visual analysis of timing, axis of motion) Ability to hold isometric contractions (timed) or number of repetitions Achieving a targeted position for a length of time Amount of feedback and correction needed Pain responses Functional tasks requiring sustained positioning Oswestry, NDI
Improve ability to withstand external forces and avoid reaching extreme end range	Promote neuromuscular control using motor control principles Multiple forms of sensory input Progress to eccentric control	Slow progression into controlled end range Eccentric control to limit end range Progress to higher loads, low repetitions (isometric or isotonic)	Achievement of targets (% of successful trials) Amount of feedback and correction needed Functional outcome measures: self-reports (NDI, Oswestry, Patient Specific Functional Scale) or objective measures such as lifting tolerance, sit-to-stand tests, squats
Improve neuromuscular coordination and response time for functional requirements	Promote neuromuscular control using motor control principles	Reaction time and controlled movement	Achievement of targets Amount of feedback and correction needed Speed: change of positions, weight transfer or weight transference for single-leg stance, standing lunge tests, lower extremity symmetry and balance tests)

from education and reassurance of recovery and from multimodal interventions including exercise (muscle endurance and strengthening, flexibility, postural reeducation, coordination, aerobic and functional training) and manual therapy.[14] There is weak evidence that patients with chronic movement coordination deficits will benefit from the same combination of education, mobilization, and exercise (including progressive submaximal muscle endurance, strengthening, flexibility, coordination), along with cognitive behavioral therapy if needed.[14] The Low Back Pain guidelines published in 2012 found strong evidence that patients who fit the neuromuscular coordination impairments practice pattern may benefit from trunk muscle coordination, endurance, and strengthening exercise for subacute and chronic conditions (including those patients who have had microdiscectomy).[15]

General exercise concepts for neuromuscular coordination exercises include:

1. Initiate muscle activation of local stabilizers in neutral or midrange of joints, progressing to global stabilizers *OR* position that is least painful.
2. Progress from supported to unsupported positions.
3. Challenge spinal position with upper extremity or lower extremity motion using anticipatory spinal position control prior to limb motion or balance responses.
4. Provide additional sensory feedback (taping, visual input, tactile).
5. Oscillatory challenges, isometrics, small-range motion, and unstable surfaces provide opportunities to initiate neuromuscular control and protective neuromuscular reactions of the stabilizing muscles.
6. Promote distribution of forces throughout the spine and emphasize use of lower extremities for functional activities.
7. Teach stabilization, neuromuscular control, and coordination of the spine to withstand external loads.
8. Modify activities of daily living and movement transitions, including weight transfer in standing.
9. Monitor for exacerbation of local, neurological, or referred symptoms as well as loss of neuromuscular control or coordination (fatigue, compensations).

See Magee,[1] Magee and Sueki,[23] and Cleland[24] for more detailed description of available tests and measures, interpretation, and psychometric properties.

CONTRAINDICATIONS AND PRECAUTIONS

Specific precautions are also listed with individual exercises (see Magee[1] for precautions and contraindications related to red and yellow flags).

- Intensity, difficulty, and level of exercise depends on severity, irritability, and if the symptoms are acute.
- Protect passive structures from excessive stress or strain; limit end ranges and amount of stress.
- Avoid excessive range (may be specific direction).
- No stretching.
- Pain responses and muscle spasm can mask underlying hypermobility; caution with active range of motion control may be necessary once pain decreases.
- Sensory input is often impaired with hypermobility, and patients may not be able to monitor position or range limits without additional feedback (tactile, verbal, or visual).
- Ligamentous laxity, previous whiplash or trauma, and presence of symptoms indicating neural compromise indicate the need for ligament stability tests prior to exercise. Any indications of possible vertebral artery symptoms or for patients at risk of vertebral artery compromise should also be screened prior to treatment.

COMPENSATIONS AND TOLERANCE OF STABILITY EXERCISE

- The primary objective is to provide active neuromuscular support in the area of concern. It is also important to observe and maintain overall alignment at proximal and distal areas influencing the forces on the joint.
- Observe for loss of position or muscle activation with fatigue.
- Use supported positions (prone, supine, side-lying, four-point kneeling over an exercise ball) if the patient is unable to control multiple regions with adequate neuromuscular coordination or if there is a need for additional proprioceptive input.
- Ask patients to report any discomfort during and after the exercise.
- Use additional sensory and proprioceptive input to limit compensations.

EXERCISES

EXERCISE DESCRIPTIONS

LOCAL STABILIZER ACTIVATION TO SUPPORT A NEUTRAL OR MID-POSITION LORDOSIS

11.19.   Local Stabilizer Activation: Neutral Cervical Lordosis

See Fig. 11.19.

Purpose
- Activate local stabilizers and improve kinesthetic awareness of mid-cervical position

Position
- Supine, head supported, if needed, particularly with forward head or thoracic kyphosis postures
- Place a partially inflated blood pressure cuff under the cervical spine to provide feedback (tactile and visual) (Fig. 11.19A).

Action (Video 11.19)
1. Activate the deep neck flexors by gently nodding the head, dropping the chin downward (upper and mid cervical flexion) toward the mid-position of the cervical lordosis.
2. The pressure in the cuff should increase by 2 mm Hg.
3. Maintain the pressure at the new reading, using the gauge to provide feedback.

Advantages
- Head is supported in the supine position.
- Blood pressure cuff provides feedback to teach kinesthetic awareness of neutral cervical position and motor control.

Teaching tips
- Instruction examples:

- "Drop your focus slightly on the ceiling, then maintain the position, keeping the needle on the pressure gauge (on the blood pressure cuff) still. Release. Try to reproduce the movement so that you get a similar reading on the gauge."
- "Nod your chin slightly and lengthen the neck gently into the cuff."
- Common errors to correct:
  - Avoid full flattening of the cervical spine or maximal upper cervical flexion.
  - Avoid excessive use of global muscles to substitute for the local stabilizers (sternocleidomastoid) to create the cervical flexion.
  - Watch for excessive tension in the trapezius, pectoralis, or sternocleidomastoid. If the patient has a thoracic kyphosis or forward head, small props can be used to decrease muscle tension.

Alternatives
- Use towel rolls to support lordosis instead of blood pressure cuff as a progression or if blood pressure cuff is not available.
- Use a partially deflated ball to provide an unstable surface.

Progression
- After correct muscle activation has been achieved, progress to multiple repetitions with short holds, followed by maintaining the position for prolonged periods of time.
- Progress to maintaining the head and cervical position while challenging with arm movements (Fig. 11.19C, D).
- Add weights to the arm movements to challenge stability of the head and cervical position (Fig. 11.19C, D).
- Use an unstable surface such as a partially inflated ball. (Fig. 11.19E).

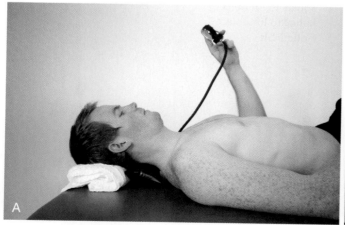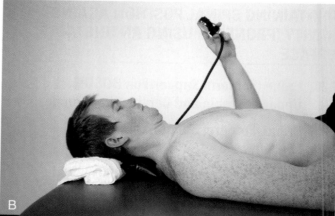

Fig. 11.19 (A and B) Use of a blood pressure cuff to monitor position of neutral cervical lordosis with deep neck flexor activation.

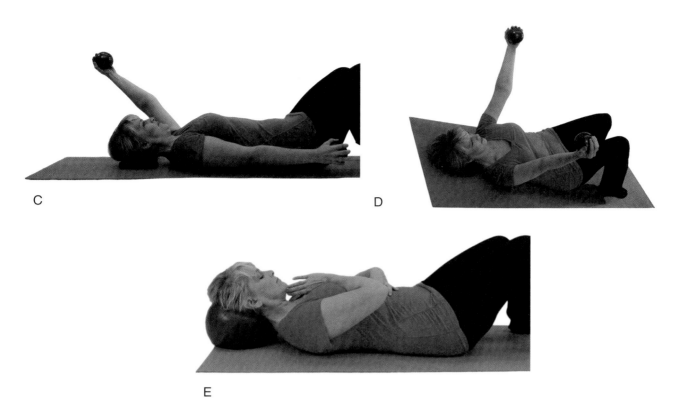

C

D

E

Fig. 11.19, Cont'd Challenge for maintaining a neutral cervical position with upper extremity movement (C and D) or using a partially inflated ball (E).

11.20. Local Stabilizer Activation: Neutral Lumbar Lordosis

See Fig. 11.20.

Purpose

- Engage deep stabilizing muscles in a mid-position (deep transverse abdominals, deep local extensors)

Position

- Supine, hips and knees flexed in hook-lying position, feet hip distance apart (Fig. 11.20A)
- Head supported to minimize stress on cervical and thoracic region

Action

1. Tilt the pelvis back and forward to find a neutral lumbar mid-position.
2. Monitor for neutral alignment of the lumbopelvic region mid-way between a full anterior and posterior tilt position. The pubic symphysis and anterior superior iliac spines should be in the same horizontal plane (Fig. 11.20B).
3. Engage the deep transverse abdominals by gently flattening the abdominal wall " like a corset" from the spine toward the midline of the abdominal wall (Fig. 11.20C).
4. Engage the pelvic floor muscles to assist creating support for the entire lumbopelvic "box" or container (Fig. 11.20D).
5. Challenge maintaining the position and awareness of the lumbopelvic position during inhalation and exhalation. The rib cage expansion and diaphragmatic action should not influence the lumbar spine position (Fig. 11.20 E).

Advantages

- Supported position, so patient does not need to maintain balance or upright position
- The sacrum provides tactile feedback to help develop awareness of the neutral lumbar position

Teaching tips

- Instruction examples:
  - To find neutral lumbar position: "Rock your pelvis back and forth until you find a position somewhere in between all the way flat and fully arched, and a point where your pelvis is level."
  - "You should have a small space under your lower back and some weight across your sacrum."
- To engage the transverse abdominal muscles: "Without moving your spine, compress your abdominals, as if creating an hourglass shape with your waist."
- "Deepen your abdominal and pelvic floor muscle contractions toward the center of your spine."
- To engage the pelvic floor:
- "Think about the pelvic floor as the bottom of a box, lift the muscles gently. If you were in an elevator you would be lifting up one floor, not all the way to the top floor."
- " Think about walking into a cold lake, the pelvic floor and abdominal muscles pull toward the center of your body."
- "If you had to stop a stream of urine, the same muscles help with supporting your spine."
- Common errors to correct:
  - Using the superficial muscles (typically the rectus abdominis) without the transversus abdominis, will result in the abdomen bulging rather than flattening.
  - Avoid using the hip extensor muscles to move the pelvis and completely flattening the lumbar spine.
- Method to address or prevent compensations:
  - The patient can use the hands on the pelvis or under the lumbar spine to help develop positional awareness of the neutral lumbar spine position.

Alternatives

- A blood pressure cuff placed under the lumbar spine can be used to reflect the degree of engagement and ability to maintain the neutral lumbar position.
- The legs can be supported on a bolster or exercise ball if the patient is working extremely hard to support the leg weight.
- Four-point kneeling can be used to encourage abdominal activation to lift the weight of the abdomen, especially when lying supine is not possible, such as after the second trimester during pregnancy (Video 6.16).

Progression

- Once the patient is activating the muscles correctly, advance to multiple repetitions with short holds, followed by maintaining the position for prolonged periods of time.
- Progress to maintaining active force closure with leg challenges or arm challenges (Exercise 11.21 or 11.22).
- Progress to finding the neutral lordosis in four-point kneeling, sitting, or standing and incorporating before and during movements such as forward hinging (Fig. 11.20F).

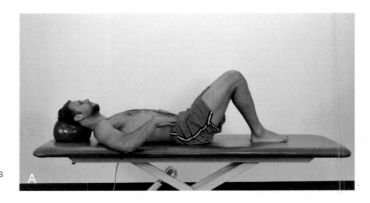

Fig. 11.20 (A) Neutral lumbar lordosis and activation of stabilizing muscles is easiest to teach in supine.

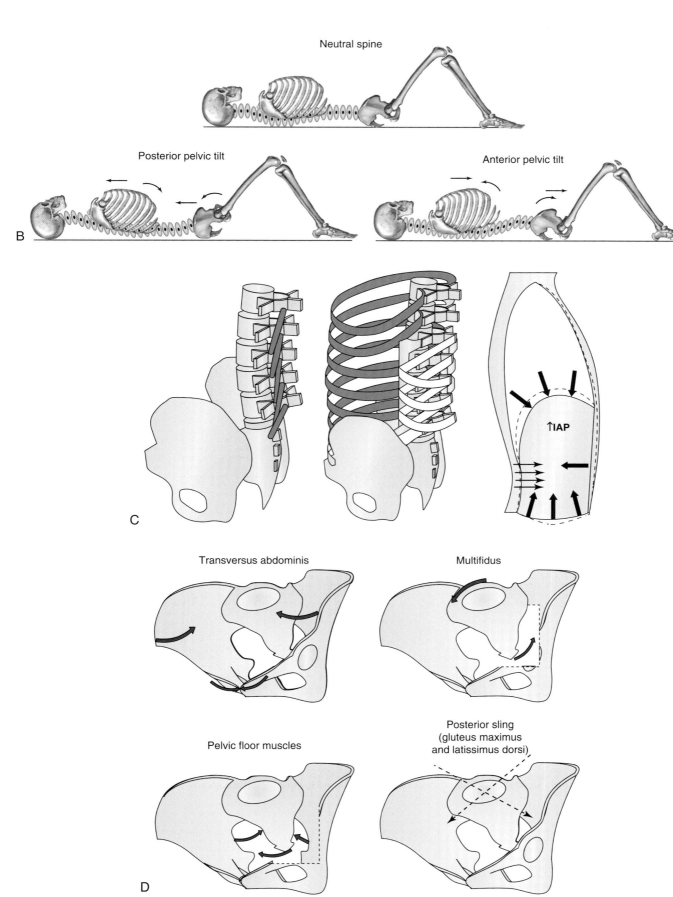

Fig. 11.20, cont'd Pelvic tilting to find a mid-position neutral spine (B), with illustrations of the contributions of the abdominal muscles, spinal extensors, diaphragm and fascia (C), pelvic floor, and gluteal muscles (D). (C to E courtesy of Professor Paul Hodges, The University of Queensland.)

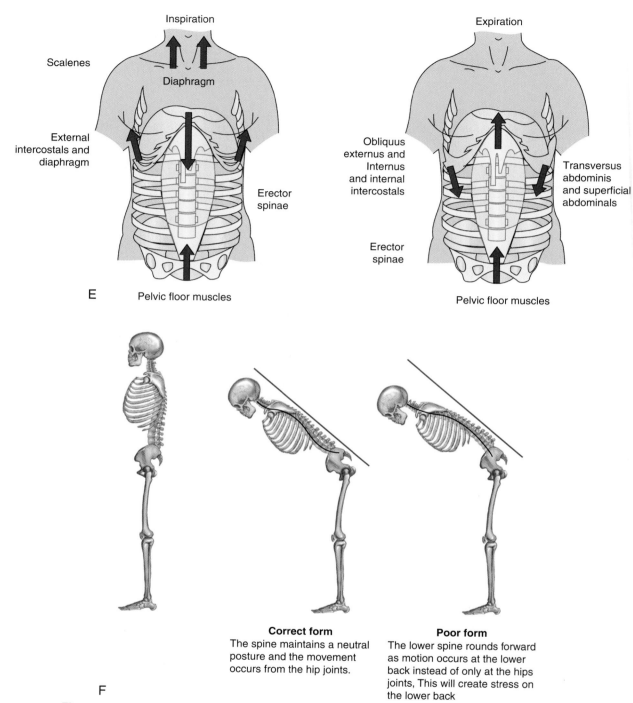

E

Inspiration

Scalenes

Diaphragm

External intercostals and diaphragm

Erector spinae

Pelvic floor muscles

Expiration

Obliquus externus and Internus and internal intercostals

Transversus abdominis and superficial abdominals

Erector spinae

Pelvic floor muscles

Correct form
The spine maintains a neutral posture and the movement occurs from the hip joints.

Poor form
The lower spine rounds forward as motion occurs at the lower back instead of only at the hips joints, This will create stress on the lower back

F

Fig. 11.20, cont'd (E) The intrabdominal pressure and overall stability is also affected by the thoracic pressures, diaphragm movement, and spinal movements. (F) Teaching the patient to maintain muscle support should be progressed to activation and support before and during movement.

CHALLENGES TO MAINTAIN NEUTRAL POSITION

11.21. Lower Extremity Challenge for Neutral Spine: Supine Leg Lifts

See Fig. 11.21.

Purpose
- Improve spinal stabilizer neuromuscular control and coordination (muscle timing and sequencing)

Position
- Supine
- Hips and knees flexed in hook-lying, feet hip-width apart
- Head is supported to minimize stress on the cervical and thoracic region

Action
1. Activate the deep stabilizing muscles in the lumbar region (see Exercise 11.20) and cervical region (Exercise 11.19).
2. Once neutral position is established, lift one leg from the floor, maintaining the lumbopelvic and spinal position (Fig. 11.21A; Video 11.21A).
3. Return to the floor, reset stabilizing muscles, and lift opposite leg.

Advantages
- Stable, supported position for the spine
- The weight of the leg and hip flexors pulling on the lumbar spine can result in spinal rotation if the transverse abdominals and obliques are not adequately opposing the movement. The patient should be able to monitor and correct the activation to oppose the load.

Teaching tips
- Instruction example:
  - "Stabilize your pelvis using your deep abdominal muscles."
  - See instructions for Exercises 11.19 and 11.20.
- Common error to correct:
  - Observe the abdominal muscles to ensure that the transversus abdominis stays active when the leg lifts occur. If the abdomen bulges out when trying to support the weight of the lifted leg, the lumbopelvic area has limited support from the "corset" of the deep muscles.
- Methods to address or prevent compensations:
  - At first, the patient may need to gently press his or her arms and/or the opposite foot into the ground before starting to lift the foot off the ground for additional feedback and muscle support.

- An inflated blood pressure cuff can be placed under the lordosis to monitor position and provide visual feedback.
- The therapist can place a hand underneath the lordosis for tactile feedback, instructing the patient to "avoid lifting your lower back away from my hand as you lift your leg."
- Emphasize that the transverse abdominal contraction should occur prior to the leg lift. The timing of the therapist's instructions should reinforce the sequence of events: "Engage your abdominals and *then* lift one leg."
- The patient can use the hands on the front of the pelvis and abdomen to monitor pelvic rotation (Videos 11.21B and 6.17).
- The goal of this exercise is to stabilize the lumbopelvic region against the weight of the lifted leg. Emphasize the importance of stability before mobility: "Think more about keeping your spine supported actively than what is moving."

Alternatives
- Support one or both legs on a large bolster or on an exercise ball to decrease range of the leg lift and the leverage created by the weight of the leg and the pull from the hip flexor (Fig. 11.21B, C; Video 6.17).
- Repeat the exercise with the same leg rather than alternating legs to decrease the challenge of rapid changes in activation from side to side.
- Use a strap behind the leg to assist with lifting or lowering to decrease forces from the leg weight

Progression
- Increase the speed of alternating movements.
- Increase the number of repetitions.
- Progress to lifting one leg, deepen the abdominal contraction, then lift the second leg to hold both legs in the air (Fig. 11.21D; Video 11.21B).
- Lift the arms while lifting one or both legs to the 90-degree position. This will increase the challenge to stabilize the lumbosacral area by decreasing upper extremity support.
- Alternating bicycle with head support (Exercise 11.23)
- Upper extremity challenge for neutral spine on the foam roller (Exercise 11.22)

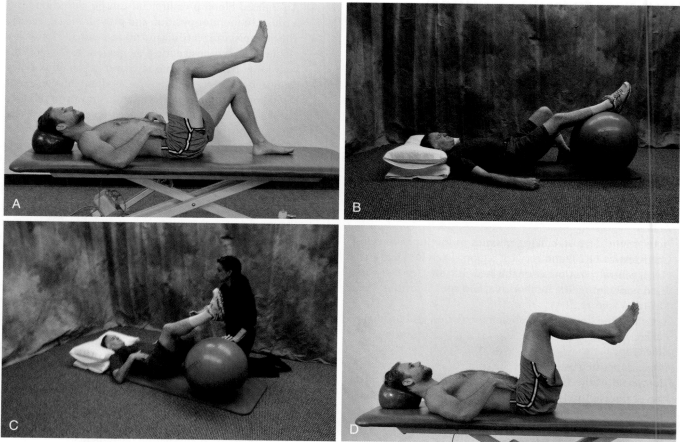

Fig. 11.21 Lower extremity challenge for neutral spine with single-leg lifts to 90 degrees of hip flexion (A), exercise ball roll-outs if the patient is having difficulty with the leg lift (B), progression to leg lifts off the ball (C), or sequential leg lifts to both legs in the air (D).

11.22. Upper Extremity Challenge for Neutral Spine on Foam Roller: Arm Movements

See Fig. 11.22.

Purpose
- Challenge the ability to maintain neutral spine position
- Promote spinal stabilizer control
- Spinal muscle neuromuscular coordination
- Spinal muscle endurance

Precautions
- Place the foam roller on a stable surface.
- Use caution and guard the patient if the foam roller is used on a raised surface such as a treatment table.
- Patients may be hesitant to lie on the foam roller and require assistance to slowly recline or roll onto the roller.

Position
- Lying supine on the foam roller, legs are hip-width apart, feet on the floor (Fig. 11.22A)
- Small pillow or towel under the head, if needed, to support head position

Action
1. Activate deep stabilizing muscles in the cervical region (Exercise 11.19) and lumbar region (Exercise 11.20).
2. Once neutral position has been established and set, lift upper extremities into slight scaption.
3. Connect the scapula to the thoracic spine using upward rotation (Exercise 10.14).
4. Alternate shoulder flexion and extension in the scaption plane or elbow flexion and extension in small ranges while maintaining spinal position (Fig. 11.22B)

Advantages
- The unstable surface and alternating arm movement facilitates rapid and timely stabilizing postural muscle function.
- The unstable surface also provides immediate feedback if excessive motion occurs.

Teaching tips
- Instruction example:
  - "Lift your arms toward the ceiling, scooping up from the shoulder blades keeping your hands wide apart. Once you feel stable, try scissoring one arm up overhead and the other arm down toward your hips."

Alternatives
- Perform alternating arm motion without the foam roller if the patient lacks the agility to safely mount the foam roller or balance reactions
- Progress from a half foam roller (flat side down for less challenge), to a half foam roller (flat side up for more challenge), to a full foam roller.
- Ipsilateral upper extremity movement: one arm moves through flexion and extension while the opposite side is held stationary.

Progression
- Increase arm range of motion.
- Increase speed of alternating motion.
- Use small hand weights.
- Asymmetrical challenge: use a weight in one hand.

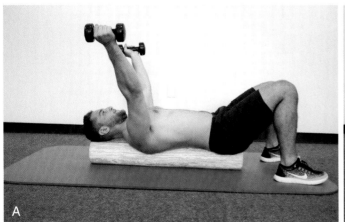
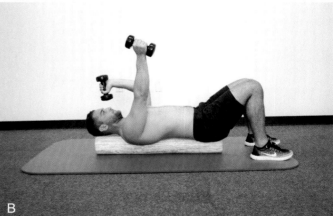

Fig. 11.22 (A and B) Upper extremity challenge for neutral spine on foam roller.

11.23.   Bicycling with Head Support

See Fig. 11.23.

Purpose

- Challenges the ability to maintain spinal position and spinal stabilizer control with additional challenge from leg weight and alternating motion

Position

- Supine, hips and knees flexed, feet hip-width apart.
- Head supported to minimize stress on cervical and thoracic region

Action

1. Activate deep stabilizing muscles in the lumbar (Exercise 11.20) and cervical regions (Exercise 11.19).
2. Once neutral position has been established, lift one leg from the floor while maintaining spinal position.
3. Deepen the abdominal contraction and lift the opposite leg without excessive movement of the lumbopelvic position.
4. Once able to maintain the position, extend the hip and knee of one leg, and then return to the starting position (90 degrees hip and knee flexion) (Fig. 11.23).
5. Repeat on the other side.
6. Alternate leg motion as long as lumbopelvic position is maintained.
7. Return to the floor, one foot at a time, while maintaining lumbopelvic stability.

Advantages

- Spinal stabilization requiring higher level of abdominal activation to support spine is challenged by the weight of the lower extremity weight.

Teaching tips

- Instruction examples:
  - "Deepen your abdominal contraction as you reach out your leg. The further away you reach your leg, the more your abdominals have to work to support the weight of your leg."
  - To assume starting position: "Press one foot into the ground, then lift the other leg off the ground without allowing your low back to move."
  - "Stabilize your spine before you move your leg."

Alternatives

- Ipsilateral movement with increased support: use exercise ball or bolster to support the leg that is moving.
- Ipsilateral movement: only extend one leg while other remains stable (on the ground or off the ground).
- Decrease the range by not fully extending the leg to decrease the length of the lever arm.

Progression

- Increase speed of movement.
- Increase length of time with both legs in the air.
- Increase range of extremity motion.
- Reciprocal leg movement: one leg is flexing while the other leg is extending.

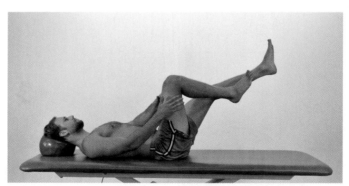

Fig. 11.23 Bicycling action with head support, alternating legs while maintaining lumbar spine position.

CLOSED CHAIN LEG EXERCISES WITH A STABLE LUMBOPELVIC REGION

Closed chain exercises may be indicated for patients who require additional lower extremity muscle force closure (particularly hip muscle strengthening) or who need to train symmetrical weight-bearing with lumbopelvic control. Patients with low back pain often present with hip weakness resulting in increased motion or concentration of forces in the lumbar spine during movements. Closed chain strengthening helps train the neuromuscular coordination needed for functional activities. Bilateral leg isometric activity in closed chain positions is also a possible starting point for patients with sacroiliac joint hypermobility.

11.24. Bilateral Hip Abduction with External Rotation: Elastic Resistance Band

See Fig. 11.24.

> *Purpose*
- Challenge the ability to maintain spinal position and spinal stabilizer control
- Activate and strengthen bilateral hip abductors and external rotators, distribute forces, and support the lumbosacral, sacroiliac, and pelvic complex

> *Position*
- Supine, hips and knees flexed in hook-lying, feet hip-width apart (Fig. 11.24A)
- Elastic band is tied around upper thigh with some tension on the band (Fig. 11.24A, B).
- Head is supported to minimize stress on cervical and thoracic region (Fig. 11.24A).

> *Action (Video 11.24A)*
1. Activate the deep stabilizing muscles in the lumbar region (Exercise 11.20).
2. Once neutral position is established and set, abduct and externally rotate hips against elastic band.
3. The position can be held isometrically or moved through a small range.

> *Advantages*
- Bilateral leg muscle activity promotes overall stabilization and is useful for generalized hypermobility and pelvic hypermobility (such as postpartum).
- Bilateral leg muscle activity places less asymmetrical shear stress on the pelvis than unilateral challenges.
- Closed chain position increases proprioceptive input, and the elastic resistance provides additional feedback for muscle recruitment and stabilization.
- External rotator activation is particularly important when addressing sacroiliac joint hypermobility or when hip or lower extremity stabilization is also needed.

> *Teaching tips*
- Instruction examples:
  - "Think about keeping your spine and pelvis still before and during the leg movement. Build up the resistance slowly without letting the spine move."
  - "Push your thighs into the band without letting your spine move."
- Common error to correct:
  - Watch for lumbopelvic rotation. This often occurs if the patient initiates the movement with one leg before the other or is not moving symmetrically and evenly with both legs.
- Method to address or prevent compensations:
  - Remind the patient that while she can feel the hip muscles working against the band, the primary intent of the exercise is to stabilize the spine.

> *Alternatives*
- Isometric adduction against a small ball between the legs provides a similar centralized stabilization.

> *Progression*
- Increase dosage (reps, sets, hold for isometric contractions).
- Increase band resistance.
- Perform the movement with one leg while stabilizing with the other leg (Video 11.24B).
- Standing with isometric hip abduction and external rotation against band when upright neutral spine position is possible.

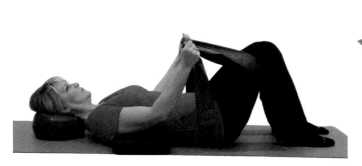

A

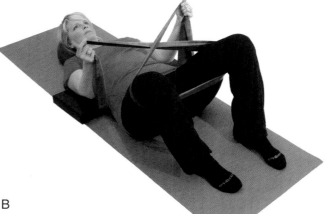

B

Fig. 11.24 (A and B) Bilateral hip abduction with external rotation against elastic resistance band in hook lying.

11.25.   Bridging with Trunk Support: Exercise Ball

See Fig. 11.25.

Purpose

- Challenge ability to maintain a neutral spinal position, stability, and control while using lower extremities
- Dissociate hip motion from lumbopelvic motion
- Strengthen hip and knee muscles while supporting the trunk

Position

- Patient is sitting with the trunk supported by the ball; the ball is resting against the wall or supported by therapist while the patient moves into the bridge position.
- Legs are slightly apart with the knees flexed and feet firmly anchored on the ground.
- Arms can be held next to the body or reaching forward in scaption.

Action (Fig. 11.25)

1. Activate deep stabilizing muscles in the lumbar (Exercise 11.20) and cervical regions (Exercise 11.19).
2. Once neutral position has been established and set, use hips and knees to lift the pelvis and torso from the floor without changing the spinal position.
3. The cervical and upper thoracic regions are supported by the ball.
4. Return to the floor, maintaining neutral spinal position throughout.

Teaching tips

- Instruction example:
  - "Once you have engaged your muscles to stabilize your spine, lift the body in one piece from the hips without losing the muscle support in moving your spine."
  - "Let your head and neck rest on the ball while you lift your pelvis from the ground."
- Common errors to correct:
  - Patients tend to initiate movement at the spine rather than stabilizing the trunk first, then using the lower extremities to lift the body.
  - Allowing the lumbar or thoracic spine to extend as the patient lifts the pelvis
  - Losing the neutral position or allowing the pelvis to hike or tilt posteriorly

- Releasing the spinal stabilization on the return
- Not keeping the pelvis level, allowing the pelvis and spine to rotate to one side
- Laterally flexing the spine (this will occur if the ball rolls to one side)
- Methods to address or prevent compensations:
  - "Use your legs to lift, without arching your back."
  - "Keeping the ball from rolling side to side will help keep your pelvis stable."

Advantages

- Stable, neutral spine while using legs leg to move
- Teaches patient to dissociate spinal movement from hip movement, which will be required for proper body mechanics during activities of daily living such as transfers or lifting.
- The exercise ball provides more instability in the frontal and transverse planes, thus increasing the challenge to control lumbopelvic rotation and lateral flexion.
- The ball position provides some proprioceptive input and support for the cervical and thoracic extensors, further providing cues for trunk extensor control.

Alternatives

- Support the trunk on an exercise foam wedge or BOSU with the feet on the ground. Lift the pelvis with the legs.
- Change the angle of the trunk or the amount of support from the ball by changing the size of the ball or the amount of inflation.

Progression

- Slower speed or eccentric control
- The further the exercise ball is placed from the hips, the greater the muscular challenge for the hip extensors to lift the body and the spinal stabilizers to maintain the position.
- Once in the supported bridge position, transfer weight toward one side while maintaining lumbopelvic position, not allowing the pelvis to drop or rotate.
- Progress to transferring weight to one leg. Lift the opposite heel then the whole foot off the ground. The single-leg lifts in a bridge position require extensive frontal and transverse plane control of the supporting leg from the hip abductors, adductors, and rotators.

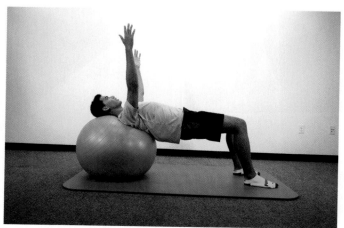

Fig. 11.25 Bridging with the trunk supported by the exercise ball.

MAINTAINING SPINAL POSITION AGAINST GRAVITY (PRONE) OR ON AN UNSTABLE SURFACE

11.26. Prone (Forearm Support) on BOSU: Upper Thoracic and Cervical Endurance

See Fig. 11.26.

Purpose

- Challenge cervical spine stabilization against gravity and promote upper thoracic extensor activation and endurance
- This exercise is a progression from Exercise 11.6.
- To reduce lower cervical anterior translation or step-off at the cervicothoracic junction, a common site for cervical hypermobility that often causes radiculopathy
- To challenge localized endurance of the cervical muscles against the weight of the head

Position (Fig. 11.26A)

- Start in prone with apex of BOSU (dome side up) under the mid-thoracic region with the head starting on the surface.
- Arms wider than the body with the hands wider than shoulder width, forearms on the surface

Action (Video 11.6A)

1. Gently nod the chin to engage the deep cervical flexors, then maintain the cervical position and lift the back of the head and neck toward the ceiling using the spinal extensors, still maintaining a neutral lordosis (Fig. 11.26B).
2. Initiate the movement with the upper thoracic and lower cervical extensors.

3. The therapist can guide the head position or the thoracic muscle activation using tactile cues (Fig 11.26 C, Video 11.6 C).
4. Gently engage the scapula stabilizers to maintain light pressure on the elbows.
5. Maintain the position against gravity for as long as possible.

Advantages

- Moving against gravity will train the upper thoracic extensors to support the weight of the head. (These muscles are often inactive during prolonged sitting or slumped positions.)

Teaching tips

- Instruction example:
  - "Nod your chin slightly, then lift the back of your neck toward the ceiling so that you are looking toward the floor."
- Common errors to correct:
  - Avoid overextending the cervical region (looking forward rather than down).
  - Correct the forward head positioning, checking cervicothoracic alignment from the side.
  - Ensure that the back of the head is lifted beyond the level of the thoracic spine. The posterior cervical and upper thoracic extensors should be active and counterbalanced by the deep neck flexors.

Alternatives

- Use foam pads under forehead to decrease range.
- Use a partially deflated ball under forehead and maintain position rather than lifting head against gravity.

Progression

- Increase time held in position.
- Progress to adding leg lifts while maintaining head position (Exercise 11.27).

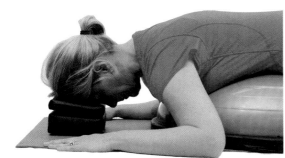
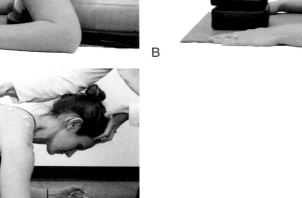
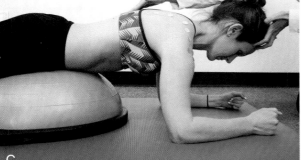

Fig. 11.26 Prone (forearm support) on BOSU for upper thoracic and cervical endurance against gravity with deep neck flexor activation to maintain a neutral cervical position (A and B) and with progression to less body support showing tactile feedback (C).

11.27. Prone (Forearm Support) on BOSU: Leg Lifts

See Fig. 11.27.

Purpose

- Increased generalized spinal extensor endurance
- Increased challenge of spinal stabilizers
- Provide spinal extensor isometric bias

Position

- Prone with apex of BOSU (dome side up) under mid-thoracic region (mid-sternum)
- Arms wider than body, head facing down for the starting position
- Foam pad or towel can be used to support the forehead

Action

1. Establish a neutral position (Exercise 11.19 and 11.20 but in prone).
2. Nod the chin and lift the head weight using process described in Exercise 11.26, maintaining a neutral position.
3. Use the forearm support to assist with maintaining the upper body position (Fig. 11.27A).
4. Engage the abdominals and spinal extensors to stabilize the neutral spine and pelvis position.
5. Lift one leg and slowly return to the ground, re-establish stability, then lift the other leg (Fig. 11.27A).

Advantages

- The BOSU is a supportive but unstable surface that facilitates proprioceptive input and feedback when undesired spinal motion occurs.
- Extensor muscles are working against gravity, which facilitates neuromuscular recruitment of the opposing muscles.
- Prone position over BOSU allows sequential posterior lower extremity muscle training.
- The position is useful if tight hip flexors make it difficult to lie prone without an anterior pelvic tilt or increased lordosis.

Teaching tips

- Instruction example:
  - "Engage your abdominals keeping your pelvis stable on the BOSU, lengthen one leg and lift it without moving anything else."
  - "Think more about keeping the pelvis still rather than the leg moving."
  - "Stability before mobility."
- Common errors to correct:
  - Initiating the movement by extending the spine rather than the hip

- Rotating or allowing the spine or pelvis to move in any plane of motion
- Correct scapula winging. Do not allow the rib cage to "sink" between the scapula.
- Methods to address or prevent compensations:
  - The patient can help stabilize and monitor the position of the pelvis on the BOSU by gently pressing the anterior iliac spines and pubic region into the BOSU.
  - Establish and maintain scapulothoracic connection (Exercise 10.14) to correct scapula winging.

Alternatives

- Substitute a large bolster or multiple pillows for the BOSU if more stability is needed.
- Keep the head supported if the patient is unable to maintain the unsupported head position (Fig. 11.27B).
- Four-point kneeling over an exercise ball; this position places the hamstrings and gluteals in midrange for individuals with limited hip extension, but the exercise ball is less stable than the BOSU (Exercise 11.28).
- If the patient has difficulty getting into prone or onto the floor, the patient can start in standing and lower his or her torso onto a plinth in a hip hinge position. One foot is kept on the ground (hip and knee flexed) and the unsupported leg is lifted while the lumbar spine is maintained in neutral on the plinth.

Progression

- Position the pelvis closer to the BOSU or exercise ball to shift the support from the BOSU to the upper extremities and increase the challenge to the spinal stabilizers by reducing the support underneath the body.
- Progress to four-point kneeling: leg lifts.
- Swimming action on a BOSU: lie prone over the BOSU, supporting the upper body weight on the forearms with the apex of the BOSU lower on the torso. Deepen the abdominals, lift one leg, and then the other so that both legs are suspended parallel to the ground. Keep the trunk stable while alternating the legs in a reciprocal "swimming" action.
- Progress to prone on elbows plank position starting from the BOSU (Fig. 11.27C), which increases the load and challenge for mid-position stabilization. Feet are hip-width apart with the toes in contact with the ground for support. Initiate the movement using scapula protraction and engage the abdominals in preparation for lifting into a plank position. Straighten the knees and use the abdominal muscles, upper body, and isometric support from the leg muscles to lift the body off the BOSU in a line from the head to the ankles.

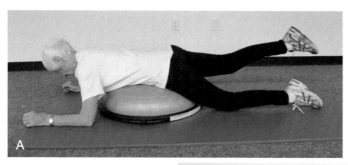 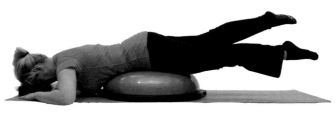

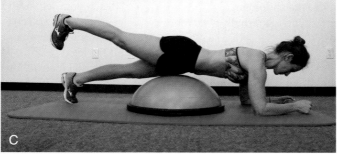

Fig. 11.27 Prone over the BOSU with single-leg lifts from a forearm support position (A), alternating leg extension scissor action with the head supported on foam pads (B), and progression to forearm plank position lifting from the BOSU with single-leg extension (C).

11.28.   Four-Point Kneeling Over Ball: Weight Shifting, Alternating Arm/Leg Lifts

See Fig. 11.28.

Purpose
- Increase generalized spinal extensor endurance
- Challenge for spinal stabilization with weight shift
- The exercise ball provides support for the body weight and proprioceptive input to assist the patient who has difficulty stabilizing the spine.

Position
- Four-point kneeling with ball under the abdomen
- Arms wider than body, shoulders slightly externally rotated at less than 90 degrees of flexion
- Hands on the floor

Action (Video 6.18)
1. Gently nod the chin to engage the deep cervical flexors, then maintain the cervical position and lift the back of the head and neck toward the ceiling using the spinal extensors, still maintaining a neutral lordosis (Exercises 11.6 and 11.26).
2. Establish and maintain scapulothoracic connection to stabilize upper body position.
3. Shift the body weight slightly to one side (Exercise 10.24).
4. Engage abdominals and stabilize pelvis and spinal position while lifting one leg, then shift to the opposite side before lifting the opposite leg (Fig. 11.28A, B).

Advantages
- Exercise ball offers support but is unstable, providing immediate proprioceptive input and feedback when undesired motion occurs.
- The quadruped position allows the lower extremities to move through larger ranges.
- An exercise ball is less stable than a BOSU but provides feedback for the abdominal area and can be used to assist with training weight-shifting.

Teaching tips
- Instruction example:
  - "Keep the ball and your spine still as you extend one leg behind you."
- Common errors to correct:
  - Avoid lifting the leg prior to stabilizing the lumbar spine.

- Avoid extending, rotating, or laterally flexing the lumbar spine while lifting the leg.
- Watch for excessive hip extension and rotation as the patient attempts to maximize the range.
- Methods to correct or prevent compensations:
  - Observing the lumbar spine axis and overall leg alignment may require observation from above as well as from the side.
  - Instructing the patient to press the front of the pelvis onto the ball may help with limiting early extension and rotation.
  - "Reach your leg away from your body rather than lifting your leg high" will encourage the patient to engage the hip extensors rather than overusing the lumbar extensors to lift the leg.
  - Sequential instructions to move the ball slightly, stabilizing the trunk and only then lifting the limb, may assist early or uncontrolled spinal motion.

Alternatives
- Prone on forearm over BOSU with leg lifts for cervical, thoracic, and lumbar spine challenge (Exercise 11.27). The BOSU is more stable than an exercise ball.
- If the patient has wrist discomfort in this postion, use a closed fist for upper extremity support (Fig. 11.28D) or place wrists on a small exercise ball or block (Fig. 11.28E).
- Adjust the arm position wider than shoulder distance apart if the patient has a large valgus angle.
- Use a bigger ball if the patient is tall or has long arms.
- Use arm lifts instead of leg lifts (Fig. 11.28C).
- Use a closed fist for upper support if full wrist extension is painful.

Progression
- Move further over the exercise ball so that the ball is closer to the pelvis, shifting the weight from the exercise ball to the upper extremities to further challenge spinal stabilization.
- Progress to four-point kneeling leg lifts without an exercise ball (Fig. 11.28C).
- Alternate opposite arm and leg (Fig. 11.28F).
- Progress to less supported positions in kneeling (Fig. 11.28G) and stride-standing (Fig. 11.28H).

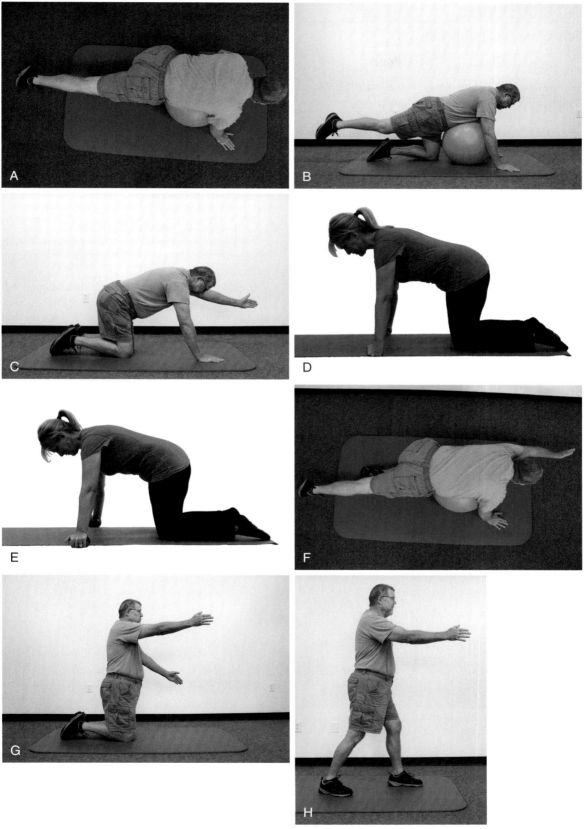

Fig. 11.28 Leg lift challenges in four-point kneeling over an exercise ball (A and B), arm lifts without an exercise ball (C), modifications if there is wrist discomfort (D and E), alternating arm and leg lifts (F), kneeling (G,) and stride-standing (H) positions.

SIDE-LYING CHALLENGES

11.29. Side-Lying Quadratus Lift

See Fig. 11.29.

Purpose

- Challenge rotatory and lateral flexor spinal stability using local and global stabilizers in a less stable, side-lying position

Position

- Side-lying with the head supported and aligned with the thorax (Fig. 11.29A)
- Head is aligned with thorax and supported with a pillow.
- Neutral anterior-posterior spinal curvatures and lumbopelvic relationship without rotation
- Hips and knees are flexed to 45 degrees.
- Top hand resting on mat for support

Action (Video 11.29)

1. Engage transverse abdominals and pelvic floor, lift waist and bottom ribs off the supporting surface with the quadratus lumborum and oblique muscles. This will place the lumbar spine in midline, or neutral in the frontal plane (Fig. 11.29B).
2. Maintain the neutral spinal position.

Advantages

- This exercise can be used to teach spinal alignment for side-lying sleeping positions.
- Relatively supported position but more challenging than supine or prone for rotatory stability with limb motion.

Teaching tips

- Instruction example:
  - "Lift your lower ribs off the table; you should be able to slide a hand underneath your waist."

- Common errors to correct:
  - If the torso is rotated in the starting position (torso or pelvis rotated forward or backward), there is a greater risk of increased rotation throughout the exercise, and rotation may be concentrated in the thoracolumbar junction.
  - If the head is anterior to the torso or allowed to side bend, the upper thoracic spinal position may cause compensations in the lumbar region.
- Methods to address compensations:
  - Correct the head and spinal alignment before asking the patient to lift the waist and ribs.
  - Ensure that the pillow fills the distance from the shoulders to the head to place the head in midline.
  - If the shoulder width is larger than the hip width or the hip width is much larger than the shoulder width, a small pillow can be placed under the pelvis (wider shoulders) or under the rib cage (wider pelvis).

Alternatives

- Straighten both legs to increase the challenge by decreasing the base of support.
- If the patient's shoulders are wider than the hips, a pillow may be needed under the pelvis.

Progression

- Lift the top hand off the floor to decrease the base of support and increase the challenge.
- Side-lying hip abduction or flexion/extension (Exercises 9.26 and 11.31)

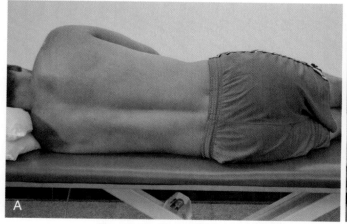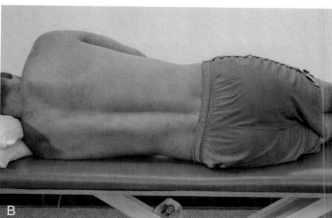

Fig. 11.29 (A and B) Side-lying quadratus lift to support the lumbar spine with active control.

11.30. Side-Lying Arm Lifts

See Fig. 11.30.

Purpose

- Spinal stability using local and global stabilizers with arm challenge for cervical and thoracic rotatory and lateral flexion stability challenge

Position

- Side-lying, pillow under head, with the head in midline in the frontal plane.
- Head is lined up with the thorax, with neutral (anterior-posterior) spinal curvatures (Fig. 11.30A).
- Hips and knees flexed to 45 degrees
- Both arms are flexed in front of body (Fig. 11.30A).

Action (Video 11.30)

1. Quadratus lift (see Exercise 11.29) to provide active spinal stabilizer engagement.
2. Hold the spine position using quadratus lumborum, then horizontally abduct the arm from its starting position (parallel to the floor) toward the ceiling (Fig. 11.30B).

Advantages

- Relatively supported position but more challenging than supine or prone for rotatory stability to oppose the forces from the limb motion

Teaching tips

- Instruction example:
  - "Gently lift your lower ribs off the mat, then hold the position while you lift your top hand toward the ceiling."
  - "Lift your hand toward the ceiling without moving your trunk."
- Common error to correct:
  - Torso or pelvis rotated in the starting position
- Methods to correct or prevent compensations:
  - "Your hips and shoulders should be stacked on top of each other."
  - "Focus on keeping your spine still while you move your arm rather than how much or how fast you can move your arm."

Alternatives

- Pillows between knees
- Start with the top arm resting on the top side of body and abduct the shoulder from next to the body to 90 degrees (toward the ceiling) and return.
- Side-lying hip abduction (see Exercise 9.26) or side-lying hip flexion/extension (Exercise 11.31)

Progression

- Legs extended (smaller base of support)
- Rotate the cervical spine, looking at the hand. The cervical rotation challenges distal spinal stability, or the progression can be used to challenge cervicothoracic muscle activity and sequencing (Fig. 11.30C).
- Add small hand weights, if the patient is able to stabilize spine and there is no discomfort (Fig. 11.30D).
- Increase speed in small ranges.
- Small-range rapid motion oscillations or circles to further challenge alternating control of spinal segments

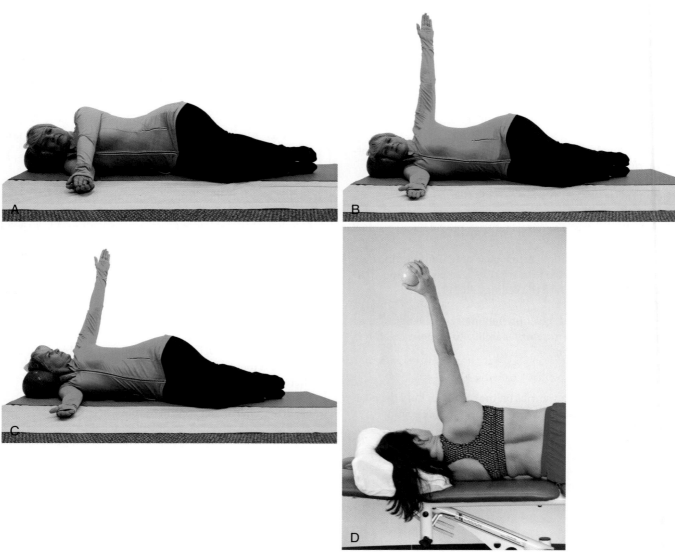

Fig. 11.30 Side-lying arm lifts follow an active quadratus lift to stabilize the spine (A and B) with adequate cervical support. Progression options include upper thoracic and cervical rotation (C) or addition of weights in different ranges (D).

11.31. Side-Lying Hip Flexion and Extension

See Fig. 11.31.

Purpose

- Challenge pelvic and spinal stability in all three planes of motion using local and global stabilizers in a less stable, side-lying position

Position

- Side-lying with head supported (Fig. 11.31A)
- Head is aligned with thorax on a pillow.
- Neutral anterior-posterior spinal curvatures and no spinal or pelvic rotation
- Bottom hip and knee flexed, top leg straight
- Top hand resting on mat for support

Action (Video 11.31)

1. Engage transverse abdominals and pelvic floor, lift waist and bottom ribs off the supporting surface with the quadratus lumborum and oblique muscles (Exercise 11.29). This will place the lumbar spine in midline, or neutral in the frontal plane.
2. Maintain the neutral spinal position and abduct the top leg until it is parallel with the floor (Fig. 11.31A).
3. Keep the spine and pelvis neutral and flex, then extend the hip (Fig. 11.31B).

Advantages

- Relatively supported position but more challenging than supine or prone for stability in the frontal and rotational planes
- Trains the patient to dissociate hip flexion and extension from pelvic anterior and posterior tilting
- Working the obliques and quadratus lumborum against gravity (global stabilizers) is a good starting point for teaching patients to engage these muscles consistently.

Teaching tips

- Instruction examples:
    - To attain starting position: "Lift your ribs to increase the space from the table; you should be able to slide a hand under your waist."
    - For the hip flexion and extension: "Keep your spine still as you can while you bring your leg forward."
    - "Use your abdominal muscles more to stop your pelvis moving as you reach your leg back."
- Common errors to correct:
    - If the torso or pelvis is rotated in the starting position, there is a greater risk of increased rotation throughout the exercise, and rotation may be concentrated at the lumbothoracic junction.
    - Keep the pelvis and lumbar spine neutral as the leg comes forward.
    - Watch for anterior tilting and lumbar spine extension as the hip extends.

Alternatives

- Leg circles: circumduct the hip while side-lying: "Keeping your leg lifting and your pelvis still, make a small circle with your leg."

Progression

- Extend the bottom leg in line with the body to reduce the base of support and increase the challenge to maintain stability.
- Lift the top hand off the floor to decrease the base of support and increase the challenge.

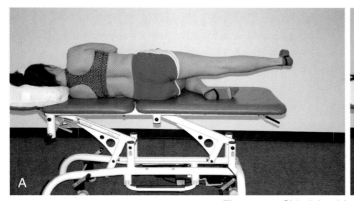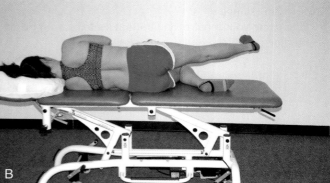

Fig. 11.31 Side-lying hip flexion and extension.

11.32.   Side-Plank: Partial or Full

See Fig. 11.32.

Purpose

- Stabilize spine using global stabilizers in side-lying position to challenge rotatory and lateral flexion stability with body weight resistance

Contraindications and Precautions

- This exercise may increase shoulder pain in the supporting arm.
- This exercise is very challenging for patients with shoulder instability. The exercise is only indicated for patients with shoulder hypermobility after the patient has demonstrated tolerance and control in bilateral closed chain exercises for the upper extremities (e.g., prone on elbows plank off BOSU [Exercise 11.27]). If the patient has any history of shoulder problems, shoulder alignment and stabilization should be monitored throughout the exercise and the exercise discontinued if there is discomfort.

Position

- Side-lying with the head lined up with the thorax
- Neutral spine and hip position with the knees flexed to 45 degrees
- The body is propped up on the forearm to establish scapular and shoulder activation before lifting into the plank position.
- The hip abductors in the bottom leg assist with lifting the pelvis off the floor.

Action

- Engage the transverse abdominals and pelvic floor, lift the waist and ribs to place the lumbar spine in midline (partial side plank) (Fig. 11.32A).

Advantages

- More challenging than side-lying exercises and requires oblique, quadratus lumborum, and latissimus dorsi activity in addition to local stabilizer function.

Teaching tips

- Instruction examples:
  - "Press into your forearm and bottom leg to lift your pelvis off the floor."
  - "Engage the muscles on the underside of your body to lift your body weight off the floor."
- Common errors to correct:
  - Do not allow the pelvis or rib cage to "sag" toward the floor.
  - Do not allow the shoulder to elevate in the side plank position.
  - Avoid rotating the body in either direction.
  - Watch for scapula winging.
- Methods or address or prevent compensations:
  - Ensure that the patient performs side-lying quadratus lift (Exercise 11.29) correctly prior to prescribing this exercise.
  - Use tactile cues to lift pelvis or waistline if the spine is "sagging" toward the floor.
  - If the shoulder girdle is elevated or winging is present as the patient lifts the pelvis, instruct the patient to stabilize the shoulder first: "Lift up underneath your shoulder as you press up into a side plank position. Keep the connection between your ribs and the shoulder blade."
  - Emphasize scapular stabilization. Using the latissimus dorsi on the bottom arm will stabilize the scapula from elevating as well as assist with lifting the body into the plank position.

Alternatives

- Use foam pillows, BOSU, or bolsters under the pelvis to decrease distance to lift pelvis to achieve full side plank alignment (Fig. 11.32B).
- Use the top hand to assist with the partial side plank.

Progression

- Bottom leg extended, top leg flexed and crossed over the bottom leg with foot on the floor to assist with side plank lift
- Both legs extended supported on the forearm (Fig. 11.32C; Video 6.24)
- Extend the supporting elbow (Fig. 11.32D).
- Increase hold or add movement of upper arm with weights (Video 6.24).

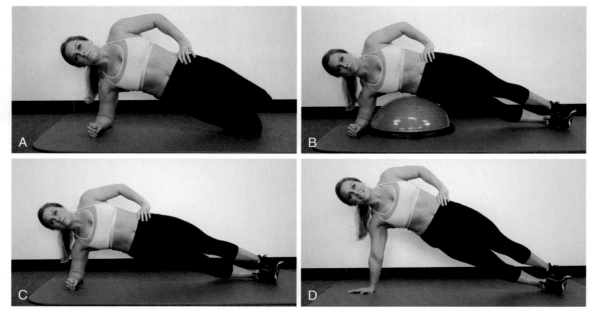

Fig. 11.32 Partial side-plank (A), with options to decrease the distance lifted (B), progression to full side-plank with forearm support (C), and full side-plank with elbow extension (D).

PROGRESSIVE RESISTANCE: GLOBAL STABILIZER FUNCTION, ABDOMINAL EXERCISES AGAINST GRAVITY

11.33.   Abdominal Curls

See Fig. 11.33.

Purpose
- Strengthen the abdominal global movers, superimposed over local and global stabilizer activation

Contraindications and precautions
- This exercise is not indicated for patients with cervical pain until the patient is able to stabilize the cervical region on an unstable surface (ball or foam roller) with upper extremity challenge.
- The alternatives are useful starting positions for individuals with neck pain.

Position
- Supine, hook-lying (Fig. 11.33A)
- Feet flat on the floor, hip-width apart
- If forward head or thoracic kyphosis is present, place a pad under the head to decrease stress on the cervical spine

Action (Video 6.22)
1. Engage the transverse abdominis and pelvic floor muscles to stabilize the lumbopelvic region and the deep neck flexors to stabilize the cervical region.
2. Curl up toward the pelvis, bringing the head and arms with the rib cage (Fig. 11.33A).
3. The pelvis and lumbar spine do not move; some weight should remain on the sacrum.

Advantages
- Flexing the thoracic spine while stabilizing the pelvis and lumbar spine in neutral limits stress on the lumbar spine.

Teaching tips
- Instruction example:
  - "Keep some space under your lower back while you curl your upper back off the mat."
  - "Keep your pelvis still and level and move your rib cage toward your pelvis."
  - "Using your abdominals, slide your ribs toward your pelvis. Keep your pelvis neutral and still."
- Common errors to correct:
  - Thoracic flexion should occur without flattening the lumbar lordosis or tipping the pelvis back.

- Avoid leading with the head (overflexing the cervical spine) or jutting the chin forward (losing cervical stabilization and extending the cervical spine).
- Using the arms (pectoralis major) or momentum to lift the upper body.
- Methods to address or prevent compensations:
  - If the patient concentrates on keeping the pelvis balanced and in contact with the mid-portion of the sacrum without tipping or rocking the pelvis backward, it is easier to maintain the counterbalanced activity of the lumbar extensors and deep abdominal muscles.
  - "Try to keep some pressure on the mid portion of your sacrum. Slide your ribs toward the pelvis without rocking your pelvis backwards. Your upper body should curl up without folding like a book."
  - The focus should be on using the abdominals to flex the thoracic spine while stabilizing a neutral lumbopelvic region. If the patient is overflexing the neck, encourage the patient to: "Support the weight of your head with your fingers and allow your head to rest back into your hands. Then use your abdominals, not your arms, to lift your upper body."
  - "Keep your neck long or some space between your chin and your upper body (to maintain cervical stabilization). Look toward your knees as you curl up, not toward the ceiling (to avoid extending the cervical spine as the thoracic spine flexes)."

Alternatives
- Lean back against a BOSU or foam wedge to assist with thoracic flexion and to decrease stress on cervical region.
- Support the head weight using a towel under the head (Fig. 11.33B; Video 6.23).
- Use a foam bolster or BOSU to support legs.

Progression
- Flex thoracic spine and hold, then lift one leg to 90 degrees of hip and knee flexion.
- Lift one leg to 90 degrees, deepen abdominal engagement, then lift the other leg, followed by thoracic flexion. (Support both legs on an exercise ball or one leg on the ball if unable to maintain transverse abdominal or oblique engagement during curls; Fig. 11.33C.)

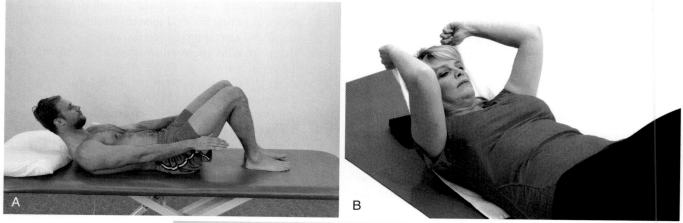

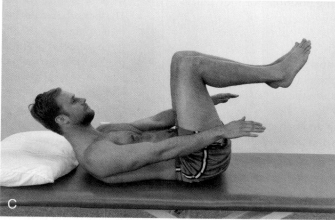

Fig. 11.33 Abdominal curls with the feet on the mat (A), with the head weight supported using a towel (B), and progressed to a curl with both legs in the air (C).

11.34. Diagonal Curl-ups

See Fig. 11.34.

Purpose

- Strengthen the abdominal global movers, focusing on the obliques, superimposed over local and global stabilizers
- Flex and rotate the thoracic spine while maintaining the pelvis and lumbar spine neutral
- Progression from abdominal curls (Exercise 11.33)

Contraindications and Precautions

- This exercise is not indicated for patients with cervical pain until the patient is able to stabilize the cervical region on an unstable surface (ball or foam roller) with upper extremity challenge.
- The alternatives are useful starting positions for individuals with neck pain.

Position

- Supine, hook-lying, feet hip-width apart
- Fingertips behind head, gently supporting weight of the head
- If forward head or thoracic kyphosis is present, place foam pad under the head to decrease cervical lordosis and stress on the anterior neck muscles.

Action

- Similar action to abdominal curls (Exercise 11.33).
1. Engage the transverse abdominal and pelvic floor muscles to stabilize lumbopelvic region and deep neck flexors to stabilize cervical region.
2. Once the lumbar spine is stable, curl the rib cage gently toward the pelvis.
3. Rotate torso toward opposite side of pelvis while further flexing the thoracic spine (Fig. 11.34).
4. Pelvis and lumbar spine do not move.

Advantages

- Head weight is supported by hands
- Spinal rotation is required for most functional movements.

Teaching tips

- Instruction example:
  - "Engage your abdominal muscles to stabilize your low back and the muscles in your neck to stabilize the neck. Curl up slightly off the mat, and then rotate your upper body toward one side. Keep looking toward the opposite knee."
- Common errors to correct:
  - Thoracic flexion should occur without flattening the lumbar lordosis or tipping the pelvis posteriorly.

- Avoid leading with the head (overflexing the neck) or jutting the chin forward (overextending the neck) or overrotating the head and neck (substituting for thoracic rotation).
- Overrotation is very common; 45 degrees or less is sufficient.
- Avoid using the arms to create the movement.
- Methods to address or prevent compensations:
  - If the patient concentrates on keeping the pelvis balanced and in contact with the mid-portion of the sacrum without tipping or rocking the pelvis backward it is easier to maintain the counterbalanced activity of the lumbar extensors and deep abdominal muscles.
  - "Try to keep some pressure on the mid portion of your sacrum. Slide your ribs toward the pelvis without rocking your pelvis back. Your upper body should curl up without folding like a book."
  - The focus should be on using the abdominals to flex the thoracic spine while stabilizing a neutral lumbopelvic region. If the patient is overflexing the neck, encourage the patient to: "Support the weight of your head with your fingers and allow your head to rest back into your hands. Then use your abdominals, not your arms, to lift your upper body."
  - "Keep your neck long or some space between your chin and your upper body (to maintain cervical stabilization). Look toward your knees as you curl up, not toward the ceiling (to avoid extending the cervical spine as the thoracic spine flexes)."
  - "Look at your knee, not past your body."
  - "Curl your upper body up before you rotate."

Alternatives

- Use BOSU or foam wedge to assist with thoracic flexion and decrease stress on cervical region.
- Use foam bolster or BOSU to support legs.

Progression

- Lift one leg to 90 degrees of hip and knee flexion and hold during thoracic flexion and rotation toward the leg in the air. Repeat on the opposite side.
- Lift one leg then the other to 90 degrees and hold both legs in the air, followed by thoracic flexion and rotation to alternating sides.
- Support one or both legs on an exercise ball if unable to maintain transverse abdominal or oblique engagement during curls.

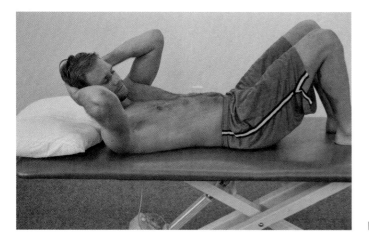

Fig. 11.34 Diagonal curl-ups with the feet supported on the mat.

POSTURAL CHALLENGE FROM LIMB MOTION AGAINST RESISTANCE

11.35. Seated Neutral Alignment: Upper Extremity Challenge

See Fig. 11.35.

Purpose

- Challenge spinal postural reactions to maintain spinal position in response to changes in arm weight and motion
- Focuses on stabilizing the cervical and thoracic regions

Position

- Sitting in supported, spinal neutral posture (Fig. 11.35A)
- Upper extremities positioned in front of the body, in scaption, with or without small weights

Action (Video 11.35A)

- Maintain stable posture while alternating arm motions.

Advantages

- This exercise can be performed in any setting: home or work environment.
- Postural position and endurance challenges are required for everyday activities.

Teaching tips

- Instruction example:
  - "Lift your arms out wide in front of your body. Keep your body still while making small movements with your arms."

- Common errors to correct:
  - Avoid hiking the shoulders to lift the arms.
  - Losing the spinal postural alignment (thoracic or cervical; Video 11.35B) or shoulder hiking may be the first sign of fatigue.
  - Observe for scapula winging, elevation, or lack of upward rotation and correct mechanics.
- Methods to address or avoid compensations:
  - Use a scaption position and ensure proximal upper quarter alignment prior to lifting the arms.

Alternatives

- Any arm movements can be used with various ranges of shoulder flexion and abduction (elbow flexion/extension, wrist flexion/extension, shoulder internal/external rotation).
- Maintain one arm in a stable position (isometric opposition) while the other arm moves.

Progression

- Increase external resistance with elastic resistance bands or heavier free weights.
- Small range progressing to larger range.
- Increase speed of alternation.
- Sitting on exercise ball to increase balance challenge facilitates postural muscle activity (Fig. 11.35B; Videos 11.35C and 6.26).

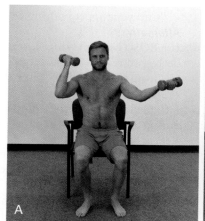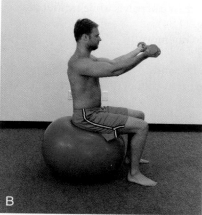

Fig. 11.35 Seated alignment and postural endurance with upper extremity challenge in a chair (A) and on an unstable exercise ball to facilitate balance responses (B).

FUNCTIONAL TRAINING, MOVEMENT REEDUCATION

11.36. Functional Movement Reeducation: Hip Rotation Drivers (Pulleys)

See Fig. 11.36.

Purpose

- Reduce localized stress in the lumbar region by training neuromuscular coordination and sequencing using hip rotation

Position (Fig. 11.36A)

- Standing with hips flexed to 30 degrees, sideways to pulley
- Both hands hold pulley handle and a pole provides visual input. Hold the wooden pole vertically in front of the body with the hands to provide visual feedback to guide synchronized spinal position.

Action

1. Stable neutral spine position, with isometric engagement of upper extremities
2. Initiate rotation from the hips; moving the pelvis and torso as one unit on the legs (Fig. 11.36B).
3. Maintain abdominal and spinal muscle support without twisting while moving from the hips and legs.

Advantages

- Functional requirement for pulling activities or sports that involve rotation such as golf, racquet sports, and swimming

Teaching tips

- Instruction example:
  - "Keep your hands in the middle of your body and rotate your pelvis and shoulders as one unit as you turn away from the pulleys."
  - "Let your hips move: you should see a crease in the hip area."
- Common errors to correct:
  - Rotating from the spine or initiating the rotational movement from the arms rather than the pelvis
  - If the pelvis and hips are "locked," the motion will take place in the spine.
  - Tilting the pelvis posteriorly will limit the amount of hip rotation.
  - The natural lower leg alignment (mid-position) is needed to maximize the amount of hip rotation. Check the mid-position and bony alignment in supine prior to standing.

Alternatives

- Cross arms with hands on shoulders, holding wooden pole across top of shoulders to provide visual feedback about rotation. The pole should not rotate further than the pelvis.

Progression

- Remove the pole and use both hands on the pulley handle (Fig. 11.36C) or only one hand (Fig. 11.36D) to challenge synchronous rotation without the feedback.
- Sports-specific ranges of motion or positions (e.g., golf or tennis back swing) (Fig. 11.36D)
- Change the plane of movement (Fig. 11.36E, F).
- Increase speed.
- Progress to transferring weight from foot to foot along with the rotation (Fig. 11.36E, F).

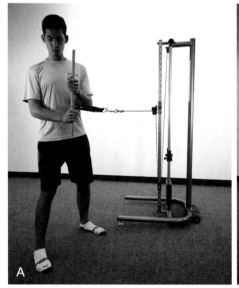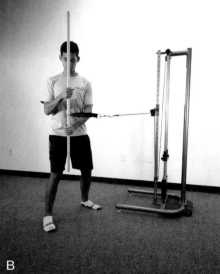

Fig. 11.36 (A and B) Functional movement reeducation using hip rotation to drive or initiate motion with less spinal rotation.

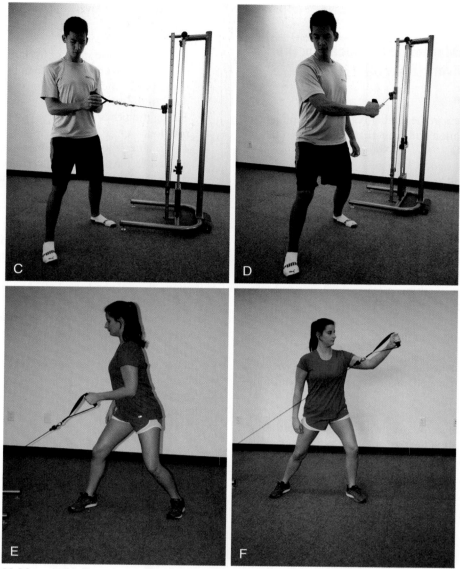

Fig. 11.36, cont'd Functional movement reeducation using the pulley handle (C and D), mimicking sports requirements for a backhand (D), and diagonal movements with weight transfer (E and F).

CASE STUDY 11.2: LUMBAR HYPERMOBILITY (NEUROMUSCULAR COORDINATION DEFICITS)

This case illustrates the choice of exercises for lumbar hypermobility with neuromuscular coordination deficits, progressing the difficulty and load while using motor control concepts and functional movement strategies to distribute forces.

A 24-year-old female undergraduate student with a history of back pain presents with lumbar pain after moving a heavy couch 4 weeks ago. She works part-time as a waitress and is studying to be a primary school teacher. She reports 3–4 episodes of low back pain a year with mild to moderate symptoms, sometimes with gluteal and leg pain and no tingling, numbness, or weakness. The previous episodes usually dissipated after 1–2 weeks. She is concerned because this episode has lasted longer than normal.

Functional Status and Goals

She is attending lectures and planning to return to work for shortened shifts after taking 2 weeks off after the injury. She relies on her income from her restaurant job and is concerned that her back pain will limit her productivity and will not allow her to tolerate lifting trays and standing for up to 4 hours at a time. She must climb three flights of stairs to her apartment and walks five blocks to the bus (carrying a backpack). She has access to the college gym, and her apartment complex has some exercise equipment. She also has a foam roller, an exercise ball, and weights at home. Her disability is moderate (Oswestry 17/50; 34%).[46,47] She would like to decrease the pain, return to her full duties as a waitress, start to work out in the gym in her apartment complex, and prevent future episodes of acute pain.

Subjective Complaints

- *Severity*: Initially pain was severe (7/10) with some leg pain (3/10) and lasted for 3 days. Pain has progressively decreased since the first visit and now the patient complains of constant, aching pain in lumbar region, 2/10. Pain increases to 3/10 with prolonged positioning, especially sleeping or extreme movements. She has no referred pain, tingling, or numbness (Box 11.4).

BOX 11.4 Interpretation of Subjective Complaints for Objective Examination Choices

Severity has decreased to LOW and irritability is minimal. Examination will need to establish the extent of hypomobility or hypermobility, neuromuscular coordination, and any other contributing impairments. She has no neurological symptoms and no distal referral at present, decreasing the indication for neural testing.

- *Irritability*: Pain increases to 3/10 with prolonged positioning, especially sleeping. Pain does not last for long and is relieved with movement.
- *Nature*: Subacute mechanical pain related to lifting
- *Stage*: Subacute, Phase II

Objective Findings

- *Posture*: She stands with knee hyperextension and an increased lumbar lordosis; the lordosis decreases if she unlocks her knees.
- *Range of motion*: See Table 11.7.
- *Muscle activation*: She has difficulty engaging the transversus abdominis and has difficulty lifting the upper body off the mat with the arms extended (poor grade) for the isometric abdominal endurance test.[1] The test is repeated with her back supported at 60 degrees from horizontal and the feet supported, but she is still unable to clear and hold the position.[48] Abdominal muscles activation is delayed and stabilization compromised with single-leg lifts (hip and knee flexion) in supine. Using the modified Biering-Sorenson test over a BOSU, she is able to achieve a neutral alignment of the upper body for 13 seconds (fair).[1,49,50] Trunk lateral flexion endurance is also fair (L = 14 seconds; R = 17 seconds).[49] Lumbar paraspinal activation is delayed with single-leg lifts in (prone over the BOSU).
- *Muscle length*: Very flexible; straight-leg raise 110 degrees of hip flexion with full knee extension
- *Special tests*: Beighton scale 8/9,[51,52] positive prone instability test[23,24,53]
- *Palpation and joint mobility*: Pain was reproduced with posterior-anterior glides L3, L4, L5.[53] Muscle guarding and spasm in the low lumbar paraspinals and gluteals.

TABLE 11.7 Lumbar and Thoracic ROM (Double Inclinometer)

	Range	Symptoms and Observation
Flexion	0–64 degrees	Pain increases to 3/10 at 40 degrees, and aberrant motion is observed on the return (uses hip and thoracic motion to return) Motion occurs in the lumbar spine
Extension	0–40 degrees	No increase in pain, limited thoracic extension
Lateral flexion R	0–35 degrees	Axis of motion at L4, pulling on L, increases to 3/10
Lateral flexion L	0–35 degrees	Axis of motion at L4, pulling on R, increases to 4/10
Rotation R	0–28 degrees	Axis of motion in low lumbar spine, increased pain to 4/10
Rotation L	0–25 degrees	Axis of motion in low lumbar spine, increased pain to 4/10

Evaluation

- *Physical therapy diagnosis*: Hypermobility, subacute low back pain with neuromuscular coordination deficits[15] (subacute exacerbation of recurring low back pain, symptoms increase with end range and provocation of lumbar segments, late muscle activation of transversus abdominis and spinal extensors, decreased endurance, and altered neuromuscular timing)
- *Contributing impairments*: Postural habits in standing, inefficient lifting techniques, and inefficient neuromuscular coordination leading to concentration of forces in the lumbar region, generalized hypermobility
- *Implications of evaluation for exercise choices:* See Box 11.5.

Precautions

- Avoid lumbar end range rotation, lateral flexion, flexion.
- Avoid increasing pain symptoms.
- No stretching.

Prognosis

The patient's pain severity and relative disability has steadily decreased, increasing the prognosis for full pain and disability resolution. Her positive attitude, strong desire to return to work, and high expectations for recovery also suggest that there is a good prognosis for a positive outcome.[15] Her overall hypermobility indicates the need for neuromuscular training and postural awareness training in multiple areas,[54] but the initial treatment will focus on the lumbar spine. A reduction of 10 points in Oswestry scores is needed to exceed minimal clinically important differences and is likely to be achievable.[55] Specific neuromuscular coordination training with an emphasis on restoration of timing and activation of the local stabilizers and progressive endurance training has been found to improve the overall prognosis for preventing recurrence of pain after the first episode of acute pain. Hides et al.[56] reported a lower rate of recurrence of low back pain after the first episode (30% at 1 year, 35% at 3 years) after 4 weeks of stabilization exercises and neuromuscular coordination training of the lumbar spine local stabilizers (transversus abdominis and multifidi) compared to a control group who demonstrated an 84% recurrence at 1 year and 75% at 3 years.

Exercise Choices

See Box 11.5 for implications of the evaluation and Table 11.8 for related exercise choices. Descriptions of the use of motor control concepts for the patient (Box 11.6), the use of exercise to promote functional alignment and force distribution (Box 11.7), the progression of exercises (Box 11.8), and the controversy surrounding the effectiveness of interventions for neuromuscular coordination deficits (Box 11.9) follow.

BOX 11.5 Implications of Evaluation for Exercise Treatment

The patient's symptoms fit with the clinical prediction rule for higher likelihood of a positive response to a stabilization exercise response: younger than 40 years, straight leg raise of greater than 90 degrees, presence of aberrant movements, a positive prone instability test,[57] and the refined version of the rule (aberrant movements and positive prone instability test.[58] She does have a history of generalized hypermobility and a positive Beightons test. Midrange and closed chain positions may be useful to prevent excessive stress and promote proprioceptive feedback to recruit muscles around the joint.[54,59] Initial pain severity has decreased from moderate-to-severe to mild, with mild-to-moderate disability.[46,47] Phase II exercise will target addressing the impairments; specifically neuromuscular coordination deficits. The physical therapy diagnosis and classification of subacute low back pain with neuromuscular coordination deficits indicates using trunk coordination, endurance, and strengthening approaches in midranges that do not increase symptoms (Tables 11.8 and 11.9).[15]

TABLE 11.8 Exercise Choices, Parameters, Modifications, and Rationale: Case 11.2

	Parameters	Monitoring During Exercise, Modifications	Rationale
General Endurance			
Bike (Exercise 11.41)	15 minutes at Level 3 on stationary bike using the random program and a, target heart rate of 60–80%	Cycling position reeducation using feedback; mirror to reach active spinal support, initially in a vertical position, later with a slight incline to target the spinal extensors. Seat height is set at a level to limit hip flexion and maintain a neutral spinal lordosis.	Generalized muscle and cardiovascular endurance to promote spinal muscle support Dynamic alignment during endurance activity Include exercise as part of normal hobbies (cycling). Aim for 150 minutes per week total cycling and walking time. Progress to stair climber (she has access to both in her apartment complex).

TABLE 11.8 Exercise Choices, Parameters, Modifications, and Rationale: Case 11.2—cont'd

	Parameters	Monitoring During Exercise, Modifications	Rationale
Neuromuscular Coordination and Lumbar Stabilization[a]			
Local stabilizer activation: Neutral lumbar lordosis (Exercise 11.20) and single-leg lifts (Exercise 11.21)	Muscle activation in the neutral position using a blood pressure cuff to maintain stable pressure for 20 seconds or more	Visual feedback while engaging transversus abdominis and local spinal extensors to maintain engagement	Teach muscle activation with visual feedback. Blood pressure cuff is used to provide feedback to monitor changes in activation. Goal is to decrease amount of variability and anticipatory sequencing. Progress to leg lifts. Progress to foam roller stabilization with arm challenges.
Local stabilizer activation; neutral spine positioning with arm challenges on foam roller (Exercise 11.22)	Supine with the spine supported on the foam roller, arms in scaption with alternating shoulder flexion/extension. Multiple repetitions using motor control concepts; recording time maintaining stability of the foam roller	Avoid excessive thoracic extension with shoulder flexion or rotation of the lumbopelvic region or motion of the foam roller.	The unstable base initiates balance responses and provides an extrinsic focus with immediate feedback and knowledge of results. The patient is able to monitor successful exercise performance immediately without verbal feedback from therapist. Progress using small weights and adding different arm challenges, still maintaining the arms in front of the body. Progress to thoracic flexion with stable lumbar spine. Progress from supported supine with visual feedback, leg lift challenge to unstable base providing external focus, abdominal curls.
Abdominal curls (Exercise 11.33)	Thoracic flexion able to perform 12 repetitions prior to losing transversus abdominis engagement	Watch for loss of transversus abdominis "flattening." Cue to avoid pulling her upper body into flexion with the arms or initiating the movement from the cervical region, jutting the chin forward or jamming the chin into chest.	Abdominal strengthening
Prone four-point kneeling arm and leg lifts (Exercise 11.28) Progression without exercise ball	Arm lifts only, leg lifts only, then alternating movement. Teach weight shift prior to lifts. Accuracy and control of sequencing is the primary goal and determines the number of repetitions.	Observe for timing and ability to maintain both abdominal engagement and spinal extensors. Limit lumbar spine rotation and encourage keeping the pelvis level before lifting the arm or leg.	Neuromuscular coordination with anticipatory timing. The position requires an emphasis on the spinal extensors and the alternating movement is used to teach sequencing of the spinal stabilizers prior to the lifts. This exercise is more challenging without the exercise ball to provide support and feedback. Use the ball if the patient is unable to achieve stability. Progress to alternating arm and leg lifts then to planks.
Planks (Exercise 10.46)	Starting position over a BOSU, lifting the body from a forearm support position.	Watch for sagging into the lumbar spine, losing the cervical spine alignment or scapulothoracic connection.	Lifting off the BOSU places less stress on the lumbar spine than lifting directly from the floor. Generalized strengthening for upper extremities and trunk. Progression from four-point kneeling arm or leg lifts
Lower Extremity Strengthening With Lumbopelvic Stabilization for Force Distribution and Stabilization Challenge			
Side-lying hip abduction with quadratus lifts (Exercise 9.26B)	Side-lying position with quadratus lift is maintained for as long as possible. Specific hip abductor fatigue is reached at 8 repetitions; strengthening dosage for the hip abductors. Three sets of 6–8 repetitions is used for the initial dosage.	Exercise is discontinued if the spine position is not maintained or when there is hip abductor fatigue.	Side-lying position is more challenging to maintain than supine positions and requires co-activation of the local stabilizers in the lumbar spine. Hip abduction strengthening is needed to support the lumbopelvic region during standing. Progress to standing hip abduction against elastic resistance to challenge single-leg standing balance.
Leg press/total gym (Exercise 9.19)	High repetitions, low load initially with the lumbopelvic region in neutral position or with limited pain exacerbation	Resistance is chosen based on ability to maintain lumbar spine position with some leg fatigue (endurance dosage >20 repetitions). Monitor equal weight-bearing.	Teach hip and trunk dissociation while strengthening legs. Promote distribution of forces to lower limbs. Progress to single-leg press and increase load.

Continued

TABLE 11.8 Exercise Choices, Parameters, Modifications, and Rationale: Case 11.2—cont'd

	Parameters	Monitoring During Exercise, Modifications	Rationale
Stabilization and Spinal Endurance in Positions Required for Functional Activities			
Maintain neutral spinal positions; seated on exercise ball with arm challenge (Exercise 11.39)	Closed chain for feedback and proprioceptive input	Use feedback from resistance band around the legs to facilitate with hip muscle activation to provide distal support. If patient is not actively stabilizing the spine, can use manual cueing, instruct to "lift up off the ball," or hold a wooden pole behind the patient's back.	Motor learning Kinesthetic awareness of position with feedback Mimics position required for sitting in daily lectures Progress speed of arm movement and add arm weight, then to maintaining the trunk position for longer time frames and adding progressive sets of different arm exercises. Progress to hinge positions in standing.
Hinge position with single-arm weights (shoulder extension, triceps extension; Exercise 11.37)	Arm weights are set to fatigue posterior arm muscles without 10–15 repetitions	Dosage set based on ability to maintain the spine alignment.	Forward hinge position and single arm exercise challenges endurance of the spinal extensors. Progression to functional movement training. Progression from sitting on the ball to hinge positions in standing.

aSee Box 11.6 for application of motor control concepts.

TABLE 11.9 Functional Movement Strategies to Distribute Forces

Functional Movement	Parameters	Monitoring	Rationale
Functional Movement Training (See Box 11.7)			
Double-leg squats to lift objects (Exercise 11.43) Stride lunge to lift objects (Exercise 11.44)	Small squat to lift light loads placed at hip height and move to another surface. Initial dosage is light to train the movement, followed by repetition and carrying objects over a distance.	Avoid flexing the lumbar spine to lift the objects. Watch for extending the spine during the lift rather than using legs.	Teach appropriate movement strategies with force closure and support of the lumbopelvic region for lifting techniques similar to work activities.
Single-leg stance with arm challenges (Exercise 9.24) Step-ups (Exercise 9.31)	Maintain position for at least 30 seconds with slow arm challenges without weight. 4-inch step, forward step-ups, initial emphasis on neuromuscular coordination; lumbopelvic alignment during movement. Feedback using a mirror, concentrating on the position of the pelvis in space using the hands on the iliac crests	Watch for loss of pelvis position (drop, hiking, rotation) or excessive lumbopelvic motion.	Train neuromuscular coordination with a smaller base of support and using balance reactions to promote muscle activation and endurance for the hip abductors and adductors and rotators. Step-ups and -downs also challenge the vertical motion and alignment of the pelvis. Progress to light hand-held weights.
Reversal from flexed positions (Exercise 11.38)	Neuromuscular coordination; sequencing from distal to proximal using the hips on return to vertical	Avoid starting the movement using lumbar extension.	Teach the patient to use hip extension to initiate reversal from a flexed position rather than early lumbar extension (distal to proximal sequencing) to avoid excessive stress in the lumbopelvic region.
Rotation (hip drivers) using pulley (Exercise 11.36)	High repetition (20–30 repetitions) in 5-minute periods. Three sets of 30 for home exercise using elastic sports cord (secured with harness around pelvis)	Trunk and hip dissociation to allow reaching Focus on movement quality, coordination, blocked to random practice for direction. High repetition with mastery	Teach the patient to use hip rotation with a stable trunk to avoid excessive stress in the lumbopelvic region and anticipatory timing.

BOX 11.6 Application of Motor Control Concepts for Neuromuscular Coordination Deficits

- Addressing the patient's neuromuscular coordination patterns requires altering movement patterns and movement strategies to promote muscle control to avoid excessive stress on the lumbar spine (see Chapter 7). Her increased flexibility and mobility also contribute to inaccurate proprioceptive awareness of positions and late reactions when moving through full range.
- A blood pressure cuff can be used to teach early anticipatory abdominal and spinal extensor muscle activation before and during arm or leg lifts. The cuff provides external feedback about transversus abdominis and spinal extensor activation, and a change in pressure would indicate a change or loss of active lumbar support and stabilization.
- Once the patient is able to achieve the appropriate muscle activation sequence, the exercise can be progressed by using an unstable surface such as a foam roller. The external focus to keep the foam roller allows the patient

- to develop the sequencing while fine-tuning and correcting the performance with feedback and error detection.
- The training of anticipatory postural adjustments and reactions[60,61] is necessary in preparation for higher loads and more complex tasks simulating her work activities.
- Once the movement performance is optimized, practice is needed to reinforce and change patterns, with progressive fading of feedback from the physical therapist. Only after the patient masters an exercise should it be added to the home exercise program to ensure that the patient is not practicing and reinforcing faulty movement patterns at home.
- After the patient is able to perform the movement in a more autonomous manner and without requiring significant concentration, the exercise complexity, speed, and timing can be progressed toward functional movement training.

BOX 11.7 Using Specific Exercise to Train Functional Alignment and Force Distribution

- Lifting training is included because her job as a waitress and to prevent recurrence because she injured herself moving a heavy couch.
- Reinforcement of the neuromuscular coordination concepts including progressive recruitment of local and global stabilizers with appropriate force closure and early anticipatory postural adjustment is included in lifting tasks.[61]
- Single-leg balance is introduced to both advance neuromuscular coordination training with a smaller base and to prepare for standing and walking. Maintaining the lumbopelvic relationship in single-leg stance with vertical movement, and during step-ups, walking, and eventually running require refined sequencing and control.
- Teaching the patient to use the hip muscles to return the trunk to vertical while maintaining the trunk and lumbar spine in a neutral position is an

- alternate strategy to distribute forces throughout the spine rather than concentrating the force in the symptomatic area. The reversal strategy is used along with a hip hinge (initially taught during Phase II) and reinforced during the lifting techniques.
- Hip rotation is taught as a strategy for work activities to distribute forces and allow reaching and turning. The majority of functional movement including walking and running requires generalized rotation.
- Even if the patient is able to perform specific neuromuscular coordination exercises, functional movement reeducation is complex and requires time, feedback, and practice. Integrating the strategies into normal activities of daily living also requires practice in the patient's daily environment.

BOX 11.8 Progression of Exercise

Once she is able to activate the lumbopelvic stabilizers, the exercise program will be progressed to include lower extremity and spinal muscle strengthening and endurance in standing positions. Weight-bearing symmetry,[62] endurance,[63] alignment,[63] and neuromuscular coordination to control the end range movements should be emphasized and trained in preparation for functional retraining. Lifting, bending, and twisting, and upper extremity challenges similar to her work tasks will be included in the program. Specifically, the patient will be taught to actively support and control the mid-range lumbar lordosis with her stabilizing muscles while using the hip global movers to dissociate hip from lumbopelvic movement.[63] Proprioceptive awareness is important to limit motion to midrange while balance responses will be used to assist with stabilization responses.[54] Adjusting her daily activities and movement strategies, including lifting and rotary tasks, is also indicated, with progressive load, speed, and range challenge.[15] The inclusion of more complex and challenging exercises and tasks will be based on her responses to exercise during and after exercise sessions. Higher load exercise is also appropriate based on her age, desire to start working out in the gym, her job as a waitress, and future profession as a kindergarten teacher. In one study of patients with generalized chronic mechanical low back pain, high-load lifting and low-load motor control interventions were both effective for pain and disability reduction in short (2 months) to long term (12 and 24 months).[64] There were no differences between the interventions, although

there were no attempts made to classify the impairments related to mobility limitations or excessive hypermobility.

Individualized and supervised exercise programs have been reported to have greater pain reduction and small gains in function compared to unsupervised home programs for nonspecific low back pain, and a high frequency of supervised treatment is more effective than lower frequency of exercise.[65,66] The ideal frequency of exercise may not be possible if there are insurance limitations. Under these circumstances, individualized exercise sessions can be distributed over time with the aim of advancing exercise dosage and choices and a home program to practice movement strategies. Home programs may be monitored by having the patient videotape her exercises, with the exercises then reviewed with her physical therapist every session. Exercises are monitored and loads and repetitions progressed as soon as the patient can tolerate the exercise load without pain and is able to control the movement without reaching end range or demonstrating aberrant movements. In addition, efficient functional activity is practiced to distribute forces using therapist feedback, mirrors, and videotaped evaluation of performance. While addressing movement control has not been shown to have superior results compared with general exercise,[67] short-term results for pain reduction and improvements in disability has been reported to be slightly better when movement reeducation was the primary intervention.[67] In this study, the active exercises were chosen to address pain-provoking postures or movements where compensations were observed.[68–70]

BOX 11.9 Controversy Related to the Effectiveness of Exercise Approaches for Neuromuscular Coordination

There is conflicting evidence supporting the effectiveness of stabilization exercises versus other interventions. A vast number of approaches have been reported and include varying definitions of "stabilization" or "motor control" interventions. Research studies have included specific, very localized exercises without progression, postural correction, strengthening, aerobic training, and correction of provocative or compensatory motor patterns, all grouped as motor control exercise. The number of overlapping exercise types makes research difficult to interpret and apply for providing general guidelines for patient management. Stabilization exercise has been found to provide small reductions in pain and disability compared to no intervention and general exercise, but not more than manual therapy.[72,73] Systematic reviews of studies tend to show sparse support for stabilization exercise for chronic low back pain if individuals with nonspecific pain without specific subgroups are included.[74] However, when only patients with instability or hypermobility have been studied, results have shown greater support for use of stabilization exercise to reduce pain and disability at least in the short term.[57,75–78] Of note, there are only a small number of high-quality randomized controlled trials where the interventions do not overlap and have large enough sample sizes to account for the wide variety of complex factors.

SECTION 3: REPETITIVE STRAIN AND POSTURAL SYNDROMES

The types of exercise used for repetitive strain injuries are described in Chapter 6 and a review of the goals, methods, parameters, and measurements is included in Table 11.5. The priority for repetitive strain injuries is to adjust the movement biomechanics while allowing tissue recovery. The overall goals are to distribute forces to avoid excessive force on inflamed, irritated, or degenerated tissue, promote alignment, optimize biomechanical efficiency, and promote symmetrical and efficient muscle function. In order to address other contributing factors, improving flexibility and length of restricted soft tissue or joint motion and promoting overall endurance are also part of the intervention strategies. If hypermobility is present, the goals for hypermobility take precedence over those for hypomobility, and additional care to avoid stresses on the area of concern is needed (Table 11.10).

CONTRAINDICATIONS AND PRECAUTIONS

- Avoid combined forces resulting in microfailure (specific directions, or type of forces, ranges, specific movements, or adjusting biomechanical factors).
- Avoid angulation or rotation in extreme ranges combined with high loads (see stress-strain curve in Chapter 2).
- Specific precautions for:
- *Spondylolysis* (stress fracture of the pars interarticularis) or spondylolisthesis (bilateral stress fractures, congenital abnormalities, or laxity resulting in anterior subluxation of the cranial vertebra on the caudal segment): Avoid end-range rotation and extension, especially with combined movements and high speed/force.
- *Compression fractures*: Avoid excessive load or vertical impact.
- *Acute disc lesions*: Avoid prolonged compressive forces (flexion, sitting, standing); avoid combined flexion and rotation with load or leverage.
- *Chronic disc degeneration*: Follow hypermobility precautions.
- *Osteoarthritis*: Avoid high weight-bearing forces.
- *Neural irritation or compression*: Avoid positions or movements that increase neural compression symptoms, monitor pain or neural irritation symptoms, and choose intensity of exercise reproducing symptoms.
- *Cervical pain*: Monitor for headaches.
- *Cervical region*: Check for vertebral artery symptoms.
- *Scoliosis*: Avoid excessive motion in transition zones where the scoliotic curves change direction (often at lumbosacral, thoracolumbar, and cervicothoracic junctions).
- *Kyphosis*: Avoid spinal flexion, support cervical spine using pillows or pads if kyphosis is severe and causing cervical stress.
- *Osteoporosis*: Completely avoid exercises involving spinal flexion for Grade III or Grade IV osteoporosis, use care with spinal flexion exercises against load, prolonged flexion exercises, and upper extremity load in a seated, flexed position.

GENERAL PARAMETERS

- Correction of the biomechanical alignment and force distribution is a priority.
- Ability to achieve optimal position determines the dosage, as does fatigue or symptoms.
- Progress supported to unsupported positions.
- Use closed chain exercises to promote a centralized axis of motion, open chain if restoration of range, or flexibility is desired.
- Dosage starts with low loads and high repetitions (>25) or low loads and prolonged holds for isometric contractions prior to fatigue. Emphasize on appropriate timing, sequencing, and targets for muscle activation and endurance.
- Dosage progresses to higher load and lower repetitions (<15) after the patient has demonstrated the ability to maintain positions or repeat movements.
- Neuromuscular coordination focus is used throughout the treatment progression with high specificity, achievement of targets, and correction of movement patterns.
- Progressing the range is based on functional requirements or alleviation of contributing factors without increasing symptoms.

TESTS AND MEASURES

See Magee,[1] Magee and Sueki,[23] and Cleland[24] for more detailed description of available tests and measures, interpretation, and psychometric properties.
1. Pain reports
2. Functional movement outcome measures for endurance or strength
3. Movement observation (qualitative)
4. Functional outcome measures for symmetry, repetition, or functional requirements
5. Ability to perform activities without compensations or home programs independently
6. Functional capacity evaluation
7. Oswestry, Neck Disability Index

OBSERVATION FOR COMPENSATIONS AND RESPONSES

- The first priority is to avoid compensations in the area of concern, but also observe overall alignment at proximal and distal areas influencing the forces on the joint.
- Observe for excessive or early movement (axis of motion).
- Monitor proximal areas and adjust position and muscle activation to address moment arms as well as excessive angulation or rotation.
- Observe for loss of position or muscle activation with fatigue and monitor symptom reproduction.
- Use supported positions if needed.
- Ask patients to report any discomfort during or after the exercise.
- Monitor for delayed-onset muscle soreness, increased effusion, or edema after treatment.

TABLE 11.10 Goals, Methods, Parameters, and Measurement When Repetitive Strain Is the Primary Mechanism of Injury

Goals	Methods	Parameters	Assessment/Measurement
Distribute forces to avoid excessive strain on inflamed, irritated, or degenerated structures	Muscle activation and endurance exercise for areas surrounding the affected region	Open chain or isometric activity around affected area Resistance applied in appropriate locale and intensity to avoid stress on affected region Start with movements in other planes of motion or use other joints rather than affected region Specific muscle activation and timing prior to generalized motion Low load, high repetitions without pain responses from affected area Range depends on the functional requirements and the ranges where stress is likely to be placed on other structures. Isometric or isotonic	Pain responses after exercise (delayed-onset muscle soreness) Specific muscle function capabilities (amount of load and repetitions prior to fatigue) Movement patterns during exercise and functional tests Functional tests
Address causative factors increasing forces on structures and impairments resulting from compensations			
Decreased joint mobility or muscle flexibility	Muscle flexibility (stretching) Joint mobility focus	End range (joint or muscle) Low loads with sustained holds Maximal length of affected tissue Progress time of hold or load Allow some time to accommodate to new lengths prior to progressing load Goals to achieve functional range	Pain responses during, and after exercise (delayed-onset muscle soreness) Range of motion (goniometric or functional tests) End feel (especially for muscle guarding)
Address muscle imbalances (decreased muscle activation, endurance or strength)	See section on distributing forces to avoid excessive forces on inflamed, irritated, or degenerated structures as applied to surrounding regions and to affected area		
Training factors	Adjust training intensity, frequency, or type to decrease local stress while maintaining conditioning Alternate exercise selected (cross-training) Cardiovascular or muscle endurance exercise	Deloaded positions RPE 11–13 if possible without increasing symptoms Multiple repetitions, low load if possible without increasing symptoms	Pain responses during and after exercise (delayed-onset muscle soreness) Time prior to onset of symptoms Functional measures DASH Time or intensity for endurance exercise
Adjust dynamic biomechanical alignment	Promote neuromuscular control using motor control principles Multiple forms of sensory input (visual, tactile including taping) Progress to eccentric control Progress to dynamic motion and balance	Slow progression into ranges where biomechanical stress is more likely Lower loads than normal functional requirements with high repetitions (supported or unsupported) Progress to higher loads, low repetitions (isometric or isotonic) in pain-free ranges	Achievement of targets (% of successful trials) Amount of feedback and correction needed Pain responses or movement quality through range or with repetitions Dynamic movement assessment
Improve neuromuscular coordination and response time for functional requirements	Promote neuromuscular control using motor control principles Closed chain or open chain dependent on functional requirements and stage of recovery Feedback for adjusting movement strategies (auditory, visual, tactile, including taping)	Supported positions progressing to unsupported, movements dependent on functional requirements Multiple repetitions after desired movement strategy has been achieved Parameters progressed based on motor learning to maintain position or controlling range without exacerbating symptoms	Biomechanical analysis (observe and analyze timing and axis of motion) Ability to perform movement correctly (timed) or % of repetitions performed prior to fatigue or compensation Amount of feedback and correction needed % of targets reached Functional capacity tests Self-reported functional outcome measures (Oswestry, NDI)

DASH, Disabilities of the arm, shoulder, hand symptom scale; *NDI,* neck disability index; *RPE,* rating of perceived exertion.

EXERCISES

FUNCTIONAL TRANSITIONS

PROGRESSIVE UPRIGHT ENDURANCE

LIFTING REEDUCATION

EXERCISE DESCRIPTIONS

FUNCTIONAL TRANSITIONS

11.37.   Hinge Positions: Upper Extremity Challenge

See Fig. 11.37.

Purpose
- Challenge spinal endurance
- Neuromuscular coordination
- Promote hip and knee muscle balance in the sagittal plane

Position
- Standing, flexed forward at the hips, trunk stabilized with neutral lumbar lordosis, knees flexed (hip hinge position) (see Exercise 9.34)
- Cervical, thoracic, and lumbar extensor muscles are used to support neutral spinal curves.
- Hold a light weight in each hand.

Action
- Extend shoulder while maintaining spinal support until the spinal muscles fatigue (Fig. 11.37A).

Advantages
- Hip hinge position is used for teaching alternate coordination and sequencing for reaching or lifting objects as well as functional activities such as cooking or housework.
- The position requires isometric and alternating spinal extensor activation with arm challenge, providing an option to target local stabilizer activation.
- Hip hinge position allows static stabilization and endurance without extremes of lower extremity movement.

Teaching tips
- Instruction example:
  - "Establish an active standing posture using the neutral lumbar position that you have practiced, then hinge forward at the hips. Keep your arms next to your side. Then extend one arm straight behind you while maintaining your body alignment, lower it to your body, then lift the other arm."
- Common error to correct:
  - Watch for signs of fatigue: decreased range of motion, increased speed, substituting cervical muscles for shoulder muscles.
- Method to address or prevent compensations:
  - "You should feel the back of your arms working to lift the weights. If you start to feel you neck muscles working to help lift the weight, stop and rest."

Alternatives
- No hand weights
- Different degrees of hip flexion or knee flexion
- Alternate arms
- Use a triceps extension exercise rather than shoulder extension.
- Use a forward incline sitting position instead of standing (Fig. 11.37B).

Progression
- Increase weight.
- Increase sets.
- Increase time held in position.
- Increase lower extremity hip and knee flexion.
- Lift one arm or alternate arms while stabilizing hip hinge and spinal positions.

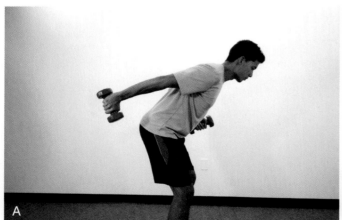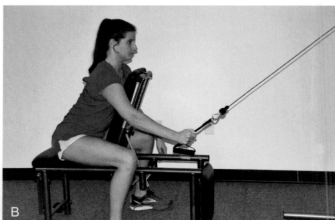

Fig. 11.37 Hinge in standing (A) or forward incline in sitting (B) with shoulder extension challenge.

11.38. Neuromuscular Reeducation: Reversal from Flexed Position

See Fig. 11.38.

Purpose

- Distributed active spinal extension to train and promote spinal movement from flexed positions
- Functional movement to train cervical, thoracic, or lumbopelvic movement coordination in the presence of combinations of hypomobility and hypermobility or overuse of a specific axis
- Useful for individuals who need to attain a supported spinal position with active muscle control prior to endurance training or as an exercise to break up prolonged periods of sitting for work or hobbies

Position

- Seated without the back resting against a chair back, the feet on the floor
- Legs are comfortably apart and supporting some weight
- The spine and head are aligned over the pelvis

Action

1. Flex the spine, starting from the head and neck, cranial to caudal direction (Fig. 11.38A).
2. Spend enough time in each section of the spine to curve the spine forward without hinging at any one point.
3. Once fully flexed, engage the transverse abdominals and pelvic floor muscles to initiate spinal support, then reverse the spinal position by extending the spine in the caudal to cranial direction (Fig. 11.38B).

Advantages

- Seated position allows the patient to focus on the motion without concerns of standing (balance)

Teaching tips

- Instruction example:
  - "Start by nodding your chin and looking downward, then continue to flex your spine one vertebra at a time. When you return to vertical, start by stacking the spine up from the bottom to the top of your spine."
- Common errors to correct:
  - Overflexing the cervical spine, jamming the chin to the chest
  - Overextending the lower thoracic or cervical spine (allowing the lower rib cage to move forward or overextending the neck; Video 11.38A and B [shown in standing])
  - Only extending at the spinal curve junctions (cervicothoracic junction, thoracolumbar junction, or lumbosacral junction—typical areas of hypermobility)
- Method to address or prevent compensations:
  - Provide tactile feedback using a wooden pole or foam roller to guide or limit the flexion or extension for the patient to be aware of how much flexion is occurring and where to return the spine.

Alternatives

- Use tape on the patient's back to limit full flexion and to provide proprioceptive feedback.
- The exercise can be performed with the back against an exercise ball or the wall.
- Standing exercise: Initiate the extension by using the hip extensors to posteriorly tilt the pelvis, followed by the spine reversing after the center of mass is over the base to a neutral standing position (Video 11.38C).

Progression

- Increase range.
- Increase speed.
- Remove feedback.

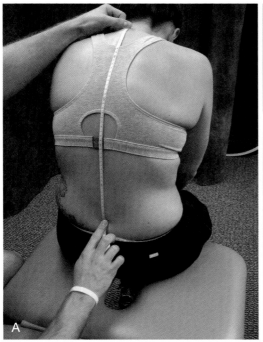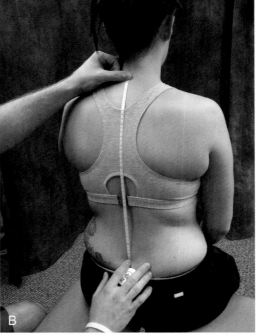

Fig. 11.38 (A and B) Reversal from flexed position in sitting.

PROGRESSIVE UPRIGHT ENDURANCE

11.39.   Seated Upright Posture Challenges: Pulleys

See Fig. 11.39.

Purpose
- Challenge seated postural endurance with resisted bilateral or unilateral upper extremity movements

Position
- Sitting on exercise ball, facing away from pulleys, holding the pulley handles below shoulder height (Fig. 11.39A)
- Upright active posture with some weight supported by the feet but with the trunk lifted off the ball slightly

Action
1. Maintain upright, seated posture.
2. Pull the handles toward the body, maintaining an upright posture (Fig. 11.39A) or use one hand to challenge rotational stability (Fig. 11.39B).

Advantages
- Unstable support requires more spinal muscle activity and promotes early activation of spinal stabilizers.
- Single-arm work requires spinal stabilization while the upright position is maintained (Fig. 11.39B).
- Exercise can be used for initial spinal muscle activation, endurance, or challenge with extremity motion.

Teaching tips
- Instruction example:
  - "Keep the ball and your body supported while moving your arms."
- Common errors to correct:
  - Do not allow the resistance from the pulleys or arm movements disturb the upright posture.
  - Losing the spinal alignment during or between alternating arm motion
  - Allowing the scapula to tip during the movement
- Methods to address or avoid compensations:
  - Ensure sitting balance on the ball before adding challenge of upper extremity movements or resistance from pulleys.
  - Provide verbal cueing for spinal posture and shoulder position prior to arm motion and in between arm movements.

Alternatives
- Facing away from the pulleys, punches (Exercise 10.24 [in sitting])
- Sideways to pulleys, single-arm adduction to challenge unilateral stability (Exercise 10.31 [on exercise ball])

Progression
- Increase time in sitting.
- Increase speed of arm movement.
- Increase resistance in small ranges.
- Rapid alternation of arm movement.

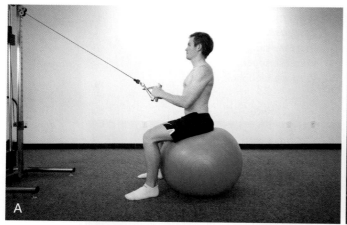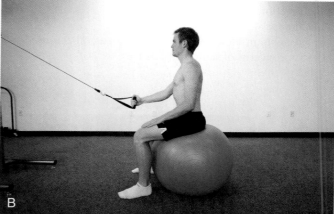

Fig. 11.39 Seated upright posture double-arm (A) and single-arm (B) challenges with pulleys on an exercise ball.

11.40. Graded Exercise Progression: Upper Extremity Challenge with Weights

See Fig. 11.40.

Purpose
- Uses incremental resistance to allow patient to accommodate to movement, resistance, and pain
- Graded exercise approaches are used when psychological contributions are influencing patient tolerance to activity (see Chapters 3, 5, 6, and 7).

Position
- Standing

Action
1. Use any arm movement against resistance (e.g., Fig. 11.40A, B).
2. Set resistance below patient's tolerance with multiple repetitions and sets.
3. Progressively and incrementally increase resistance while maintaining spinal posture and muscle activation.

Advantages
- Wide variety of exercise options that can be performed at home or at a gym for a home program or discharge

Alternatives
- Elastic resistance or pulleys instead of free weights
- Alternate areas of resistance to allow recovery

Progression
- Increase repetitions and weight

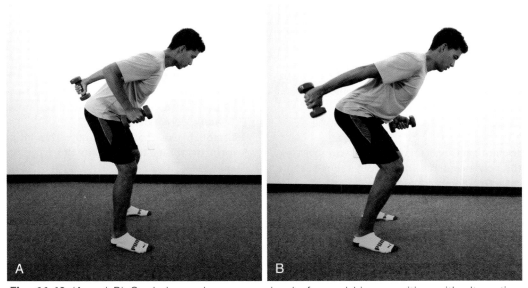

Fig. 11.40 (A and B) Graded exercise progression in forward hinge position with alternating elbow extension against free weight resistance.

11.41. Generalized Aerobic Exercise: Treadmill, Elliptical, or Stair-Climber

See Fig. 11.41.

Purpose

- Increase muscle and cardiovascular endurance using functional aerobic activity
- Challenge ability to maintain spinal posture for prolonged upright positions and during exercise
- Improve general fitness level
- Provide aerobic stimulus for addressing pain responses (endorphins)
- Use before other motor control exercise to enhance neuromuscular coordination benefits

Precautions

- Confirm the patient's cardiovascular status and monitor vital signs before, during, and after the exercise.
- Weight-bearing symmetry is required for even distribution. Other aerobic equipment (bike, recumbent bike, UBE), may be more appropriate if the patient is unable to attain (and maintain) equal weight distribution between legs while standing.
- If the patient lacks hip or knee extension, seated equipment may be more appropriate until the patient is able to extend the hip to neutral or beyond.
- Not indicated for patients with sacroiliac instability

Action

1. Standing on the elliptical (Fig. 11.41A) or stair-climber (Fig. 11.41B) with the pelvis centered in between the feet and a relatively neutral active alignment, use a small step excursion to alternate motion.
2. Use medium resistance to limit the step excursion for the stair climber.

Advantages

- Elliptical or stair-climber machines challenge the patient's ability to manage vertical forces and transfer of forces to the spine with hip extension but without jarring or high loading forces.
- Treadmill can be used to increase aerobic capacity or functional reeducation for ambulation and progressed to running.
- Closed chain
- All aerobic machines are valuable to address biomechanics and neuromuscular coordination for functional requirements.

Teaching tips

- Instruction examples:
  - "Engage your abdominal muscles feeling as if you are lifting your spine away from your legs before you start to change your weight from one foot to the other."
  - "Allow one pedal to move downward slightly then shift your weight to the other side, keeping your trunk supported (on stair-climber)."
  - "Keep your pelvis level and allow your legs to move underneath you."
- Common errors to correct:
  - Letting the pedals move the legs without stabilizing the spine (stair-climber)
  - Rotating or laterally flexing the spine excessively
  - Allowing the spine to absorb forces at one axis, particularly transition zones where there are changes in the curvature.
- Methods to address or prevent compensations:
  - Observe the patient's spine for localized or excessive lumbar spine motion (from the back).
  - Observe the patient's pelvic rotation and symmetry from the side and front.
  - Use a mirror to assist with corrections.
  - Encourage equal use of the legs and a smaller rather than large stride or leg reach, especially in front of the body: "Think about staying lifted and supported through your spine rather than trying to reach your legs forward."
- Monitor for fatigue and set time based on loss of spine position and/or cardiovascular responses.

Specific parameters

- Establish time based on subjective fatigue or on loss of form or ability to maintain the trunk position with the exercise.
- Cardiovascular responses can be based on heart rate or perceived exertion if there are no cardiovascular precautions. Blood pressure and heart rate responses must be monitored along with symptoms if there is any history of cardiovascular problems.
- Gait velocity, 2-minute walk test, or 6-minute walk test can be used to monitor endurance improvements.
- Timed up-and-go, 5× sit-to-stand, or step-up tests are appropriate to evaluate the ability to perform vertical transfers.
- Pain or disability related to prolonged positions on self-report measures (NDI, Oswestry)

Alternatives

- Walking on level surfaces
- Airdyne bike, bike, or recumbent bike

Progression

- Increase time.
- Increase speed.
- Increase resistance.
- Alternate speed or resistance using equipment programs.

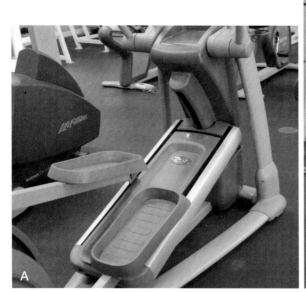
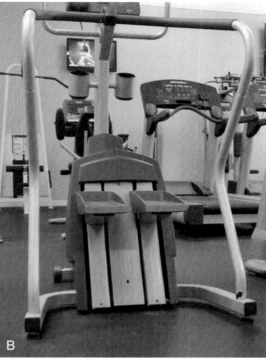

Fig. 11.41 Elliptical (A) or stairclimber (B) machines can be used for general aerobic stimulus for addressing pain responses.

11.42.   **Functional Capacity Graded Exposure**

See Fig. 11.42.

Purpose

- Gradually introduce functional activities, broken down into achievable tasks in order to avoid excessive stress
- Progressively introducing functional tasks can assist with reintroduction of movement that the patient is avoiding in the presence of fear avoidance or kinesophobia.

Position

- Varies, according to occupation or functional deficits

Action

1. Exercises mimic aspects of occupation or activities of daily living requirements that the patient is avoiding or considers painful (Fig. 11.42A–F).
2. Teaching the correct mechanics is a prerequisite to testing load (see movement reeducation for lifting, Exercises 11.43–11.45).
3. Start with low loads and slowly increase load and complexity of movements without avoiding pain.
4. Test the optimal dosage, and set dosage below levels of fatigue and/or excessive pain exacerbation.

5. Loads may be established with patient input on his or her tolerance *OR* expectations of the loads that patients anticipate will be difficulty or increase symptoms (especially if the patient is presenting with high fear avoidance, anxiety, or catastrophizing).
6. Slowly increase dosage based on pre-established goals and observed tolerance. Subjective pain responses are not used to set the progression.

Advantages

- Slowly increasing dosage provides an opportunity to accommodate to stress and adjust psychological expectations.
- Starting with low dosage helps address the fear avoidance components.
- Functional capacity testing informs overall work or activity modifications with progressive goals to return to work or resume functional activities.

Progression

- Increase in duration, sets.
- Increase in complexity.
- Increase in load.

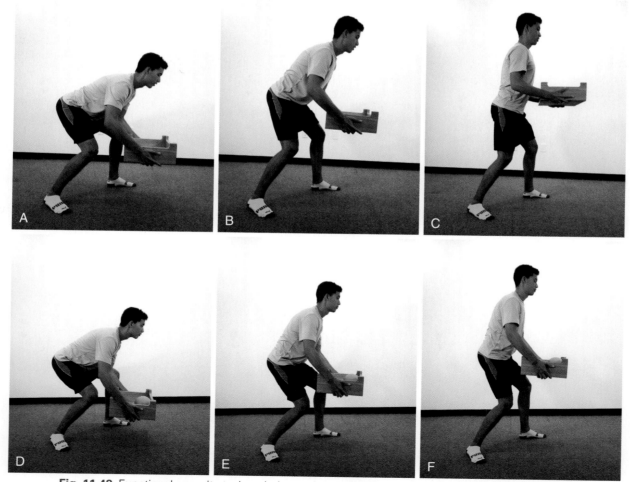

Fig. 11.42 Functional capacity tasks mimic requirements for occupation and activities of daily living with progressive loads, repetitions, and duration of the tasks perceived as painful or difficult.

LIFTING REEDUCATION

11.43. Double-Leg Squat to Lift Object

See Fig. 11.43.

Purpose
- Teach lifting techniques for objects that can be held close to the body
- Neuromuscular coordination and power for lifting using lower extremities for vertical motion

Position
- Standing, feet hip-width or slightly wider apart, natural mid-position of the hip alignment or externally rotated
- Neutral spine with engaged abdominal, back extensor, and pelvic floor support. Position object to be lifted within patient's base of support.

Action
1. Squat down close to object, keeping core muscles engaged and neutral spine (Fig. 11.43A).
2. Engage abdominals prior to pulling object in toward body and deepen level of activation prior to lifting.
3. Hip hinge forward to get closer to the object and bring object closer to the body prior to standing up.
4. Use the legs to stand up; straighten up and extend the hips toward the end of the lift without overextending the spine (Fig. 11.43B).

Advantages
- Functional activity training including lifting laundry baskets, groceries, and smaller objects (Fig. 11.43A, B)
- Lumbar stabilization training while using lower extremities through range of motion

Teaching tips
- Example instruction:
  - "Set your feet as close as you can to the object. Bend your hips and knees while hinging at your hips like you just practiced. Before you lift, re-engage your abdominal muscles and prepare your spine. Lift the object inside your base, then use your legs to stand up."
- Common errors to correct:
  - Lifting from the arms or the legs without engaging the core muscles first

- Extending the spine early or without using hip extension
- Methods to address or prevent compensations:
  - Ensure that the patient understands and can demonstrate dissociating hip flexion from lumbopelvic motion when squatting as well as the hip hinge before prescribing this activity.
  - Teach and ensure proper squatting mechanics (Exercise 9.30) and resolve strength and range deficits before adding a load to lift (Fig. 11.43F–H).
  - Some objects can be tipped to rest on a corner or edge. This elevates the object, reducing the depth of the squat required to lift the object from the floor and allows the patient to bring the object closer to the body.

Alternatives
- Use objects of different sizes or load (Fig. 11.43A–E).
- Stride lunge lift (Exercise 11.44) or golfer's lift (Exercise 11.45). If patients lack adequate closed chain dorsiflexion or knee flexion, they will not be able to squat low enough to the ground to pick up the object and will flex at their spines instead to reach it. A stride lunge lift does not require as much dorsiflexion in the rear leg because the heel lifts off the ground as the patient lowers into the lunge position and does not require as much knee flexion as squatting.
- Start lifting objects elevated on a chair or low bench and progress to lifting from the floor.
- Tipping the object on an edge or corner will effectively elevate it and make it easier to grasp the underside of the object.

Progression
- Increase weight.
- Adjust range of motion for squat or for lifting from different heights.
- Change object shape.
- Add lifting and placement of objects on higher surfaces without excessive lumbar extension.
- Add moving objects over greater distances.
- Increase speed of lift.
- Functional capacity training with multiple tasks, multiple repetitions, and longer time frames

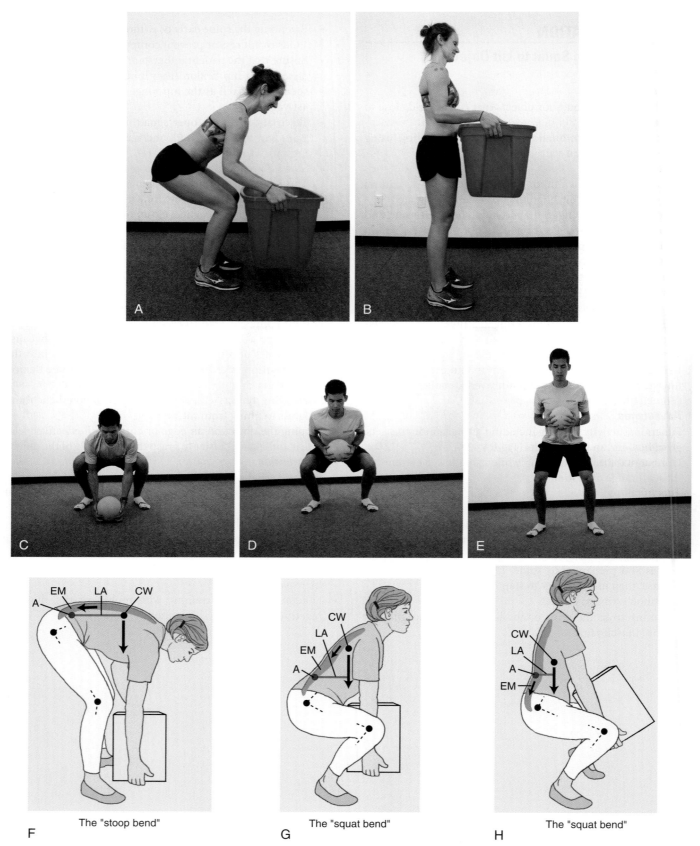

Fig. 11.43 Double leg squat to lift objects such as laundry baskets (A,B), weighted balls from the floor (C–E). Ideally the stoop bend should be avoided (F) with a greater moment arm than the squat lift (G,H) . The closer the object to the patient's center of mass, the smaller the moment arm on the axis of movement (*red dot* A). *CW,* Center of trunk weight; *EM,* extensor muscle force; *LA,* lever arm. (F to H from Muscolino JE. *Kinesiology.* 2nd ed. St. Louis, MO: Mosby; 2011.)

The "stoop bend"

The "squat bend"

The "squat bend"

F

G

H

11.44. Stride Lunge to Lift Object

See Fig. 11.44.

Purpose

- This lifting technique is effective for objects with a wider base in the sagittal plane or for larger, light objects.
- The technique also allows patients with limited knee flexion or dorsiflexion to lower closer to the ground with less compensations than a double-leg squat lift.
- Neuromuscular coordination for lifting using the lower extremities

Position

- Standing, feet hip-width or slightly wider apart, one foot forward in front of the body, one foot behind the body (sagittal plane), natural mid-position of the hip alignment, ankle plantarflexed, and the back heel lifted (Fig. 11.44A)
- Neutral spine with abdominal, back extensor, and pelvic floor muscles engaged for support
- Position the object to be lifted within the base of support.

Action

1. Lower the body close to object, keeping the core muscles engaged and neutral spine.
2. The stride lunge position allows for more weight to be placed on the front leg if needed.
3. Engage abdominals prior to pulling object in toward body and deepen level of activation prior to lifting.
4. Bring object closer to body prior to standing up, using the legs.
5. Straighten up and extend the hips toward the end of the lift without overextending the spine.

Advantages

- Functional activity training including lifting laundry baskets, groceries, and larger light objects
- Lumbar stabilization training while using lower extremities through range of motion

- The rear heel can lift when squatting down (accommodates for limited dorsiflexion range of motion)

Teaching tips

- Methods to address or prevent compensations:
  - Ensure that the patient understands and can demonstrate dissociating hip flexion from lumbopelvic motion before prescribing this activity.
  - Practice lunges without lifting an object first (Exercise 9.49).
  - Address mobility or strength impairments prior to introducing lifting with loads.
  - Start lifting objects resting on top of a chair or low bench before progressing to lifting from the floor.
  - Tipping the object on an edge or corner will effectively elevate it and make it easier to grasp the underside of the object.

Alternatives

- Squat lift (Exercise 11.43)
- Golfer's lift (Exercise 11.45)

Progression

- Increase weight.
- Adjust range of motion for squat.
- Practice with objects of different sizes and shapes.
- Lift and place objects on higher surfaces without excessive lumbar extension.
- Move objects over greater distances, at different angles or positions (Fig. 11.44B–D).
- Increase speed of lift.
- Functional capacity training with multiple tasks, multiple repetitions, and longer time frames
- Place objects in positions requiring rotation by taking steps or rotating using the hips to place object in desired location (Fig. 11.44B–D).

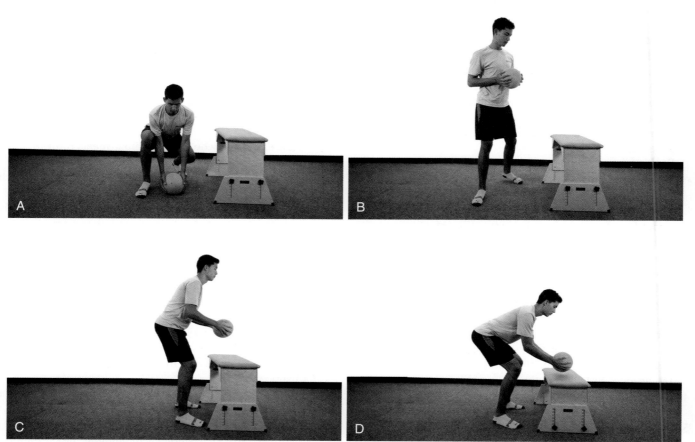

Fig. 11.44 Stride lunge position to lift objects (A) with progressive steps to rotate (B) and place object on surfaces of different heights (C and D).

11.45. Golfer's Lift

See Fig. 11.45.

Purpose

- Teach lifting techniques for lightweight objects which are further away from the body or in awkward positions

Position

- Standing, weight is on one leg, one leg is free to move, natural mid-position of the hip alignment
- Neutral spine with engaged abdominal, back extensor, and pelvic floor support

Action

1. Hinge at the hip of the supporting leg (Exercise 9.34), keeping core muscles engaged and neutral spine. The opposite leg slides back on the floor or can lift off the floor to counterbalance the upper body reaching toward the floor (Fig. 11.45A, B).
2. Hinge position allows reaching forward to lift light objects that are further in front of the body without tilting the pelvis (Fig. 11.45A–C).
3. Engage abdominals prior to lifting object in toward body and deepen level of activation prior to lifting.
4. Return the body to the upright position by extending the hip of the supporting leg and allowing the posterior leg to return to the ground.
5. Avoid rotating or twisting the spine during the movement.

Advantages

- Functional activity training including objects out of the trunk of a car, from a top-loading dryer, or over obstacles
- Lumbar stabilization training while using lower extremities through range of motion
- Good option for patients who lack adequate lower extremity range of motion and neuromuscular control to squat or lunge.

Teaching tips

- Example instruction:
  - "Keep your back straight as you reach to pick up the object. You can slide your back leg back as you pitch forward from your hip. Only use this technique to pick up light objects."

Alternatives

- Squat lift (Exercise 11.43)
- Stride lunge lift (Exercise 11.44)
- Strengthening in a hinge position (Exercise 11.37)
- Sliding the rear foot on the floor requires less balance than lifting the rear leg off the floor.

Progression

- Increase weight.
- Lift from different heights. The smaller the object, the further the patient has to flex at the hips to get to the ground.
- Lift objects placed further away.
- Increase speed of lift.
- Functional capacity training with multiple tasks, multiple repetitions, and longer time frames

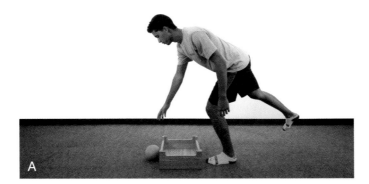

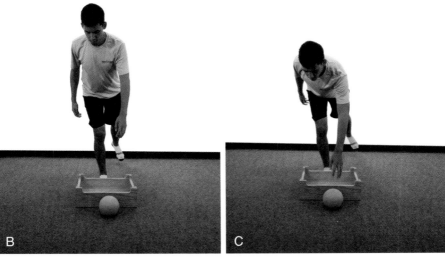

Fig. 11.45 (A–C) Golfer's lift for smaller, lighter objects at a distance from the body.

◎ CASE STUDY 11.3 REPETITIVE STRAIN: SPONDYLOLYSIS IN AN ADOLESCENT ATHLETE

Krissa Gorman, PT, DPT

This case illustrates concepts related to (1) repetitive strain injury management for a patient with acute low back pain (Phase I management); (2) precautions based on evaluation; (3) evaluation of progress and symptoms during treatment with consideration of possible structural pathology; (4) exercise choices for contributing impairments and primary neuromuscular coordination deficits, along with progression of exercise choices from Phase I to Phase III; and (5) use of functional outcome measures.

A 15-year-old female track-and-field athlete is referred to physical therapy by her primary care physician for complaints of low back pain. She is a relative novice in competitive sprinting and hurdling, competing very successfully at the state level over the past year. Her left leg is her lead leg over hurdles. She started experiencing low back pain after increasing the intensity of weight training and conditioning 6 weeks ago. The program included floor core training, shoulder weighted squats, dead lifts, and bench press. She has no significant past medical history or comorbidities.

Functional Status and Goals

She reports constant pain with intermittent, sharp pain on the right side of her lower back during sprinting and hurdling. She has difficulty participating in her track conditioning program and has problems sitting for more than 15 minutes. She also reports pain and "popping" in her lower back during sit-to-stand transitions. Her goal for therapy is full return to sport and to decrease pain with daily activities.

- Functional outcome measures:
  1. Medical Outcomes Study Short Form 36 (SF-36): 51, bodily pain; 52, general health perception; 50, role limitations due to physical problems; 80, physical functioning; 84, mental health.[79]
  2. Oswestry Disability Index (ODI) 15.6%[47]
  3. Lower Extremity Functional Scale (LEFS): (39/80)[80]
  4. Patient Specific Functional Scale (PSFS)[81]: The PSFS requires patients to rate a minimum of three activities they feel are the most difficult on a scale from 0 to 10 (inability to complete task = 0; ability to perform activity at same level prior to injury = 10). The patient reported difficulty with running (2/10), lifting (0/10), turning (0/10), bending (0/10), and jumping (0/10).

Subjective Complaints

- *Severity*: She reports intermittent right lumbar pain levels of 6–8/10 with spinal movement; pain increases with sprinting, hurdling, lifting weights, and sit-to-stand transitions. Her pain also increases with prolonged sitting.
- *Irritability*: Pain limits her sitting for longer than 15 minutes. Increased pain with sprinting decreases back to baseline after 15 minutes.
- *Nature*: Mechanical, repetitive strain, structural microtrauma (spondylosis) needs to be considered
- *Stage*: Acute; Box 11.10

BOX 11.10 Interpretation of Subjective History and Complaints

The patient's high severity of symptoms, Oswestry, PSFS, and physical scale of the SF-36 reflect major limitation of daily function. The acute onset of the pain, history of increased physical activity, and young age indicate the need for caution and full screening for structural damage. The incidence of low back pain in competitive adolescent athletes is higher than in age-matched controls.[82] Spondylolysis is the most common source of back pain in young athletes, with a prevalence of 8–15% in competitive adolescent athletes and 8% in track-and-field athletes.[83] Spondylolysis (fracture of one or both of the pars interarticularis) in young athletes is typically caused by repeated stress or an acute overload. Repeated high loads in extension and/or with spinal rotation, such as landing after clearing hurdles or lack of stabilization during dead lifts in this case, increase risk for both spondylolysis and spondylolisthesis.[83,84] The patient's training (high-load weight-lifting) and athletic training (hurdles) with pelvic and lumbar extreme rotation followed by landing increase the risk for specific localized forces contributing to spondylolysis.[85]

Growth spurts also increase the risk of sufficient repetitive stress on the spinal structures, especially if there are muscle flexibility limitations and muscle function imbalances. Lower extremity flexibility should be assessed for limitations contributing to early or greater rotation, or angulation during landing. During the evaluation, the therapist should consider spondylosis as one of the hypotheses, along with low back pain with neuromuscular coordination deficits or mobility deficits.[15] Training patterns and biomechanical contributions, as well as movement patterns, should also be evaluated.

Objective Findings

- *Posture/alignment*: Excessive lumbar lordosis, sway back posture, bilateral pes planus with increased pronation left foot greater than right, and a left navicular drop
- *Range of motion*: The patient complained of pain with initial ranges of trunk extension active ROM. In addition, she reported pain with lumbar flexion, left thoracolumbar rotation, and bilateral thoracolumbar lateral flexion. Right thoracolumbar rotation was pain-free, and mobility appeared to be within normal limits.
- *Muscle length*:
  - Slightly decreased flexibility of the hip extensors (0–10 degrees hip extension in prone, 0 degrees in Thomas test position), and moderate flexibility limitations of the quadriceps (R 0–45 degrees L 0–60 degrees knee flexion in Thomas test position)
  - Decreased dorsiflexion: Limited to 5 degrees of plantarflexion bilaterally
  - Slightly decreased flexibility piriformis (pain and muscle spasm, passive internal rotation on the right 15 degrees, left 25 degrees); gluteal muscle flexibility restricted slightly and painful.
  - Hamstrings within normal limits on average, but less than desirable for hurdles (30 degrees of knee flexion in 90/90 test). Some pain reproduction in the right leg, more than in the left posterior leg.
- *Muscle function: Activation:*
  - Difficulty activating the transversus abdominis: Unable to obtain more than 4 mm Hg change in pressure on the blood pressure cuff for more than 5 seconds and unable to lift her head and upper body off the mat without pain

- Unable to activate the small spinal extensors in the low lumbar region with leg slides in quadruped. She is not maintaining her pelvis and lumbar position, allowing the pelvis to rotate during the movement.
    - Premature thoracolumbar extensor activation with arm lifts, and she is unable to maintain a neutral position (lumbar spine "sags" toward the plinth).
- *Muscle function: Strength:*
    - Moderate strength deficits (3/5) for hip extension and abduction (bilateral), abdominal strength, and lumbar stabilizers.
- *Special tests*: Positive prone instability test[24,86]
- *Palpation and joint play*: Minimal muscle tenderness and myofascial restriction in lumbar paraspinals found during palpation. She reported pain at all levels of lumbar spine and lower thoracic spine with posterior-anterior glides with more intense pain reported at L3–L5. There were no specific areas of restriction.
- *Movement assessment*: The patient demonstrated further increase in her lumbar lordosis during squats past 30 degrees of hip flexion. Jumping or running was not tested secondary to the acute nature of condition.

Evaluation

- *Initial medical diagnosis*: Low back pain
- *Primary physical therapy diagnosis*: Low back pain with movement coordination impairments.[15] The possibility of spondylosis or spondylolisthesis could not be excluded at initial evaluation.
- *Contributing impairments*:
    1. Moderate hip and core muscle weakness possibly related to pain, below expected levels for an athlete.
    2. There are thoracolumbar active ROM deficits secondary to pain with lumbar spine hypermobility and a positive prone instability test supporting form closure deficits.
    3. Hip muscle flexibility deficits bilaterally may be related to pain (gluteals and piriformis) but will need to be evaluated once the pain has decreased to determine if cautious stretching is indicated.
    4. Mild hip flexor and quadriceps (R>L) and bilateral gastrocnemius flexibility limitations are present.
    5. Movement coordination is impaired, with an early axis of motion and concentration of movement in the lumbar spine during functional activities and range of motion.
    6. Training loads and frequency were increased rapidly over a short period, and weight lifting form may have contributed to concentration of forces. Defer observation and assessment of weight lifting form until the patient has progressed to Phase II and pain has decreased.

Precautions

- Based on history, symptoms, and objective findings, spondylolysis or spondylithesis should be considered and has not been ruled out by medical imaging.
- Avoid extreme ranges of motion (flexion, extension, bilateral lateral flexion, left rotation) and prolonged sitting until pain levels and irritability have decreased.

- Avoid athletic training including, weight-lifting and running until pain levels have decreased.

Prognosis

There are conflicting factors influencing her prognosis. Her age, motivation, and overall athletic goals indicate a good prognosis for functional recovery as long as contributing factors, including training and movement modifications, are addressed. She understands the need to rest from practice, conditioning, and sports competition but is highly motivated to recover and return to sport. Another positive prognostic indicator is her high-level athletic ability. However, adolescent growth spurts and limited flexibility increase the risk of concentrated forces on the spine. The history, contributing factors, and presentation suggest the possibility of spondylolysis. If present, stress fractures of the pars interarticularis diminish her prognosis with a higher risk of chronic lower back pain and difficulty with sporting activities.[84]

Treatment and Exercise Choices

See Box 11.11 for implications of evaluation for exercise choices.

Weeks 1–2

1. Manual therapy:
    - Soft tissue mobilization to lumbar paraspinals, quadratus lumborum for pain and muscle spasm relief
    - Posterior-anterior glides, thoracic spine
2. Exercise emphasis during the first 2 weeks is on neuromuscular coordination, with a stable lumbopelvic position and balance activities to promote midrange lumbopelvic responses (Tables 11.11 and 11.12). Goals are to decrease pain and pain-related muscle spasm as well as to improve neuromuscular activation and sequencing.

BOX 11.11 Implications of Evaluation for Exercise Choices

- Although the majority of back pain in athletes resolves within 4–6 weeks,[87] the relative severity, acuity, and irritability of her symptoms require rest from sport and suggest caution with the aggressiveness of treatment. The initial treatment should follow Phase I principles for exercise and neuromuscular coordination deficits.
- During treatment the potential for underlying structural stress fractures needs to be considered and responses monitored closely.
- The patient's athletic goals drive long-term goals to achieve sufficient flexibility, muscle endurance, and strength for her hobbies but should also include movement reeducation and neuromuscular coordination to limit localization of stress. Exercises will eventually mimic sports-specific movements; however, in the early phases the acuity, severity, irritability, and the potential of spondylosis all require a more specific impairment-based approach. Basic functional requirements for activities of daily living (sitting, sit-to-stand, walking) need to be addressed to decrease pain.
- Training patterns and movement will need to be addressed during Phase II and III.

TABLE 11.11 Exercise Progression

Exercise Phase I/Early Phase II	Progression (Phase II/Phase III)
General Aerobic Exercise (Warm-Up, Pain Relief)	
Exercise 11.41: Recumbent bike, progress to walking on treadmill starting at slow speeds 2.5 mph, progress speed in weeks 4–6	Warm-up: walking on treadmill, self-selected speed Interval running: jogging at 6 mph × 1 min, walk × 1 min (5 rounds)
Muscle Activation and Endurance: Core Stabilization Exercises	
Exercise 11.20: Local stabilizer activation	Exercise 9.26: Clam shells and hip abduction
Exercise 11.21: Leg lifts	Exercise 10.46: Plank
Exercise 11.22: Stabilization on foam roller	Exercise 11.31: Side-lying hip flexion and extension
Exercise 11.23: Bicycle	Exercise 11.32: Side plank
Exercise 11.28: Four-point kneeling with weight shift, alternating arm lifts	Exercise 11.33: Abdominal curls
Exercise 11.29: Side-lying quadratus lift	Exercise 11.34: Diagonals
Promote Balance and Symmetry (Core Engagement Focus)	
Exercise 9. 24: Single-leg balance, uneven surfaces (foam)	Exercise 9.35: Star balance (week 6)
Lower Extremity Muscle Strengthening to Promote Optimal Biomechanics	
Exercise 11.24: Bilateral hip abduction and external rotation against elastic resistance	Exercise 9.28: Side-stepping elastic resistance (small steps) with moderate resistance at ankle
Exercise 9.19: Reclined squats on total gym	Exercise 9.30: Mini squats
	Exercise 9.49: Lunges onto BOSU (small range), then increased depth of lunge
Muscle Flexibility (Delayed Until Pain Decreases and Core Control Improves)	
	Exercise 9.8: Hip flexor stretch
	Exercise 9.10: Gluteal stretch
	Exercise 9.11: Piriformis stretch
	Exercise 9.13: Gastrocsoleus stretch
Teach Biomechanical Adjustments	
Exercise 9.30: Mini-squats (small range)	Exercise 9.31: Step-ups
Exercise 11.46: Log-rolling	Exercise 9.49: Progressive lunges
Exercise 11.47: Supine to sitting	Exercise 11.37: Hinges with upper extremity challenge
Exercise 11.49: Sit-to-stand	Exercise 11.43: Squat lift
	Exercise 11.44: Stride lunge to lift
	Exercise 11.45: Golfer's lift
Sports-Specific Exercise Introduction and Progressions (Delayed Until Pain Decreases and Core Control Improves)	
	Exercise 9.36: Running
	Exercise 9.52: Agility drills: ladders, modified hurdle drills over low obstacles
	Exercise 11.36: Hip rotation drivers

See Table 11.13 for progression by visit and weeks.

TABLE 11.12 Graded Exercise Parameters and Dosage Example for Squat Lifts

	Initial test	Day 1	Day 2	Day 3	Day 4	Day 5	Day 6	Day 7	Day 8	Day 9	Day 10
Range	Partial range (50%) (Fig. 11.42A–C)				Partial range (75%) (Fig. 11.42D–F)						
Load	Empty box							2 lbs (Fig. 11.42D–F)			
Reps	15 prior to loss of spinal position	8	10	12	8	10	12	8	10	12	12
Sets		3						2			3
Rest period		2 min									

New Symptoms at Visit 3

On her third visit the patient reported tingling in her low back traveling up the spine with prolonged standing , and by the fifth visit, the frequency of the sensation had increased and was experienced with movement. By early week 3, she was experiencing intermittent stinging and shooting pain with trunk movement (flexion or rotation) going down the back of the legs. She stated the pain was alleviated within 2 minutes and tingling was alleviated almost immediately after the movement.

Adjustment in Management From Weeks 3–5 (Box 11.12)

Due to the new neurological symptoms and referred pain, the treatment intensity was modified to limit stress and shear forces in the lumbar spine and care was taken to avoid any forces concentrated in the low lumbar region. Neuromuscular coordination, stabilization, and balance exercises were continued, but the therapist monitored the lumbar spine carefully throughout each exercise to ensure that the patient was able to maintain a neutral lumbar spine position without compensations. Balance exercises in standing were discontinued at week 3 and only resumed with care at the end of week 5 (Table 11.13). The loss of local stabilizer activation, early motion in the lumbar spine, or loss of lumbopelvic alignment in standing exercises was used to determine the stop point for the exercise rather than pushing the patient to achieve higher repetitions or load. Rotation or extreme ranges were avoided, and the patient was encouraged to maintain midrange as much as possible during functional activities.

At the beginning of week 3, the patient reported high resting pain levels as she started her treatment, but pain levels decreased to 0/10 by the end of the session.

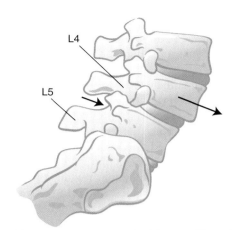

From Salvo SG. *Mosby's Pathology for Massage Therapists*. 3rd ed. St. Louis, MO: Elsevier; 2014.

By week 4, resting pain had decreased significantly, and she reported 0/10 pain at the beginning of treatment. Difficulty, repetitions, and overall complexity of the core stabilization was progressed. Endurance was challenged using timed side planks and planks once she was able to maintain a neutral position at week 5.

BOX 11.12 **Evaluation of New Symptoms and Referral for Medical Consultation and Imaging**

The patient's new complaints of neurological symptoms, the severity of pain with movement, and the potential for underlying pathology led the therapist to refer her back to her primary care physician to be evaluated for spondylosis. Unfortunately, difficulty with insurance approval delayed the radiography appointment ordered by her primary care physician until week 6. The radiographic report was not available until week 8. In the meantime, the treatment was performed using the same criteria to limit stresses in the lumbar spine area with additional care to limit movement to within a range that did not reproduce severe pain or tingling.

TABLE 11.13 **Interventions from Week 1–8**

	WEEK	1		2		3		4		5		6		7		8
	Visit	1	2	3	4	5	6	7	8	9	10	11	12	13	14	15	16
Manual therapy		●		●	●			●	●		●						
Core stabilization and neuromuscular coordination		●	●	●	●	●	●	●	●	●	●	●	●	●	●	●	●
Balance			○			○	○	○	○	○	○	○	○	○	○	○	○
Lower extremity strengthening		●	●	●	●	●	●	●	●	●	●	●	●	●			
Functional movement retraining[a]		○	○	○								●	●	●	●	●	●
Sports specific												○		○	○	○	○
Lower extremity flexibility												●		●		●	

[a]Early functional movement training focused on sitting posture, log rolling and supine to sit, sit-to-stand transitions, (visit 2) and integration of core activation and neutral position into activities of daily living. Late functional movement retraining included step ups, squats, lunges, hinges with upper extremity challenge.

Weeks 6–8 and Return to Athletic Practice

At her twelfth visit (week 6), her pain had decreased to 0/10 (no pain) for both resting pain and with movement. The 6-point change exceeded the minimally clinically important difference (MCID) in NPRS (2.2 points at 4 weeks of physical therapy).[88] At this point, the patient was able to tolerate functional training and strengthening (step-ups, lunges, hinges, squats, lifting techniques with low load) (see Tables 11.10 and 11.11). Modified sports-specific exercises, such as interval running, negotiating low obstacles, and progressive sports-specific strengthening, were added at this visit. The intensity, range, and frequency of her sports-specific drills was increased slowly from week 6 to week 8. Flexibility exercises were delayed until her fourteenth visit in order to limit stress in the lumbar region, although gastrocnemius stretches were included earlier in the treatment.

The patient only received the radiographic report and radiographs at visit 16 (week 8), confirming bilateral healed L5 pars interarticularis fractures (spondylolysis) without separation or spondylolisthesis. The orthopedic physician instructed the patient to avoid any weight-lifting activities for 6 months. At this point her symptoms had improved enough to start with a return to her running program. She returned to team practice starting with walk/run training on alternate days, progressing to speed before distance (no hurdles). The therapist videotaped her running mechanics on the treadmill, then reviewed the videos with the patient and provided feedback to improve cadence and decrease overstriding. Frequency of physical therapy treatment was reduced to once a week from week 8 to week 12, and the patient continued to progress sports-specific training, flexibility, and functional strengthening. She was discharged at week 12 after returning to full track practice (no hurdles) without low back pain or any tingling sensations. Since discharge, she completed the remainder of her athletic season and participated successfully in two competitive meets.

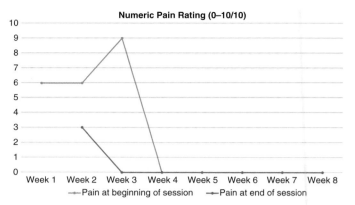

Outcomes

Pain decreased in the lumbar spine to 0/10 by visit 8 (week 4; Table 11.14). At visit 11 in week 5, she no longer reported tenderness on PA glide, lumbar paraspinal palpation, or trunk active ROM. Scores on ODI, SF-36, LEFS, PSFS, Focus on Therapeutic Outcomes (FOTO), pain intensity level, and prone instability were documented on visits 1, 12 (week 6), and 16 (week 8). Due to the patient's athletic goals, single/triple hop distance was measured at weeks 12 and 16 when lower extremity functional activities and sports-specific training were introduced. By visit 16 (week 8), the patient reported a 15.6% improvement in the Oswestry score, which exceeded the MDC (5.94%) and the MCID for low back pain (12.8%).[89,90] She also demonstrated meaningful improvement in all SF-36 subcategories from visit 1 to visit 16.[90] By visit 12 (week 6) she achieved the maximum score of 100 for physical functioning, and, by visit 16 (week 8), the maximum 100 was reported for the bodily pain section reflecting improvement in daily function, including sitting, lifting, and participating in sports-specific activities. Her functional improvements were also reflected in the changes in PSFS for running, lifting, turning, bending, and jumping, exceeding the MCID for PSFS of 2–3 points[81] by visit 12 (see the patient-specific functional scale graph later in the case study).

TABLE 11.14	Severity, Irritability, Nature, Stage (SINS) for Visits 1, 6, and 16			
	Visit 1	**Visit 3/4 (Week 2)***	**Visit 8 (Week 4)**	**Visit 12 (Week 6)**
Severity	Resting pain 6/10	Resting pain 7/10	Resting pain 0/10	Resting pain 0/10
	Pain with movement 8/10	Pain with movement 8/10	Pain with movement 4/10	Pain with movement 0/10
Irritability	Moderate irritability	Moderate irritability	Low irritability	None
Nature	Mechanical minor referred pain	Mechanical, some neural symptoms	Mechanical, no neural symptoms	Mechanical, spondylolysis confirmed
Stage	Phase I acute/worsening	Phase I acute/worsening	Phase II subacute/improving	Phase III

*Referral to primary care physician for further evaluation

BOX 11.13 Prognosis for Long-Term Functional Outcomes

- The healing time for spondylosis can vary by classification of injury: a single-level, unilateral defect has greater healing potential than chronic lesions with separation or multilevel injuries.[84] This patient did have bilateral defects, but there was no slip or separation. Estimated healing time for spondylosis is approximately 3–6 months, with 3 months of rest or longer providing favorable odds for an excellent short-term outcome.[84] Most patients who are compliant with PT and rest from sport demonstrate good short-term outcomes; however, only 81% maintain full participation in their sport at follow-up (1.5–5.6 years post initial diagnosis).[84] Selhorst,[84] using a logistic regression model to investigate factors associated with poor prognosis, found female sex, adverse reactions during care, and multilevel injury to be significant predictors of poor long-term outcome with recurrence of low back pain requiring care. The patient participates in a low-contact sport and responded very well to neuromuscular coordination training and stretching. Continued avoidance of weight-lifting and care with slow progression of training along with appropriate form were recommended based on the potential for recurrence.

- The radiographs showed bilateral healed spondylolysis without separation or slip, although radiographic healing does not necessarily equate to clinical outcomes.[84] The patient's improvements in pain and disability (see graphs) and functional capabilities upon discharge (she returned to running and hurdles) indicated a good prognosis for long-term outcomes.

- The patient's improved performance with core stability exercises, general neuromuscular coordination, and compliance with home exercise program, along with addressing possible contributing factors (lower extremity flexibility) contributed to her overall improvement.

- Functional performance retraining was also progressed to include sports-specific activities. Although the spondylolysis was not identified until after the completion of treatment, this case illustrates a good clinical outcome of acute low back pain in an adolescent athlete, with reliance on clinical reasoning, SINS factors derived from patient complaints (Table 11.14), an emphasis on caution, and continuous re-evaluation.

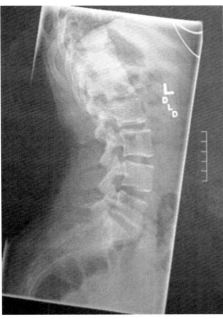
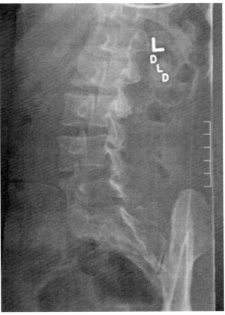

Lateral and oblique radiographs taken at week 8 showing spondylolysis. Note the increased lordosis and lumbosacral angle contributing to the anterior shear forces in the low lumbar region and compression of the L5–S1 joints. The a classic "collar" around the neck of the "scotty dog" indicates sclerosis is visible at the L5 pars interarticularis. There is no obvious gap or anterior slip.

Although the LEFS is not currently validated for use in the low back pain population, the measure was used to track functional ability with lower extremity sports activities. The patient reached the maximum score of 80/80 by visit 12 (week 6), an improvement of 41 points, greatly exceeding the MCID of 9 points for various lower extremity injuries.[91] Her single-leg hop and triple hop tests were not tested on visit 1, but at week 12 symmetry was relatively equivalent (Tables 11.15 and 11.16). Her triple hop distance improved slightly from week 12 to week 16.

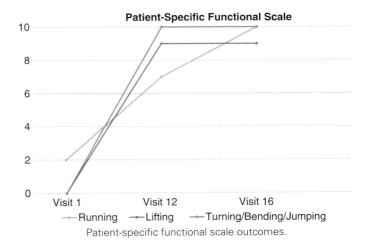

Patient-specific functional scale outcomes.

TABLE 11.15 Functional Outcome Measures

	Visit 1	Visit 12	Visit 16
Oswestry	15.6%	0%	0%
LEFS	39	80	80
SF-36			
Bodily pain	51	62	100
Physical functioning	80	100	100
Role: physical limitations	50	100	100
General health	52	47	62
Mental health	84	100	100
PSFS			
Running	2	7	10
Jumping	0	10	10
Turning	0	10	10
Bending	0	10	10
Lifting	0	9	9

TABLE 11.16 Impairment-Based Outcome Measures

	Visit 1	Visit 12 (Wk 6)	Visit 16 (Wk 8)
Prone instability	Positive	Negative	Negative
Pain (NPRS)	6	0	0
Pain with lumbar motions	6	0	0
Single hop distance*		R 156.85 cm L 133.98 cm	R 158.75 cm L 143.51 cm
Triple hop distance*		R 480.7 cm L 480.7 cm	R 518.16 cm L 510.54 cm

*Not tested on first visit secondary to acuity/SINS.

SECTION 4: POSTSURGICAL MANAGEMENT

GENERAL TREATMENT APPROACHES

The immediate priorities after surgery or trauma are to protect the injured or surgically repaired structures from excessive force and tension, while slowly and progressively introducing forces suitable for tissue healing and regeneration. Treatment follows principles for phases of management with different timelines based on the type of tissue, surgical incisions, and type of surgery. Early exercise will focus on preventing and minimizing atrophy during weight-bearing or movement restrictions. Postsurgical management will progress from protective management and resolving range of motion in the healing phase to restoring motion, strength, and function as the healing constraints and postsurgical protocol allows. Principles outlined in the preceding sections may be appropriate to regain sufficient range of motion or flexibility (Section 11.1); promote muscle activation, endurance, and strength related to limited structural stability (Section 11.2); and address contributing factors such as biomechanical alignment and neuromuscular coordination or impairments related to prolonged immobilization or weight-bearing restrictions (Section 11.3).

Typical postsurgical diagnoses in this category for the spine include:

- Discectomy
- Fusion
- Laminectomy
- Scoliosis fusion
  Trauma diagnoses:
- Conservative fracture management

CONTRAINDICATIONS AND PRECAUTIONS

During the early phases of healing, spinal movement may be limited (especially flexion and rotation) or completely avoided (see Chapter 2). Forces are introduced slowly once intial healing has occurred. Postsurgical precautions can range from 6 weeks to 3 months, depending on the surgical fixation; fracture fixation precautions can extend longer, depending on bone healing. Precautions to avoid extremes of range, combined movements, and impact are set by the surgeon. Spinal orthoses, soft lumbar braces, and hard or soft collars are used to assist with controlling the amount of range. After the braces are discontinued, muscle control of the region should be retrained in single planes and supported positions before increasing range and external loads.

GOALS

- Promote force closure around surgical site to distribute forces and allow healing
- Address any possible causative factors (impairments and movement patterns) that were related to presurgical dysfunction
- Restore functional range of motion
- Restore muscle activation, endurance, strength, and power after muscle and neuromuscular adaptations related to weight-bearing or movement precautions
- Promote functional return and neuromuscular coordination while following healing precautions
- Address psychological components (fear avoidance beliefs and pain behavior)

TESTS AND MEASURES

See Magee,[1] Magee and Sueki,[23] and Cleland[24] for more detailed description of available tests and measures, interpretation, and psychometric properties.

1. Pain reports (with movement, functional activity or positions)
2. Functional movement outcome measures for endurance, strength, neuromuscular coordination (symmetry, repetition, timed tests): single-leg standing balance, sit-to-stand, ambulation or distance, symmetry, speed
3. Movement observation (qualitative)
4. Ability to perform activities without compensations or home programs independently
5. Oswestry, Neck Disability Index

OBSERVATION FOR COMPENSATIONS AND RESPONSES

- Monitor the plane, specific ranges, and directions involving the injured or surgically repaired structure.
- Limit motion resulting in accumulation of force or high stress/strain on the injured structures while allowing motion in other planes.
- Keep the area of concern supported with active neuromuscular control as the first priority, but observe for overall alignment at proximal and distal areas influencing the forces on the joint.
- Monitor proximal areas and adjust position and muscle activation to address moment arms as well as excessive angulation or rotation.
- Observe for loss of position or muscle activation with fatigue and monitor symptom reproduction.
- Use supported positions when needed.
- Ask patients to report any discomfort during or after the exercise.

METHODS

- Phase I: Teach functional activities while adhering to healing precautions
- Promote neural mobility
- Phases II and III: Promote return to function with progressive strengthening and movement reeducation
- Address fear avoidance behaviors and pain behavior during exercise management using cognitive-behavioral techniques, graded exercise exposure, and/or progressive exercise for muscle activation, strengthening, and endurance.
- Address cardiovascular and specific muscle endurance deficits.
- Address contributing factors.
- Promote functional return through movement reeducation and training.
- Address hypomobility and lack of flexibility in other regions to address possible causative factors.
- Promote strengthening of extremities and spinal muscles (Phases II and III) (Table 11.17)

TABLE 11.17 **Postsurgical Management Precautions, Exercise Choices Following Fracture Stabilization or Fusion**

Spine: Postsurgical Management	Precautions	Choices of Exercises
Fracture stabilization or fusion	Avoid motion in surgical region in all planes until sufficient bone healing. Avoid motion at fusion site or immediately around fusion site until sufficient bone healing. Balance precautions if necessary (muscle weakness, sensory deficits, or difficulty with reactions due to orthoses)	Stabilization and neuromuscular coordination around site (especially for local spinal extensors which are often incised or atrophied after the surgery) Teach functional transitions (log-rolling, side-lying to sitting, sit-to-stand, gait reeducation, and progressive weight-bearing, squats).
Compression fractures	Avoid high-impact vertical forces Avoid flexion, especially sustained flexion or high loads. Avoid flexion and rotation.	Exercise in supine, prone, or four-point kneeling once cleared. No abdominal flexion exercises until full healing (12 weeks+).

EXERCISES

PREOPERATIVE OR IMMEDIATE POSTOPERATIVE FUNCTIONAL TRAINING

- Muscle recruitment, coordination, and stabilization techniques (see Section 11.2)

NEURAL MOBILITY

- Alignment and force distribution (Section 11.3)

- Chronic pain approaches (graded exercise exposure) (see Section 11.3)
- Functional movement reeducation (see Section 11.3)
- Progressive lower or upper extremity strengthening (Sections 9.2, 9.3, 10.2, 10.3, 11.2, and 11.3)
- Generalized endurance (Sections 9.3, 10.3, and 11.3)
- Address contributing factors

EXERCISE DESCRIPTIONS

PREOPERATIVE OR IMMEDIATE POSTOPERATIVE FUNCTIONAL TRAINING

11.46.   Log-Rolling

See Fig. 11.46.

Purpose

- Stabilization of the trunk while rolling in bed or as a transition to move from side-lying into sitting
- This is an important skill that should be taught early in the rehabilitation process.

Precautions

- After spinal surgery, log-rolling is taught to protect the surgical site or fracture from isolated rotation or increased rotational stresses. The normal axis of motion when moving in bed or from supine to sitting is in the lumbar spine, especially if the arms and legs are moved at different times.
- Engaging the abdominal muscles helps maintain the core position, while moving the shoulders and pelvis at the same time helps distribute forces.
- The movement can be performed in a brace.
- If the patient is getting up from the bed for the first time, orthostatic hypotension precautions are important after the log-rolling (Exercise 11.47).

Position

- Supine

Action

1. Maintaining an active abdominal engagement and neutral spine position, flex one hip to 45 degrees followed by the second limb.
2. Maintain a neutral position in the lumbar spine.
3. Brace the spine and allow the body to roll on to the side, with simultaneous upper and lower spinal motion (Fig. 11.46A, B).

4. Reach the arm as the body starts to roll, keeping the thoracic spine moving with the lumbar spine and pelvis. The upper extremity motion should be synchronized with the lower extremity movement.

Advantages

- Important to teach the patient how to avoid excessive rotation in the lumbar spine or an unsupported axis of motion in the postsurgical region to decrease strain on the incised structures

Teaching tips

- Instruction examples:
  - "Engage your abdominal muscles to connect your pelvis and rib cage. Keeping your back in the same position bend one knee at a time. Keeping your abdominal muscles engaged, roll your body onto one side."
  - "Your shoulders and pelvis should roll at the same time."
- Common error to correct:
  - Avoid twisting the spine by only reaching with the arms or allowing either the arms or the legs to lead the movement without moving the spine at the same time (this will result in spinal rotation).
- Methods to address or avoid compensations:
  - Brace with the core muscles prior to starting to move the legs or arms to avoid rotating the spine.
  - Have the patient turn the head in the direction that he or she wants to move at the same time as rolling the body.

Alternatives

- The movement can be performed, holding a pillow over the stomach or using an elastic binder to help with proprioceptive input.
- Therapist assistance for timing of movement
- Sequential rolling with pillows propped behind the body if necessary

Progression

- Increase speed of movement.
- Decrease feedback.

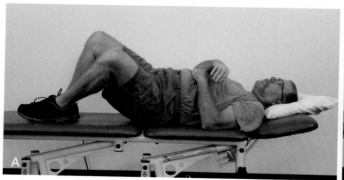 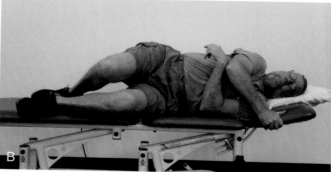

Fig. 11.46 Log-rolling from supine to side-lying.

11.47.   Side-Lying to Sitting

See Fig. 11.47.

Purpose
- Stabilization of the trunk to move from side-lying into sitting

Precautions
- Ensure that the patient is not too close to the side of the bed when rolling or about to move to sitting.
- Monitor for postural hypotension (dizziness, lightheadedness). Allow the patient to pause once in the sitting position and perform ankle pumps to recirculate the blood back toward the head.
- Guard the legs and ensure that height of the bed allows the patient to place the feet firmly on the ground.

Position
- Supine

Action (Video 11.47)
1. Roll from supine to side-lying using a log-rolling action with active abdominal engagement (Exercise 11.46).
2. Maintaining an active abdominal engagement and neutral spine position, use the (top) free arm to assist pushing up onto the elbow on the underside.
3. Stabilize with the core muscles, lower the legs off the edge of the bed as the arms simultaneously push the body up to sitting (Fig. 11.47A–D).

Advantages
- Important skill to avoid excessive rotation or side-bending while pushing up to sitting

Teaching tips
- Instruction examples:
  - "Roll to your side. Brace with your core muscles and carefully push up onto your elbow. Lower your feet off the side of the bed and as your feet lower, push yourself up to sitting."
  - "When your feet lower, use your arm to help your upper body to lift off the bed at the same time."
  - "Time the movement of your upper body (moving up) and legs (going down)."

Alternatives
- Holding a pillow over the stomach or using an elastic binder to help with proprioceptive input.
- Therapist assistance for timing of movement

Progression
- Increase speed of movement.
- Decrease feedback or assistance.

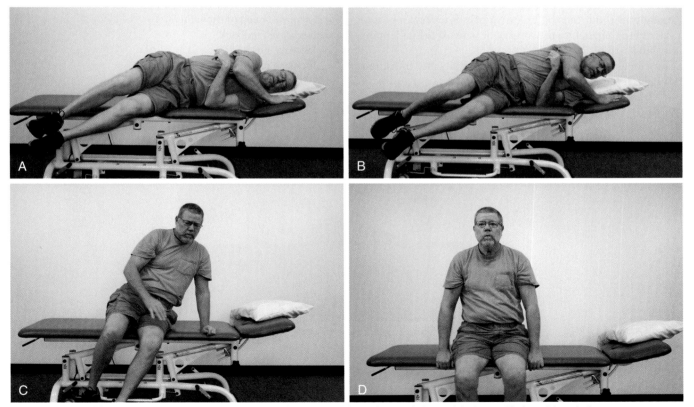

Fig. 11.47 Progressive movement from side-lying (A) to sitting with feet off the side of the table (B–D).

11.48.   Bridging with Lateral Transfer for Bed Mobility

Purpose

- Stabilization of the trunk to move around in bed, prior to transferring from supine to sitting
- Training or preparation for transitional movements

Precautions

- Avoid excessive lumbar extension.
- Monitor for spinal movement or muscle fatigue.
- Monitor timing of trunk muscle activation.

Action

1. Stabilize the lumbar spine by engaging the deep abdominal muscles after establishing a neutral lumbar curve.
2. Lift the pelvis, maintaining the lumbar spine muscle stability (Fig. 11.48).
3. Move the trunk to one side, then lower the pelvis to the bed.
4. Lift one leg and move it in the direction of the pelvis and place it down, then repeat with the other leg.
5. If the movement is followed by a transition from supine to sitting, repeat the movement until the body is close enough to the edge of the bed to roll to the side before sitting up (Exercise 11.46).

Advantages

- Necessary to avoid excessive rotation in the lumbar spine or creation of an unsupported axis of motion in the postsurgical region with stretch on the incised structures
- If the patient is spending more time in bed than usual, bed mobility without causing excessive pain is a very important activity to train before the surgery or to assist the patient in a hospital setting.
- Functional activity required for bed mobility and transitions

- This exercise can also be used to assist patients with high pain levels after fractures or other spinal pathology such as metastatic cancer or osteoporosis.

Teaching tips

- Instruction example:
  - If the patient is having difficulty bridging without pain, the global stabilizers can be used to help stabilize spine at first: "Press your arms down onto the bed before lifting your pelvis, this should help you lift without increasing your pain. Keep your abdominal muscles tight as you lift."
- Common errors to correct:
  - Twisting or rotating the spine at the same time as the bridging
  - Excessive extension only occurring in the lumbar spine
- Methods to avoid or correct compensations:
  - Ensure that the patient is able to engage the abdominal muscles and find a neutral spine position prior to lifting.
  - Small movements to the side or vertical movements in the bed are easier to perform and are less likely to cause loss of trunk stability.

Alternatives

- The movement can be performed in a brace if the patient has had a fusion requiring external support as part of the spinal precautions.
- Therapist assistance for timing of movement
- Small lift off from the surface
- Vertical movement

Progression

- Increase speed of movement.
- Decrease feedback.
- Increase range.
- Increase repetitions.

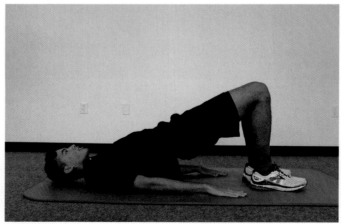

Fig. 11.48 Bridging prior to a lateral shift required for bed mobility.

11.49. Sit-to-Stand

See Fig. 11.49.

Purpose
- Muscle stabilization of the trunk to move from sitting to standing
- Timing and motor training to avoid initiating movement using spinal extension at a specific axis
- Lower extremity strengthening with trunk stabilization

Precautions
- Ensure that the patient is not too close to the side of the bed when about to move to sitting.
- Monitor for postural hypotension (dizziness, lightheadedness).
- Guard the legs and ensure that height of the bed allows the patient to place the feet firmly on the ground.
- Follow any spinal precautions.

Position
- Sitting, choose the chair height appropriate for the patient's height

Action (Video 6.15)
1. Maintaining an active abdominal engagement and neutral spine position, scoot the pelvis toward the front edge of the bed or chair.
2. Maintain a neutral position in the lumbar spine and hinge forward at the hips.
3. Lean the body forward until the center of gravity is over the base, then use the hips and knees to lift the body off the chair in a vertical direction (Fig. 11.49A, B).
4. Trunk extension should occur either after or as the hips and knees begin to extend but not before the legs start to lift the body.
5. The hands can be used on the chair to help with balance and to assist with vertical propulsion.

Advantages
- Important functional skill that should be taught preoperatively or in the early postoperative recovery to avoid excessive flexion or extension in the lumbar spine or creating an unsupported axis of motion in the postsurgical region

Teaching tips
- Instruction example:
  - "Bring your hips toward the front edge of the chair and make sure your feet are underneath your body. When you are ready to stand up, engage your abdominal muscles, lean forward over your feet. Use your hips and knees and push down into your legs to stand up. Before you straighten up, bring your hips underneath your body, keeping your abdominal muscles engaged."
- Common errors to correct:
  - Extending the spine early
  - Looking up as the patient stands up can result in early lumbar and cervical extension
  - Placing the feet too far forward (outside base of support)
  - Keeping one hand on the chair causes spinal rotation
- Methods to address or prevent compensations:
  - Looking forward and allowing the eye gaze to slowly change as the trunk straightens
  - Ensuring that the feet are close to the chair and under the body
  - Using both hands on the edge of the chair initially for guidance, but reaching forward past the feet with the arms if possible

Alternatives
- Holding a pillow over the stomach or using an elastic binder can help with proprioceptive input.
- Starting from a higher surface than a standard chair seat height will decrease the range required.
- A staggered stance with the legs (with stronger leg back) will help accommodate strength or range of motion deficits in the forward leg.

Progression
- Increase speed of movement.
- Decrease feedback.

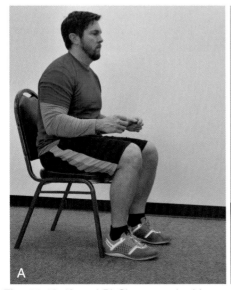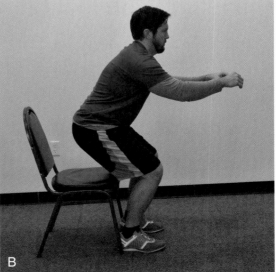

Fig. 11.49 (A and B) Sit-to-stand without arm support. Note that the center of mass is moving towards the base and the feet are close to the chair.

NEURAL MOBILITY

The neural mobility exercises may be indicated for individuals with only mild to moderate irritability or after spinal surgery. The goal of neural "flossing" or motion after surgery is to move the neural structures to avoid fibrosis or adhesion formation, particularly in areas where surgical interventions have relocated or stressed surrounding structures or the nerve itself. For patients with a history of previous surgery, trauma, or chronic problems, adhesions and connective tissue adaptations can contribute to pain or difficulty with movement. Moving the nerve is also thought to improve circulatory responses and address fear avoidance early in the postsurgical time frame. The therapist can perform the movements at first, then train the patient to perform the exercises as a home program.

11.50.   Lower Limb Neural Gliding

See Fig. 11.50.

Purpose
- Mobilize neural structures

  Contraindications and precautions
- Use extreme care and limit movement to distant areas if the neural symptoms are easily reproduced or highly irritable.
- If the patient's symptoms are moderately irritable, use caution when progressing neural mobility exercises.
- Symptoms should not be exacerbated during or after the exercise.

  Position
- Supine, hook-lying

Action
1. Maintaining neutral spine position, flex one hip and knee to 90 degrees, supporting the leg with the hands or ask the patient to support the thigh using a strap (Fig. 11.50A–C).
2. The patient straightens the knee actively until lower extremity symptoms are reproduced, followed by releasing the position and flexing the knee slightly to a point where symptoms are not experienced.
3. Dorsiflexion of the ankle can be added to produce a caudal glide of the sciatic nerves (Fig. 11.50B). Inversion and plantarflexion can be used to provide further gliding of the tibial and peroneal nerves (Fig. 11.50D).

   Advantages
- Support of the spine and the knee position prevents compensatory movement at the proximal regions.

  Alternatives
- Maintaining the ankle in a dorsiflexed position, create the gliding by extending and flexing the knee through a small range, short of the full stretch.

  Progression
- Increase range of oscillations.
- Increase range to reach the range where symptoms are reproduced but move out of the end range immediately.
- Maintain position for short holds of 5–10 seconds.
- Use a slump position in sitting to lengthen the entire proximal neural system. Trunk flexion and cervical flexion can be used as a starting position followed by hip flexion and knee extension, with or without ankle motion (Fig. 11.50E–G).
- Mobility of the femoral nerve complex can be performed using hip extension and knee flexion in prone (Fig. 11.50H).

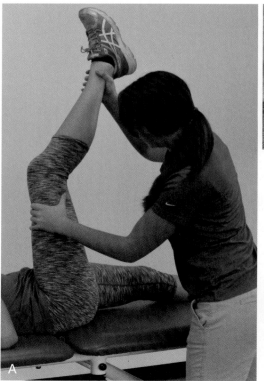
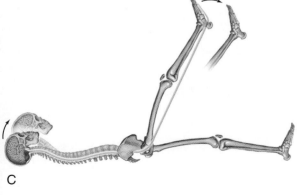
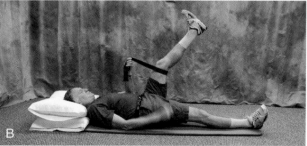

Fig. 11.50 Neural gliding in supine with hip flexion, knee extension provided by the therapist (A) or actively by the patient (B). Dorsiflexion (B) or cervical flexion (C) can be added for further neural motion.

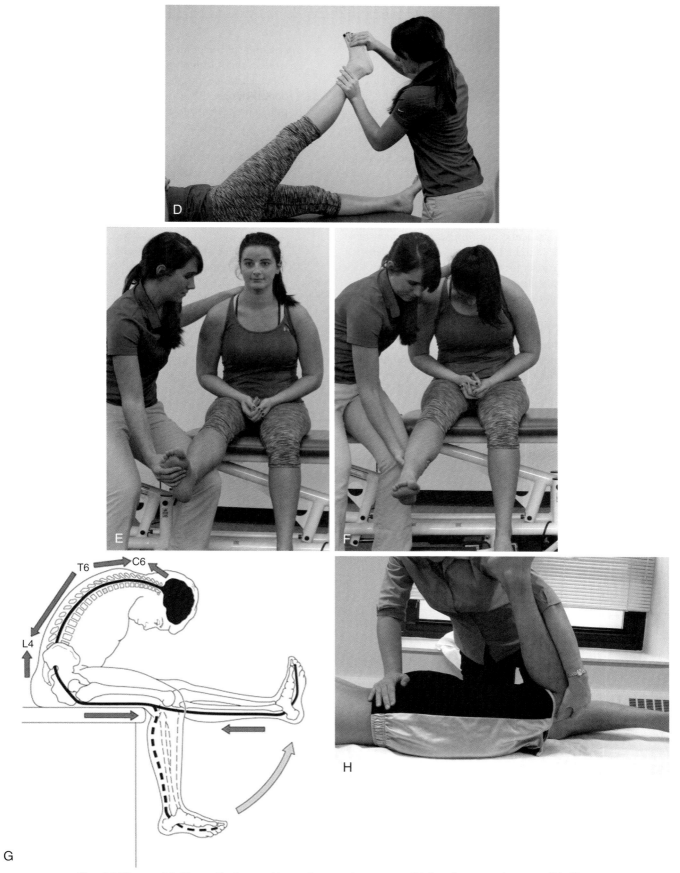

Fig. 11.50 cont'd Plantarflexion and inversion used to target tibial and peroneal nerves (D). Sitting slump position for proximal motion (E and F), with (E) or without (F) distal ankle motion. The maximal stretch of the entire complex is usually not necessary to reach full length of the neural complex (G). Femoral nerve mobility is targeted in prone with hip extension and knee flexion (H). (C and G from Cameron MH, Monroe LG. Physical Rehabilitation. St. Louis, MO: Mosby; 2007.)

11.51.   Upper Limb Neural Gliding

See Fig. 11.51.

Purpose

- Increase or maintain mobility of neural structures

Contraindications and Precautions

- Use extreme care and limit movement to distant areas if the neural symptoms are easily reproduced or highly irritable.
- If the patient's symptoms are moderately irritable, use caution when progressing neural mobility exercises.
- Symptoms should not be exacerbated during or after the exercise.

Position

- Supine, neutral cervical spine position with sufficient head support to avoid stress on the head, neck, and shoulders
- Maintain scapula position in slight depression using a block or ball, or the therapist limits the movement by holding his or her fist above the shoulder.

Action

- *Upper limb tension 1 for median nerve[1]* (Fig. 11.51A, B)
  1. Abduct the shoulder to between 70 and 110 degrees with full shoulder external rotation with the elbow flexed to 90 degrees. Shoulder and upper arm can be supported on a towel or small pillow if necessary to avoid symptom reproduction.
  2. Extend the elbow with the forearm supinated.
  3. Extend the wrist and fingers (including the thumb), short of excessive pain or neural symptoms.
- *Upper limb tension position 2 for median nerve*
  1. Abduct the shoulder to 10 degrees, externally rotate the shoulder with the elbow flexed to 90 degrees. Shoulder and upper arm can be supported on a towel or small pillow if necessary to avoid symptom reproduction.
  2. Extend the elbow with the forearm supinated.
  3. Extend the wrist and fingers (including the thumb), short of excessive pain or neural symptoms.

- *Upper limb tension position 3 for radial nerve* (Fig. 11.51C, D)
  1. Abduct the shoulder to between 70 and 110 degrees with medial rotation and the elbow flexed to 90 degrees. Shoulder and upper arm can be supported on a towel or small pillow if necessary to avoid symptom reproduction.
  2. Extend elbow with the forearm pronated and wrist in ulnar deviation.
  3. Flex the wrist and fingers (including the thumb), short of excessive pain or neural symptoms.
- *Upper limb tension position 4 for ulnar nerve* (Fig. 11.51E, F)
  1. Abduct the shoulder to between 10 and 90 degrees, extend the shoulder with lateral rotation, elbow extended. Shoulder and upper arm can be supported on a towel or small pillow if necessary to avoid symptom reproduction.
  2. Forearm supinated or pronated and wrist in radial deviation.
  3. Extend the wrist and fingers, short of excessive pain or neural symptoms.

Advantages

- Supported position for the spine and the shoulder position help prevent compensatory movement in the proximal regions.
- Active motion can be controlled by patient.

Alternatives

- Decrease the range of the shoulder, elbow, or wrist to decrease tension on the neural structure.
- Maintain the wrist position and move the elbow.

Progression

- Increase range of oscillations.
- Increase range to reach the range where symptoms are reproduced but move out of the end range immediately.
- Maintain position for short holds of 5–10 seconds.
- Add cervical spine lateral flexion away from the moving arm (Fig. 11.51G, H).

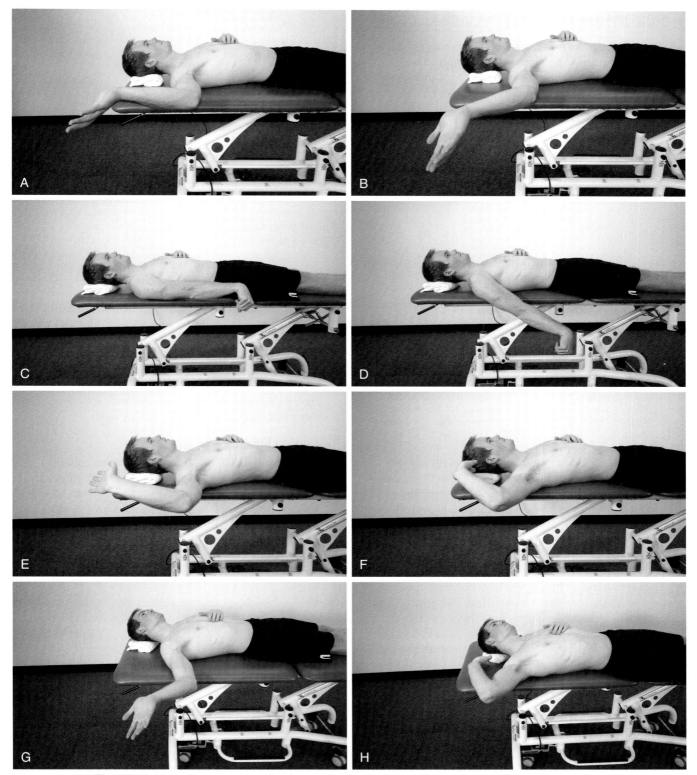

Fig. 11.51 Upper limb neural gliding for median nerve (A and B), radial nerve (C and D), and ulnar nerve (E and F), with cervical positioning for additional tension (G and H).

◎ CASE STUDY 11.4: POST PELVIS FRACTURE

This case study illustrates implications of chronic pain post trauma, when yellow flags require application of psychological concepts for therapeutic exercise choices, delivery, and progression.

A 45-year-old man sustained a left ilium and sacral fracture 3 years ago in a motor vehicle accident. The fractures were treated with external fixation and bedrest initially, followed by internal fixation.

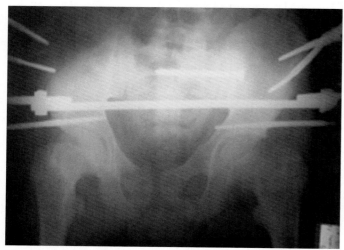

(From Borozda IV, Ganzhurov NA, Kapustyansky AA, et al. Step-by-step external fixation of unstable pelvis with separate anterior and posterior modules. *Asian Pac J Trop Biomed.* 2016.)

He was allowed to start weight-bearing 8 weeks after the surgery. He has had chronic lumbar pain with radiating pain down the left leg since the accident. He was a construction worker prior to the injury but is now on disability, and he is married with three children. He is using oxycodone for pain relief.

Functional Status and Goals

He reports difficulty with dressing and showering secondary to being unable to stand on his left leg. He is currently the primary caregiver for his children and is able to drive, but is he unable to tolerate household chores or assist around the house. He is unable to sit or stand for more than 10 minutes, unable to stand on his left leg or walk more than 10 meters without increasing pain. He is unable to lift objects. His goals are to be able to walk around the house without pain and to decrease pain in sitting and standing. He would like to be able to play basketball with his son. His Oswestry score is 68% (severe disability),[47,90] and fear avoidance behaviors questionnaire scores are very high 80/96.[92,93]

Subjective Complaints

- *Severity*: High; reports 8/10 pain and flexion or rotation increases his pain; sitting, standing or walking are also more painful.
- *Irritability*: High; the patient reports pain levels of 8/10 when sitting and standing for more than 5 minutes and when walking more than 10 meters. If he does stand or walk for more than 5 minutes, the pain only returns to baseline (5/10) after 15 minutes or more. The longer he stands or walks, the longer it takes

for the pain to decrease. Although is pain is lowest when lying down, is unable to sleep for more than 2 hours at a time. He reports throbbing and burning pain in his left sacral area, low lumbar spine, and down the back of the left leg (also constant).
- *Nature*: Post trauma, left pelvis fracture with surgical fixation, deconditioning, chronic pain; low back pain with radiating pain, high fear avoidance, chronic pain (Box 11.14)
- *Stage*: Chronic

Objective Findings

- *Posture*: Sway back position, increased extension in sitting and standing, weight-bearing asymmetry standing on right, pelvis rotated toward right
- *Range of motion*: All active movements are guarded, and he reports increased pain to 8/10 from a baseline 5/10. He stops the movement after 20 degrees of flexion, 10 degrees of extension, 5 degrees of lateral flexion to the left, and 12 degrees to the right. Rotation is limited to 15 degrees on both sides.
- *Neural examination*: Reflexes are normal. He is hypersensitive to touch on the left side in the L4, L5, and S1 dermatomes. Myotomal testing is limited by hypersensitivity and pain reports.
- *Muscle length*: Neural tension testing reproduces lower extremity pain with knee extension at 45 degrees of knee flexion and at 90 degrees of hip flexion.
- *Functional testing*: 10-meter walk increases pain to 8/10, gait speed 1.8 m/sec. Antalgic gait and positive Trendelenburg sign on left, asymmetrical with shorter stride on right. Uses a cane for longer distances.
- *Balance*: Single-leg standing balance on right leg 20 seconds, unable to stand on left leg secondary to pain and fear of weight-bearing.

Evaluation

- *Medical diagnosis*: Post pelvic fracture, chronic pain
- *Physical therapy diagnosis*: Postsurgical management pelvis fracture, chronic pain; low back pain with psychological contributions

- *Contributing impairments:*
  1. Deconditioning and decreased cardiovascular endurance
  2. Chronic pain: Altered pain sensitivity, avoidance left weight-bearing, fear avoidance behavior, possible secondary gain
  3. Decreased flexibility gluteals, left neural mobility
  4. Decreased muscle activation, endurance, and strength all left hip muscles, abdominal, and trunk muscles
  5. Poor neuromuscular coordination lumbopelvic stabilizers
  6. Postural compensations and asymmetry contributing to localization of forces

Precautions

- Limit exacerbating excessive radiating pain, *but* use graded exercise to slowly introduce exercise and movement.
- Use balance precautions.
- Address fear avoidance.

Prognosis

Although there are limited descriptions of long-term outcomes after pelvic fractures requiring surgical fixation, Gabbe[109] reported that 77% of 114 patients with severe pelvic ring fractures were living independently and 59% had returned to work after 2 years. Fracture type and management did not predict recovery, although higher severity had a lower odds of return to work. Patients with chronic low back pain and psychological distress have a five times greater risk of a poor outcome for disability compared to other patients.[110] This patient had a severe injury and has not worked in his physically demanding job since the injury more than 2 years ago, and he is seeking disability—poor indicators for return to work and for full recovery. His Oswestry score shows severe disability and Fear Avoidance Beliefs Questionnaire (FABQ) scores are high.[93,94] His prognosis for full resolution of pain and disability is therefore poor without intervention aimed at both psychological and physical impairment resolution.[94,111] The extent of his disability and FABQ suggest that regular frequent individualized treatment would be optimal, supplemented by a program of self-management strategies and psychological support.[103,111,112] A systematic review of management programs for chronic low pain using cognitive-behavioral approaches concluded that approximately 26 sessions would be appropriate to address the need for progressive increases in exercise quotas and patient education tailored to each individual's specific needs (Box 11.15).[111]

BOX 11.15 Impact of Psychological Contributions for Exercise Testing and Choices

Goals are to assist the patient with managing his pain and restoring some level of function, rather than completely alleviating the pain or disability. A graded exercise approach is chosen to introduce progressive quotas (repetitions and time) within a tailored general activity program.[104,107,108,111] George et al.[106] found no difference between the efficacy of physical therapy management supplemented with either graded exercise approaches or graded exposure. In a systematic review, Macedo[108] reported small effects for graded activity over minimal interventions for pain and disability reductions. This patient was used to athletic training and has indicated a desire to play basketball with his son; therefore, the graded exercise approach was chosen to match his personal factors. While graded exposure is indicated for patients with high pain-related fear and would have been appropriate for this patient, the approach places higher emphasis on psychological intervention to address depression and maladaptive behavior and less emphasis on physical activity.[103]

Baseline exercise was established by evaluating his ability to perform exercise without compensations such as symmetrical weight-bearing, rather than on avoiding pain. The initial exercise testing took place over 2–3 sessions, during which movement patterns and tolerance were assessed while early education and strategies to address his fear were introduced.[97] Encouraging the patient to progressively increase his movement tolerance and activity involved both cognitive (education, explanations)[98–100] and behavioral approaches (goal-setting, rewards when he was able to finish the exercise quotas, distraction).[94,104,106] Obtaining buy-in throughout the process was a key factor; the patient was asked

to prioritize exercise goals and given options for his preferences for exercises and order of exercises.[112] A few of the exercises (bridging, single-leg slides on the exercise ball, four-point kneeling over the ball with weight shift) provided some pain relief (Table 11.18). These exercises were interspersed with the more difficult activities once he was able to progress to practicing sit-to-stand and log-rolling.

Supported recumbent positions were *less* painful (not necessarily pain-free), and exercises were performed in these positions first to introduce movement without discouraging the patient from continuing to exercise.[112] As the patient was able to tolerate more exercise, the weight-bearing exercises were slowly introduced. Functional movement reeducation was integrated into transitions between positions, and pacing was introduced. Educating the patient about the physiology of pain and assisting the patient to reshape his beliefs and behaviors related to the fracture and his approach to movement was integrated into the sessions. The breaks between exercises were used to provide information and to assist the patient to set goals related to participating with his family and children and specific exercise quotas.[114,101] The emphasis on pain was shifted to self-management and progressive activity despite the severity of his pain reports.[96] He was also taught to perform relaxation and breathing techniques while focusing on his achievements for the session. The discussion of his fears and beliefs related to pain and movement and reintroducing movements associated with pain was slowly progressed while providing activity guidance.[94,106,113]

TABLE 11.18   Exercise Choices and Modifications for Case 11.4: Initial Visit

Exercise and Purpose	Parameters	Monitoring During Exercise, Modifications	Rationale and Goals
Stabilization and Neuromuscular Coordination			
Neutral spine position activation of transversus abdominals (Exercise 11.20)	Engagement of stabilizers with feedback from blood pressure cuff, mid-position neutral spine position, no increase in symptoms	Education about pain responses and self management is introduced during stabilization techniques and awareness of breathing. Ability to maintain neutral position	Recruit local stabilizers. Awareness of position. Introduction of breathing techniques and self-monitoring of position for symmetry in supported position
Lumbopelvic Stabilization, Neuromuscular Coordination, and Hip Muscle Strengthening			
Bilateral hip abduction and external rotation against elastic resistance band (Exercise 11.24)	Neutral spine position, anticipatory local stabilizer engagement followed by bilateral small range hip motion holding elastic band (low load). Able to perform 12 repetitions prior to fatigue of left leg, dosage set to 3 sets of 10 with lighter resistance band.	Monitor neutral lumbopelvic position. Symmetry of hip range and activation. Monitoring for fatigue and symmetry. Dosage is based on muscle fatigue rather than pain symptoms.	Activate hip muscles (hip deep external rotators, gluteus medius, minimus). Symmetry and alignment reeducation
Neural Mobility			
Supine knee extension with hip at 90 degrees (Exercise 11.50)	Short of the available range with short hold. High repetition. Early home program	Range that allows motion of the nerve without symptoms or muscle spasm	Improve mobility and gliding of the neural and surrounding structures, as well as desensitization
Muscle Flexibility Without Stress on Region			
Gluteal stretching supine (Exercise 9.10)	End range; start by reaching end range but no hold, progress to short hold, then slowly increase to 15- to 20-second hold	Avoid spinal motion while stretching	Increase muscle flexibility
Self-Management Pain Control			
Pelvic tilt (Exercise 11.8) Segmental flexion with legs supported on an exercise ball. (Exercise 11.9) Oscillations: rotation in supine hook-lying or on exercise ball (Exercise 11.9 alternative: rotation)	Midrange, small movement with neutral spine position and engagement of stabilizers. Multiple repetitions	Used if there is excessive pain exacerbation during treatment and as a home program, avoid excessive range	Provide an active self-management method for method of pain modulation. Used to assist with cognitive elements of the patient's ability to control responses and encourage continuation of exercise once pain modulation has been achieved (Box 11.16).
Functional Training, Symmetry, and Hip Strengthening			
Bridging (Exercise 9.21)	Double-leg bridging with emphasis on stable pelvis and equal weight-bearing. Repetitions until weight shift to R leg is noticed. Initial exercise evaluation – able to perform 8 repetitions prior to shift, home program set at 6 repetitions with 2 sets, progressing repetitions to allow 15-20 repetitions	Progressive repetitions and then range once symmetrical. Monitor symmetry and teach patient to monitor pelvis position and pressure on both feet to limit weight shift to the right. Educate on excessive compensations. Use of local stabilizers prior to movement (anticipatory) to maintain neutral spine position	Functional training with distribution of forces and force closure around lumbopelvic region. Strengthening of hip extensors. Neuromotor coordination and symmetry, and proprioceptive awareness
Alignment, Neuromuscular Coordination, Proprioceptive Awareness			
Weight shift in four-point kneeling on exercise ball (Exercise 11.28)	Education of coordination of weight shift with tactile and verbal feedback. Concentration on weightbearing shift and feedback from upper extremities and ball motion. Multiple repetitions	Motor control concepts with awareness of goals, sensory feedback	Retraining of symmetry and ability to accept weight in unloaded position. Four-point kneeling provides congruent position for hip joint which promotes stabilizing function of the hip muscles attaching to the pelvic region. Exercise ball provides feedback and support for lumbar spine neutral position. Weight shift promotes activation of spinal extensors.

TABLE 11.18 Exercise Choices and Modifications for Case 11.4: Initial Visit—cont'd

Exercise and Purpose	Parameters	Monitoring During Exercise, Modifications	Rationale and Goals
Neuromuscular Coordination and Stabilization Techniques			
Four-point kneeling supported on an exercise ball: hip extension and knee extension slides (Exercise 9.45)	He was able to manage the exercise well (18 repetitions) using the support of the exercise ball. Dosage for home program (quadruped without lifting the leg off the surface) was set as 2 sets of leg slides for 15 repetitions, with relaxation in between sets	Avoid arching or allowing an axis of motion in the spinal region (extension or rotation)	Promote local stabilizer activation, Promote activation of local and global stabilizers
Four-point kneeling single-leg lifts on exercise ball (left side only) (Exercise 11.28)	Only able to perform 8 repetitions prior to fatigue (hip extensors). Required more feedback to maintain position on the exercise ball for the single-leg hip extension against gravity; not used as a home program for first visit.	Monitor pelvis position, avoid rotation or extension in lumbar spine Adjust hip extension range to allow open chain motion without lumbar spine movement Feedback to use posterior hip muscles while maintaining pressure of pelvis on exercise ball to maintain alignment	Posterior hip muscle focus including gluteus maximus and hamstrings for hip extension Lumbar spine stabilization with limb motion to train proximal stability
Functional Training			
Log-rolling (Exercise 11.46)	Movement reeducation included during exercise session for position transitions	Education of simultaneous motion of upper and lower body for neuromotor coordination training	Functional training to distribute motion while moving from supine to sitting
Sit-to-stand (Exercise 11.49)	He was able to perform the movement 10 times but started to complain of radiating pain after 7 repetitions and shifted his weight to the right leg. He was asked to practice the movement when standing up with further movement reeducation and training planned for the next visit.	Monitoring for weight shift, excessive trunk extension instead of using legs Reeducation using hip and knee extension rather than trunk extension Exercise needs to be monitored at next visit, with plan to introduce mirror or video feedback for knowledge of results	Functional training with distribution of forces Incorporated into daily routine

BOX 11.16 Cognitive-Behavioral, Pain Education, and Motivational Approaches

Cognitive-behavioral concepts are used during the initial evaluation and exercise to introduce expectations for progressive exercise.[102,103] The patient's athletic history and his desire to return to playing basketball with his son provides an opportunity to compare progressive exercise to training for competitive sports (ICF personal factors; see Chapter 3) and establish specific goals using the SMART guidelines (see Chapter 7).

During the session, the patient asked if he should get a magnetic resonance imaging (MRI) study to see if the fracture has healed. The therapist took the opportunity to explain that bone healing typically takes 3 months for pelvic fractures and that, if he has been cleared by the orthopedic surgeon, strengthening the muscles around the area to support and distribute forces is the most important priority at this stage. The therapist also took the opportunity to educate the patient about sources of chronic pain using pictures and providing timelines about tissue healing. Clear expectations were established prior to asking the patient to perform each exercise by outlining the purpose of the exercise and explaining the likelihood that pain may be present or increase during the exercise.

While a progressive graded approach was applied, if the patient reported increased pain (especially referred down the leg or >6/10), the movement and the exercise choices were still adjusted, further cues provided for timing or symmetry, and the patient was allowed to rest in the first session. However, the therapist took the time during the rest break to provide education about pain responses and to persuade the patient to try the exercise again, while explaining the goals to continue with the exercise and develop strategies to continue to move despite the pain.

If the patient did respond by continuing the exercise despite the pain, the therapist provided positive reinforcement without perseverating on the pain location, intensity, or negative emotions. While the symptoms were severe and irritable, the psychological characteristics and the chronic nature of the pain indicated a slow progressive introduction of quotas rather than limiting or avoiding movement completely. The positive reinforcement aimed to reinforce healthy attitudes and behaviors, conditioning the patient to develop mechanisms to deal with his pain.[97,103]

In addition, if the patient did exhibit any negative emotions, the therapist worked with him to counteract these maladaptive patterns.[103,105] The patient was able to use breathing techniques to address his pain responses and images of preparing for basketball training. Redirecting his attention to the moment and his exercise form also helped.

He was also given the opportunity to choose exercises that he felt he could perform at home to initiate self-efficacy and personal involvement: bridging, pelvic tilts, hip external rotation against the band, and gluteal stretching. He was asked to record the number of times he works on the specific exercises.

REFERENCES

Introduction

1. Magee DJ. *Orthopaedic Assessment*. 6th ed. St. Louis, MO: Saunders Elsevier; 2014.

2. Neumann DA. *Kinesiology for the Musculoskeletal System*. 3rd ed. St. Louis, MO: Elsevier; 2017.

3. Simoneau GG, Heiderscheit BC. Kinesiology of walking. In: Neumann DA, ed. *Kinesiology for the Musculoskeletal System*. 3rd ed. St. Louis, MO: Elsevier; 2017:654–705.

4. Rozumalski A, Schwartz MH, Wervey R, et al. The in vivo three-dimensional motion of the human lumbar spine during gait. *Gait Posture*. 2008;25:378–384.

5. Heiderscheit BC, Simoneau GG. Kinesiology of running. In: Neumann DA, ed. *Kinesiology for the Musculoskeletal System*. 3rd ed. St. Louis, MO: Elsevier; 2017:706–727.

6. Bruijn SM, Meijer OG, van Dieen JH, et al. Coordination of leg swing, thorax rotations, and pelvis rotations during gait: the organization of total body angular momentum. *Gait Posture*. 2008;27:455–462.

7. Ralston HJ. Effects of immobilization of various body segments on energy cost of human locomotion. *Ergon Suppl*. 1965:53.

8. Magee DJ, Zachazewski JE. Principles of stabilization training. In: Magee DJ, Zachazewski JE, Quillen WS, eds. *Scientific Foundations and Principles of Practice in Musculoskeletal Rehabilitation*. St. Louis MO: Saunders Elsevier; 2007:388–413.

Section 1: Hypomobility

9. Hunter SK, Brown DA. Muscle: the primary stabilizer and mover of the skeletal system. In: Neumann DA, ed. *Kinesiology of the Musculoskeletal System: Foundations for Rehabilitation*. 2nd ed. St. Louis, MO: Mosby Elsevier; 2010:47–76.

10. Brennan GP, Fritz JM, Hunter SJ, Thackeray A, Delitto A, Erhard RE. Identifying subgroups of patients with acute/subacute "nonspecific" low back pain: results of a randomized clinical trial. *Spine (Phila Pa 1976)*. 2006;31:623–631.

11. Browder DA, Childs JD, Cleland JA, Fritz JM. Effectiveness of an extension-oriented treatment approach in a subgroup of subjects with low back pain: a randomized clinical trial. *Phys Ther*. 2007;87:1608–1618.

12. Fritz JM, Delitto A, Erhard RE. Comparison of classification-based physical therapy with therapy based on clinical practice guidelines for patients with acute low back pain: a randomized clinical trial. *Spine (Phila Pa 1976)*. 2003;28:1363–1371.

13. Long A, May S, Fung T. The comparative prognostic value of directional preference and centralization: a useful tool for front-line clinicians? *J Man Manip Ther*. 2008;16:248–254.

14. Blanpied PR, Gross AR, Elliott JM, et al. Neck pain: revision 2017. Clinical practice guidelines linked to the international classification of functioning and health from the Orthopaedic Section of the American Physical Therapy Association. *J Orthop Sports Phys Ther*. 2017;47(7):A1–A83.

15. Delitto A, George SZ, Van Dillern L, et al. Low back pain: clinical practice guidelines linked to the international classification of functioning, disability, and health from the orthopaedic section of the American Physical Therapy Association. *J Orthop Sports Phys Ther*. 2012;42(4):A1–A57.

16. Macdermid JC, Walton DM, Avery S, et al. Measurement properties of the neck disability index – a systematic review. *J Orthop Sports Phys Ther*. 2009;39(5):400–417.

17. Vernon H, Mior S. The neck disability index: a study of reliability and validity. *J Manip Physiol Ther*. 1991;14:409–415.

18. Szeto GPY, Straker LM, O'Sullivan PB. Neck-shoulder muscle activity in general and task-specific resting postures of symptomatic computer users with chronic neck pain. *Man Ther*. 2009:339–345.

19. Kuo YL, Tully EA, Galea MP. Video analysis of sagittal spinal posture in healthy young and older adults. *J Manip Physiol Therap*. 2009;32(3):210–215.

20. Dunleavy K, Goldberg A. Comparison of cervical range of motion in two seated postural conditions in adults 50 or older with cervical pain. *J Man Manip Ther*. 2013;21(1):33–39.

21. O'Leary S, Falla D, Jull G. The relationship between superficial muscle activity during the craniocervical flexion test and clinical features in patients with chronic neck pain. *Man Ther*. 2011:452–455.

22. Jull G, O'Leary S, Falla DL. Clinical assessment of the deep cervical flexor muscles: the craniocervical flexion test. *J Man Manip Ther*. 2008;31(7):525–533.

23. Magee DJ, Sueki D. *Orthopedic Physical Assessment Atlas and Video*. St. Louis, MO: Elsevier Saunders; 2011.

24. Cleland JA, Koppenhaver S, Su J. *Netter's Orthopaedic Clinical Examination: An Evidenced Based Approach*. 3rd ed. Philadelphia, PA: Saunders Elsevier; 2016.

25. Childs JD, Cleland JA, Elliott JM, et al. Neck pain: clinical practice guidelines linked to the international classification of functioning, disability and health from the Orthopaedic Section of the American Physical Therapy Association. *J Orthop Phys Ther*. 2008;38(9):A1–A34.

26. Jull G, Trott P, Potter H, et al. A randomized controlled trial of exercise and manipulative therapy for cervicogenic headache. *Spine*. 2002;27(17):1835–1843.

27. Fritz JM, Brennan GP. Preliminary examination of a proposed treatment-based classification system for patients receiving physical therapy interventions for patients receiving physical therapy interventions for neck pain. *Phys Ther*. 2007;87:513–524.

28. O'Leary S, Falla D, Elliott JM, Jull G. Muscle dysfunction in cervical spine pain: implications for assessment and management. *J Orthop Sports Phys Ther*. 2009;39(5):324–333.

29. Hoving JL, Koes BW, de Vet HCW, et al. Manual therapy, physical therapy or continued care by a general practitioner for patients with neck pain: a randomized controlled trial. *Clin J Pain*. 2006;22(4):370–377.

30. Karlberg M, Magnusson M, Eva-Maj M, Elander A, Moritz U. Postural and symptomatic improvement after physiotherapy in patients with dizziness of suspected cervical origin. *Arch Phys Med Rehab*. 1996;77:874–882.

31. Miller J, Gross A, D'Sylva J, et al. Manual therapy and exercise for neck pain: a systematic review. *Man Ther*. 2010;15:334–354.

32. Gross A, Kay TM, Paquin JP, et al. Exercises for mechanical neck disorders. *Cochrane Database Syst Rev*. 2015;1:CD004250. https://doi. org/10.1002/14651858.CD004250.pub5.

33. Gross AR, Goldsmith C, Hoving JL, et al. Conservative management of mechanical neck disorders: a systematic review. *J Rheumatol*. 2007;34:1083–1102.

34. Varatharajan S, Ferguson B, Chrobak K, et al. Are non-invasive interventions effective for the management of headaches associated with neck pain? An update of the bone and joint decade task force on neck pain and its associated disorders by the Ontario protocol for traffic injury management (OPTIMa) collaboration. *Eur Spine J*. 2016;25:1971–1999.

35. Bertozzi L, Gardenghi I, Turoni F, et al. Effect of therapeutic exercise on pain and disability in the management of chronic nonspecific neck pain: systematic review and meta-analysis of randomized trials. *Phys Ther*. 2013;93:1026–1036.

36. O'Riordan C, Clifford A, Van De Ven P, Nelson J. Chronic neck pain and exercise interventions: frequency, intensity, time, and type principle. *Arch Phys Med Rehabil*. 2014;95:770–783.

37. Quek J, Pua YJ, Clark RA, Bryant AL. Effects of thoracic kyphosis and forward head posture on cervical range of motion in older adults. *Musc Science Pract*. 2013;18(1):65–71.

38. Soo Park M, Moon SH, Lee JM, et al. related changes in cervical sagittal range of motion and alignment. *Global Spine J*. 2014;4(3):151–156.

39. Falla D, Jull G, Hodges P, Vicenzino B. An endurance-strength training regime is effective in reducing myoelectric manifestations of cervical flexor muscle fatigue in females with chronic neck pain. *Clin Neurophysiol*. 2006;117:828–837.

Section 2: Hypermobility

40. Costa LO, Maher CG, Latimer J, et al. Motor control exercise for chronic low back pain: a randomized placebo-controlled trial. *Phys Ther*. 2009;89:1275–1286.

41. Hodges PW, Richardson CA. Inefficient muscular stabilization of the lumbar spine associated with low back pain: a motor control evaluation of transversus abdominis. *Spine*. 1996;21:2649–2650.

42. Hodges PW, Richardson C. Relationship between limb movement speed and associated contraction of the trunk muscles. *Ergonomics*. 1997;40:1220–1230.

43. Hodges PW, Richardson CA. Feedforward contraction of the transversus abdominis is not influenced by direction of arm movement. *Exp Brain Res*. 1997;114:362–370.

44. Hodges PW, Richardson CA. Delayed postural contraction of the transversus abdominis in low back pain associated with movement of the lower limb. *J Spinal Disord*. 1998;11:46–56.

45. Hodges PW, Ferreira PH, Ferreira M. Lumbar spine: treatment of instability and disorders of movement control. In: Magee DJ, Zachazewski JE, Quillen WS, eds. *Pathology and Intervention in Musculoskeletal Rehabilitation*. St. Louis, MO: Elsevier; 2007:389–425.

46. Changulani M, Shaju A. Evaluation of the responsiveness of Oswestry low back pain disability index. *Arch Orthop Trauma Surg*. 2009;129:691–694.

47. Fairbank JC, Pynsent PB. The Oswestry disability index. *Spine (Phila PA 1976)*. 2000;25:2940–2952.

48. McGill S. *Low Back Disorders: Evidence-Based Prevention and Rehabilitation*. Champaign, IL: Human Kinetics; 2002.

49. McGill SM, Childs A, Liebenson C. Endurance time for low back stabilization exercise: clinical targets for testing and training from a normal database. *Arch Phys Med Rehabil*. 1999;80:941–944.

50. Jorgensen K, Nicolaisen T. Trunk extensor endurance: determination and relation to low-back trouble. *Ergonomics*. 1987;30:259–267.

51. Naal FD, Hatzung G, Muller A, Impellizzeri F, Leunig M. Validation of a self-reported Beighton score to assess hypermobility in patients with femoroacetabular impingement. *Int Orthopaed*. 2014;38(11):2245–2250.

52. Hermanns-Le T, Reginster MA, Pierard-Franchimont C, Delvenne P, Pierard GE, Manicourt D. Dermal ultrastructure in low Beighton score members of 17 families with hypermobile-type Ehlers-Danlos syndrome. *J Biomed Biotechnol*. 2012:878107.

53. Hicks GE, Fritz JM, Delitto A, Mishock J. Interrater reliability of clinical examination measures for identification of lumbar segmental instability. *Arch Phys Med Rehabil*. 2003;84:1858–1864.

54. Celenay ST, Kaya DO. Effects of spinal stabilization exercises in women with benign joint hypermobility syndrome: a randomized controlled trial. *Rheumatol Int*. 2017. https://doi.org/10.00.1007/s00296-017-3713-6. Published online.

55. Ostello RW, Deyo RA, Stratford P, et al. Interpreting change scores for pain and functional status in low back pain: toward international consensus regarding minimal important change. *Spine (Phila Pa 1976)*. 2008;33:90–94.

56. Hides JA, Stokes MJ, Saide M, Jull GA, Cooper DH. Evidence of lumbar multifidus muscle wasting ipsilateral to symptoms in patients with acute/subacute low back pain. *Spine (Phila Pa 1976)*. 1994;19:165–172.

57. Hicks GE, Fritz JM, Delitto A, McGill SM. Preliminary development of a clinical prediction rule for determining which patients with low back pain will respond to a stabilization exercise program. *Arch Phys Med Rehabil*. 2005;86:1753–1762.

58. Rabin A, Shashua A, Pizem K, Dickstein R, Dar G. A clinical prediction rule to identify patients with low back pain who are likely to experience short-term success following stabilization exercises: a randomized controlled validation study. *J Orthop Sports Phys Ther*. 2014;44(1):6–18.

59. Russek LN, LaShomb EA, Ware AM, Wesner SM, Westcott V. United States Physical Therapist's knowledge about joint hypermobility syndrome compared to fibromyalgia and rheumatoid arthritis. *Physioth Res Int*. 2016;21:22–35.

60. Hines C, Mercer V. Anticipatory postural adjustments: an update. *Neurol Report*. 1997;21(1):17–22.

61. Toussaint JM, Dianne AC, Commissaris M, Hoozemans JM, Ober MJ, Beek PJ. Anticipatory postural adjustments before load pickup in a bi-manual whole body lifting task. *Med Sci Sports Exer*. 1997;29(9):1208–1215.

62. Childs JD, Piva SR, Erhard RE, Hicks G. Side-to-side weight-bearing asymmetry in subjects with low back pain. *Man Ther*. 2003;8(3):166–169.

63. Hides JA, Stanton WR, McMahon S, Sims K, Richardson CA. Effect of stabilization training on multifidus muscle cross-sectional area among young elite cricketers with low back pain. *J Orthop Sports Phys Ther*. 2008;38(3):101–108.

64. Michaelson P, Holmberg D, Aasa B, Aasa U. High load lifting exercise and low load motor control exercises as interventions for patients with mechanical low back pain: a randomized controlled trial with 24-month follow-up. *J Rehab Med*. 2016;48(5):456–463.

65. Hayden JA, van Tulder MW, Malmivaara A, Koes BW. Exercise therapy for treatment of non-specific low back pain. *Cochrane Database Syst Rev*. 2005:CD000335. https://doi.org/10.1002/14651858.CD000335.pub2.

66. Hayden JA, van Tulder MW, Tomlinson G. Systematic review: strategies for using exercise therapy to improve outcomes in low back pain. *Ann Intern Med*. 2005;142:776–785.

67. Saner J, Kool J, Sieben JM, Luomajoki H, Bastiaenen CHG, De Bie RA. A tailored exercise program versus general exercise for a subgroup of patients with low back pain and movement control impairment: a randomized controlled trial with one-year follow-up. *Man Ther*. 2015;20:672–679.

68. O'Sullivan P. Diagnosis and classification of chronic low back pain disorders: maladaptive movement and motor control impairments as underlying mechanism. *Man Ther*. 2005;10(4):242–255.

69. Dankaerts W, O'Sullivan PB, Straker LM, Burnett AF, Skouen JS. The inter-examiner reliability of a classification method for non-specific chronic low back pain patients with motor control impairment. *Man Ther*. 2006;11(1):28–39.

70. Luomajoki H, Kool J, de Bruin ED, Airaksinen O. Reliability of movement control tests in the lumbar spine. *BMC Musculskel Disord.* 2007;8:90–101.

71. Gomes-Neto M, Lopes JM, Conceicao CS, et al. Stabilization exercise compared to general exercise or manual therapy for the management of low back pain: a systematic review and meta-analysis. *Phys Ther Sport.* 2017;23:136–142.

72. Gomes-Neto M, Lopes JM, Conceicao CS, et al. Stabilization exercise compared to general exercise or manual therapy for the management of low back pain: a systematic review and meta-analysis. *Phys Ther Sport.* 2017;23:136–142.

73. Macedo LG, Maher CG, Latimer J, McAuley JH. Motor control exercise for persistent, nonspecific low back pain: a systematic review. *Phys Ther.* 2009;89:9–25.

74. Colle F, Rannou F, Revel M, Fermanian J, Poiraudeau S. Impact of quality scales on levels of evidence inferred from a systematic review of exercise therapy and low back pain. *Arch Phys Med Rehabil.* 2002;83:1745–1552.

75. Hides JA, Richardson CA, Jull GA. Multifidus muscle recovery is not automatic after resolution of acute, first-episode low back pain. *Spine.* 1996;21:2763–2769.

76. Hides JA, Jull GA, Richardson CA. Long-term effects of specific stabilizing exercises for first-episode low back pain. *Spine.* 2001;26:E242–E248.

77. O'Sullivan PB, Phyty GD, Twomey LT, Allison GT. Evaluation of specific stabilizing exercises in the treatment of chronic low back pain with radiologic diagnosis of spondylolysis or spondylolisthesis. *Spine.* 1997;22:2959–2967.

78. Fritz JM, Whitman JM, Childs JD. Lumbar spine segmental mobility assessment: an examination of validity for determining intervention strategies in patients with low back pain. *Arch Phys Med Rehabil.* 2005;86:1745–1752.

Section 3: Repetitive Strain

79. McHorney CA, Ware Jr JE, Lu JF, Sher-bourne CD. The MOS 6-item short-form health survey (SF-6): III. Tests of data quality, scaling assumptions, and reliability across diverse patient groups. *Med Care.* 1994:40–66.

80. Binkley JM, Stratford PW, et al. The Lower Extremity Functional Scale (LEFS): scale development, measurement properties, and clinical application. North American Orthopaedic Rehabilitation Research Network. *Phys Ther.* 1999;79(4):371–383.

81. Horn KK, Jennings S, Richardson G, Vliet DV, Hefford C, Abbott JH. The Patient-Specific Functional Scale: psychometrics, clinimetrics, and application as a clinical outcome measure. *J Orthop Sports Phys Ther.* 2012;42(1):30–42.

82. Schmidt CP, Zwingenberger S, Walther A, et al. Prevalence of low back pain in adolescent athletes—an epidemiological investigation. *Int J Sports Med.* 2014;35:684–689.

83. D'Hemecourt PA, Micheli LJ, Fields KB, Grayzel J. Spondylolysis and Spondylolisthesis in Child and Adolescent Athletes. *Clinical Presentation, Imaging, and Diagnosis.* 2016. UpToDate https://www.uptodate.com/contents/spondylolysis-and-spondylolisthesis-in-child-and-adolescent-athletes-clinical-presentation-imaging-and-diagnosis#H1053052.

84. Selhorst M, Fischer A, Graft K. Long-term clinical outcomes and factors that predict poor prognosis in athletes after a diagnosis of acute spondylolysis: a retrospective review with telephone follow-up. *J Orthop Sports Phys Ther.* 2016;46(12):1029–1036.

85. Gurd DP. Back pain in the young athlete. *Sports Med Arthrosc.* 2011;19(1):7–16.

86. Alqarni AM, Schneiders AG, Cook CE, Hendrick PA. Clinical tests to diagnose lumbar spondylolysis and spondylolisthesis: a systematic review. *Phys Ther Sport.* 2015;16:268–275.

87. Stuber KJ, Bruno P, Sajko S, Hayden JA. Core stability exercises for low back pain in athletes: a systematic review of the literature. *Clin J Sport Med.* 2014;24(6):448–456.

88. Childs JD, Piva SR, et al. Responsiveness of the numeric pain rating scale in patients with low back pain. *Spine (Phila Pa 1976).* 2005;30(11):1331–1334.

89. Dawson AP, Steele EJ, et al. Utility of the Oswestry Disability Index for studies of back pain related disability in nurses: evaluation of psychometric and measurement properties. *Int J Nurs Stud.* 2010;47(5):604–607.

90. Copay AG, Glassman SD, et al. Minimum clinically important difference in lumbar spine surgery patients: a choice of methods using the Oswestry disability index, medical outcomes study questionnaire short form 36, and pain scales. *Spine.* 2008;8(6):968–974.

91. Yeung TS, Wessel J, et al. Reliability, validity, and responsiveness of the lower extremity functional scale for inpatients of an orthopaedic rehabilitation ward. *J Orthop Sports Phys Ther.* 2009;9(6):468–477.

Section 4: Trauma and Psychological Factors

92. Swinkels-Meewisse EJ, Swinkels RA, et al. Psychometric properties of the Tampa Scale for kinesiophobia and the fear-avoidance beliefs questionnaire in acute low back pain. *Man Ther.* 2003;8(1):29–36.

93. George SZ, Fritz JM, et al. Fear-avoidance beliefs as measured by the fear-avoidance beliefs questionnaire: change in fear-avoidance beliefs questionnaire is predictive of change in self-report of disability and pain intensity for patients with acute low back pain. *Clin J Pain.* 2006;22(2):197–203.

94. George SZ, Stryker SE. Fear-avoidance beliefs and clinical outcomes for patients seeking outpatient physical therapy for musculoskeletal pain conditions. *J Orthop Sports Phys Ther.* 2011;41(4):249–258.

95. Cleland JA, Fritz JA, et al. Psychometric properties of the fear-avoidance beliefs questionnaire and Tampa scale of kinesiophobia in patients with neck pain. *Am J Phys Med Rehabil.* 2008;87(2):109–117.

96. George SZ. Pain management: road map to revolution. *Phys Ther.* 2017;97:217–226.

97. Foster NE, Delitto A. Embedding psychosocial perspectives within clinical management of low back pain: integration of psychosocially informed management principles into physical therapist practice: challenges and opportunities. *Phys Ther.* 2011;91:790–803.

98. Louw A, Diener I, Butler DS, Puentedura EJ. The effect of neuroscience education on pain, disability, anxiety, and stress in chronic musculoskeletal pain. *Arch Phys Med Rehab.* 2011;92:2041–2056.

99. Louw A, Diener I, Landers MR, Puentedura EJ. Preoperative pain neuroscience education for lumbar radiculopathy: a multi-center randomized controlled trial with 1 year follow up. *Spine (Phil PA 1976).* 2014;39:1449–1457.

100. Moseley GL. Reconceptualizing pain according to modern pain science. *Phys Ther Rev.* 2007;12:169–178.

101. Moseley GL. Evidence for a direct relationship between cognitive and physical change during an education intervention in people with chronic low back pain. *Eur J Pain.* 2004;8:39–45.

102. Vlaeyen JW, Haazen JW, Schuerman JA, Kole-Snijders AM, van Eek H. Behavioural rehabilitation of chronic low back pain: comparison of an operant treatment, an operant-cognitive treatment, and an operant-respondent treatment. *Br J Clin Psychol.* 1995;34(1):95–118.

103. Brunner E, De Herdt A, Minguet P, Baldew S, Probst M. Can cognitive behavioral therapy based strategies be integrated into physiotherapy for the prevention of chronic low back pain? A systematic review. *Disab Rehab.* 2013;35(1):1–10.

104. George SZ, Zepperieri G, Cere AL, et al. A randomized trial of behavioral physical therapy interventions for acute and subacute low back pain. *Pain.* 2008;140:145–157.

105. Turner JA, Jensen MP. Efficacy of cognitive therapy for chronic low back pain. *Pain.* 1993;52:169–177.

106. George SZ, Wittmer VT, Fillingim RB, Robinson ME. Comparison of graded exercise and graded exposure clinical outcomes for patients with chronic low back pain. *J Orthop Sports Phys Ther.* 2010;40(11):694–704.

107. Staal JB, Hlobil H, Twisk JW, Smid T, Koke AJ, van Mechlen W. Graded activity for low back pain in occupational health care: a randomized controlled trial. *Ann Intern Med.* 2004;140:77–84.

108. Macedo IG, Smeets RJ, Maher CG, Latimer J, McAuley JH. Graded activity and graded exposure for persistent nonspecific low back pain: a systematic review. *Phys Ther.* 2010;90:860–879.

109. Gabbe BJ, Hofstee DJ, Esser M, et al. Functional and return to work outcomes following major trauma involving severe pelvic ring fracture. *ANZ J Surg.* 2015;85(10):749–754.

110. Main CJ, Wood PL, Hollis S, Spanswick CC, Waddell G. The Distress and Risk Assessment Method. A simple classification to identify distress and evaluate the risk of poor outcome. *Spine.* 1992;17:42–52.

111. Nicholas MK, Linton SJ, Watson PJ, Main CJ. The "Decade of the Flags" working group. Early identification and management of psychological risk factors ("yellow flags") in patients with low back pain: a reappraisal. *Phys Ther.* 2011;91:737–753.

112. Beattie PF, Silfies SP, Jordon M. The evolving role of physical therapists in the long-term management of chronic low back pain: longitudinal care using assisted self-management strategies. *Braz J Phys Ther.* 2016;20(6):580–591.

113. Hodges PW, Smeets RJ. Interaction between pain, movement and physical activity. Short-term benefits, long-term consequences and targets for treatment. *Clin J Pain.* 2015;31(2):97–107.

114. Sueki DG, Dunleavy K, Puentedura EJ, Spielholz NI, Cheng MS. The role of associative learning and fear in the development of chronic pain – a comparison of chronic pain and post-traumatic stress disorder. *Phys Ther Rev.* 2014;19(5):352–366.

Note: Page number followed by "f" indicates figures, by "t" tables, and by "b" boxes.